OXFORD MEDICAL PUBLICATIONS

Sexual Deviation

Sexual deviation

Second edition

Edited by Ismond Rosen, M.D., F.R.C.PSYCH., D.P.M.

Chairman and Consultant Psychiatrist,
Paddington Centre for Psychotherapy, London

Emphasis on castrating mother
cases, men, seducing sons.

1978

OXFORD UNIVERSITY PRESS

Oxford   New York   Toronto
1979

Oxford University Press, Walton Street,
Oxford OX2 6DP

OXFORD LONDON GLASGOW NEW YORK
TORONTO MELBOURNE WELLINGTON IBADAN
NAIROBI DAR ES SALAAM LUSAKA CAPE TOWN
KUALA LUMPUR SINGAPORE JAKARTA HONG KONG
TOKYO DELHI BOMBAY CALCUTTA MADRAS
KARACHI

© Oxford University Press 1979

First Edition (published as *The pathology and treatment of sexual deviation*) 1964
Second Edition 1979

British Library Cataloguing in Publication Data
The pathology and treatment of sexual deviation.
—2nd ed.
1. Sexual deviation
I. Rosen, Ismond
616.8'583 RC557 78–40262

ISBN 0–19–263208–6

Printed in Great Britain by Thomson Litho Ltd.,
East Kilbride, Scotland

Preface

The most pertinent single statement one may make about perversion is that events in the real world as well as within the psyche take on a symbolic and provocative meaning. When I was engaged in the final preparation of the earlier edition of this book the very last reference that I edited happened to contain the name 'Phoenix'. I was struck by the symbolism that a new book would one day arise from the ashes of a work not yet in print, yet it has come to pass, fifteen years later.

These two editions have in common a shared methodological approach to the study of perversion. The first edition was purely by British authors and covered a slightly wider field, whereas the second has an international authorship of the highest calibre, and deals in depth with the growth of knowledge in each area discussed. The links between the two editions are therefore of a traditional kind: each author has been chosen for his wide clinical or practical experience as well as for his theoretical knowledge, and many have made leading contributions to the world literature. The two editions complement one another in having varying viewpoints, in addition to being successive.

The chapters are intended to express individual points of view on major issues rather than to comprise a systematic textbook account. Ideally, many chapters taken together, or the book as a whole, will provide the best rounded view of particular syndromes.

Anthony Wakeling first presents the problems facing the general psychiatrist dealing with sexual deviation, the choice of treatments, and an expert view on the use of hormones in these conditions.

My own Chapters 2 and 3 should be taken together, and deal with general psycho-analytical theory. Preference has been given to views expressed in the literature, and comments are made where appropriate, using my own clinical material. Chapter 3, on perversion as a regulator of self-esteem, has been presented separately because this subject has not yet received appropriate discussion in the literature. The chapter has been kept brief to retain a scientific elegance, but is capable of much further elaboration.

We are much indebted to Phyllis Greenacre, the foremost modern thinker on fetishism, for collating her views on the subject especially for Chapter 4 of this volume. Robert Stoller's renowned work on sex and gender is providing us with new perspectives with which to view all sexual deviation. His clear exposition on the gender disorders in Chapter 5 is a welcome contribution from California. Chapter 6, on exhibitionism and voyeurism, dealing with phenomenological as well as treatment aspects, has been updated from the earlier edition, because of its systematic and historical basis.

Three chapters, 7, 8, and 9, deal exclusively with homosexuality. All the authors have extensive clinical experience treating such patients analytically, in itself quite a rare phenomenon. The reader may compare the theoretical approaches and classifications used in Britain, France, and the USA, and discover the many similarities and points of difference. Dr. Limentani continues the psychoanalytically eclectic tradition of the Portman Clinic, of Glover and of Rubinstein and of other esteemed colleagues who are now deceased. Their work remains for us to build on, in grateful salutation. Joyce McDougall brings a fresh viewpoint into female homosexuality, and adds Gallic insight where it is most needed. Charles Socarides outlines the psychology of male homosexuality from the developmental and treatment points of view, aspects he has helped to determine. Other chapters are rich in specific references to homosexuality, and the subject is dealt with much more extensively than in the earlier volume. Mervin Glasser, in Chapter 10, has drawn on his wealth of clinical experience treating both sexual deviants and delinquents at the Portman Clinic, as a guide in formulating his ideas on the role of aggression in sexual deviation. He has avoided the usual approaches to this difficult relationship (which are in any case provided in other chapters) and has forged ideational links between the most recent analytical thinking and clinical practice.

Murray Cox's chapter is culturally erudite and illustrates his skill as a group therapist with the most difficult of sexual problems, the incarcerated sexual offender. Chapter 11 provides evidence of how warmth, humanity, and sensitive group-analytical insights may penetrate therapeutically to the being inside the rapist and the sexual murderer.

Michael Gelder, as one of the fundamental researchers into behaviour therapy, as well as head of a large academic general psychiatric unit, is well placed to evaluate the merits of behaviour therapy in Chapter 12. Michael Freeman is a barrister with wide experience at the Bar, who is also a sought-after academic teacher. His treatise on the law and sexual deviation deals with British and American law, and apart from providing the legal facts, discusses the principles and issues that lie behind their formulation, in a critical and highly informed manner.

In Chapter 14 Richard Michael, assisted by Doris Zumpe, has enriched his original historical account of the biological factors underlying sexual behaviour by describing in detail the experimental work of the last decade on the endocrine role in behavioural interactions between the higher primates. This work, emanating mostly from his own department, enables us to understand better the 'chain of causation' between biological factors and sexuality.

So much for the present volume. I think the reader will hopefully find much to ponder over that is helpful or enlightening. Whether a wished-for successor to this volume should appear, in series, the future will determine. More important is it for us to share and I hope enjoy the fruits of our present labours.

I.R.

July 1978

Acknowledgements

Chapter 7 is an abridged version of a paper published in the *British Journal of Medical Psychology* under the title 'The differential diagnosis of homosexuality' (1977) **80**, 209–16 and appears with the permission of the Cambridge University Press. Permission to use the following illustrations which appear in Richard Michael's chapter is gratefully acknowledged:
Fig. 14.1: *Journal of Reproduction and Fertility*; Fig. 14.2: *Nature*; Figs. 14.3 and 14.4: *Science*.

The editor would like to express his gratitude to the staff of the Oxford University Press for their help and encouragement during the production of this book.

Contents

Contents

List of contributors

Murray Cox, M.A., M.R.C.PSYCH., D.P.M.
Consultant Psychotherapist, Broadmoor Hospital; Hon. Lecturer in Psychotherapy, The London Hospital Medical College.

M. D. A. Freeman, LL.M.
Of Gray's Inn, Barrister; Lecturer in Laws, University College, London.

Michael Gelder, D.M., F.R.C.P., F.R.C.PSYCH.
Handley Professor of Psychiatry, University of Oxford.

Mervin Glasser, F.R.C.PSYCH., D.P.M.
Chairman and Consultant Psychotherapist, Portman Clinic, London; Member, British Psycho-Analytical Society.

Phyllis Greenacre, M.D.
Member of Faculty of the New York Psychoanalytic Institute; Clinical Professor of Psychiatry (Emeritus), Cornell Medical College, New York.

A. Limentani, M.D., F.R.C.PSYCH., D.P.M.
Consultant Psychotherapist, Portman Clinic, London; Training Analyst, British Psycho-Analytical Society.

Joyce McDougall M.A., D.ED.
Psychoanalyst; Training and Supervising Analyst, Institut Psychoanalytique de Paris, Paris.

Richard P. Michael, M.D., D.SC., PH.D., D.P.M., F.R.C.PSYCH.
Professor of Psychiatry and Anatomy, Emory University School of Medicine and Director, Biological Psychiatry Research Laboratories, Georgia Mental Health Institute, Atlanta, Georgia.

Ismond Rosen, M.D., F.R.C.PSYCH., D.P.M.
Chairman and Consultant Psychiatrist, Paddington Centre for Psychotherapy, London; Member, British Psycho-Analytical Society.

Charles W. Socarides, M.D.
Professor of Psychiatry, State University of New York, Downstate Medical Center, New York; Member, American Psychoanalytic Association

Robert J. Stoller, M.D.
Professor of Psychiatry, University of California at Los Angeles School of Medicine; Member, Los Angeles Psychoanalytic Society and Institute.

Anthony Wakeling, PH.D., M.R.C.PSYCH., D.P.M.
Senior Lecturer in Psychiatry, Royal Free Hospital Medical College, London.

Doris Zumpe, PH.D.,
Associate Professor of Psychiatry, Emory University School of Medicine, Atlanta, Georgia.

1 A general psychiatric approach to sexual deviation

Anthony Wakeling

Introduction

In recent years there has been a resurgence of interest in sexual behaviour. Changes in social attitudes have led to a more tolerant and less inhibited approach to sexuality. Such changes have helped to create a climate where sexual behaviour in all its aspects is recognized as a legitimate field for serious and scientific study. The important studies of Kinsey and his group (Kinsey, Pomeroy, and Martin 1948; Kinsey, Pomeroy, Martin, and Gebhard 1953) and Masters and Johnson (1966; 1970) have helped to shape this change, and have provided important knowledge concerning the taxonomy of human sexual behaviour and the psycho-physiological aspects of the sexual act. Rapid advances in the field of neuro-endocrinology have raised the hope that we are on the verge of further understanding of the biological aspects of sexual behaviour. Of particular importance have been the discovery of roles for prenatal endocrine factors in the subsequent sexual dimorphism of behaviour, and findings highlighting the complexity of the reciprocal interaction between hormones and behaviour. In addition, increasing sophistication in psychological and social research methods has enabled studies to yield new information about many aspects of human sexual behaviour. The effect of all these endeavours has been to underline further the complexity and multi-variate nature of the factors that shape human sexual behaviour.

In the present social climate, there is a more open and, to some extent, more informed discussion of sexual behaviour. People who are distressed by their sexual lives are more likely to identify themselves and to seek help. This is certainly the case where the difficulties involve failure of function. There has been a burgeoning of clinics and centres purporting to provide treatment for such conditions, which most commonly include erectile impotence and premature ejaculation in the male and varieties of orgasmic failure in the female. This growth area stems directly from the innovatory research of Masters and Johnson and their reports of successful treatment of such disorders by behavioural techniques. While such methods are undoubtedly successful in a proportion of cases, the therapeutic euphoria generated by this movement should be viewed with caution and scepticism. There is, as yet, a complete absence of proper evaluation of these methods. The more thoughtful practitioners in this field are more cautious in their claims for successful intervention and recognize that simple behavioural techniques do not meet with success in every individual. This is particularly so when the sexual dysfunction is but one aspect of more generalized personality disorder or neurotic illness. As Bancroft (1977) has pointed out the importance of these new directive treatment methods has been the recognition that some individuals can suffer from sexual symptoms in the absence of profound neurotic disorder.

Similar factors can be discerned when one turns to the other major class of sexual disorders: the sexual deviations. Changes in social attitude have led to an apparently more open-minded and tolerant view of diverse forms of sexual behaviour. There is a growing awareness of the wide variety of sexuality and sexual behaviour both between and within different societies. There is an increasing tendency for sexual deviants to identify themselves, either to seek help or to join a relevant sub-cultural group. There has been for some time a substantial and varied homosexual sub-culture (Hooker 1965). However, in keeping with greater social tolerance, other forms of deviance which hitherto had been invariably of the individual type are beginning to form their own sub-culture. Transsexuals, transvestites, fetishists, and paedophiles are now openly organizing themselves in this way. Identification with such a sub-culture mitigates some of the effects of stigma and undoubtedly plays an important role in the shaping of life and sexual relationships. It is, of course, individuals outside the sub-culture who are more likely to seek help. A whole complex of factors will determine whether or not an individual seeks help but it is likely that only a small proportion of sexual deviants do so. Whether this proportion is increasing or decreasing is uncertain, but there has certainly been an increase in therapeutic optimism over the last decade. This stems in part from numerous recent reports that deviant sexual behaviour can be modified in some individuals by both psychoanalytically-oriented treatment and by behavioural treatments.

Definition

As awareness of the variability and complexity of sexual behaviour increases, the boundaries between normal and deviant sexual behaviour tend to become more blurred. However, there are certain forms of sexual behaviour that are generally held to be deviant in our society. Scott (1964, p.88) adumbrated those features which basically characterize such behaviour.

The elements of a comprehensive definition of sexual perversion should include sexual activity or fantasy directed towards orgasm other than genital intercourse with a willing partner of the opposite sex and of similar maturity, persistently recurrent, not merely a substitute for preferred behaviour made difficult by the immediate environment and contrary to the generally accepted norm of sexual behaviour in the community.

This definition emphasizes that it is the persistent and compulsive substitution of some other act for heterosexual genital intercourse which chiefly characterizes the behaviour called sexual deviation. Sexual deviations are usually separated into categories according to the predominant or outstanding sexual behaviour. These categories include homosexuality, sexual activity with immature partners of either sex (paedophilia), dead people (necrophilia), animals (bestiality), or inanimate objects (fetishism). Also included are sado-masochism, sexual violence, rape, incest, exhibitionism, voyeurism, and transsexualism.

Although generally classified in this way it is clear that these categories are not discrete phenomena. There is usually considerable overlap between them in that more than one deviation may be present in an individual, although one may predominate. Moreover, within each category will fall individuals with a wide range of deviant behaviour, differing in terms of personality structure and development, fixity and strength of deviant behaviour, attitude to deviant behaviour, co-existence of other forms of sexual behaviour, and so on.

Clinically, deviant sexual behaviour is often associated with an impairment of the ability to achieve mutually satisfying relationships with adults of the opposite sex, and with the retention of childlike patterns of relating to others. In contrast to normal sexual behaviour, deviant behaviour is often associated with strong affects of guilt and hate. Whereas normal sexual behaviour is more likely to occur in a setting of affection and mutual sharing, of equal giving and receiving of pleasure, deviant behaviour frequently occurs without discrimination as to partner, and without consideration of the feelings of others. It appears to be dictated more by neurotic or non-sexual than by erotic needs, which leads to a large element of compulsiveness and risk-taking associated with the behaviour. As sexuality is intimately interwoven throughout all aspects of personality, it is to be anticipated that deviant sexual behaviour will frequently co-exist with profound personality maladjustment, severe neurotic difficulties, and fears of heterosexuality. However, sexual deviation is also compatible with adaptive social functioning and with elements of relatively normal heterosexual functioning. Some individuals do pass through a phase of homosexuality or bisexuality to a satisfactory and persisting hetero- sexual role and others pass in the opposite direction. Fetishism and exhibitionism, for instance, can co-exist with heterosexual behaviour. This is again to emphasize the tremendous variability of sexual behaviour and those aspects of such behaviour labelled deviant. There will be an immense gulf between individuals at one end of a spectrum who have never passed beyond an infantile level of psychosexual development, and those well-adjusted individuals at the other end who revert to deviant sexual behaviour only under the impact of severe physical or psychological stress.

Aetiology

Whilst recognizing recent research advances, there is still a profound lack of precise knowledge regarding the factors involved in the deri- vation of sexual behaviour in all its forms. The determinants of gender identity, gender role behaviour, sexual preference, and sexual behav- iour are still largely unknown. Unifying theories of varying degrees of complexity of the aetiology of sexual deviation have been constructed in terms of psychoanalytic theory (see Chapter 2), and behaviour or learning theory (Maguire, Carlisle, and Young 1965). Such theories, of course, provide very useful models, particularly when formulated in such a way that they have heuristic value, and are important guides to understanding and treatment. However, at the present stage of know- ledge, these theories should be regarded as hypotheses to be tested and modified by further research and experience.

A wide range of factors is likely to operate in the shaping of sexual behaviour. The aetiology of sexual deviation will, therefore, be multi- factorial, representing a sequence of related and interacting pheno- mena within and outside the individual's body. These factors can be separated artificially into intrinsic and extrinsic groups. The intrinsic factors will be those related to heredity and constitution; the extrinsic ones those referring either to some form of physical damage or to some experiential interaction with the environment. The present section will not attempt an exhaustive review of aetiology but will focus on some recent attempts to illuminate the roles of suggested intrinsic and extrinsic aetiological factors.

Intrinsic Factors

In recent years, paralleling the rapid development of modern genetics and neuro-endocrinology, attempts have been made to examine whether there might be some genetic or hormonal predisposition towards certain forms of sexual deviation.

Genetic studies. Genetic factors have been investigated primarily through twin studies in homosexuals. The earliest and best-known study was that of Kallman (1952) who reported 100 per cent concordance for homosexuality in a total of 37 pairs of monozygotic twins compared with 12 per cent in a total of 26 pairs of dyzygotic twins. This suggested that genetic factors played an important role in the origin of homosexuality. Other workers, notably Rosenthal (1970), drew attention to serious methodological errors in Kallman's study and cast substantial doubts on the validity of his findings. Subsequently several authors have reported pairs of monozygotic twins discordant for homosexuality (Rainer, Mensikoff, Kolb, and Carr 1960; Klintworth 1962; Parker 1964). Heston and Shields (1968) presented data concerning the twin pairs in the Maudsley twin register. Twelve male twins with a diagnosis of homosexuality included five who were monozygotic. Of these, three were concordant and two were discordant. Of the seven dyzygotic twins only one was concordant, six were not. As Heston and Shields found the same overall incidence of homosexuality in their monozygotic and dyzygotic twin population, it is unlikely that it is monozygocity *per se* rather than genetic factors that renders monozygotic twins more likely to become homosexual.

No firm conclusions can be drawn from these studies. A higher concordance rate for homosexuality in twins is not necessarily due to genetic factors, but may result from factors such as intense identification or specific environmental factors related to twinships. However, the generally higher incidence of concordance in monozygotic than in dyzygotic twin pairs provides some tentative support to the suggestion that genetic factors are involved in the genesis of homosexuality. Such factors could operate through a process of predisposing or sensitizing the individual to particular environmental influences.

Perinatal endocrine factors. Interest in the possibility of an innate constitutional or biological base for some forms of deviant sexual behaviour has been revived recently by findings in the field of neuro-endocrinology. It is now known that in lower animals the actions of foetal hormones, particularly androgens, acting in minute amounts at particular phases of development, play an important role in subsequent adult sexual functioning. A wide variety of experiments has shown that deprivation of foetal androgen in the male animal at the critical period of development will predispose to the expression of female sexual behaviour under the influence of male hormone in adult life. This occurs without the development of any abnormality in the external genitalia.

There is also evidence to suggest that sexually dimorphic behaviour in primates is influenced by the early perinatal endocrine environment. Infant male and female rhesus monkeys differ with respect to such behaviours as rough-and-tumble play, threat, and aggressivity. These differences have been clearly linked with differences in perinatal androgen levels (Young, Goy, and Phoenix 1964). One should not, of course, extrapolate findings in laboratory animals and primates to humans. Nevertheless, such studies at least point to the possibility that the endocrine environment at critical phases of development may influence the direction of sexual drive and sexually dimphoric behaviour in humans. Some tentative support for such a hypothesis derives from studies on females with the adreno-genital syndrome, where excessive amounts of adrenal androgen is produced *in utero*. In comparison to their non-affected sisters, the affected girls have been described as showing less interest in doll play, playing with infants, and wearing dresses, and are more often described as tomboys (Ehrhardt, Epstein, and Money 1968).

Green (1977) has indicated how differences in rough-and-tumble behaviour and aggressive play, which may be influenced by perinatal androgen levels, could affect psychosexual development adversely. A low level of aggressivity in a boy, for instance, might affect in a variety of ways his relationships with both his peers and his parents. There is, however, no direct evidence to link perinatal hormonal environment and subsequent behaviour patterns in humans. There are formidable hurdles to overcome before the perinatal hormone environment in humans can be assessed reliably. When this can be accomplished it should be possible to mount longitudinal studies to test some of these hypotheses.

Other endocrine factors. The recent development of specific and sensitive hormone assay procedures has revived interest in a possible association between homosexual behaviour in the adult and circulating hormone levels. Earlier studies in this area had failed to detect any difference in hormonal profiles between heterosexuals and homosexuals. However, in 1970, Margolese studied the breakdown products of testosterone in 24-hour samples of urine in a group of homosexual and a group of heterosexual males. He demonstrated a clear difference in the ratio of two metabolites, androsterone and etiocholanolone, between the two groups. Loraine, Ismail, Adamopoulos, and Dove (1970) reported low 24-hour urinary testosterone levels in two male homosexuals and high levels in four female homosexuals, in comparison with relevant controls. These studies await replication with larger groups and with proper attention to all the relevant control factors.

Measurements of plasma levels of hormones have given conflicting results. Thus, Kolodny, Masters, Hendryx, and Toro (1971) reported finding lower plasma testosterone levels in a group of 30 homosexuals in comparison with a control group of heterosexual males. Three subsequent studies (Tourney and Hatfield 1973; Barlow, Abel, and Blanchard, 1974; Pillard, Rose, and Sherwood 1974) failed to replicate these findings, whilst another study (Brodie, Gartrell, Doering, and Rhue 1974) found higher testosterone levels in homosexuals than in heterosexuals. Yet another study, although finding no difference in testosterone levels, reported significantly higher levels of plasma oestradiol in homosexuals in comparison with a group of heterosexuals (Doerr, Kockott, Vogt, Pirke, and Dittmar 1973).

Obviously no firm conclusions can be drawn from this data. Further studies in this area will require more sophisticated methodology. It is known that hormone levels and particularly androgen levels are affected by both physical and emotional stress (Rose, Bourne, and Poe 1969; Kreuz, Rose, and Jennings 1972), sexual activity (Fox, Ismail, Love, Kirkham, and Loraine 1972), and the ingestion of drugs such as marihuana (Kolodny, Masters, Kolodner, and Toro 1974).

Extrinsic factors

Parent–child relationships. Psychoanalytic theory emphasizes that the conditions which determine the development of sexually deviant behaviour are laid down in early childhood experiences. Disturbances in parent–child relationships, particularly mother–child relationships, as would be predicted from Oedipal theory, were stressed in classic psychoanalytic expositions (Fenichel 1945). There have been a number of studies undertaken to investigate the early family backgrounds of sexual deviants, but those that have used any form of control group have been confined to homosexual populations. The most famous study is perhaps that by Bieber, Dain, Dince, Drellich, Grand, Gundlach, Kremer, Rifkin, Wilbur, and Bieber (1962), which appeared to produce experimental evidence for the psychoanalytic view of the origin of sexual deviation. This study collected information from 77 psychoanalysts regarding the retrospective accounts of the family background of 106 male homosexuals and 100 male heterosexuals, who were undergoing psychoanalysis. The mothers of the homosexuals were reported as more often close-binding and intimate, and more often controlling and demanding, than those of the heterosexuals, whilst the fathers of homosexuals were often detached and more often hostile and indifferent. Most of the homosexuals' parents had poor marital relationships and, in comparison with the heterosexual group, the homosexuals had more abnormal upbringings. Although the group recognized variations of this pattern, it was concluded that a family constellation of detached, hostile father and close-binding, intimate mother contributed to the homosexual preference. Support for this hypothesis came from West (1959) and O'Connor (1964) who both studied groups of homosexuals from clinic populations in comparison with heterosexuals from clinic populations. These studies are open to a number of criticisms, one of which is that it is unwarrantable to generalize findings from homosexuals in psychiatric treatment to all homosexuals. However, Evans (1969), using a questionnaire based on that used by Bieber *et al.*, studied a large group of non-patient, predominantly exclusive, male and female homosexuals and reported findings in broad agreement with those of the Bieber study. Nevertheless, Evans placed a different interpretation on his findings; he stated that the triangular family constellation was not necessarily a cause of homosexuality but perhaps resulted from the effect of the child's early 'abnormal' behaviour on the attitudes and behaviour of the parents.

Bene (1965a), also studying family backgrounds of non-patient groups of homosexuals in comparison with heterosexuals, afforded some further support for the Bieber hypothesis at least in terms of the fathers' behaviour. Her findings regarding mother–child relationships were, however, contrary to those of Bieber. Thus, male homosexuals tended to have weak, ineffectual fathers but not especially domineering mothers. She concluded that lack of good relationships between father and son facilitated the development of homosexuality. In a similar study with female homosexuals, Bene (1965b) concluded again that it was the father–daughter relationship which appeared the most significant.

In the most recent important study in this area, Siegelman (1974) compared the family backgrounds of a group of 138 male heterosexuals with a group of 307 exclusive, or predominantly exclusive, male homosexuals. These were non-patient groups and care was taken to match the groups on social, educational, and other factors. About one-half of the homosexuals were drawn from an American homosexual organization. For the whole group, the homosexuals described both their fathers and their mothers as less loving and more rejecting, and their relationship with their fathers as less close than did the heterosexuals. The homosexuals did not differ from the heterosexuals in measures purporting to assess closeness to mother, mother versus father dominance, and parental protective and demand behaviour. Interestingly when comparisons were made between homosexuals and heterosexuals scoring low in neuroticism, as measured by a psychological test, there were no differences between the two groups in their perception of their parents. Siegelman concluded that his findings cast serious doubt on the assumption that negative parental behaviour, particularly on the part of the mother, played a critical role in differentiating the backgrounds of homosexuals and heterosexuals.

A number of general points can be made about the body of data summarized in this section. Much of it is unsatisfactory for a variety of reasons. First, there are the problems of obtaining a representative sample, and this is formidably difficult when one is studying deviant behaviour. Homosexuals who go to a psychiatrist, for example, are clearly not representative of homosexuals generally. The problems of selection continue to operate, of course, when non-patient populations are studied. Here one relies on volunteers and recourse is frequently made to organized minority groups, who may constitute a relatively well-adjusted group, or be intent on presenting a particular view or image of themselves. Secondly, all these studies relied on retrospective data, which have been shown to have rather low reliability and important biases (Yarrow, Campbell, and Burton 1970). No study looked at the parents of homosexuals in an attempt to corroborate the retrospective information. Thirdly, although control groups were used these were usually poorly matched on many variables. Siegelman's findings attest to the importance of careful consideration to the characteristics of the control group. Fourthly, it should be emphasized that these studies were correlational, and it is erroneous to draw firm conclusions as to cause and effect from such studies. Little consideration has been given in these studies to the fact that parental behaviour has been shown to be affected by the infant (Bell 1968). Nevertheless, in spite of these objections, and although the data are inconsistent, some trends can be discerned. In most studies, the fathers of homosexuals appear as more distant and rejecting than those of heterosexuals. Mothers appear either over-protective and intimate, or rejecting and hostile. The family backgrounds of homosexuals do often appear disrupted but a variety of patterns have been described. The usual description of the parental background of homosexuals found in standard texts is obviously an over-simplified stereotype and it is a disservice to perpetuate it. It might usefully be added here that there have been clinical accounts of the family backgrounds of individuals with other types of sexual deviance which point to rather similar abnormal parental relationships. There is, however, a shortage of well-designed studies, with adequate controls, of the families of these other varieties of deviance, which mitigates against drawing any firm conclusions.

Disturbances in parent–child relationships and pathological family constellations would, however, be regarded generally as important in the shaping of personality and psychosexual development. It is possible that certain types of parent–child interaction, an absent father, or a particular family constellation, may predispose to the development of sexual deviation. Moreover, specific deviations may derive from specific family patterns. Nevertheless, as Feldman (1973) has pointed out a greater sophistication of research techniques concerned with child-rearing practices is required before there can be a proper evaluation of the influence of family environment on sexual development. Although disturbances in family experience may play a necessary role in the aetiology of sexual deviance in many cases, such factors cannot be regarded as sufficient in themselves. The various pathological factors incriminated in the backgrounds of sexual deviants have all, of course, been detected in the backgrounds of adult heterosexuals. They can properly be seen therefore only as predisposing factors.

Early social learning experiences. In addition to the psychoanalytical theory of psychosexual development, there are several other major hypotheses which might be subsumed under the rubric, social learning theories. These theories attach prominence to such processes as observational learning, and various modelling and cognitive processes in the development of a child's sex role.

Sexual identity consists first of the self-concept of being male or female; secondly, of sex-linked behaviour and attitudes; and thirdly of genital sexual orientation (Green 1977). There is now a considerable body of evidence to suggest that the most important factor bearing on the acquisition of gender role – that is whether a person feels himself to be male or female – is the sex that the child is assigned to by his parents and thus the sex in which he is brought up (Hampson and Hampson 1961; Money and Ehrhardt 1973). Such data suggest that sex-role identity is becoming well established by the age of three years. Sex differences in children's behaviour and attitudes are also evident from early childhood and quite marked at age four to five years although differences continue to increase up to eight or nine years (Kagan 1964). Social learning theories assert that this early development of gender identity and sex-linked behaviour occurs primarily on the basis of social reinforcement and conditioning patterns. One theory emphasizes praise or discouragement. Thus gender identity and sex-typed behaviours are learned in the same way as any other sort of behaviour by selective parental responses and reinforcements. Parents and others reward and praise boys for boy-like behaviour, and actively discourage them from behaviours thought to be feminine (Mischel 1967; Bandura 1969). Other theories emphasize imitation, whereby children choose same-sex models especially the same-sex parent and use these models for developing and shaping their own behaviour. This, of course, includes the process of identification with the same-sexed parent (Kagan 1964). That this latter process cannot in itself be an adequate explanation for the development of gender identity is suggested by the fact that sex-role identity is well established by the age of four, when both sexes probably still identify with the mother. Bandura (1969) has argued that children can develop normal sex-role identity, in the absence of a same-sexed parent, by interaction with a variety of adult and peer models. Recent research has demonstrated that the child's attention and motivation to specific models depend upon such factors as the model's power, status, and nurturance (Maccoby and Jacklin 1975). Yet another theory (Kohlberg 1967)

emphasizes the process of self-socialization in psychosexual development. This is a cognitive developmental process, where the child
gradually develops concepts of masculinity and femininity from what
he has seen and what he has been told. He then attempts to fit his own
behaviour to his developing concept of what behaviour is sex-
appropriate. Such a process would be seen as part of cognitive
development and would follow the same motivational and learning
processes shown by other aspects of cognition.

All these social learning theories relating to the development of
gender identity and sex-typed behaviours have some experimental
support, but there is insufficient data to decide between them. It is
likely, as suggested by Maccoby and Jacklin (1975), that there is an
interaction between all these processes, but whether such processes in
themselves are sufficient to explain adequately all the complexities of
psychosexual development is doubtful. Nevertheless, such theories
suggest hypotheses about the development of deviant sexual behaviour.
It might be expected that such behaviour would be more likely to occur
on the basis of the childhood acquisition of disturbed or faulty gender
identity and inappropriate sex-typed behaviours. There is evidence to
suggest that some children do indeed fail to learn appropriate sex-typed
behaviours and preferences (Mischel 1970). Does this occur commonly
in the backgrounds of sexual deviants? Bene (1965a), Evans (1969),
and Gundlach (1969), in their studies on the early life of groups of
homosexuals, all reported that many of their subjects who had no
gender identity disturbance nevertheless saw themselves as lacking in
appropriate sex-typed skills and interests as children. Bieber *et al.*
(1962) reported that about one-third of 100 male homosexuals recalled
preferring girls as playmates during boyhood compared with 10 per
cent of the heterosexual control group, and less than 20 per cent of the
homosexuals took part in competitive games as against 63 per cent of
the heterosexuals. In a more recent study of non-patient homosexuals,
Saghir and Robins (1973) reported that two-thirds of a large group
of homosexual males described themselves as having been 'girl-like' in
childhood compared with only 3 per cent of the heterosexual control
group. A majority of those who were 'girl-like' recalled having no male
friends, avoiding boys' games, and having played mainly with girls.
They recalled in addition being regarded as effeminate and being
teased as a consequence.

These studies indicate that certain behaviours, culturally deemed
feminine or non-masculine, appear to characterize the early life of

many homosexuals. Atypical sex-role behaviour in childhood may thus persist as atypical sex-role behaviour during adult life. Studies on transsexuals also demonstrate that disturbed gender role behaviour in boyhood foreshadows atypical adult sexuality (Green 1977). In addition, Prince and Bentler (1972) have reported that many trans- vestites demonstrate an early onset of atypical sexual behaviour. In their study of 500 transvestites, approximately half recalled the onset of cross-dressing prior to puberty.

In addition to this retrospective data, there is some, albeit limited, direct empirical evidence from prospective studies that links childhood learning of inappropriate gender identity and sex-typed behaviour to later adult deviant sexual behaviour (Zuger 1966; Lebovitz 1972; Green 1977).

This body of data suggests that specific behavioural interactions between a child and his parents and his environment play a role in shaping psychosexual development. It also suggests the possibility that therapeutic intervention at an early stage in those children showing abnormal psychosexual development, such as gender identity disturb- ances and inappropriate sex-linked behaviour, might prevent the emergence of deviant sexuality in later life.

Later specific learning experiences. Maguire, Carlisle, and Young (1965) have put forward a theory of sexual deviation which emphasizes the importance of learning experiences not in early life but associated with the first sexual experience, usually during adolescence. They postulate that the nature of the first sexual experience followed by orgasm is critical for the establishment of sexual orientation. The learning takes place after the initial experience, which is seen as playing a role in pro- viding a fantasy for subsequent masturbation. Thus deviant behaviour is maintained by masturbation to the deviant fantasies. It is suggested that the individual masturbates to his particular deviant fantasy rather than to thoughts, say, of heterosexual intercourse, because the precipi- tating incident of a deviant nature, which preceded the initial orgasm, was of a particularly strong stimulus value. This stimulus becomes sex- ually more exciting through association with masturbation, and hetero- sexual stimuli are extinguished through lack of reinforcement. Such a process might be more likely to occur if the individual had experienced early aversive heterosexual experiences or feelings of inadequacy. Such a theory would appear too simplistic to be accorded much weight although, to its merit, it does generate some testable hypotheses.

It is possible that a complex variety of early experiences may predispose an individual to sexual deviation but that, given favourable adolescent experiences with his peer group, a satisfactory heterosexual adjustment will result. Conversely, adverse sexual circumstances during adolescence may tip the balance the other way with the onset of deviant behaviour. Whether this is continued will then depend upon a complex of factors, which will include the personality attributes of the individual himself, his attitude to the deviant behaviour, and the various rewards and contingencies associated with the deviant behaviour. Whether there are specific aspects of pubertal and adolescent experience that are of importance in the aetiology of sexual deviation is unknown. Both West (1968) and Green (1977) have drawn attention to the paucity of research in this area.

Conclusions

The major aetiological theories of sexual deviance differ in the particular emphasis they attach to specific aetiological factors. Some theories emphasize genetic or constitutional factors. Psychoanalytic theories emphasize early infantile experiences such as pre-Oedipal and Oedipal conflicts. Social learning theories attach prominence to general learning processes during childhood, whilst some behavioural theories emphasize the importance of events associated with the onset of sexual behaviour at puberty or during adolescence. The most comprehensive theories are undoubtedly those derived from psychoanalysis. Nevertheless, precise knowledge about aetiology is very limited. It would seem prudent, therefore, in the clinical situation to allow for a number of causal factors, each contributing to a varying degree to the genesis of sexual deviation, and to anticipate that different factors may operate at different strengths in different individuals.

Treatment

The prevalence of sexual deviance within our culture is unknown. It would be assumed, however, that most sexual deviants do not seek treatment and those that do constitute an unrepresentative sample of the whole. For example, many sexual deviants accept their deviant behaviour to varying degrees, and lead more or less satisfying and productive lives. Others may function in a more limited, but still adequate, fashion by organizing their lives so that their deviant behaviour can remain concealed. Such people may never seek help, or they may do so only under specific circumstances. Yet others are distressed by their deviant behaviour and seek help, in some cases, in a conscious attempt to understand and thus derive a greater feeling of personal autonomy. They may seek help to control their deviant urges, and this may or may not be combined with a desire to attempt to change sexual preferences. In others who seek help, their compulsive and obligatory sexual urges may bring them into conflict with the law, may harm others, or threaten so to do. The clinician is concerned with those individuals who seek help.

It will be clear that in the writer's view the pathways to sexual deviation are multiple and, although the roots are most likely to be found in the vicissitudes of childhood experience, a variety of other life events and experiences operate to initiate, shape, and maintain sexual behaviour. There is, therefore, an enormous diversity in the type of sexually deviant behaviour and its meaning to the individual, and in the personality of the individual himself. In the absence of a full understanding of aetiology, there are no specific treatments for particular conditions, no penny-in-the-slot diagnostic and treatment formulations. As it is also clear that, in most cases, sexual deviation arises out of experiential events and is not behaviour that is consciously chosen by the individual, the main arm of treatment will be psychotherapeutic. In an individual patient, this may mean psychoanalysis or analytically-orientated psychotherapy, individual supportive therapy, or group therapy: these may or may not be supplemented by other treatments such as specific counselling, social case-work, behaviour therapy, and physical therapies. This is to emphasize that treatment must be fitted to the individual, and not the individual to the treatment. Such a general psychiatric treatment approach is essentially eclectic and borrows in a non-scientific way from diverse disciplines. This is not to decry those therapists working within specific disciplines and attempting to further understanding of aetiology and treatments within the frameworks of those disciplines; such work is essential if further progress and understanding is to occur. But in the present state of knowledge, there are no clear guidelines from the literature as to the most effective treatment approaches for particular conditions. The place of most treatments still depends more on clinical opinion than on scientific fact. In these circumstances, the management of the individual becomes a matter of balanced clinical judgement. Treatment will be based on a thorough assessment of the individual and will be formulated as a treatment plan that will be relevant and realistic for the individual. Treatment will rarely be limited to one specific approach, although of course the emphasis will vary from individual to individual.

Assessment

This entails a full consideration of the essential and idiosyncratic features of the individual, and the circumstances in which he finds himself. It is important initially to identify as clearly as possible the individual's motives for seeking help and what he is hoping for from treatment. Motives and expectations are often mixed and complex. Deviant sexual behaviour is not concerned solely with sexual gratification, but is often used to defend against unpleasant feeling states of anxiety and depression. It usually provides, however, some means of obtaining sexual gratification and relief, which often leads to a degree of ambivalence towards changing the behaviour.

It is important to ascertain whether the individual has sought help himself or mainly to please others; whether he is genuinely concerned to involve himself in treatment or whether he is involving himself to please others. These factors should be teased out, as motivation plays a vital role in treatment and outcome. Equally, it is important to ascertain at this stage what particular help the individual is seeking. He may be quite explicit about this: he may ask for help in suppressing unwanted deviant behaviour without being interested in alternative forms of sexual release; he may ask for help to be able to achieve and enjoy a heterosexual relationship. Alternatively, he may seek help to enable himself to adjust better in his deviant behaviour. The individual may be genuinely ignorant about what help is available and not have formulated clearly what precise help he is seeking, apart from relief from his compulsive and obligatory sexual urges. Again, motives and expectations may not be apparent until a full assessment has been made and a therapeutic relationship established. In some cases, a full exploration of such matters may end the contact at this point.

The next stage is a systematic psychiatric history with a review of the family background, early life, personal history and development, social, interpersonal, and occupational history. Particular attention should then be paid to obtaining a full sexual history and a comprehensive appraisal of personality attributes.

The sexual history includes details of sexual development, early sexual education and experiences, gender identity and gender-appropriate behaviour. A detailed inquiry into the type and quality of each sexual relationship is essential, as are details related to past and current sexual fantasy, sexual preferences and dislikes. A careful assessment should be made of the onset and subsequent course and nature of the deviant behaviour, its strength and the factors that influence its expression. The individual's attitudes towards his deviant behaviour and the extent to which this is ego-dystonic or ego-syntonic are of importance. If he is engaged in a current sexual relationship the partner should, if possible, be seen together with the patient. It is, of course, often necessary to involve the partner in any therapeutic programme.

A proper assessment of personality factors involves appraisal of the capacity for forming relationships, the quality of relationships, the modes of relating to others, social skills and assets, cognitive strengths, and other facets of temperament. In addition, complete mental status and physical examinations should be carried out.

After such an assessment a diagnostic formulation is made. This will indicate whether or not there is a primary physical or psychiatric disorder and will include a phenomenological diagnosis of the sexual disorder, together with an account of those factors assumed to be of importance in the initiation and maintenance of the deviant behaviour. On the basis of this a treatment programme is drawn up, which will have to take account both of what it is possible to achieve and the availability of treatment facilities.

Treatment of primary condition

Primary physical and/or psychiatric disorders should, of course, be treated initially wherever possible. Sexually deviant behaviour can occur on the basis of impaired cerebral functioning; in such cases there will usually be other signs and symptoms of the specific disorder. Often it will be obvious that there has been a regression from previously normal sexuality; this is an aspect of impaired cerebral functioning, which may lower self-control to allow the expression of more infantile forms of sexual behaviour that the individual may have left behind or previously entertained in fantasy. Such regression might occur at the onset of a dementia, or in association with cerebrovascular disease, epilepsy, alcoholism, or cardiovascular disease. Any disorder in which there is impairment, either transient or permanent, of cerebral functioning might release such behaviour.

Deviant sexual behaviour can similarly arise in association with severe functional psychiatric disorder. Psychosexual confusion and deviant behaviour may occur with the onset of a schizophrenic illness. Severe depressive illness can, in some individuals, release sexually deviant behaviour. There are patients who are troubled with deviant fantasies which may be expressed only at the time of severe depressive-mood swings. Another aspect of depressive illness concerns those individuals who express marked feelings of guilt about their deviant behaviour only at times of depression: thus, the reasonably well-adjusted homosexual may present for help, with a request to change his sexual preference, whilst in the throes of depressive illness. In all these cases treatment is initially that for the primary condition. In some cases, subsequent treatment for the sexual symptoms will be required.

General treatment

For the majority of individuals seen in the clinic, the diagnostic assessment will focus specifically upon the relationship of the sexually deviant behaviour to the rest of the personality. In many, sexual deviance will form just one aspect of profound personality disorder. This category will include personality disorders of all kinds, from severely inhibited and withdrawn individuals, to those with poor impulse control and marked psychopathic personalities. Others will have more effective personality structures where deviant sexual behaviour may form only part of the sexual life, or may dominate it in a compulsive, obligatory way. Others may have regressed to deviant behaviour under specific stresses. In all these cases, the basis of the treatment plan will be psychotherapy which depends on the direct and personal relationship between the patient and the doctor. On a basis of understanding and acceptance, the doctor attempts to provide a rationale according to which the patient can begin to understand himself, and a framework within which he can gradually change.

In adolescents of relatively sound personality, who present with anxiety about deviant fantasies or the onset of deviant practices, short-term psychotherapeutic intervention may be appropriate. Such treatment would emphasize emotional support, together with education, counselling, and guidance.

In those adult sexual deviants with the necessary degree of motivation and capacity to respond to insight and to work within a psychotherapeutic context, intensive psychotherapy of the analytic kind is probably the treatment of choice. It must be recognized that such a view is based on clinical opinion and that the facilities for such intensive, time-consuming treatment are limited. It might be that less intensive treatment programmes, based on directive and behavioural methods, will be as effective for these individuals. This remains a matter for the future to be resolved by systematic research.

There will, of course, be great variation in the capacity for reality testing, in motivation, and in personality strengths, among those individuals seeking treatment. Treatment resting solely on individual intensive psychotherapy would be inappropriate and unrealistic in many of these individuals. Here, within the therapeutic alliance, the doctor attempts to utilize what strengths the patient has to encourage self-reliance and autonomy, and to encourage positive change. In those individuals with the co-existence of normal and deviant sexual behaviours, emphasis is placed on understanding those factors which prevent the full expression of healthy sexual behaviour rather than on suppressing the unwanted behaviour. By and large, the greater the severity of the personality disorder, the less likelihood there is of radically affecting the deviant behaviour. In such individuals involvement in a treatment setting with clearly-defined aims, for long periods of time may be envisaged. Emphasis here may initially be placed upon measures to increase self-control, this will perhaps entail repeated examination with the patient of those events and circumstances which appear to trigger off deviant acts. Focusing in such a way upon these precipitating events, and working out with the patient more appropriate ways of reacting to them, can be beneficial. In some individuals with severe arrest of psychosexual development and marked personality limitations, some increase in self-control might be all that can be achieved. In many, however, the capacity for some degree of personality maturation with time will be present. A measure of self-control may be important in allowing this process to proceed. Where possible the doctor will attempt to foster positive change. This may be brought about by examining those anxieties and behaviours that prevent the development of satisfactory relationships. There may be marked social anxieties and inhibitions, poor social skills, lack of sexual knowledge and awareness, which will all require attention within the treatment process. Where possible a spouse or partner will be brought into treatment. The help of an experienced social worker is often called for and specific efforts may be directed at environmental or occupational change. Specific behavioural and physical treatments may be utilized to achieve particular goals within the treatment programme. The aim always is to help the patient within the treatment alliance to increase his understanding of himself, to help him more effectively confront his difficulties, and to achieve a more mature and satisfying interpersonal, social, and sexual adjustment. The treatment aims must be realistic and be geared to the patient's needs and abilities, and must be such as not to bring harm to him.

Behaviour therapy

There are, of course, treatments for sexual deviations devised within the framework of learning theory and method (see Chapter 12). Whilst in the past, behaviour therapists emphasized the application of specific techniques in a precise way, current practitioners adopt a more flexible approach and devise wide-ranging treatment programmes (Bancroft 1977). The emphasis is placed not on suppressing unwanted behaviour, but on encouraging, through a variety of behavioural techniques, more satisfying and adaptive sexual behaviour. Attention to cognitive change and to the development of social skills is emphasized, as is a recognition of the importance of the relationship between the individual and the therapist. It would seem that the independence of behaviour therapy from many forms of psychotherapy is more apparent in theory than in practice.

Behavioural treatments clearly have a role to play in the treatment of sexual deviation but what that role should be, and its extent, await the outcome of further research. Although behavioural methods have generated much research already, few clinically relevant questions have, so far, been answered (Bancroft 1977). In my view specific behavioural treatments may be helpful as one aspect or part of an overall treatment programme of the sort outlined in this chapter. For instance, in an individual where importance is attached to increasing self-control over deviant behaviour, a specifically designed course of one of the aversive procedures, such as covert sensitization, may be undertaken. This would never be given alone but as a specific part of a mutually agreed treatment plan and in the context of a therapeutic alliance. Equally, on the same principle, a course of systematic desensitization might be of particular benefit where specific anxiety is preventing the expression of heterosexual behaviour. This may or may not be combined with a course of social skills training. Such a course might well be an appropriate part of the treatment process in other individuals.

It may be that a treatment programme conceived entirely within the behavioural framework would be superior to the mixed multi-disciplinary and eclectic approach I am advocating here. The response to that would be that there is no sound evidence available to support such a contention. Treatment methods are still empirical, and in this situation the clinician will rely on those general psychiatric approaches to treatment that constitute sound clinical practice.

Pharmacological treatment

The role of hormones in the treatment of sexual deviation is limited to those substances which suppress basic sex drive. These are the so-called anti-libido agents whose use has been generally confined to the treatment of habitual sexual offenders, such as habitual paedophiliacs and rapists. Their use raises complex ethical issues (Stoller 1973). Formerly, the most commonly used hormones were the oestrogens. They undoubtedly reduce libido and thus have a profound effect on sexual behaviour in some individuals, but their use is limited by unwanted effects, such as feminization with gynaecomastia. In recent years the development of a unique class of substances, the anti-androgens, has opened up new approaches to pharmacological inter-vention in the treatment of sexual deviations. Oestrogens produce their effects by suppressing pituitary gonadotrophin secretion, and thus endogenous testicular output of testosterone. Antiandrogens suppress basic sex drive by means of specific antagonism, by a competitive blocking effect on androgens at the hormone receptor sites. Such compounds thus block the actions of endogenous androgens produced by the testes and adrenals in males and the ovaries and adrenals in females and androgen administered therapeutically.

The antiandrogen, cyproterone acetate, has been used in Europe in the last few years in the treatment of sexual offenders. This substance is an analogue of chlormadinone, a compound widely used in oral contraceptives. It posses antigonadotrophic as well as antiandrogenic properties. This confers upon it the ability to suppress libido and potency by its antiandrogenic properties, in the presence of normal pituitary gonadotrophic levels and only slightly diminished endogenous testosterone secretion. Its administration leads to atrophy of the semi-niferous tubules which is reversible after withdrawal of the drug. It does not produce physical feminization.

A number of reports of the effects of the drug when administered to sexual offenders have appeared from Europe (see Wakeling 1977 for a summary of these studies). The most comprehensive account is that of Laschet (1973) who reported on the long-term treatment effects in a group of 150 sexually deviant males of whom half were sexual offenders. These studies suggested that at a dose of 100 to 200 mg of cyproterone acetate daily there was a marked inhibition of libido and potency, within two to three weeks after administration started, in most subjects. Although the drug reduced or inhibited sexual behaviour, the direction of the sexual drive was unaffected. Male sexuality appeared to be affected by cyproterone acetate in the following order – libido, erection, orgasm – with reversibility occurring in the same order. The dose could be adjusted either to suppress libido completely or to reduce it. Reversibility of full erectile capacity may take some weeks, and reversibility of spermato-genesis inhibition up to five months, after cessation of the drug.

These studies commented upon the paucity of undesirable or unwanted psychological or physical effects. The most common psychological manifestation was some depression of mood confined to the first few weeks of the treatment. Moderate weight gain was reported in some patients after prolonged treatment, and occasionally loss of body hair and increase in head hair, and a decrease of sebaceous gland secretion, were noted.

These studies all commented upon the positive therapeutic effects of the reduction of libido in the majority of cases. It is difficult to evaluate these claims because of the poor design of many of the studies and the lack of clinical detail presented. Double-blind techniques and objective methods for assessing change in sexual behaviour during antiandrogen administration were absent from these studies. Possible placebo effects were rarely ascertained and most of the studies up to now have utilized subjects either in prison or in other institutions, which would cast some doubt on the veracity of self-reports of change. There are a variety of objective methods for assessing change in different aspects of sexual behaviour (Bancroft 1974), but until rigorous studies utilizing such procedures have been undertaken, the precise effects of cyproterone acetate on sexual behaviour, and the specific characteristics of patients most likely to benefit from the drug, must remain in doubt. It is clear that the drug is likely to affect only sexual behaviour that is androgen-dependent and associated with a strong sex-drive. Much sexually deviant behaviour would not, of course, fall into this category.

Until more is known about the precise effects of antiandrogens on sexual behaviour, its use in the treatment of sexual deviation, like that of oestrogens, will be limited. It may be of use as part of the treatment programme in those sexually deviant individuals with high sex-drives, intense preoccupation with sexual fantasy, and poor ability to control deviant sexual urges. In such individuals the use of anti-androgens to produce a sexual 'calm' should always be combined with psychotherapeutic and other treatments. It may be that such treatment would be given over brief periods of time, to help the individual over particularly difficult or stressful life events when control over deviant behaviour might be further impaired. In other cases it might be administered over a longer period with the aim of inducing a sexual 'calm' whereby the individual might become more accessible to general psychotherapeutic treatments, perhaps combined with social-skills training in more appropriate sexual conduct. The drug would then be withdrawn whilst the other treatments continued.

In every case such treatment should only be used with the full consent of the patient. He should be fully informed of the nature of the treatment, its complications, its possible effects, and the possibility of its producing improvement. He should consent to treatment, and see that it is his decision to continue or otherwise. It is perhaps sensible initially to administer the treatment for a limited period of time within the context of a defined treatment programme.

If used in this way, cyproterone acetate (Androcur) is administered in an initial daily dose of 100 mg until libido has been decreased or inhibited. If there is no response after four weeks the dose is increased to 200 mg daily, and can be increased to 300 mg daily for short periods. After libido suppression has been accomplished a daily maintenance dose of 25 to 50 mg is usually sufficient. This can if necessary be adjusted to allow some degree of sexual activity.

The effects of treatment

Some success has been claimed for many different types of treatment, and for most types of sexual deviance. However, the task of assessing critically the effects or efficacy of specific treatments, aimed at modifying deviant sexual behaviour, is formidable. Single case reports or reports of a small, selected series of patients submitted to a particular treatment have little value – except to indicate that the condition is treatable under certain instances. Individuals who present with the same deviation differ enormously in a variety of other ways. In order to be able to assess the effects of specific treatments for particular types of deviation, it is necessary to know the outcome without treatment, and to know those prognostic features which might have a bearing on such an outcome. There is very little precise knowledge about the natural history of these conditions. Patients who improve or appear to respond to one particular form of treatment may be patients with particular features which might indicate a favourable outcome without specific treatment.

Most of the studies reported in the literature concerned with assessing the efficacy of particular treatment methods are difficult to evaluate. The clinical, psychological, and sexual characteristics of the subjects are often scantily and poorly delineated. The specific treatments used are frequently imprecisely defined, and there is usually a lack of clear-cut specific criteria to measure improvement. In some, success is determined by a reduction in deviance, in others by an increase in normal heterosexuality, and in many no specific criteria for assessing improvement are stated. Because of these variations, it is difficult to draw any comparisons between studies. There is, in addition, the problem of patient selection. Thus doctors working within different frameworks or treatment centres are likely to attract to themselves, or to have referred to them, pre-selected groups of those individuals seeking help. Referrals to a psychoanalyst are likely to differ in a great variety of ways from those referred to a behaviour therapist or a general psychiatrist; yet a different population would probably be seen by a forensic psychiatrist. Comparisons of the effects of different treatments in carefully matched, large groups of patients, with careful attention paid to measures of outcome, and with adequate length of follow-up are sadly lacking in this field.

Nevertheless, there are a number of studies, reporting the effects of various kinds of psychotherapeutic and behavioural treatments in series of patients, from which a few general points regarding outcome and prognostic features can be drawn. Most of these studies are concerned with attempts to modify homosexual behaviour, but it is possible that specific prognostic factors have relevance whatever the type of sexual deviance. The overall reported improvement rate for homosexuals treated with behaviour therapy is of the order of 30 to 40 per cent and this is strikingly similar to that reported using psychotherapeutic techniques (Bancroft 1974, p.148). The general prognostic factors indicating favourable outcome are similar in the two groups of studies.

Thus, strong motivation, a positive desire for change, and a willingness to work towards it are undoubtedly of importance. Some degree of heterosexual behaviour or interest prior to treatment appears to increase the likelihood of a successful outcome. Age also appears to be a factor, albeit an uncertain one; the general view being that people above the age of 35 are less likely to change their sexual behaviour. Good intelligence and a personality structure with features associated with the ability to achieve satisfaction in interpersonal relationships, also seem to be good prognostic indicators. The more the individual is integrated within his deviant subculture, and the more his deviance is ego-syntonic, perhaps the less is the likelihood of change. All studies have shown that, for many individuals, the direction of homosexual drive cannot be substantially altered with current treatment methods. In general it appears that the more arrested the personality structure and the psychosexual development, the less chance there is of substantially changing sexual behaviour. Clinical experience, however, attests to the value of therapeutic intervention for many sexual deviants. It also emphasizes that, in our current state of limited knowledge, it is impossible to predict the outcome to a course of treatment in the individual case.

There are, as yet, no firm guidelines from the literature as to the choice between different treatment techniques for any particular type of deviant sexuality, and no firm indications of the success rate for any specific kind of treatment. I have advocated a general clinical approach, essentially multidisciplinary and eclectic in nature, to the treatment of these disorders. Such an approach is based upon a framework of accumulated clinical experience rather than theoretical assumptions about aetiology, and would obviously be modified in the light of further research findings and experience.

References

Bancroft, J. H. J. (1974). *Deviant Sexual Behaviour: Modifications and Assessment*. Oxford.

—— (1977). The behavioural approach to treatment. In *Handbook of Sexology, Section XVI* (ed. J. Money and H. Musaph). Amsterdam and London.

Bandura, A. (1969). Social learning theory of identificatory processes. In *Handbook of Socialization Theory and Research* (ed. D. A. Goslin). Chicago.

Barlow, D., Abel, G. G., and Blanchard, E. (1974). Plasma testosterone levels and male homosexuality: a failure to replicate. *Arch. Sex. Behav.* **3**, 571.

Bell, R. Q. (1968). A reinterpretation of the direction of effects in studies of socialization. *Psychol. Rev.* **75**, 81.

Bene, E. (1965*a*). On the genesis of male homosexuality: an attempt at clarifying the role of the parents. *Brit. J. Psychiat.* **111**, 803.

—— (1965*b*). On the Genesis of female homosexuality. *Brit. J. Psychiat.* **111**, 815.

Bieber, I., Dain, J. H., Dince, P. R., Drellich, M. G., Grand, H. G., Gundlach, R. H., Kremer, M. W., Rifkin, A. H., Wilbur, C. B., and Bieber, T. B. (1962). *Homosexuality: A psychoanalytic study*. New York.

Brodie, H. K. H., Gartrell, N., Doering, C., and Rhue, T. (1974). Plasma testosterone levels in heterosexual and homosexual men. *Am. J. Psychiat.* **131**, 82.

Doerr, P., Kockott, G., Vogt, H. G., Pirke, K. M., and Dittmar, F. (1973). Plasma testosterone, estradiol and semen analysis in male homosexuals. *Arch. Gen. Psychiat.* **29**, 829.

Ehrhardt, A., Epstein, R., and Money, J. (1968). Fetal androgens and female gender identity in the early treated adrenogenital syndrome. *Johns Hopkins Med. J.* **122**, 160.

Evans, R. (1969). Childhood parental relationships of homosexual men. *J. Consult. Clin. Psychol.* **33**, 129.

Feldman, M. P. (1973). Abnormal sexual behaviour – males. In *Handbook of Abnormal psychology* (ed. H. J. Eysenck). London.

Fenichel, O. (1945). *The psychoanalytic theory of neurosis*. New York.

Fox, C. A., Ismail, A. A. A., Love, D. N., Kirkham, K. E., and Loraine, J. A. (1972). Studies on the relationship between plasma testosterone levels and human sexual activity. *J. Endocrinol.* **52**, 51.

Green, R. (1977). Atypical psychosexual development. In *Child psychiatry: modern approaches* (ed. M. Rutter and L. Hersov). Oxford.

Gundlach, R. H. (1969). Childhood parental relationships and the establishment of gender roles of homosexuals. *J. Consult. Clin. Psychol.* **33**, 136.

Hampson, J. L. and Hampson, J. G. (1961). The ontogenesis of sexual behaviour in men. In *Sex and internal secretions* (ed. W. C. Young) (3rd edn.). Baltimore.

Heston, L. L. and Shields, J. (1968). Homosexuality in twins. *Arch. Gen. Psychiat.* **18**, 149.

Hooker, E. (1965). Male homosexuals and their worlds. In *Sexual inversion* (ed. J. Marmor). New York.

Kagan, J. (1964). Acquisition and significance of sex typing and sex role identity. In *Review of Child Development Research, Vol. 1* (ed. M. L. Hoffman and L. W. Hoffman). New York.

Kallman, F. J. (1952). Comparative twin study on the genetic aspects of male homosexuality. *J. Nerv. Ment. Dis.* **115**, 283.

Klintworth, G. K. (1962). A pair of male monozygotic twins discordant for homosexuality. *J. Nerv. Ment. Dis.* **135**, 113.

Kinsey, A. C., Pomeroy, W. B., and Martin, C. E. (1948). *Sexual behaviour in the human male.* Philadelphia.

——, ——, ——, and Gebhard, P. H. (1953). *Sexual behaviour in the human female.* Philadelphia.

Kohlberg, L. (1967). A cognitive-developmental analysis of children's sex role concepts and attitudes. In *The Development of Sex Differences* (ed. E. E. Maccoby). London.

Kolodny, R. C., Masters, W. H., Hendryx, J., and Toro, G. (1971). Plasma testosterone and semen analysis in male homosexuals. *New England J. Med.* **285**, 1170.

——, ——, Kolodner, R. M., and Toro, G. (1974). Depression of plasma testosterone levels after chronic intensive marijuana use. *New England J. Med.* **290**, 872.

Kreuz, L. E., Rose, R. M., and Jennings, J. R. (1972). Suppression of plasma testosterone levels and psychological stress. *Arch. Gen. Psychiat.* **26**, 479.

Laschet, V. (1973). Antiandrogens in the treatment of sex offenders: mode of action and therapeutic outcome. In *Contemporary sexual behaviour: critical issues in the 70's* (ed. J. Zubin and J. Money). Baltimore.

Lebovitz, P. (1972). Feminine behaviour in boys—aspects of its outcome. *Am. J. Psychiat.* **128**, 1283.

Loraine, J. A., Ismail, A. A. A., Adamopoulos, D. A., and Dove, G. A. (1970). Endocrine function in male and female homosexuals. *Br. Med. J.,* (**iv**), 406.

Maccoby, E. E. and Jacklin, C. N. (1975). *The psychology of sex differences.* London.

Maguire, R. J., Carlisle, J. M., and Young, B. G. (1965). Sexual deviation as conditioned behaviour: a hypothesis. *Behav. Res. Ther.* **2**, 185.

Margolese, S. (1970). Homosexuality: a new endocrine correlate. *Horm. Behav.* **1**, 151.

Masters, W. H. and Johnson, V. E. (1966). *Human sexual response.* London.

—— and —— (1970). *Human sexual inadequacy.* London.

Mischel, W. (1967). A social learning view of sex differences in behaviour. In *The development of sex differences* (ed. E. E. Maccoby). London.

—— (1970). Sex typing and socialization. In *Manual of child psychology, Vol. 11* (ed. P. H. Musson). New York.

Money, J. and Ehrhardt, A. (1973). *Man and woman; boy and girl.* Baltimore.

O'Connor, J. (1964). Aetiological factors in homosexuality as seen in Royal Air Force psychiatric practice. *Brit. J. Psychiat.* **110**, 381.

Parker, N. (1964). Twins: a psychiatric study of a neurotic group. *Med. J. Austral.* **2**, 735.

Pillard, R., Rose, R. M., and Sherwood, M. (1974). Plasma testosterone levels in homosexual men. *Arch. Sex. Behav.* **3**, 577.

Prince, V. and Bentler, P. (1972). Survey of 504 cases of transvestism. *Psychol. Rep.* **31**, 903.

Rainer, J. D., Mensikoff, A., Kolb, L. C., and Carr, A. (1960). Homosexuality and heterosexuality in identical twins. *Psychosom. Med.* **22**, 251.

Rose, R. M., Bourne, P. G., and Poe, R. O. (1969). Androgen response to stress, *Psychosom. Med.* **31**, 418.

Rosenthal, D. (1970). *Genetic theory and abnormal behaviour.* New York.

Saghir, M. and Robins, E. (1973). *Male and female homosexuality.* Baltimore.

Scott, P. D. (1964). Definition, classification, prognosis and treatment. In *The pathology and treatment of sexual deviation* (ed. I. Rosen). London.

Siegelman, M. (1974). Parental background of male homosexuals and heterosexuals. *Arch. Sex. Behav.* **3**, 3.

Stoller, R. J. (1973). Psychoanalysis and physical intervention in the brain: the mind body problem again. In *Contemporary sexual behaviour: critical issues in the 70's* (ed. J. Zubin and J. Money). Baltimore.

Tourney, G. and Hatfield, L. M. (1973). Androgen metabolism in schizophrenics, homosexuals, and controls. *Biol. Psychiat.* **6**, 23.

Wakeling, A. (1977). Antilibido agents. In *Psychotherapeutic drugs Part II:— Applications* (ed. E. Usdin and I. S. Forrest). New York.

West, D. J. (1959). Parental figures in the genesis of male homosexuality. *Int. J. Soc. Psychiat.* **5**, 58.

—— (1968). *Homosexuality* (3rd edn), London.

Yarrow, M. R., Campbell, J. D., and Burton, R. V. (1970). Recollections of childhood: a study of the retrospective method. *Mon. Soc. Res. Child. Develop.* **35**, No. 5 (Serial No. 138).

Young, W. C., Goy, R. W., and Phoenix, C. H. (1964). Hormones and behaviour. *Science* **143**, 212.

Zuger, B. (1966). Effeminate behaviour present in boys from early childhood. *J. Pediatr.* **69**, 1098.

2

The general psychoanalytical theory of perversion: a critical and clinical review

Ismond Rosen

Introduction

This chapter reviews the psychoanalytical literature on the general theory of perversions, emphasizing the contributions from the last fifteen years. For an historical review of the preceding period, see Gillespie (1964). The term perversion covers a vast field of human experience in what is now a widely expanding area of psychoanalytic knowledge. Whereas no succinct, generally-accepted theory of the perversions has emerged, notable contributions have been made by many analysts, working individually or in research groups. Our understanding of the general theory of the perversions has been furthered by detailed investigations into special areas of interest. Many authors are either contributors to this volume, or their work is referred to in it. May I express my appreciation of the work of all these analysts, whose ideas will be credited where they are either original, expressed in a novel way, or appropriate to illustrate developments in thought or observation.

Definition of perversion

We live in an era of increasing tolerance of all forms of individual sexual expression and identity. Accordingly, terms such as perversion and sexual deviation are regarded as unnecessarily pejorative, degrading to self-esteem, and better replaced by less specific phraseology, if referred to at all. Let us remember that acceptance of sexuality in all its forms received its main impetus this century from Freud. Psychoanalysts still follow his tradition, and treat patients, teach, and research into sexual problems with tolerance and respect (see also Wiedemann's comments in Panel Report 1977, p.183). Analytic authors have preferred to retain the term perversion in their writings, using sexual deviation as an optional alternative. The basis for this retention is that perversion denotes a group of clinical and

29

psychopathological entities in which common features can be eluci-
dated. Perversions may be distinguished from neuroses, psychoses, and
character disorders, although aspects of these latter conditions may
coincide with established perversions, or interact dynamically with
them. Understanding the dynamics of perversion as an entity improves
the ability to treat the condition.

Features common to all perversions were clarified by Freud in his
'Three essays on the theory of sexuality' (1905). With certain modifications they still hold good. Deviant or perverse sexuality denotes a
sexual preference which departs from the accepted norm of heterosexual coitus with orgasm. It is as if part of sexual foreplay had grown
in intensity and importance so as to take over the role of genitality
itself. Such an act or preoccupation might be the need to look at or to
exhibit the sexual organs, to experience or inflict pain, as the prerequisite to the attainment of sexual satisfaction. The preferred sexual
mode derives from any of the basic drives or objects (part-object,
transitional object, whole-object) experienced in childhood – sucking,
excreting, masturbation, or identifying with behaviour usually regarded as belonging to the opposite sex. As a result, actual genital
behaviour in intercourse becomes either impossible, unsatisfying, or
facilitated only by the perverse act.

A distinction must be made between behaviour that is perverse, and
the pathological syndrome of perversion. In both, the sexual behaviour
derives from infantile sexuality, where single components, or alternating polymorphous perverse elements, become predominant. In
perversion, there is the characteristic of repetitive fixed behaviour
which leads to orgasm, and which facilitates potency.

Freud's libido theory distinguished between disorders of aim
(perversion) from disorders of subject choice (inversion – a term which
is rarely used now). Perversion needs to be understood now from many
points of view. The drives, libidinal and aggressive; the ego functions,
gender identity, and super-ego effects upon both the drives and the
ego-ideal; the object relationships which have been formed in early life
with partial and whole objects, and with other persons during later
development; the internalized representations of the self and the objects
and the relationships between them; and finally the inner and outer
world's effects on the personality as a whole, and the whole-self's
response expressed as the sense of self-esteem.

Clinical features in the definition of perversion

The drives: perversion and genitality

The elements of compulsion and fixity in perversion are well known. Recent authors have reiterated these facts. McDougall (1972) extended their scope in her definition. 'One factor which would appear to characterize the pervert...is that he has no choice; his sexuality is fundamentally compulsive'. 'The erotic expression of the sexual deviant is an essential feature of his psychic stability and much of his life revolves around it'. She added that in perverse character traits there was a concious erotization of the defences.

Freud's theory of sexual development was that the partial instincts of earliest infancy became integrated initially under the influence of genital primacy in the phallic phase preceding latency, and permanently organized from puberty onwards. It cannot be stressed sufficiently that perversion is the interference with integrated genital sexuality by a component drive. This is revealed in maturity where one aspect of foreplay predominates in pleasure over the sexual act itself. Fenichel (1945) following Freud, postulated that perversion was due to a disturbance of genital primacy for which the partial component instict was a substitution. He sought to determine the nature of the disturbance of genital primacy. As genital primacy commenced at the time of the phallic phase and oedipal complex, he postulated that it was the accompanying castration anxiety which undid the integrating genital primacy. Anxiety led to regression to pre-oedipal infantile sexuality because genital enjoyment had become too threatening and therefore impossible. The infantile component chosen was determined by previous fixations, and he largely discounted the influence of constitutional factors. Alexander (1965) thought perversion could result either from the fixation of partial drives, or be due to regression where disintegrative forces led to the genital patterns of psychic function breaking down into their components.

Balint (1965) writing on 'Perversions and genitality' pointed out that all perversions have genital pleasure as their final aim, although the perversion was usually concerned with the quality of experience gained from the object in foreplay. During coital orgasm, all persons required the capacity and the willingness to allow themselves to regress emotionally. This mature regressive capacity was the prerequisite for sexual gratification, plus the resulting tranquil contentment and sense of well-being. The achievement of this regression presupposed a well-integrated ego which had mastered castration anxiety. All perverts avoided this regression due to their ego weakness, lack of integration, faulty mastery over anxiety (especially castration anxiety), and their faulty sense of reality, which was similar to that found in neurotics but defended against in a different way.]

Ostow and his group (1974) found significant differences in the role of the genitals in defining perversion, 'perverse behaviour usually occurred in two distinct phases; the specific perverse activity, followed by apparently normal intercourse in which the person's potency was augmented by the antecedent perverse behaviour'. They also believed that the occurrence of normal intercourse did not invalidate the diagnosis of perversion. In their experience it was common to find married persons with perverse patterns expressing the perverse sexuality extra-maritally, while continuing a 'lack-lustre and per-functory' sex-life, which appeared normal, within the marriage. Such cases are known to most workers within this field. In my clinical experience, sexual excitement remains attached to the perverse object and practice, and normal intercourse may not occur, or be emotionally irrelevant, in keeping with a pseudo-genitality.

There seems general agreement that in the perversions, whatever the source of the initial erotic stimulation, which is where the height of gratification may lie, the final common pathway of sexual discharge is genital orgasm. Impotence or inadequacy of genital discharge in the absence of the perverse mechanism being exercised, is a hall mark of perversion.

The libidinal aspects of the perverse, or infantile, sexual-wishes have long been stressed. Fenichel regarded the original childhood sexual fixations as having been chosen for their reassuring effect against fear, having been experienced in childhood as providing feelings of security, which warded off the anxiety of castration and therefore made genital functioning possible again. Later in the chapter we shall deal with the origins of the hyper-libidinization, or hypertrophy of the libidinal aspects of the component infantile sexual drives. The hyper-libidinization provides the intense pleasure in the practice of the perversion, which, flooding the ego, reassures against castration anxiety, and makes the perverse act realizable even at the cost of inappropriate behaviour, which is out of keeping with reality.

Aggression

A growing body of evidence is now confirming the role of aggression in the aetiology of perversion. Childhood frustrations and traumas lead to an intensification of the aggressive drives in the child, which increases the sadism of the oral and anal phases, as well as the phallic castration anxiety. This will be discussed in detail later. For the clinical aspects of aggression, libido, and perversion, see Chapter 11.

Stoller has selected aggression, in the form of hatred, to be one of the major elements in his definition of perversion. In his book *Perversion: the erotic form of hatred* (1975a), he regards hostility as the primary motive in perversions, which 'takes form in a fantasy of revenge hidden in the actions that make up the perversion and serve to convert childhood trauma to adult triumph'. The trauma according to Stoller is always aimed at the sense of gender. Stoller's examination of the meaningfulness of the trauma and revenge theme in terms of the self and its narcissistic evaluation are valuable, because this theme is found in all perversions to some degree. Because of the small size of the sample of cases studied by Stoller, who were mainly gender disorders, it is doubtful if the valuation placed by him on these factors regarding aetiology is generally valid.

Ego aspects

Perversion usually implies a sexual act of some kind which is insistent and gratifying. This behaviour may be ego-syntonic, that is freely acceptable by the self, or, quite often after the event, ego-dystonic, experienced as unacceptable. It is frequently the threat of discovery or police arrest which makes the person request for help. Running risks introduces the element of excitement which raises self-esteem.

Object relationships

Perversion always takes as its object something representing a primary object, usually the mother, The sexual object may be some feature of the self; it may be symbolized by some material if the use of the material is necessary for sexual fulfilment; or some other person may play a carefully defined role. However, where there are strong narcissistic elements in the personality a partner may be dispensed with, and the perversion may be indulged in a solitary fashion. The function of perversion for narcissistic purposes has been stressed by Greenacre, while Rosen (1964, 1968) explored the idea of perversion as a regulator of self-esteem (see Chapter 3).

In those cases where the criteria for the presence of perversion are met, there are often additional signs of mental disturbances. Mention has been made too of the concurrence of psycho-somatic disorders in homosexuality, as evidence of the early disturbances in body-ego function. See also Sperling (1968), McDougall (1972).

Homosexuality as perversion. The question of whether homosexuality deserves to be classified as a perversion is dealt with in Chapters 7, 8, and 9.

Balint (1965) placed homosexuality among the perversions on the basis of 'the atmosphere of pretense and denial that is so characteristic of the other group of perversions'. 'This overemphasis is in order to deny – what they all know – that, without normal intercourse, there is no real contentment'.

Ostow's group considered perversion and homosexuality as two aspects of the same disorder because of their frequent association. They justified this approach on the grounds that:

(1) the developmental arrest required for one appeared to favour the other;
(2) both phenomena represented infantile fixations, with respect to the object in homosexuality and to the aim in perversion;
(3) narcissism, infantilism, and acting-out were common to both perversion and homosexuality; and
(4) homosexuality was sometimes used as a defense against other forms of sexual deviation which would become predominant in heterosexual relationships if they were permitted.

They qualified their view by the statement that homosexual behaviour need not be perverse under certain social conditions, and where there is no 'quality of compulsion and fixity'.

The importance of compulsion and fixity of homosexual behaviour would appear to be supported by the work of Limentani (1976) in his study 'Object choice and actual bisexuality'. He presented cases which revealed a protracted capacity for both heterosexual and homosexual relationships. These people commonly had borderline and narcissistic states. Their underlying psychopathology included a tendency to be caught up between anaclitic and narcissistic types of object choice. Their bisexual involvement was basically illusory, as the two objects, male and female, with whom they were involved were a cover up for splitting of the original love-object together with a severe preoedipal disturbance. See Chapter 7, page 202.

In this regard, Balint made an important point about object

relationships in the perversions. Such people remained fixated in their loving to what he called 'primary love' – a partnership where only one partner may have desires, wishes, and interests. This diminished capacity for object relationship will be examined later, but it is as well to point out here that in the extreme case the fetishist may come to rely on an object that is not only symbolic but purely inanimate. Balint asserted that in perversion there was an escape from the necessity of the work of conquest with the partner, where initial indifference was changed into a cooperative genital sexual partnership. This raises important issues of classification where permissive attitudes towards sexuality may have led to increased promiscuity. Promiscuity, like the professional counterpart, prostitution, is a disorder of object relationships. The degree to which character disorder, neurosis, or sado-masochism plays a part must be determined in each case. Promiscuity as a perversion depends on the degree to which the behaviour is compulsive, necessary for the attainment of satisfactory orgasm, and fixed to a violation of cultural attitudes, plus the association of overt perverse practices which are disguised because of the sado-masochistic features.

Not all sado-masochistic relationships are perverted and therefore must be separated from true perversions. In the former the sexual and social conquest has been made, but the relationship in its basic sexual and social meaningfulness has regressed and withered leaving the elemental battle for control over one partner, or over each other, based on emotional blackmail. Such relationships I would more properly regard as 'cruelty relationships' because of the libidinal de-cathexis of the relationship leading to hard-hearted indifference, denial of the feelings of the partner or of both, and the accent on cruel attitudes and personal gratification at the expense of the partner, who remains under subtle control and trapped in the situation. Some people cruelly use multiple objects to gratify separate urges – for sex, for domestic purposes, for comfort against loneliness. In the cruelty relationship, the aim of the sado-masochism is not sexual gratification leading to orgasm, but a raised self-esteem from controlling the object and inflicting punishment in lieu of the primary frustrating and controlling mother.

Aetiology of the perversions

In this review chapter there is an advantage in presenting the theoretical view of perversion which pertained in the early nineteen sixties followed by an account of the evolution in psychoanalytic thinking leading to present day understanding.

Gillespie's general summary of the psychoanalytic theory of perversion (1964) was as follows.

The essence of the theory is still to be found in Freud's *Three Essays on the Theory of Sexuality*. It is impossible to begin to understand sexual perversions without a knowledge of infantile sexuality, of its peculiar features, its development and vicissitudes, and of the transformations which it normally goes through at puberty before emerging as adult sexuality.

Nevertheless, what we encounter clinically in cases of perversion is by no means, or only rarely, a simple continuation into adult life of all the elements of infantile sexuality. On the contrary, most clinical perversions are highly specialized and specific; that is, only very limited ways remain open to the adult pervert for achieving sexual excitement, discharging sexual tension and establishing a sexual object relationship. A clinical perversion of this kind has a very obvious defensive function, with the aim of warding off anxieties concerned with the Oedipus complex, and especially castration anxiety. It is, therefore, in the nature of a compromise between instinctual impulse and ego defence, and in this way closely resembles a neurotic symptom.

The defences adopted in perversion involve regressions of various kinds – regression of libido to pregenital levels, and regression too in the aggressive impulse: together this leads to an increase in sadism, which gives rise to further anxieties specific to the dangers both to the object and to the self which are inherent in sadism, and to consequent defences designed to ensure the safety of both.

The behaviour of the ego in perversion is especially characteristic; instead of an attitude of hostility to the instincts, dictated by super-ego pressure (as in neurosis), the ego adopts as its own one particular piece of infantile sexuality, and this helps it to oppose the rest. The result depends on a super-ego which is tolerant of this specific aspect of sexuality. Splits in the ego and in the object make possible attitudes to reality, confined to the sexual sphere, which, if more widespread, would lead to a psychosis.

Reference to the wide-ranging developments during the past fifteen years in psychoanalysis in general, and the perversions in particular, may be made by following Greenacre (1968), who listed the areas best studied to enlarge our knowledge of the perversions:

(1) Theories of aggression.

(2) Studies of ego maturation and function.

(3) Studies of separation and individuation.

(4) Stages of object relationship.

(5) Body-image development.

(6) Early body-ego formation.

(7) Development of self-representation.

(8) Problems of identity.

Particular reference to these areas will be made in the study of the aetiology of perversion, which will be under four headings:

(a) Factors contributing to the formation of the perverse drive component.

(b) Early development factors.

(c) Ego mechanisms and organization.

(d) Perversion as a regulator of self-esteem (see Chapter 3).

Formation of the perverse drive component

Aetiological factors in perversion are best studied by examining major elements in development in isolation, and then trying to understand how they interact to produce psychic organization of structure and function. These are charted in Fig. 2.1.

Infantile sexuality has a polymorphous perverse quality, which may lead to many different perverse aims being present in an organized perversion. Usually there is the intensification of only a single or partial drive which becomes the core of the perverse strivings. The drive intensification, according to the literature, stems from a combination of constitutional and environmental factors. Constitutional elements were considered by Freud: (i) as a general cause of perversion and neurosis, where both were found to occur in the same family (1905); (ii) as precursors of the weakness of the urge towards the normal sexual aim; and (iii) in the person's final attitude to sex not being determined until puberty. Bisexual tendencies were regarded as having a constitutional basis, as was the capacity for sexual pleasure from parts of the body other than the genitals.

Constitutional factors are not much better understood now, though we prefer to regard them as biological or hereditary. The biological factors underlying sexuality are dealt with in Chapters 1 and 14. On the hereditary side, there are several reports of perversions occurring within the same family – transsexualism (Hore, Nicolle, and Calnan 1973; Stoller and Baker 1973; Hoenig and Duggan 1974), masochism

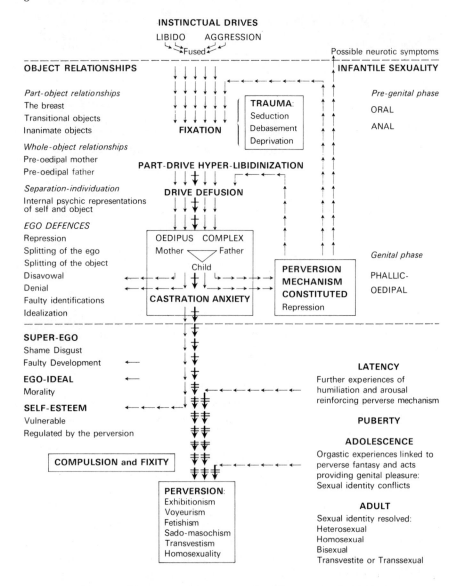

INSTINCTUAL DRIVES
LIBIDO   AGGRESSION
Fused

Possible neurotic symptoms

OBJECT RELATIONSHIPS

INFANTILE SEXUALITY

Part-object relationships
The breast
Transitional objects
Inanimate objects

Pre-genital phase
ORAL
ANAL

TRAUMA:
Seduction
Debasement
Deprivation

FIXATION

Whole-object relationships
Pre-oedipal mother
Pre-oedipal father

PART-DRIVE HYPER-LIBIDINIZATION

Separation-individuation
Internal psychic representations
of self and object

DRIVE DEFUSION

EGO DEFENCES
Repression
Splitting of the ego
Splitting of the object
Disavowal
Denial
Faulty identifications
Idealization

OEDIPUS COMPLEX
Mother   Father
Child

CASTRATION ANXIETY

PERVERSION
MECHANISM
CONSTITUTED
Repression

Genital phase
PHALLIC-
OEDIPAL

SUPER-EGO
Shame Disgust
Faulty Development

EGO-IDEAL
Morality

SELF-ESTEEM
Vulnerable
Regulated by the perversion

COMPULSION and FIXITY

LATENCY
Further experiences of
humiliation and arousal
reinforcing perverse mechanism

PUBERTY

ADOLESCENCE
Orgastic experiences linked to
perverse fantasy and acts
providing genital pleasure:
Sexual identity conflicts

PERVERSION:
Exhibitionism
Voyeurism
Fetishism
Sado-masochism
Transvestism
Homosexuality

ADULT
Sexual identity resolved:
Heterosexual
Homosexual
Bisexual
Transvestite or Transsexual

Fig.2.1   Diagrammatic representation of perversion formation.

(de M'Uzan 1973). Genetic factors in transsexualism were examined by Wålinder and Thuwe (1977) who studied 61 cases of transsexualism in Sweden, where excellent records exist for family relationships dating back to the seventeenth century. No case of cousin marriages was disclosed, although there was a normal assumption of 1–2 cousin marriages per 100 marriages in Sweden. This was against the hypothesis of recessive genes playing a part in the causation of transsexualism. Genetic influences in homosexuality have been reviewed by Bancroft (1975) for males, and Kenyon (1975) for females. The conclusions they drew were that genetic factors in some cases sensitized the individual to certain environmental influences, but did not necessarily influence the direction of the libido directly. Stoller (1975*b*) concurred that biological potentialities were subject to environmental influences for realization. Hereditary, as well as normal factors, producing variable drive intensities are discussed by Dr Wakeling in Chapter 1. In general the effect of biology on drives and in perversion in particular remains unresolved, and clinical analysts still think in terms of a constitutional and environmental interaction producing psychic determinism.

The psychological reasons advanced for increased drive intensity in perversion are based on childhood sexual trauma due to seduction and deprivation, singly or in combination. Freud (1905) showed that seduction had both drive and object consequences. Perverse sexuality was 'an innately human characteristic in children, brought out by seduction' (p.191). 'Seduction is confusing in that it presents children prematurely with a sexual object for which the infantile sexual instinct shows no great need.'

In early childhood, pre-genital sexual seduction is traumatic because the intensity of the experience is beyond the infant's capacity to endure it. The ego anxiety aroused by being out of control is countered by the hyper-libidinization accompanying the pleasure in the experience. The pleasure arising from the closeness and sense of togetherness of the encounters is experienced, when they cease, as loneliness and loss, which contributes to the longing to repeat the experience. Actual loss is perceived as traumatic when active separation, deprivation, or rejection follows the seductions, or is interspersed with them. The inner perceptions of the self in relation to external objects are therefore somewhat distorted in the direction of a narcissistic orientation, with the pleasure-pain modality exceptionally sensitized. Compulsive repetition of traumatic aspects of pleasure and frustration occurs as a means of gaining ego mastery of the events, as is the ego defence of turning passive experience into activity done to others. The most important result of seduction is the hyper-libidinization or erotization, which is mobilized with the defences together with the increased aggressive feelings that are engendered.

There is therefore libidinization of anxiety, ego defences, aggressive drives, as well as the accompanying affects. Libidinization of the narcissistic constellations also occurs to protect the emerging self from the traumas of being mastered, overwhelmed, and devalued, following the libidinal overvaluation from the erotic experiences.

It is generally accepted that what has been said about the aims of the drives in perversion could be equally true for neurosis. The early theoretical difference between perversion and neurosis was that the drives suffer different fates. The developmental barrier of castration anxiety led to drive repression in neurosis, but to sexual gratification of the drive in perversion. Hence Freud's 1905 dictum, 'neurosis is the negative of perversion'. Sachs (1923) was credited with having shown that perversion also has defensive organizational functions similar to neurosis, which was why symptoms of perversion and neurosis occur in the same person. Sachs described a mechanism in perversion, where the highly developed partial-drive with its powerful pregenital pleasure aspects was taken up into the ego, and used in the repression of other wishes, aggressive and libidinal, stemming from oedipal conflicts that could not pass the castration anxiety barrier. These repressed conflicts could become linked to earlier fixations that unconsciously provided a sense of comfort and security, or they could be expressed through neurotic symptom formations. The pre-genital powerful partial drive (with its object representation) passed through the Oedipus complex where it formed relationships of a special kind, which accounted for the pre-oedipal fixations manifesting as oedipal pathology. The manoevre whereby the perverse wish is taken up by the ego, and used in the service of repression of other unwelcome oedipal wishes, constitutes the mechanism of perversion from the point of view of the libido theory. The high degree of pleasure in the perverse infantile sexual component entering the ego is what enables it to pass the castration barrier, and to be further developed at puberty and adolescence into the full-scale perversion. See Fig. 2.1. on p.38.

In passing it must be stressed that perversions always contain the element of conflict. Because of the apparent freedom of action and the high degree of pleasure and urge, the view has been aired that a conflict-free aspect may exist in perversion together with the traditional conflictual basis of psychic symptomatology. Some non-analysts prefer to exclude psychic conflict in perversion, because it signifies inner motivation. This approach, for example, makes it easier to attribute homosexuality to biological or social causes, which eliminates the need for treatment due to the supposed organic or statistically acceptable aetiology. This does not fit the facts found in analytical treatment situations, where perversions including homosexuality, relate to complex defence systems dealing with the unconscious conflicts of infantile sexuality, gender identity, and object relationships, especially the separation-individuation experiences and transitional object fixations. The latter phenomena are dealt with in Chapter 4 by Phyllis Greenacre, with special reference to fetishism, but they play a significant role in perversions generally. Conflict may be considered to arise from the following sources:

(a) The libidinal and aggressive drives;

(b) Loving and hating affects in the relationships with parents and siblings at the pregenital as well as the oedipal level. The objects and the self must be protected from the aggressive and destructive wishes.

(c) Masculine and feminine identity aims, based on biological bisexuality and the later conflicts of identification with parental figures.

(d) Castration anxiety, especially the need to protect the genitals, and in the boy, the need to maintain primacy of the penis.

I now turn to aggression, which, in the period under review, has come very much to the fore in the study of perversion. Distinction must be made between aggression as a drive, and aggression as hostility derived from frustration (see Chapter 10). Freud regarded libido and aggression as the two basic drives normally existing together in a fused state, which gave to sexuality the impulse for mastery over the object of desire. What was fused together could conversely undergo various degrees of defusion. The sadistic aspects of the normal pregenital phases, oral and anal, were accompanied by the ambivalent loving and hating attitudes towards the same object. These disparate tendencies only became integrated later, during the phallic or genital phases. The drive regressions due to castration anxiety led, in the perversions, to an increase in instinctual defusion. The degree of defusion was reflected later in the variable intensity of sado-masochism in the perverse sexual and emotional life. Pronounced sado-masochism featuring as the major characteristic in a perversion resulted from the aggregation of several additional factors.

One case of sado-masochism reported by Ostow was described as having the aggression 'commingled' rather than completely fused with the erotic elements, so that there was no attenuation of each other. Instinctual fusion-defusion is a continuum, with the sadism of normal infantile phase development at one end, the developed sado-masochistic perversion at the centre, and at the other extreme, uncontrolled acts of violence and destruction which could be sexualized, as in rape or sexual murder. In general, the high degree of libidinization in perversion serves to bind the increased aggression and hostility, so that physical damage is rarely done to others. Danger occurs when the perversion fails, that is to say there is insufficient libido to contain the aggression, the perverse mechanisms are deficient, or there has been hyperabundant aggression aroused by threats to the self and its preservation in reality.

In masochistic perversions, there is a conflict between the hostile wish and the placatory expiation of guilt to preserve the loved object. There appears to be a relation between the severity of the adult perversion and the severity of the traumatic experiences in childhood. The following clinical vignette exemplifies this and many other features of a perversion which will serve as an introduction to the next sections on object relationships and identification.

The patient had a life style of a masochistic surrender of assets and opportunity. His sexual gratifications were perverse and required him to be beaten by prostitutes. He had idealized fantasies of loving and possessing beautiful young women, which he felt to be impossible to realize, but he was tempted to make sexual advances to very young girls which he feared would lead to his arrest. Most of his earnings went in supporting an alcoholic ex-prostitute, and he cared for her every want. He was a well-educated mild-mannered and softly spoken person, who lived alone. In childhood his identical twin brother died of illness. The triumph of his normal twin-rivalry death-wish was short-lived. He was present at a prestigious consultation where his parents were told he too was not expected to live – an attitude descriptive of his life thereafter in a masochistic sense. His mother who had previously been very close became withdrawn, and his oedipal conflicts and father rivalry were accentuated. He responded to all of this with passivity, unconsciously atoning and surviving by refusing to live. The aggression in the underlying conflict was turned against himself and libidinized. The masochism was also a defence against the underlying sadness and loss of the attachment to the brother. The conflicts he had experienced about actual closeness between himself, his twin, and his mother, were enacted in his symbiotic 'life-saving' dealings with the prostitute, where he reversed the roles of mother and child, turned passive into active, and exercised his primary identification with the feeding mother, and a dual identification with father and mother at the oedipal level.

This case is instructive for many reasons. It demonstrates the fact that beneath masochism there is an opposite unconscious fantasy of omnipotent mastery, which gains pleasurable gratification through suffering. The patient's sexual impulses and their being granted satisfaction in reality, signified the possibility of suffering and punishment, whether there was orgasmic relief or not. His main source of fulfilment was compliance-defiance, with his inner super-ego dominance, and a merging narcissistic submission to demands. Falling in love with a girl at work resulted in his losing his job. His basic aim in treatment was not to obtain relief, but to gain help in avoiding impulsive acts towards young girls. During treatment, aggressive impulses with masochistic aspects predominated, but were bound by the hyperlibidinization. Pre-oedipal fears of annihilation served to augment his castration anxiety, and a massive regression ensued. Frankly paranoid ideas emerged which supported Kohut's idea that if a great variety of polymorphous perverse acts presented in the perversion, a borderline condition lay underneath. The perversion assisted in covering the flaw in his reality sense (Glover 1964). Most of the analytical material described above was uncovered only after much treatment. Lihn (1971) has described a similar case of masochism which stresses the importance of the real preoedipal experiences of traumatic suffering and erotic experiences which were repeated in a similar pattern in adulthood. The oedipal aspects were distorted, and there were regressions to the libidinized fixations. The whole complicated picture can only be understood in all such cases as having 'a constructive function – the recovery of narcissistic integrity' (de M'Uzan 1973).

This author described a case of unusually severe masochism; the patient had a masochistic cousin, whom he married, and a father who was also masochistic. Constitutional factors were indicated in this case to explain the ego's reaction to pain, which was such as to require an escalating degree of torture for the sought after sexual ejaculation to occur. The masochistic perverse sexual pleasure was secondary, however, to the main aim of humiliation. The self-renunciation and striving for total humiliation was to fulfil a uniquely intense fantasy, that in this way he could heal his underlying primordial narcissistic wound. This unique case was previously documented in French in the excellent publication *La sexualité perverse* (de M'Uzan 1972).

In these cases, the fantasies and passive experiences of being beaten corroborate recent findings in the literature. Most males with beating fantasies are likely to maintain an identification with a castrated mother, and this identification may obscure identification with, and a vengeful fury toward, the phallic mother. The accomodation becomes then, a solution of the oedipus complex in negative terms (Ostow). In the Novicks' (1972) study of beating fantasies in children, they found that in severely disturbed children, the beating fantasy could be called a 'fixed fantasy', because once formed it remained a relatively permanent part of the child's psychosexual life. The basis of such fixity lay in the early masochistic tie to the mother, together with severe wide-ranging masochistic pathology and accompanying ego disturbances. In their material 'the beating fantasy was not formed until the phallic-oedipal stage was reached, but the primary determinants of the beating wish which was discharged in the fantasy are pre-oedipal'.

The question of masochism in females has been reviewed by Blum (1977) in relation to female personality development and the ego-ideal. The conclusion was reached that female masochism was a residue of unresolved infantile conflict, and was neither essentially feminine nor a valuable component of mature female function and character. There was no evidence of any particular female pleasure in pain. It was important to distinguish between masochistic suffering as a goal in itself (which if it gives pleasure is a perversion), and tolerance for discomfort or deprivation in the service of the ego or ego-ideal.

In the march of psychological science, we are apt to give greater emphasis to more recent discoveries, especially with regard to their aetiological significance. This is particularly true with relevance to the importance of pre-genital versus phallic-oedipal factors in the genesis of perversion. Obviously both are important and contributory – we have to know how they interact and function on the lengthy organizational pathway a perversion must traverse before being fully formed. Bak's (1968) views are illuminating. He considered valid his 1956 observations of the over-excitation of the aggressive drive in infancy and its deleterious influence on all libidinal phases, which called attention to aggressive conflicts and the defences used against them, for example, the substitution of sexual – perverse – solutions via regression to safeguard this object. He felt that new discoveries had tended to shift the emphasis of aetiology of the sexual perversions away from the castration complex and the phallic phase towards pre-genital factors such as orality and separation-individuation. Bak still agreed with Freud that no percursors of the castration complex can diminish the importance of the phallic phase. He therefore attempted to integrate the interplay of castration anxiety, the aggressive conflict, and the early identifications, in his understanding of the perversions. Three main points were postulated:

(a) Common to all perversions is the dramatized denial of castration.

(b) Perverse symptoms are regressive adaptions of the ego to secure gratification without destroying the object and endangering the self which is identified with the object (Bak 1956).

(c) In all perversions the dramatized or ritualized denial of castration is acted-out through the regressive revival of the fantasy of the maternal phallus. This primal fantasy constitutes the psychological core of the bisexual identification (Bak 1968).

Because of the central position of castration anxiety in the aetiology of the perversions, and its relationship to earlier traumas, a brief description of the conflicts and phenomena underlying castration anxiety now follows.

Castration anxiety

Castration anxiety, which is clearly placed in the phallic-oedipal phase, stems from certain basic fears:

(a) The fantasized loss of the penis in the boy is given credence by his witnessing the female genital area, and the variable shock effect on finding the penis missing.

(b) The oedipal rivalry with the father for possession of mother and for intimacy with her, is accompanied by destructive wishes to castrate father and the fear of retaliation. The ensuing guilt augments the castration fear as a punishment.

(c) Other conflicts contributing to castration anxiety are bisexuality, expressed as identification with mother in the negative oedipal aspects, with father as the preferred partner; sadistic impulses towards the mother; the perversion of the earlier fantasy of the phallic mother and the presence of the maternal phallus.

Consideration of what provokes castration must be qualified by the factor of degree. The suddenness of any of these experiences, the shock effect, lack of understanding by the child, and the accompanying humiliation, overt fear, or the anxiety, are highly productive of a traumatic response. The specific traumas of the phallic phase should be considered in the light of any possible additional cumulative trauma (Khan 1963) continuing from earlier phases. The mother, instead of acting as a protective shield, subjects the child to body-ego stresses and strains emanating from their faulty relationship.

Early developmental factors

Object relationships

The traumas of seduction or humiliation in childhood which seem to form the growing points of the core of the later perverse act, are produced by or in relation to the mother, the primary object. This mother is, as we know, already possessed of a character type which, especially later in relation to father's character, will influence the child in the direction of perversion (see Chapter 1). Such scope for influence exists because of the closeness in feelings which the subsequently perverse individual develops with mother in infancy. This excessive closeness, seen best in the transsexuals described by Stoller (see Chapter 5), exists in all perversion to some degree. The origin may lie in the mother's sense of bodily inadequacy, and the exaggerated use she makes of the child and its responses. to supplement the gap in her body-ego awareness. The mother's penis-envy, which includes a grossly diminished sense of self and body-self, seeks enrichment by her in a covert, highly narcissistic manner. These mothers are greedy in the manner of a temple goddess who demands continual sacrifice to her self-esteem. The child, brought up in close proximity to this already distorted maternal narcissistic system, has its growing sense of self-awareness, body adequacy, and later self-esteem deleteriously influenced. Some authors speak of the child being susceptible to the mother's unconscious needs and conflicts. In earliest childhood, the baby gives the mother satisfaction by its presence as a product she has produced. While the child is totally under her control, an extension of her self and will, there is a symbiotic flowing of the narcissistic satisfactions between mother and child, which reinforces the 'merging' experiences commonly found in adult perversion which are both longed for and feared, especially in the regression of analytic therapy.

These symbiotic narcissistic satisfactions form the first intensive libidinization experiences for the child, and are proto-erotic, that is they are generalized and not yet specific as to organ, aim, and object. Whether this conveys itself to the visual experiences at this stage is beyond proof at present, but, as the oral stage proceeds, visual experience is patterned psychically upon oral phase percepts and modes. Where oral fixations occur, looking functions similarly to eating, and is subject to the same intensification and vicissitudes. Actual fixation upon the nipple or breast in a compulsive-erotic way would seem, in my clinical experience to result from traumas in the oral phase which were continued into the oedipal phase and beyond, where the mother frequently exposed herself in a seductive and frustrating manner. For a more complete consideration of the development of the body ego, body image, and body awareness in the child in relation to normal and traumatic stimuli, see Chapter 4.

The child's earliest experiences of humiliation occur when some break in the intense narcissistic bodily togetherness with mother, provides a sense of devaluation to the self. Whereas this happens in all narcissistic disorders, the proto-pervert has a link established with hyper-libidinized experiences which simultaneously deal with object loss and self-devaluation on a body-ego level. Somewhere in the core of every perverse act is the notion of being looked after or the failure to be looked after. This is especially so in the masochistic elements of the perversion and in risk taking. The perverse act in the adult is a plea for togetherness and help, and a sexualized attack for the failure to provide it, symbolically enacted in relation to the whole world, directed at the primary object once more, still on a part-object level, and with a disturbed orientation to reality as a result. By acting in the regressed manner of the perversion, the person can re-experience the narcissistic togetherness on a symbiotic level, which is the accompaniment, as I have said, of the prototype of hyper-libidinization. The success of the perversion is that it can proceed to a genital orgasm, that the individual has control over his sexual responses as well as the objects that arouse them, and is no longer under the control of the mother at a pre-genital level of functioning. Post-orgastic experiences differ in perversion, varying from a sense of emptiness and guilt, to sexual gratification, triumph over and contempt for the sexual object, a sense of ego-accomplishment, and ego-ideal satisfaction. In some degree there is always a sense of failure following the perverse act. As the narcissistic pleasure level falls, the sense of separateness and inner loneliness emerges once more. The outcome depends on the prevailing emotional state. Sufferers with perversions are much more at risk emotionally during episodes of object loss or depression, and these may constitute crisis conditions, such as the acute homosexual panic following the loss of a close partner. Object loss may be defended against by hyper-activity, perverse or otherwise, whereby pain of loss, shame, and guilt are avoided. Winnicott (1935) and Klein, Heimann, Isaacs, and Riviere (1952) have conceptualized such activity as a manic defence. Because perversion necessitates action, failure to libidinize the aggressive drive may lead to substitutes involving risk such as the suicidal attempt, the motor accident, or the loss of valuable objects, while delinquency, especially stealing, plays an ancillary role in many perversions. One transvestite would mysteriously rob his own house, and alarm the occupants, yet remain undetected. Fortunately these manifestations are not usually of a serious nature, as the perversion protects the self as well as the object. Where open physical violence or gross sadism occurs towards the object of sexually deviant behaviour, the diagnosis must be queried whether the perpetrator basically suffers from a character disorder, or a narcissistic personality, or is a borderline psychotic. Such people are fixated at primitive oral object-relationships, and have conflicts over controlling or being controlled by the object, with resultant rage and temper tantrums. Outbursts of rage may occur early in treatment, which then contributes a threat to the therapeutic situation (Kernberg 1975).

The father plays a crucial role in the development of perversion and may fail to protect the child against the mother's anxieties and influences. From the boy's point of view, father's adequately masculine presence is essential for him to develop his own full masculinity. Whereas in both oedipal and pre-oedipal phases the father should be emotionally and physically available for the boy to identify with, it is particularly at the time of the oedipus complex that the boy's future as a full functioning male is determined. The underlying bisexuality of a boy and his relationships with both parents is what enables him to make relationships and identifications with both parents simultaneously. Stoller, as reported in a Panel Report (1977), described how the degree of femininity in males developed in childhood mainly under mother's influence, but in essence, the development of femininity was controlled by both parents' actions in encouraging the boy to become separate from the symbiotic relationship with his mother, and to develop his own masculinity. The degree to which masculinity was obtained was determined by a host of factors, but determined in the main by the mutual interactions of the parents with the child. Stoller (1975*b*) provided the basic hypotheses that the 'degree of femininity that develops in a boy and the forms it takes, will vary according to exactly (not approximately) what is done to him in earlier childhood'. Similarly, in each of the categories where a degree of effeminacy is found, transsexuals, effeminate homosexuals, transvestites and effeminate heterosexuals, a different state of parental and personal dynamics is found. Drawing on the transsexual phenomenology Stoller postulated a very early phase in mental development which is free of conflict, during which impressions are, as it were, imprinted or conditioned on the emerging mental apparatus, which goes to form the core gender identity, or sense of maleness or femaleness. Because of the symbiotic closeness to the mother, the boy undergoes a primitive identification with her, from which he has, in Greenson's term (1968), to 'dis-identify'. Only then can he begin to be masculine. In the transsexual, the symbiosis is maintained beyond the normal phase of separation and individuation described by Mahler (1968). No masculinity is therefore developed in the transsexual, there is no fear of castration, but rather there is a fear of loss of gender identity. Stoller found a special interplay of family dynamics in the transsexuals. Very briefly the marriage was empty and distant; father merely supplied the finances and was rarely around when the son was active and awake. The mother was chronically depressed, with a history of marked masculinity before puberty, and suffered severe penis envy; the beauty these children possessed sparked off mother's reactions which led to the development of a specially intense symbiotic closeness, which was prolonged and provided a physical contact with the child in a blissful union that lasted for years. The child served the mother as the treasured phallus for which she had yearned. Such children revealed signs of femininity between the ages of one and three years, and the longer the femininity endured the less chance there was of facilitating any change towards masculinity, especially where the father had failed to disrupt the pathogenic symbiosis.

Effeminate homosexuals and fetishistic cross-dressers have conflicts concerning masculinity and femininity which preserve the underlying conflicts of the earlier experience of the wish to merge with mother at the same time as preserving themselves as separate individuals. The way the gender identity problems, together with any actual perversion, becomes enshrined in their character structure is a vital process used by them to maintain masculinity. In both these conditions the penis is preserved as an object of gratification, existing, as it were, surrounded by a threatening femininity.

For the fetishistic cross-dresser there are intense experiences of closeness, or invariable separations from the maternal object. The important additional element is the occurrence of humiliation during the overwhelming excitement of togetherness, or the intolerable separation, or both. In the history of one such patient the mother was very attractive, narcissistic, exciting sexually to the boy but somewhat emotionally out of reach as far as he was concerned. He felt alternately excited and rejected by her, and his first discoverable act of cross-dressing occurred soon after he went to boarding school aged eight. He was discovered aged fifteen squatting on the matron's bed and urinating in her knickers. Subsequently he developed a most severe and complex perversion where any frustration would lead to immediate acts of voyeurism in ladies' lavatories, stealing, and leaving erotic or shocking pictures or drawings for passers-by to see. He cross-dressed under his clothes, and was totally unable to work or form relationships. In analysis he regressed to experiences of actual baby body-ego awareness with overwhelming merging tendencies. Any separations were extremely unbearable in the transference and necessitated open access to the analyst at times. On one occasion his reality sense appeared to become altered in the direction of actual psychosis when he believed he was being penetrated, all alone in the dark in the country, spread-eagled on the bonnet of his car. In this case the father was someone with whom there was the opportunity for masculine identification as he was successful in his job and expected his son to be likewise. Unfortunately he was so engrossed in his work and his own problems that he failed to nurture any relationship with his son beyond that of providing for his material needs and expecting achievements from him. This patient suffered a handicap from physical illness in childhood, which further contributed to the interference with his masculinity.

The constellation of the parents in homosexuality has been described by Bieber, *et al.* (1962) and Socarides (1968). In general the mother is both seductive and threatening to the boy's unfolding masculinity, while father is either emotionally withdrawn or openly hostile, the boy being clumsy, shy, and fearful of games. For full details see Chapters 1, 7, 8, and 9. The father's role in the aetiology of overt homosexuality is far-ranging, extending from those fathers who, in a small minority of cases, actively seduce their sons physically or who permit or encourage homosexual relationships, to the majority who are either indifferent, absent, or cruelly hostile to their sons. In such cases, the father fails the boy as an object for masculine identification, especially during the oedipal phase when castration anxiety is at its height. The boy's failure to identify with the father deprives him of full masculinity, with the result that he is forced back to an earlier imitative identification with the father; the conflict of identifying with mother; the maintenance of castration anxiety which becomes repressed and leads to the accentuation of the phallus as an object of possession; and an increased fear of the female genitalia. Because the castration complex has not been surmounted, there remains the tendency to regress, together with the need to search for the ideal male object with whom to identify or to possess.

In the successful analysis of patients with homosexuality, the dynamic interplay between the parents and the child from earliest infancy onwards is worked through and the patient is able to establish relationships with the father that had previously been precluded by the mother's manoeuvres in isolating the father from the child, and the father's apparent willingness to accept this. In many cases, the father has not been sufficiently strong in his own sense of masculinity to prevent this. The homosexual's close loving attachment to the mother is basically ambivalent and the violent rages stored up against her require to be worked through. One such patient treated by me was extremely religious and had intense homosexual fantasies and longings which he never revealed in any way. To further repress his tendencies he unsuccessfully tried hormone treatments followed by aversion therapy which pained him considerably and left him mildly paranoid. After a long, full analysis he married and raised a family. His inhibitions exercised a passivity derived from early oral experiences where his overwhelming mother forced food into his mouth which he refused to swallow. His father was also passive emotionally and his successful treatment lay in resolving his anger and passivity towards mother and in his acceptance and identification with active masculinity in the transference, while mitigating his severe super-ego.

Recent researches based on child observation (Roiphe and Galenson (1968), Galenson and Roiphe (1974, 1976), Edgcumbe and Burgner (1975)) have produced evidence for the presence of an early genital stage, occurring between the ages of 2 and 3 years in both sexes. Roiphe and Galenson showed that castration anxiety can occur in the second year of life giving rise to problems that ante-date the oedipal phase. The relevance of this material for homosexuality has been succinctly reviewed by Payne (Panel Report 1977, p.196–7) from which I quote.

Recognition of this state means that we do not have to postulate a later oedipal revival of earlier developmental conflicts, or a regression from oedipal conflict to an earlier developmental phase in order to explain the coexistence of abandonment and engulfment fears with the overinvestment in and pre-occupation with the genitals shown by homosexual men. Instead, the anxiety that the genitals will be lost, damaged, or defective, may occur concurrently with the fear of separation and the fear of merging with the mother. The heightened narcissistic cathexis of the genitals then plays an important role in shoring up the yet unstable structure of the representation of the body image and the development of gender identity.

The significance of these remarks is discussed further by Socarides in Chapter 9. For an account of internal object and self-representations and the development of perversion, see Chapter 3.

Individuation–separation and body-image development

It has been pointed out that the disturbances of separation–individuation occur not only in perversions but also in the more frequently found narcissistic disorders and 'border-line' personalities. Pursuing the question of what distinguishes perversion from other disorders in the area further, Greenacre suggests that disturbances of individuation in itself may occur based on the experiences the child receives in its growing awareness of anatomical sexual differences between the sexes. The boy's awareness of his genitals as part of his own body-ego identity may be influenced by the degree to which he is exposed to visual perception of female genitals, his mother's or sister's. A great deal of controversy exists concerning the influence of such experiences on later development. Freud placed emphasis on boys seeing sexual differences which contributed to the castration complex; the fantasy of the phallic mother, and the need for ego splitting to contain the two ideas of the mother with and without a penis. In a study of my own at the Hampstead Clinic, all Index cases were examined, and three boys and three girls in full analysis were discovered to have parents who had a liberal attitude towards appearing nude with their children. The children became disturbed where the parents had wittingly or otherwise introduced emotional elements into the shared nudity which became overstimulating to the child, producing frustration rather than liberation, and led to oral regressions in some children. In some of the boys, there was premature libidinal development, or the excessive stimulation led to an enhancement of oedipal phase phenomena, an increased comparison and competitiveness with father, and a resulting feeling of inadequacy instead of a gain in masculine pride and identification. A greater bodily cathexis occurred, especially for the penis. The awareness of sexual differences and retaliatory fears produced a heightened castration anxiety and complex, which was associated with a wide-range of defensive processes. These defences were characterized by regression to anal and especially to oral phases; defences against perception – denial, disavowal, perceptual distortion; and increased fantasy due to the hyperlibidinization and aggressiveness. This resulted in learning and ego inhibitions. Sublimations were initially minimal in all three boys. Inhibition of any show of aggressiveness was finally the picture in all three boys. Two latency children remained sexually active in fantasy and all three developed passive, dependent positions in relation to their fathers, the older two conforming to a passive homosexual orientation.

Greenacre considers that early exposure to the child, if repeated and almost constant, can lead to attitudes of genital interest and confusion. Any conditions which interfere with the attainment of separation will intensify this genital confusion. In my experience, compulsive questioning regarding the genitals may involve other areas. For example one sado-masochistic patient with perverse character formation, who came to treatment for impotence, had a profound sense of the smallness of his penis. He also had a torturing preoccupation with the small size of his girl-friend's breasts, with whom he was otherwise well suited. The breast preoccupations were a substitutive regression from his castration anxiety, which linked with his exposure to the naked, seductive, and controlling mother beyond the normal breast-feeding phase. In this man's adolescence, his narcissistic mother would still ask him to admire her figure, and the continual arousal of his incestuous desires sharpened his sense of physical inadequacy and the unconscious oedipal rivalry. Actual incestuous relations with a sister, who practised similar breast seductions in adolescence, were only just resisted.

However, one can also quote cases in which mothers have overwhelmed infants in prolonged feeding situations and kept them in the bathroom while they bathed for many years of childhood. Such a patient revealed in analysis actual body-ego experiences of breast proximity which were highly pleasurable, but unbearably overwhelming. However overt features of perversion were missing except for masochistic needs and self-damage amounting to actual suicide attempts. Some ingredient appeared to be missing, which if present, would have led to homosexual perversion, but which was forbidden by the ego-ideal attitudes.

Perversions are disturbances in sexual development taking place in the area of ego development.

Greenacre (1968) has put the relationship between perversion and ego development most lucidly in her statement 'The defectively developed ego uses the pressures of the libidinal phases for its own purposes in characteristic ways because of the extreme and persistent narcissistic needs'. She has described two phases of phallic sensitivity. One related to the oedipal period in the fourth year, belonging to the accepted phallic phase of development. The other started much earlier, in the second year of life, and related to the sense of bodily exhilaration associated with better sphincter control and the assumption of the upright posture. Both phases contain a marked sensitivity to bodily trauma and increased fear of castration.

Greenacre has concluded that trauma is important as a predisposing factor in perversion if it occurs in the second and fourth year of life to children who are already unusually uncertain about their bodies, especially their genitals. This is especially pertinent if mutilation or bleeding is experienced or seen in others. Such events are commoner than is supposed, with evidences of menstruation, miscarriages, or accidents being seen by the child.

Trauma is of importance according to the degree to which the child is overwhelmed and resorts to fantasy or denial of reality in order to deal with the panic. The fetish fulfils these conditions admirably.

Ego defences

The ego defences found in perversions relate to the level of developmental fixation as well as to the use of particular mechanisms associated more with one type of disorder than another. For example, introjection–projection mechanisms predominate in early oral/anal conflicts. Splitting of the ego and of the object, together with denial, are found more commonly in fetishism. The reader is referred to the chapters on specific perversions for further details of mechanisms used.

Of greater interest in this section is the function of the personality as a whole in perversions, the character type of defenses so to speak. Various perverse manifestations may exist in layered fashion and in these persons denial is a particular feature.

Fenichel (1945, p.328) following the Sachs mechanism, has drawn attention to the similarity between the defense mechanism of denial, perverse symptom formation, and the psychology of screen memories. 'In perversions, as in screen memories, the work of repression is apparently facilitated through something associatively connected with the repressed being consciously stressed. The fact that certain impulses, usually forbidden, remain in consciousness [the perverse drives] guarantees the repression of the oedipus and castration complexes'. A clinical example is given below, in conjunction with an examination of the role of denial in perversion.

Denial is used when the child is continually brought face to face with an unacceptable reality over which it has no control, and may defend against unwelcome drives, object-relationships or affects.

An exhibitionist offender denied having exposed himself to some young girls, but the facts seemed incontrovertible, especially as he had a history of such exposures. In the light of the evidence, his denial seemed curious. The multifacetted reasons for it were discovered much later when he reported reluctantly that he was forced to share his mother's bed from birth up until his early twenties. Using denial he tolerated his mothers nocturnal embraces, and his waking with erections in the morning. He was a love-child to whom his mother clung tenaciously. He knew his father only briefly, from a screen memory; the father came to visit twice weekly in his childhood, when he would be sent off for a walk, while the parents had intercourse. He was expected to deny his childhood awareness of these clandestine arrangements. The exhibitionism was the uppermost of a series of defensive layers. The underlying layer was of overt homosexual behaviour of mutual masturbation with strangers in cinemas, which defended against massive hostility, intense castration anxiety, and active incestuous wishes. His pubertal masturbation fantasies centred on maternal intercourse and were repressed. Hidden by the screen memory was his love for his father. Analytically speaking, this patient's narcissistic proclivity for mastery was used in the service of the cure, the aspects described being mostly resolved.

In contrast to this case I was consulted by a man accused of exhibiting himself by alleged witnesses. He denied the accusation and sought my help to determine if he possibly could have exposed himself. Nothing in his history or recent life or psychopathology fitted with the diagnosis of an exhibitionist. It was only finally in court after witnesses (including a policeman) had testified to his guilt, that suddenly a garage attendant proved the accused was far away having his car filled with petrol when the offence – a near psychotic one – was committed. This case of mistaken identity could have disastrously ended his professional reputation, had he been found guilty of what in that court was a minor first offence punishable by a small fine. His strenuous legal defence preparations saved him, and there was no pathological denial in this very co-operative person. Examination of his psychopathology had shown a reliable witness, based on the absence of precipitating factors; healthy self-esteem amply nourished by reality attainments; satisfactory whole-object relationships of a family, sexual, and social kind; good previous response to stress, and no history of childhood or infantile traumas, seductions, or perverse activities.

Ego organization

Freud in his early writings used the word ego to connote the executive psychic apparatus of the mind, as well as the person's subjective experience usually known as the self. Hartmann (1956, 1964) made a formal distinction between the ego apparatus and the self. He defined the term ego as 'a substructure of personality defined by its functions'. Freud had already emphasized the functions of the ego as centering around the relation to reality in his remark, the 'relation to the external world is decisive for the ego' (1932, p.106). Hartmann regarded the ego as organizing and controlling motility and perception – perception of the outer world but probably also of the self. Self-criticism, while based on self-perception, was a separate function attributed to the super-ego. The ego therefore had to deal with the outer world, with id drives, the super-ego demands, and with the self.

Accepting the distinction between ego and the self, this section examines the way the ego develops specific perceptual modes and patterns of motility, in relation to particular external stimuli, which contribute to perversion. The self, which is more properly conceptualized as an inner mental representation of the self, is studied in the next section, on perversion as a regulator of self-esteem.

Disorders of perception

The ego defects found in perversion are fundamentally pre-oedipal in type. Such ego defects stem from interferences in the earliest mother–child relationships. Their exact nature depends on the fixation points which occur during the process of separation–individuation, as the child matures away from the initial symbiotic relationship with the mother (Mahler 1968). These fixation points are described differently depending on the theoretical orientation of early ego- and self-formation, see page 69 (see also Kohut 1971).

Perversions may be considered as disturbances in sexual development taking place in the sphere of a developing ego. The earliest ego perceptions appear to be that of body-ego symbiosis. Only later is there the growth of awareness of the genital body-image in the context of gender-identity – the formation of the sense of masculinity or femininity.

The clinical psychoanalytical situation provides numerous examples in perverse patients of conflicts concerning regression to early symbiotic levels. There is the conflicting wish and fear of regressing to the state of merging with the earliest part-object, the breast. This arouses defences against the fear of being overwhelmed by the actual merging experience; or against the painful loss if, in the merged state, the object suddenly disappears. The adult perverse act or character defence symbolically expresses both sides of this equation of conflict. When actual regressive experiences of a body-ego kind occur in analysis, they prove to be frightening to the patient, for example, experiencing the physical proportions of being a baby, with large head and small body: wishes and experiences in the transference of merging with the analyst in the role of the feeding mother; the anger or rage at the frustration of these wishes; or the very frightening somatic compliances symbolizing castration. Such observations, made with transvestite patients, as well as with homosexuals, bear out the contention of authors such as Socarides (1977, see Chapter 9) on the significance of merging experiences as part of early symbiotic fusion desires that are defended against in homosexuals. In Ostow (1974), Gero has elaborated on the visual aspects of merging in a homosexual patient, by which it was possible to become like his idealized athletic partner, and to possess his penis, by the patient seeing the objects of his desire. Merging through tactile experience was observed in another patient who by putting on mother's nightgown relieved the tension of separation – this went beyond the ordinary identification of wearing mother's garment.

Apart from constitutional factors, visual sensitivity in perversion has early environmental origins. One patient was referred after a long analysis because of homicidal threats to the referring therapist at the ending of fruitless treatment. He was found to have a relative impotence, great masochistic material losses, massive perverse fantasies of a defensive kind, and an inability to look at the therapist. Resolving the perverse defences enabled the visual component to be investigated. He was unable to look at nudity and especially not at nipples. There were early traumatic sights of mother's nipples through her nightgown which overwhelmed him. The libidinization and repression of seeing nipples defended against his actual visual sensitivity which had the quality of a devouring desire which was never to be fulfilled. This formed the basis of his severely masochistic instinctual life, including the initial negative therapeutic reaction. His highly narcissistic mother deprived him orally in reality. In face to face treatment, he was persuaded to 'take in' the therapist visually, resistances against this were analysed, and a meaningful relationship became established, which led to a successful result.

Some homosexuals establish an 'eye' for beauty which becomes fixated on the phallic male and cannot delight in females to the same degree. This may be difficult to alter in treatment due to the ego-ideal and ego-syntonic factors, together with the intensity of castration anxiety that is somatized, and defended against.

The high degree of libidinal cathexis invested in these visual images and abilities probably also makes it difficult for therapists using conditioning modifications on pre-orgastic fantasies in homosexuality to reduce their intensity where visual merging qualities are present (see Abel and Blanchard 1974).

There is a 'literalness' or concreteness of experience and expression in such patients which not only shows the early ego derivation, but which enters into ego perceptions of later phase developments. Mention has already been made of the importance and intensity of castration anxiety in perversion. The following example illustrates how the concreteness of body-ego and self-awareness altered the quality of castration anxiety in an already intensified oedipal rivalry. This patient had homosexual preoccupations and overt adolescent encounters. His parents were those classically described in homosexuality, and in childhood there were many primal scene experiences. In analysis he relived experiences at the age of three to four years where he said, 'I was so afraid, I *became* terror'. He reported a memory of a hand at the foot of the bed which he actually felt holding his foot; the terror of the hand reaching up and taking away his penis; or his penis was felt to become his anus – a concrete body-ego elusion. He would search the house, symbolically, to investigate every part of mother, where he thought his father or brothers had been. In the analysis, he re-experienced early psycho-somatic complaints relating to maternal dependence and the anger at separation. In the transference, he re-lived his need for physical contact, including the feeling of feminine identification in the primal scene, where he experienced being underneath the analyst. His aggression emerged against the early mother: 'You're a despicable bitch and I should cut off your tits and throw them away, take out your teeth and grind them away, and there would only be a head and a body left. Where have you gone? I can't make you come back'. He felt forced to conclude that if he admitted his inadequacy in being unable to make mother come back, 'it means I am nothing. There is nothing for you to see if you don't want to come and see me'. That is his threatened loss of self required mother's attention, in being seen. This patient set up a configuration in his world to deal with the threat of such traumatic separations whereby the representation of his mother image, was fused with his self-representation and influenced and was present at his every move. In his later fused mother-self identity he experienced the importance of seeing attractive men, or being well-dressed.

Visual concreteness or merging deals with the threat to the self which results from the loss of the early part-object at the stage of symbiotic fusion and the literal body-ego perceptual awareness. Perversion and narcissistic character disorders share much in common due to fixations at this level. The perversions are hyper-libidinized or sexualized and therefore have a greater power of binding the aggression. In the patient described above, the sexualization derived from the stimulating, exciting narcissistic mother who would rub his anus to soothe him, yet left nurse-maids to care for him.

This case illustrates the part-object need-satisfying level of relationship at which the patient remained fixated, and the mother continuing to function towards her son in a similar part-object idealized and frustrating manner. This is typical of the developed perversion. The libidinization of early mother–child experience may thus take place through actual acute seduction which is repeated, or occur as a result of the less overt maternal excitement on a narcissistic basis, but which is transmitted to the immature ego at periods of phase susceptibility.

The result is an ego capacity for high libidinal excitement, together with undue sensitivity to frustration and rejection, which are used defensively against the threat of loss of object, rejection of the self, and the accompanying frustration, hostility, and anger.

The early libidinization links with needs to regress to symbiotic closeness and omnipotent control of objects. The sequelae of these early conflicts are a fixation of ego structure and function. Sublimatory capacities are interfered with, and many patients enter treatment because of their inability to work or use their creative capacities. It is often such patients who lose perversions such as homosexuality, for which they had no wish to be treated, in the course of treatment.

Ego boundaries are also disturbed in perversion. In the safety of the analytic situation, patients experience loss of control of their thoughts; feelings of falling off the couch; and various other manifestations indicative to the individual that he is out of control in an overwhelming environment. These phenomena are usually defended against by fantasy, by passivity which is demeaning to the self, or by recourse to perverse action, or each in turn. The passivity–activity axis is one of the determinants of the perverse character style. Action serves to avoid the aloneness with its immobilizing passivity that links with early traumatic experiences of separation from mother or both parents. This loneliness and object-loss carries an underlying quality of intense fear of abandonment, which is temporarily removed by the libidinization in perversion. One patient libidinized the inner merged self-object, which masqueraded as a maternal image, which kept him company constantly. See page 210.

During the course of psychoanalytic treatment, the patient is faced with the working through of these deep conflicts of the fears of engulfment and of abandonment, the symbiotic merging with mother and the loss of ego boundaries (Person's Comments in Panel Report 1977). Primary identification with the original maternal object is maintained, increasing the bisexual conflict and the task of self-individuation. Dual identification is also a feature in any sexual or social life encounters.

The ego and motility

Because of the infantile seduction and sexualization, the adult ego is compelled to seek action in risk-taking, excitement, thrills and orgastic discharge. The tolerance for high degrees of stimulation is exemplified by some homosexuals with a high orgastic capacity and the compulsive need for casual sexual encounters amounting to hundreds annually.

The simultaneous sensitivity to humiliation and low tolerance for frustration, induces the capacity for disparate modes of functioning which is replicated in all spheres and gives to the character a quality of contradictoriness. The underlying aggression in response to over-stimulation or frustration puts the person at risk and necessitates perverse libido to counteract it. True neutralization does not occur. Voyeurs are particularly sensitive to being overstimulated by sexual scenes, and occasionally the aggression which is aroused may lead to violent attacks, for example, on couples petting in unfrequented places.

Ostow (1974) covers research on the basic mode of action in perversion. Action is a way of life which circumvents conflict, and is reinforced by a hypercathexis of perception (especially visual) at the expense of abstract thinking capacity and a tendency to seek a literal concrete experience. The perverse act occurs where fantasy gratification fails and is a repetition of childhood seduction and frustration. Based on the original object, the pleasure-giving and idealized, as well as hateful, aspects of the mother, there is a need for action as a means of solving the contradiction between the inculcated passivity and the identifications with the active stimulating, coming-and-going mother. Overactivity in childhood and infancy is reported in some perverse individuals and may be partly constitutional in origin.

The action patterns and the perverse act itself are the result of ego modifications in development, which are based on the early seduction experiences and the overcathexis of the perceptual and motor systems, which later are used to rectify anxiety, of castration in particular, by discharging it along pathways laid down in the perverse mechanism. Perverse fantasy may be used as the initial source of gratification, but where this fails, action supervenes – the fantasy is achieved in a literal way. The final form or expressions which perverse needs may actually take are determined largely by chance external events which occur in childhood, latency and especially in adolescence, when orgasm further fixates orgastic behavioural determinants of the perversion with regard to object, place and sexual act.

The next section in the logic of this presentation, perversion as a regulator of self-esteem, follows on directly in Chapter 3.

References

Abel, G. G. and Blanchard, E. B. (1974). The role of fantasy in the treatment of sexual deviation. *Arch. Gen. Psychiat.* **30**, 467.

Alexander, F. (1965). A note to the theory of perversions. In *Perversions: psychodynamics and therapy* (ed. S. Lorand and M. Balint). London.

Balint, M. (1965), Perversions and genitality. In *Perversions: psychodynamics and therapy* (ed. S. Lorand and M. Balint). London.

Bancroft, J. H. J. (1975). Homosexuality in the male. *Contemporary Psychiatry*, selected reviews from the British Journal of Hospital Medicine (ed. T. Silverstone and B. Barraclough).

Bak, R. (1956). Aggression and perversion. In *Perversions: psychodynamics and therapy* (ed. S. Lorand and M. Balint). London.

—— (1968). The phallic woman: the ubiquitous fantasy in perversions. *Psychoanal. Study Child.* **23**. 15.

Bieber, I., Dain, H. J., Dince, P. R., Drellich, M. G., Grand, H. G., Gundlach, R. H., Kremer, M. W., Rifkin, A. H., Wilbur, C. B., and Bieber, T. B. (1962). *Homosexuality*. New York.

Blum, H. (1977). Masochism, the ego ideal, and the psychology of women. In supplement—Female Psychology, *J. Am. Psychoanal. Assoc.* **24**, 5, 157.

M'Uzan, M. de. (1972). Un cas de masochisme pervers. In *La sexualité perverse*. Paris.

—— (1973). A case of masochistic perversion and an outline of a theory. *Int. J. Psycho-Anal.* **54**, 455.

Edgcumbe, R. and Burgner, M. (1975). The phallic-narcissistic phase: a differentiation between pre-oedipal and oedipal aspects of phallic development. *Psychoanal Study Child* **30**, 161.

Fenichel, O. (1945). *The Psychoanalytic theory of neurosis*. New York.

Freud, S. (1905). Three essays on the theory of sexuality. *Complete psychological works of Sigmund Freud. Standard edition.* **7**, 123. London.

—— (1932). New Introductory Lectures. *Complete psychological works of Sigmund Freud. Standard edition.* **22**, London.

Galenson, E. and Roiphe, H. (1974). The emergence of genital awareness during the second year of life. In *Sex differences in behaviour* (ed. R. C. Friedman, R. M. Richart, and R. L. Van de Wiele). New York.

—— —— (1976). Some suggested revisions concerning early female development. In Supplement—Female Psychology, *Am. J. Psychoanal.* **24**, 5, 29.

Gillespie, W. H. (1964). The psycho-analytic theory of sexual deviation with special reference to fetishism. In *The pathology and treatment of sexual deviation* (ed. I. Rosen). London.

Glover, E. (1964). Aggression and sado-masochism. In *The pathology and treatment of sexual deviation* (ed. I. Rosen). London.

Greenacre, P. (1968). Perversions: general considerations regarding their genetic and dynamic background. *Psychoanal. Study Child* **23**, 47. New York.

Greenson, R. (1968). Dis-identifying from mother. *Int. J. Psycho-Anal.* **49**, 370.

Hartmann, H. (1956). The development of ego in Freud's work. In *Essays on Ego Psychology*, p.267 (1964), New York.

—— (1964). *Essays on Ego Psychology*. London.

Hoenig, J. and Duggan, E. (1974). Sexual and other abnormalities in the family of a transsexual. *Psychiatrica Clinica* **7**, 334.

Hore, B. D., Nicolle, F. V., and Calnan, J. S. (1973). Male transsexualism: two cases in a single family, *Arch. Sex. Behav.* **2**.

Kenyon, F. E. (1975). Homosexuality in the female. In *Contemporary Psychiatry; selected reviews from the British Journal of Hospital Medicine* (ed. T. Silverstone and B. Barraclough).

Kernberg, O. (1972). Early ego integration and object relations, *Ann. N. Y. Acad. Sc.* **193**, 233.

—— (1975). *Borderline conditions and pathological narcissism*. New York.

Khan, M. M. R. (1963). The concept of cumulative trauma. In *The primacy of the self* (1974). London

Klein, M., Heimann, P., Isaacs, S., and Riviere, J. (1952). *Developments in psychoanalysis*. London.

Limentani, A. (1976). Object choice and actual bisexuality. *Int. J. Psycho-Anal. Psychother.* **v**, 205.

Lihn, H. (1971). Sexual masochism: a case report. *Int. J. Psycho-Anal.* **52**, 469.

Mahler, M. (1968). *On human symbiosis and the vicissitudes of individuation*. Vol. 1. New York.

McDougall, J. (1972). Primal scene and sexual perversion. *Int. J. Psycho-Anal.* **53**, 371.

Novick, J. and Novick, K. K. (1972). Beating fantasies in children. *Int. J. Psycho-Anal.* **53**, 237.

Ostow, M. (ed.) (1974). *Sexual deviation: a psycho-analytical approach*. New York. Participants: Ostow, M., Blos, P., Furst, S., Gero, G., Kanzer, M., Silverman, D., Sterba, R., Valenstein, A.

Panel Report (1977). The psychoanalytic treatment of male homosexuality. (reporter E. C. Payne) *J. Am. Psychoanal. Assoc.* **25**, 183.

Payne, E. C. (1977). See Panel Report above.

Reich, A. (1960). Pathological forms of self-esteem regulation *Psychoanal. Study Child* **15**, 215. New York.

Reich, W. (1949). *Character analysis*. New York.

Roiphe, H. (1968). On an early genital phase. *Psychoanal. Study Child* **23**, 348. New York.

Rosen, I. (1964). Exhibitionism, scopophilia, and voyeurism. In *The pathology and treatment of sexual deviation* (ed. I. Rosen) London.

—— (1965). Looking and showing. In *Sexual deviation and the law*. (ed. R. Slovenko). Springfield.

—— (1968). The basis of psychotherapeutic treatment of sexual deviation. *Proc. R. Soc. Med.* **61**, 793.

—— (1977). The psychoanalytic approach to individual therapy. In *Handbook of sexology*. (ed. J. Money and H. Musaph). New York.

Sachs, H. (1923). Zur genese der perversionen. *Int. Z̲. Psycho-Anal.* **9**, 172. English translation by Hella Freud Bernays, 1964, Psychoanalytic Institute Library, New York.

Socarides, C. W. (1968). *The overt homosexual.* New York.

—— (1977). See Panel Report above.

Sperling, M. (1968). Acting-out behaviour and psychosomatic symptoms, *Int. J. Psycho-Anal.* **49**, 250.

Stoller, R. J. (1975*a*). *Perversion: The erotic form of hatred.* New York.

—— (1975*b*). *Sex and gender. Vol. 2. The Transsexual Experiment.* London.

—— and Baker, (1973). Two male transsexuals in one family. *Arch. Sex. Behav.* **2**.

Wålinder, J. and Thuwe, I. (1977). A study of consanguinity between the parents of transsexuals. *Brit. J. Psychiat.* **131**, 73.

Wiedemann, G. (1977). See Panel Report above.

Winnicott, D. (1935). The manic defence. In *Collected papers.* London.

3 Perversion as a regulator of self-esteem

Ismond Rosen

Regulation of self-esteem is one of the major functions of the perversions. From a clinical point of view, patients seeking help for perversions simultaneously present complaints of a disordered narcissistic economy, with feelings of inadequacy and under- or over-assertion of themselves. They regard their perverse acts or fantasies either as a source of pleasure and pride with which they do not want to part, or of pain and diminution in their sense of self-esteem, because their actions conflict with their super-ego valuation of their ideal selves. Patients report episodes of exhibitionism, or of importuning, which were precipitated by actual trauma or by external events unconsciously signifying threats of object loss or castration, which stress they felt unable to tolerate. Whatever the source of the precipitating stress, the impact is registered on the sense of self, both consciously and unconsciously, and is experienced as humiliation, defined as being humbled or lowered in position, or internally as having a lowered sense of self-esteem. There may be a corresponding compensatory surge of perverse sexual fantasy followed by conscious perverse acts. However, the more that unconscious conflicts enter into the reactions, the more self-esteem will be lowered, and there may little or no awareness of fantasy, preceding or during the perverse act, which is performed in a manner lacking conscious awareness, that is it is a preconsciously executed act.

The preservation of the personality as an integrated whole is one of the functions of self-esteem, whose maintenance and regulation is essential to healthy psychic functioning. In order to understand the development of the integration of personality, and how perversion regulates self-esteem, we must first examine the new concepts of narcissism, the self, the ego-ideal, the super-ego and self-esteem and its regulation.

In his 1914 paper 'On narcissism', Freud said 'We have discovered, especially clearly in people where libidinal development has suffered some disturbance, such as perverts and homosexuals, that in their later choice of love-objects they have taken as a model not their mother but

65

their own selves. They are plainly seeking *themselves* as a love-object, and are exhibiting a type of object-choice which must be termed "narcissistic". In this observation we have the strongest reasons which have led us to adopt the hypothesis of narcissism'. Narcissism became defined as the libidinal investment, or cathexis, of the self-image or representation rather than the structural ego, as defined above. Jacobson (1975) refined narcissism as the 'intra-psychic cathexis of the self-representation with more or less neutralized or deneutralized libidinous or aggressive drive energy.' Stolorow (1976) succinctly stated that it is the struggle for selfhood which lies at the heart of the phenomenon of narcissism. Primary narcissism is today regarded as an ego state within the individual derived from the child's early symbiotic union with mother. Repeated over-stimulation in early infancy can intensify primary narcissism.

The self is defined in terms of its content within the mental apparatus, as a series of self-representations (as opposed to object-representations) which are located within the ego, the id, and the super-ego, see Hartmann (1953), Sandler, Holder and Meers (1963), Mahler (1968), and Kohut (1970).

An attempt to integrate these authors' views on development of the self was made by Lichtenberg (1975). He defined the self as self-experience, or sense of self, and distinguished between self-image referring to experiences, and self-representation referring to structures formed from the memory traces of the experience. Later in this section, the work of various authors will be examined in detail regarding development of the self and perversion. At this point it is useful to paraphrase Lichtenberg's summary.

In brief the self develops from the earliest stage before self-differentiation, where the infant enters the symbiotic relationship with the mother, and is endowed with a 'basic core of fundamental trends', 'object relatedness, anxiety potential and libido-aggression balance' (Weil 1970). The merging state gives rise to symbiotic dependency and islands of experience lead to the formation of ego-id nuclei (Glover 1943, 1964) of body representations. These bodily self-images later blend experientially with images of the self that have developed in relation to objects that are perceived as separate, and with images of a grandiose self associated with idealized self-objects to form a 'sense of self that has the quality of cohesion – of unity and continuity in time, space and state'.

Over-stimulation or seductions in infancy leads to fixations of the archaic and omnipotent experiences of the self. A further result is that the external self and objects may be represented in a merged undefined way, different to the later separate representations of self and objects. The quality of self-experiences in perversion may vary enormously and exist contradictorily so that a sense of inferiority (resulting from a depleted self) may supplement notions of omnipotence. The resulting sense of self-esteem may therefore be inherently unstable and the ego-ideal contains targets impossible for satisfaction or attainment.

Freud (1914) describe how 'development of the ego [self] consists in a departure from primary narcissism', 'brought about by means of the displacement of libido onto an ego-ideal imposed from without'. In growing up, the ego-ideal becomes the target of the self-love enjoyed by the ego and the early narcissism lost in childhood.

Chasseguet-Smirgel (1974) discussed the development of the ego-ideal as the heir to primary narcissism. In perversion she considered there was a disturbance of ego-ideal development mainly assisted by mother in the oedipal relationship. The pervert idealizes the partial pregenital insticts and regards them as superior to aims of genital primacy. The need for idealization which is compulsive is never directed towards objects, but only to part-objects, preferably associated with the anal-sadistic phase.

The term self-esteem, dating from 1657, is defined (Shorter Oxford English Dictionary) as the 'favourable appreciation or opinion of oneself. In phrenology it was one of the mental faculties for which a "bump" was assigned'. Freud (1914) referred to this faculty as self-regard, which was an expression of the size of the ego and derived from three main parts: the residue of infantile narcissism; the fulfilment of the ego-ideal; and the satisfaction of actual accomplishments. Lowered self-regard, or sense of inferiority was 'due to impoverishment of the ego [self] due to the libidinal cathexes which have been withdrawn from it, due, that is to say, to the injury sustained by the ego through sexual trends which are no longer subject to control'.

Recent child studies indicate that the development of self-esteem derives from early drive satisfactions, which, together with ego accomplishments, finally link with the structural development of the super-ego, ego-ideal, and sense of self. The manner in which pleasure in achievement links with the child's instinctual life is regarded by Anna Freud (1966) as unsolved. Certain operative factors seem unmistakable, such as imitation and identification in the early mother–child relationship, the influence of the ego-ideal, the turning of passive into active as a mechanism of defence and adaptation, and the inner urge toward maturation, that is toward progressive development.

Pleasure in achievement, linked only secondarily with object relations, is present in very young children as a latent capacity and is used in nursery school methods (Montessori) to 'afford the child the maximum increase in self-esteem and gratification by means of task completion and independent problem solving'. 'Where this source of gratification is not tapped at the same degree with the help of external arrangements, the pleasure derived from achievement in play remains more directly connected with praise and approval given by the object world, and satisfaction from the finished product takes first place at a later date only, probably as the result of internalization of external sources of self-esteem' (A. Freud, 1966).

Self-esteem therefore derives from many roots:

(a) Accomplishment – gratification of ego capacities in which drive activity manifestations occur as an expression of forward maturity.

(b) Imitation and identification in the early mother–child relationship.

(c) Ego-ideal influences which develop from residues of primary narcissism and the development of a healthy attainable ego-ideal.

(d) Ego-defence mechanisms as adaptational manoeuvres, for example, turning active into passive.

(e) Super-ego influences, where the idealized parental images are internalized during the post-oedipal and early latency phases.

However, as Jacobson (1975) has pointed out, in a fine review with reference to depression, *regulation* of self-esteem is a complicated mechanism which must be distinguished from the factors making for its development. The preservation of a healthy level of self-esteem depends on the inner narcissistic balance, that is the economy of libidinal cathexis of the self-representations with relatively conflict-free energies. Any conflicts or excessive drives provoked within the individual or derived externally will lead to a rise or fall in self-esteem.

Lichtenberg (1975) has emphasized the positive emotional states resulting from inner-regulation of drives at the toddler stage which stem from self-cohesion, and which 'serve as esteem-raising counterparts to feelings of anxiety, shame and guilt'. He traces the grandiose omnipotent self-images of childhood, which peak at 16 to 18 months, as the precursors of adult self-images with high self-esteem. The most vulnerable to point for self-esteem deflation is according to Mahler and Furer (1969, pp.22–23), the second eighteen months of life. This is the time of life when the maintenance of a sense of control is necessary to restore a sense of being worthwhile. This feature is actively continued in narcissistic and perverse patients. The most pathologically deflating effect on self-esteem at this period of growth is where the mother oscillates from overwhelming closeness to cold withdrawn rejection. The child, having no control over mother's behaviour or presence, varies from sharing in her omnipotence, to feeling an emptiness of his self- and object-images.

Pathological regulation of self-esteem is coincident with faulty development of the drives, self- and object-representations, ego, ego-ideal, and super-ego formation. Detailed clinical studies have been made of disturbed self-esteem regulation by A.Reich (1973) who described different types; Kohut (1971) and Kernberg (1975) in narcissistic and borderline disorders; Jacobson (1975) in depression.

Before systematically examining the developmental factors which lead to disturbed self-esteem and its regulation in perversion, it would be advantageous to examine the work of Kohut, and Kernberg, on the disorders of narcissism. These new concepts of narcissism have been critically discussed by Ornstein (1974), who has well summarized the comparisons between Kohut and Kernberg, and by Hanly and Masson (1976).

Kohut (1971) formulated certain stages in the development of narcissism, which when specifically disordered provide the nuclei for clinical disturbances such as perversion and the narcissistic disorders. Based on Kohut's concepts, Goldberg (1975) discussed the feasibility of a systematic classification of the perversions based on the fixation points of developing pathological narcissistic constellations and the affects which are sexualized. Unfortunately no such systematic studies have yet been published on these early narcissistic fixations in relation to perversion.

Kohut has postulated two stages of self-formation. An *auto-erotic* stage where, also following Glover's notions of ego-nuclei, there are disparate self-nuclei. As growth proceeds, a *cohesive self* is formed, which gives rise to grandiose-self and idealized-parental images. The formulations are most valuable because they are based on the child's relationship to the parents, especially the mother and her handling of its narcissistic needs. Thus, if the mother, because of her lack of empathy, rejects the child's narcissistic strivings subtly or overtly, these will be repressed, leading to what Kohut terms a 'horizontal split'. In adulthood, these unfulfilled archaic demands remain split off from the adult reality ego, draining off its energies.

Clinically this leaves the patient in his conscious self-perception, devoid of a sense of contentment, with low self-esteem, shame propensity and a tendency to hypochondriacal brooding.

If, on the other hand, the mother attempts to enmesh the child in her own narcissistic world and use his performance for her own narcissistic satisfactions, this will lead to a side-by-side coexistence of openly displayed infantile grandiosity coupled again with low self-esteem, shame propensity, and hypochondriacal preoccupations, maintained by the mechanism of disavowal, termed by Kohut a 'vertical split'. In the vertical split, perverse behaviour resides in a split-off sector of the psyche.

Perverse activities have been defined by Kohut in terms of sexualization of pathological narcissistic constellations, and may be used to stem regression in one of many ways: as a substitute for an absent narcissistically invested self-object; as a substitute for the non-availability of a person who was being used to represent a missing part of the self; or as a source of pathological hypercathexis of the grandiose self.

Kohut (1970 p.98) describes a patient's recall of long hours in childhood where voyeuristic preoccupations (the child searching through drawers in an empty house), led to his putting on his mother's clothes. These perverse activities became intelligible when they were understood not so much as sexual transgressions that were undertaken while external surveillance was lacking, but rather as attempts to supply substitutes for the idealized-parent image and its functions, by creating erotized replacements through the frantic hypercathexis of the grandiose self. (p.99) 'The various perverse activities which the child engages are the attempts to re-establish the union with the narcissistically invested lost object through visual fusion and other archaic forms of identification.' Compare the almost identical concrete searching for mother with my case described on page 59.

In the next case, Kohut shows how pathological sexual fantasies were used as an inner esteem-regulator, replacing a missing stable system of idealized values. This case presented for treatment because of homosexual fantasies. The fantasies were understood in the analysis as 'sexualized statements about his narcissistic disturbance', and 'stood, of course, in opposition to meaningful insight and progress since they were in the service of pleasure gain and provided an escape route from narcissistic tensions'. Kohut showed how in this case where there was no acting-out of the fantasies, the sexualization of the patient's defects was due to a moderate weakness in his basic psychic structure, resulting in an impairment of its neutralizing capacity. The fantasies themselves, which occasionally led to orgasm, were of a quasi-sadistic triumph over men of great strength and of perfect physique in which they were rendered helpless or drained of their power by him masturbating them. After the homosexual fantasies had subsided, in the analysis, Kohut used the interpretation of their meaningfulness to deal with the underlying narcissistic conflicts. This patient suffered from the 'absence of a stable system of *firmly idealized values*', one of the important sources of the internal regulation of self-esteem. He had in his sexual fantasies replaced the inner ideal with its sexualized external precursor, an athletic powerful man; and he had substituted for the enhancement of self-esteem which is experienced by living up to the example of one's idealized values and standards, by the sexualized feeling of triumph, as he robbed the external ideal of its power and perfection and thus in his fantasy acquired these qualities for himself and achieved a temporary feeling of narcissistic balance. The specific pathogenic disturbance in this patient related to the traumatic devaluation of the father-image and its idealized aspects of the beginning of latency. This occurred on an earlier basis of an assumed failure of his mother to supply proper emphatic responses to him early in life based on her unpredictability and shallowness.

According to Goldberg (1975), the object-deficits do not cause the perversion. Sexualization is used to counter the regression, as well as dealing with the overwhelming affects that accompany the lowering of self-esteem in humiliation. The sexualization itself is explained on the basis of the unavailability of the archaic object which does not allow for neutralization and produces a more primitive drive expression.

Kernberg (1972) postulated four stages of development of internalized object-relations, and correlated these with the clinical manifestations of pathological arrest or fixation at each stage. Stage 3 included borderline personality organization, including impulse neuroses, addictions, and narcissistic personalities. Character disorders seen in severe perversion would belong here. Severe chronic frustrations in early childhood were the main causative factor. The lack of impulse control stems from the ego weakness, where there is a poor integration of the 'good' self- and object-images with their corresponding 'bad' type. The defences, mainly of splitting, act to keep apart these frightening contradictory images. Kernberg postulates that 'the integration of loving and hating feelings in the context of internalized relationships with others seems to be a major precondition for neutralization of instinctual energy'. This lack of neutralization deprives the ego of sublimatory capacity. These drive vicissitudes are all the more significant in borderline patients because premature sexualization and oedipalization of the relationships with parental figures and siblings leads only to aggressive 'contamination' of these relationships.

In stage 4 are represented the neuroses, higher levels of character pathology, and depressive-masochistic characters. The major defenses are repression rather than splitting. Oedipal, genital conflicts predominate over pre-genital ones. Cases with perverse behaviour mainly of oedipal type would appear to belong to this category where there is no particular pathology of internalized object-relations, with a stable self and object representational world.

In 1975, Kernberg examined the narcissistic disorders as a spectrum of defences protecting self-esteem and the integrity of the self, which range from non-specific character traits to the specific operations of the narcissistic personality formations. He stated that pathological character traits have as one function the protection of self-esteem and, therefore, analytic efforts to modify a neurotic character structure always included the implication of a narcissistic lesion (W. Reich 1949).

Kernberg (1975) has linked oral aggression with a premature development of oedipal strivings resulting in a pathological condensation between pregenital and genital aims under the overriding aggressive aims. Such factors are important in the development of male homosexuality, where the father is submitted to sexually to obtain the oral gratifications missing from mother, who is viewed as a dangerous castrator. In the girl, oral deprivation from mother leads to positive oedipal strivings being developed prematurely. Pregenital aggression is projected on to the father, which increases the oedipal conflicts and penis envy. There may be many outcomes such as promiscuity, masochism, and homosexuality, depending on the projective–introjective use of the rage, and the internal splits and threats from the internalized mother- and father-images.

These types of perverse psychopathology are consistent with borderline personality disorder, associated with defences of splitting, primitive idealization, early forms of projection, demand and omnipotence.

Kernberg (1975) has classified three types of male homosexuality, using a continuum that differentiates the degree of severity of pathology of internalized object-relations. The first type, which has the best prognosis, is where genital oedipal factors predominate. The oedipal self is submissive towards the oedipal domineering prohibitive father and renounces the forbidden oedipal mother. The second type which is more severe has 'a conflictual identification with an image of his mother and treats his homosexual objects as a representation of his own infantile self'. These men enact the emotional tie to their mothers with their homosexual partners. However, pregenital conflicts predominate over genital ones and are consistent with findings of loving but disturbed object-relationships and possible character disorders. In a third type of homosexual relation the 'homosexual partner is "loved" as an extension of the patient's own pathological self, and hence we find the relation, not from self to object, nor from object to self, but from [pathological grandiose] self to self'. This has the worst prognosis because the homosexuality exists in the context of narcissistic personality structure proper. This does not exclude such persons from functioning well socially.

This brief survey indicates that where there is a pathological development of narcissism there is also a disordered regulation of self-esteem, with the affects, object relationships, ego and super-ego functionings being simultaneously involved. Contributing particularly to such faulty self-esteem regulation are those cases where the self- and object-images retain vague boundaries or exist in a fused state. In severe perversions, early projective and introjective identifications between mother and child are finally introjected by the child to become part of the self-image, although derived from the object. At the same time, the self-object image is filled with narcissistic self-representational material which has gained an object-representational quality. This may interfere with the affects, object relationships, ego and super-ego functioning inner self-object image is facilitated by the seductions and frustrations which occur in the symbiotic and transitional object phases. One may postulate that due to weakness of the inner boundaries, the partial drive hyper-libidinization floods the undifferentiated or fused self–object image. The excess drive becomes available for the structural part of the ego to maintain primitive splitting defences. With maturation and further cohesion of later self- and object-representations, the hyper-libidinization becomes available in the terms of Sachs' mechanism, thus transforming anxiety into pleasure by the temporary resolution of conflict, whereby the pleasure-giving self- and object-images are libidinized, and the painful aggressive and hating of the self- and object-images are either repressed, split-off or denied. This latter manoeuvre includes a swing towards pleasure in the delicate libido-aggressive balance that exists intrapsychically, thus contributing to positive inner narcissistic constellations (cathexis of the self-representations with neutralized libido and aggression). The result is a heightened self-esteem that carries, in temporary accordance, the modifying influences of the ego-ideal and super-ego.

The super-ego in perversion was previously regarded as having developed 'lacunae' towards perverse behaviour based on the tolerating attitudes in the parents (Gillespie 1964). More recent work has shown that the super-ego itself develops faults in keeping with the ego, self, and internal object disorders described above. In particular, failures of internalization of the ego-ideal, unwillingness to identify with unsuitable parents and the tendency towards merging, all militate against normal super-ego development. The type of perversion or its absence, together with the degree or quality of the perverse act, are usually determined by the demands made upon the self by the ego-ideal and super-ego.

The following clinical case study exemplifies perversion as an esteem regulator. The patient had been in treatment on and off for over fifteen years, and was first reported in some detail in Slovenko's *Sexual deviation and the law* (Rosen 1965). A compulsive voyeur and secret collector of personal pornographic material, he feared he would be discovered to his great detriment. Of use in therapy were previous drawings by a friendly prostitute of his perverse fantasies which were passive into active reversals of childhood humiliations.

The drawings were first used for masturbation and then kept locked away with a dual purpose in mind. Resource could be had to them for masturbation, and they functioned as an inanimate source of satis-faction and excitement under the patient's control. Excitement by means of seeing was a defence against the dull feelings of loss at being rejected by someone he loved, which was based on the original loss of his mother as someone of whom he had sole possession. The thought that others would be shocked at seeing the pictures made him feel audacious and raised his self-esteem. This phallic excitement defended him against his fear of regression to a state of oral dependency on mother. Opposing this was the fear that the drawings would be discovered and he would suffer humiliation and rejection by those he loved. Though these fears and feelings were quite conscious and the risks taken were calculated ones, he was still acting under a repetition-compulsion dating back to his childhood. These drawings were analogous to a drawing he had made of a 'little penis' at the age of five, when he had secretly kept this drawing in his pocket, and both wished for and feared its discovery by his mother. Possession of the drawing made him feel he was 'bad' and independent of her, as she was against such things and had deprecated his competitive urinary games with other boys. Being a 'good' boy meant he might be overwhelmed by her love and lose his sense of identity. He further never minded his mother discovering the drawing, as he then felt revealed as a sexual partner for her. He recalled his great sexual pleasure in having his penis fondled by mother at an earlier age, but also felt she coveted it. There was also an awareness of mother's sensual pleasure, both in these acts and in the fantasied mutuality of the breast feeding situation. The excitement associated with the possession of the 'little penis' drawing and the later ones, therefore expressed the mutuality of his and mother's physical pleasure both in the feeding situation and in bed at night. He had shared her bedroom for the first two years of life while his father was away, and he was unceremoniously ejected on father's return.

Already formed was the core of his perverse-mechanisms as a regulator of self-esteem. The drawing of the little penis was an ego accomplishment which gave him great pride. He could draw this in relation to mother; keep it hidden from her; and experience in anticipation the thrill of discovery and possible punishment, by which means he elevated his sense of courage as opposed to his cowardliness in having to hide it. The 'little penis' stood high in relation to father's big penis and the fetishistic aspects of the female penis by virtue of its having been drawn, which led to maturing ego sublimatory capacities. This patient never drew in later life, and possibly his talents were not up to expression in the plastic arts, or they may have been inhibited by the perverse-mechanisms. He achieved success later in other verbal sublimations. One feature that he consciously retained from childhood, apart from his compulsion to keep sexually exciting pictures, was a peculiarity of speech. A highly cultivated and articulate man, he revealed that he never used words in speech with the letter *R*. As a child he could not say *R* clearly, and on being teased, he felt humiliated and resolved never to use this letter again, nor later to reveal his intricate avoidance devices. This manoeuvre went undetected by me until he confessed after years of treatment. He could neither stand the humiliation of pronouncing a babyish *R*, nor did he want to analyse and give up the esteem-raising perverse devices. This speech disorder, while fixated on phallic and latency experiences, was based on early infantile object-dependent sources. His ego-ideal had accepted this manoeuvre as a requirement he had to pursue and maintain for gratification sake. What remained perverse were the unresolved early conflictual elements which were acted-out, thought of as perverse, kept hidden, and which if discovered would repeat the humiliation, but which gave constant gratification in the exercise of his ego capacities and their underlying sexualized aspect, that is he would remain the baby, where he was the undisputed consort of mother's sexual and emotional life. The early infantile passivity was elevated to an achieved omnipotent gratification and ideal in the perverse mechanism. The hostile elements were also mainly hidden in the patient by his excellent integrative capacities, but expressed in his fierce independence of social codes that meant acceptance. His life activities were in separate compartments maintained by splitting mechanisms, for example, a pillar of established respectability, he consorted with prostitutes all his life, and under other names was eminent in 'progressive' fields. The ability to control the blending or separateness of the contradictory areas of his life, together with his actual perverse gratifications were the major part of the patient's successful self-esteem regulation. A charming and courteous man, he had first come to treatment when his regulating system had gone out of control, and he was in danger by virtue of his voyeurism. His treatment made him capable of whole-object relationships, and therefore liable to depressions, which were his reason for later visits, following actual object loss. One feature of this case was his need for the mutuality of excitement in his perverse activities. Urinating on his penis, practised on him by his wife, left him unmoved, because she was doing it for his sake rather than for the excitement of the act, whereas his prostitutes became excited, or feigned successfully. This excitement by the object, linked with his awareness of his mother's excitement over his penis, and brought him close to the primal object, symbolized also in the drawings.

This patient demonstrates that perversions and their precursors are intimately connected with the processes of self-esteem formation and regulation. This was evident early in the mother–child emotional relationship with its intense gratifications and frustrations, which influenced the later aspects of self and ego accomplishments in both symbolic and reality activities, and his ego-ideal attainments. In this patient, as in most perverts, self estimation became linked with gender identity through his notions of masculinity. The vulnerable masculine self-esteem was revealed in his passive infantile humiliations, which were repeated in latency and adolescence, and which necessitated masculine-type symbolic or real perverse acts, sexual and otherwise, to raise his sense of inferiority, both at the time and in adult life. The regular boost to his self-esteem was secured by his capacity for active conscious control and manifestation of his perversion. Patients may first seek help as he did, where the ego control is becoming unstable, or has been overwhelmed due to traumas which repeat infantile modes of reaction, regression, and uncontrolled perverse acts.

The factors which produce perversion tend towards instability of psychic function and self-esteem. The perversion is utilized by the personality as a self-esteem regulator, where the splits within the ego and the self can temporarily gain an inner representation of wholeness or narcissistic integrity. (See also pages 312–15.)

References

Chasseguet-Smirgel, J. (1974). Perversion, idealization, and sublimation. *Int. J. Psycho-Anal.* **55**, 349.

Freud, A. (1966). *Normality and pathology in childhood*. London.

Freud, S. (1914). On narcissism: an introduction. *Complete psychological works of Sigmund Freud*. Standard edition **14**, 67. London.

Gillespie, W. H. (1964). The psycho-analytic theory of sexual deviation with special reference to fetishism. In *The pathology and treatment of sexual deviation* (ed. I. Rosen). London.

Glover, E. (1943). The concept of dissociation. In *On the early development of mind* (1956). New York.
—— (1964). Aggression and sado-masochism. In *The pathology and treatment of sexual deviation* (ed. I. Rosen). London.

Goldberg, A. (1975). A fresh look at perverse behaviour. *Int. J. Psycho-Anal.* **56**, 335.

Hanly, C. and Masson, J. (1976). A critical examination of the new narcissism. *Int. J. Psycho-Anal.* **57**, 49.

Hartmann, H. (1953). Contribution to the metapsychology of schizophrenia. *Psychoanal. Study Child* **8**, 177. London.

Jacobson, E. (1975). The regulation of self-esteem. In *Depression and human existence* (ed. E. J. Anthony and T. Benedek). Boston.

Kernberg, O. (1975). *Borderline conditions and pathological narcissism*. New York.

Kohut, H. (1970). Opening and closing remarks of the moderator in Discussion of 'The self: a contribution to its place in theory and technique'. (D. C. Levin). *Int. J. Psycho-Anal.* **51**, 176.

—— (1971). *The analysis of the self.* New York.

Lichtenberg, J. D. (1975). The development of the sense of self. *J. Am. Psychoanal. Assoc.* **23**, 453.

Mahler, M. (1968). *On human symbiosis and the vicissitudes of individuation.* Vol. 1. New York.

—— and Furer, M. (1969). London edition of above.

Ornstein, P. H. (1974). Discussion of the paper 'Further contributions to the treatment of narcissistic personalities' by O. Kernberg, both in *Int. J. Psycho-Anal.* **55**, 215 and 241.

Reich, A. (1963). Pathological forms of self-esteem regulation. *Psychoanal. Study Child* **15**, 215. New York.

Sandler, J., Holder, A., and Meers, D. (1963). The ego ideal and the ideal self. *Psychoanal. Study Child* **18**, 139. London.

Stolorow, R. D. (1976). The narcissistic function of masochism (and sadism). *Int. J. Psycho-Anal.* **56**, 441.

Weil, A. (1970). The basic core. *Psychoanal Study Child* **25**, 442. New York.

4 Fetishism

Phyllis Greenacre

Introduction

The concept of the fetish rests on a very broad base. The term seems to have originated in the 15th Century, when Portuguese explorers in West Africa applied it to carved wooden figures or stones. It was thought that the natives regarded these as having magic value, and that they might have been considered as the habitations of gods or spirits. This interpretation may have been derived in part from the regard and worship of relics of the saints or other holy persons, already familiar to the explorers. Here the part (the relic) stood for the person, who in turn represented God, and was cherished or worshipped in a kind of eternal mourning reaction. The body might be gone, but the spirit remained attached to some memento which was, or represented, a body part, or some object immediately associated with the body, of the deceased individual.

This kind of worship was probably an indication of adoration or awe, in which there was also a fear of catastrophe or ill-luck if the belief in the holy overseer was allowed to fade and slip away. The relic served as a constant reminder. At best, it might serve as an agent of an external control; in any case, it was a token or a memento, invested with various degrees of magic. This concept then became formalized in group rituals in which the original relic was replaced by a symbol. This in turn has continued in quasi adornments of group practices in many religious or secret organizations. To lose or to destroy the symbol becomes an act of hostility or treachery to the group and risks severe punishment, from either the god(s) or the mortal representatives of divine power. With the emancipation from direct dependence on divine guidance and intervention, and with the increase in authority invested in the group, the tangible symbol may take on the significance of an amulet, a charm, and gradually become little more than a decorative bangle. Frequently, however, the hint of magic-value, bringing luck, is lurking somewhere.

Similar phenomena are frequent in our own culture and form a normal part of children's play, especially in the latter half of latency. They appear in both individual and group games where special objects, ritualistic practices, or even sayings are used as protection against bad-luck. Such practices may be abandoned in puberty or converted into more socially accepted and sophisticated forms. They may also reappear in special stylistic adornment of dress or decor and in fads in adult life. While these rituals vary considerably in different locations, periods, and cultures, there are some striking similarities in the conditions which produce them. It seems to me that, in the individual life, the dependence on such interests and practices portends a struggle with hostile aggressive impulses while these are augmented by fear in anticipation of submission in sexual union, not only to the partner, but to the unique quality of helplessness in the culmination of the sexual act itself.

The specific term *fetish*, derived from the Portuguese word *fetico*, has the connotation of an object made by art and skilfully conceived, in contrast to an actual relic; thus the term is related to artifact, which also has a two-faced meaning. It is a small something, which is especially skilfully contrived, and it is also a foreign body which is objectionably intrusive and misleading in an area of investigation or study. The fetish might also be worshipped and feared as a thing in itself, not merely as a symbol or representative of an unseen power.

All these variations and shades of meaning appear in conditions of pathological fetishism, as this is encountered in individual forms (in perversions and in more-or-less normal fetishistic phenomena) in our own time and culture. My own study has been focused mainly on fetishism as a perversion, manifest in the adult psychosexual life.

Clinical remarks

In understanding the genesis of fetishism, it is useful to consider not only the fetish as it is manifested in the perversion, but also as a phenomenon of varying form and intensity in conditions which cannot be considered definitely abnormal, as it appears ubiquitously. It may indeed be part of a vivid and rich emotional life. Perhaps the most frequent normal fetishistic phenomenon of adulthood is the love-token, or memento, which enhances the courtship love-play and may find its place as a preferred, but not a necessary, contribution to the foreplay of intercourse.

Fetishism as a perversion may be described in phenomenological terms, as the *obligatory* use of some non-genital object as a part of the sexual act, without which culmination cannot be achieved. The object chosen may be some other body part, or some article of clothing, or even a seemingly impersonal object. In this latter instance however, the fetish is found to be a symbolic substitute for a body part. In most cases, the need is for the possession of the object, so that it can be seen, touched, or smelled during or in preparation for the sexual act, whether this be masturbation or some form of sexual intercourse. In some instances not only possession of the object, but its incorporation into a ritualistic performance is required (Greenacre 1953).

One of the difficulties in presenting an adequate discussion of fetishism lies in the fact that the condition is by no means a clear-cut entity. The use of the fetish in one form or another and at various times in life can be detected in very many neuroses and character disorders. It is my impression that it is also to be found in some quite regressed psychotic states. And it is encountered regularly at certain developmental stages in infancy and childhood.

Indeed there is a spectrum of fetishistic manifestations, which differ both in content and in the degree of their compelling power. At one end is the hard core perversion, in which an object is demanded which is clearly associated with and represents the genitals. It must also be immediately available, tangible, and appealing to all the senses with the possible exception of hearing – although in a few instances this is the sense most involved. In a less severely circumscribed form of fetishism, an impersonal object, actually present or insistently remembered, or a fantasy version of an old memory will suffice. In another area of the spectrum is the use of fantasy alone, sometimes in a repetitive and sterotyped fashion, to enhance sexual pleasure. Tangibility is not demanded here: in fact, the emphasis is rather on the ability to be satisfied by a private illusion.

The fetishist does not generally seek help because of his need for the fetish, but because of other neurotic symptoms which are consciously more disturbing. He is inclined to think of the use of the fetish more as an incidental personal peculiarity than a symptom. Because this state is largely ego-syntonic, its existence may be unknown to the analyst until the patient has been in treatment for some time.

The very way in which a fetish is used indicates its defensive and quasi-reparative function. It appears as a reinforcing adjunct for a penis of uncertain potency. The fetish itself may be a single object, or any one of a number of related objects, used repetitively and quickly replaced if lost. It somewhat resembles a prosthetic body part, an artificial limb or, more precisely, a crutch or a hearing aid. It does not entirely replace a lost part but serves to increase the efficiency of an organ, the penis, which does not perform well without it. While it is not actually attached to the body, it must be nearby or recently at hand to be seen, touched, or smelled in order to exert its encouraging influence. The beneficial effect of the fetish seems to result from the incorporation through the senses of the image of the fetishistic object. This can be immediately elaborated by the arousal of unconscious memories, as occurs in the process of free association. It thus gains unique significance and lends its aid as though by magic. The result appears paradoxical, in that the inert object – the fetish – is thus unconsciously animated, and can give strength to the penis.

The ability of illusion to play an activating role is further apparent in those cases, related to fetishism, in which no external tangible object is used, its place being taken by fantasy, which is often stereotyped and repetitive. Such a state may be regarded as a fetishistic phenomenon. The need for it may seem to be less essential than when an objective fetish is used; but it is difficult to assess this situation as there is an implied, but usually fallacious belief, that fantasy is more readily controlled and modified by the patient than use of a concrete external object.

The use of the actual fetish, rather than a fantasy, may be more frequent in men than in women. It was earlier thought that fetishism only occurred in men. This disparity is largely due to the influence of the anatomical differences between the sexes, which permit a woman to conceal an inadequate sexual response, from herself as well as from her mate, more readily than is possible for a man. She appears also to have less direct conflict about this hidden 'inadequacy', and it mobilizes a different set of related conflicts; whereas in the man any appreciable interference with potency is obviously and drastically crippling to sexual performance. It is well known that an illusion of having a penis may develop early in a girl child after observing the penis of a boy or a man. This illusion is related to a prefetishistic state, and if long sustained may leave a lasting influence on the child's behaviour and character. The relinquishment of such an illusion is favoured by her later development, generally decisively so with the appearance of the menses at puberty. Symptoms more directly comparable to fetishism in the male, develop only in females in whom the illusionary phallus has gained such strength as to approach the delusional. In my experience this rarely occurs except in cases in which there are other severe disturbances in the sense of reality. This is especially illustrated in cases reported by Von Hug Helmuth (1915), Sperling (1963), and Zavitzianos (1971).

Fetishism is clearly associated with a very severe castration complex. This exists as an intense, prevailing fear of castration in the male and a much more complicated, though less readily recognized, set of related reactions in the female.

The developmental background

The early psychoanalytic description of the perversion of fetishism presented this condition as essentially due to a disruption in the usual libidinal development. This was first placed at or near puberty, when the young boy was overwhelmed by the awareness that his mother lacked a penis, and dealt with this apprehension by an unconscious manoeuvre, fixating on some part of her body or its covering (clothing) which was associated with the traumatic observation of her supposed castration. The mechanism is essentially that of a beginning screening process; but differs in its further development in that the altered memory must be both further concealed and concretized. The body part (or article substituting for it) seemed thus to be a compromise defence which both indicated the mother's genital structure and gave her a 'thing' which both concealed and represented her alarming deficiency. Articles of feminine clothing, especially corsets, shoes, or panties, were recognized as the commonest fetishistic objects. Further clinical studies modified this first point of view, and recognized that the traumatic event which precipitated the manifest fetishism involved an impact on and a disturbance of ego functioning – a splitting in the ego – making it possible for two opposing reality perceptions to operate simultaneously, to make amends for the alarming demonstration of the supposedly castrated-state of the woman. The very intensity of this traumatizing observation presumed an earlier established conviction in the young boy that his mother's genital equipment was like his own. I refer here to Freud's papers (1905, 1927, 1938), and shall return to these later in dealing with the concepts of the nature of fetishism as this was influenced by and became part of the development of psycho-analytic theory as clinical investigation progressed.

We now recognize that there are disturbances in infancy, predisposing to this outcropping of fetishism, which often occurs in anticipation of or associated with puberty. The traumatic observation of the absence of the penis undoubtedly has a powerful and specific effect on the rising castration fears of the young boy. But this will not by itself be sufficient to precipitate the neurosis, unless pathogenic conditions in early infancy have already impaired the sound progress of drive development and further interfered in characteristic ways with the emerging sense of reality (Greenacre 1953, 1955, 1960*a*, 1968). It is now also recognized that some quite severe cases of manifest fetishism may be found in the young child and may continue uninterruptedly into adult life (Sperling 1963; Spiegel 1967; Winnicott 1953, 1971). The significance of such early appearances of fetishism will be discussed later in this chapter, in considering their relation to transitional objects and transitional phenomena.

During the last two to three decades, our psychoanalytic understanding has been enriched through an increased interest in the forerunners and early stages of ego development, with a special concern with its autonomous functions. This puts the early ego in quite a different position in our thinking from when it was regarded as a development from the id, involved chiefly with defences. It has also been necessary for us to recast our ideas of the origin, nature, and vicissitudes of aggression. Our enlightenment has been furthered by many research studies with long-term, nursery observations of infants, especially with regard to early infant–mother relationship. This branch of psychoanalytic research furnishes an invaluable supplement to the knowledge obtained from direct analyses of children, as well as to that gained from reconstructions in analytic work with adults. It is not my intention here to attempt the considerable task of reviewing the various theoretical conceptions with their special terminologies, which have grown out of the many, and very productive, research studies.

I would rather emphasize now that while such perversions may become manifest at various times between early childhood and young adulthood, their occurrence is more frequent and sustained in adulthood. Their development in any case regularly rests on a base of severe disturbance in infancy, that is in the first two years of life. Such disturbances may be of various kinds, but of sufficient severity and/or duration to have an impact on, and somewhat interfere with, the orderly, progressive unfolding of development, which in these early months is so impressively rapid. There is not only the increase in the actual body size of the infant; but this is involved further with changing proportions of the body parts and the internal organs in accord with maturational processes and corresponding elaborations of functions. In addition there is a reciprocal enlargement of the scope and complexity of the infant's responsiveness and developing perceptiveness of his surroundings, in which the mother plays a central role.

Here I must digress to explain that my picture of what normally takes place does not coincide in all respects with the psychoanalytic theories of early psychic development as these are frequently presented. For a detailed set of quotations from various authors dealing with this subject, see Edgcumbe and Burgner (1972). My views may be somewhat more congruent with many of the observational studies of infants in nurseries, in which the infant–mother relationship is especially studied by psychologists and others, who are concerned with the physiology of infancy and its inter-relation with the beginning of psychic reactions. I would mention especially the study by Greene (1958), and Escalona's discussion of the phenomenon of 'contagion' (1953). Such findings have often been considered as outside the field for psychoanalytic investigation, which should limit itself to the psyche alone. Even so it seems to me that psyche and soma are never completely isolated from each other; and that early infancy is a time zone during which physiological conditions may be important determinants of significant variations in the development of beginning psychic phenomena.

The early concept of fetishism took scant account of the disturbance in the role of aggression, although it was recognized implicity that the use of the fetish might be associated with, or take the place of, sado-masochistic fantasies (Payne 1939; Gillespie 1940, 1952; Glover 1953; Bak 1953). The acting-out of such fantasies in condensed ways sometimes formed the nucleus of fetishistic rituals; or they might appear as repetitive antisocial acts in certain other forms of perversion. They were regarded as resulting from very intense castration fears of the phallic and oedipal periods, with regressive components from the anal phase. But with the further direct observation of infants and young children, it has become apparent that both penis envy in girls and castration fears in boys arise before this time and may be clearly discerned in the second year of life (Galenson and Roiphe, 1971).

This expanding knowledge of infantile development, from direct observational studies, has also brought some shift in the psychoanalytic conceptualizations of the early psychic structuring. Importantly associated with these studies was Hartmann's theoretical contribution (1939), in which, among other things, he pointed out that the ego developed from an earlier time than had been conceptualized, and that its autonomous functions of control and adaption must depend on fundamental biologic roots. From these sources, certain ideas have evolved concerning the nature and timing of the beginning of the ego, which is still a moot question. The older theoretical postulate of the duality of psychic structuring by the differentiation of the ego from a primal id, has somewhat given way to the consideration that both instinctual drives (id) and primitive regulatory controls (possibly the earliest signs of ego) arise from an 'undifferentiated state'. The term 'undifferentiated' is used in various connotative references sometimes to mean that the ego is not differentiated from the id, and sometimes that the id is not differentiated by itself from some primordial biologically determined state.

An increasing number of studies of the conditions, circumstances, and early responses of the newborn have led to various points of view regarding the beginning of aggression and of the ego. Among the most important of these are the studies of M.Mahler and her co-workers; R.Spitz; S.Escalona; S.Brody; S.Provence and others at the Child Study Center at Yale; the Putnam Childrens Center in Boston; the recent work of Galenson and Roiphe; as well as the many reports of individual observers. Anna Freud (1965) has stated the postulations which she and her students have worked out at the Hampstead Clinic. She sees the ego as developing from the vicissitudes of the ongoing-relationship of the infant to the mother – shaped according to the latter's ability or failure to meet the infant's needs. According to this conception, the infant is in 'a narcissistic unity' with the mother (or a mother figure), and there is at first (which probably means at birth) no distinction between the self and the environment. The infant leans on the parents to understand and manipulate the outer world, so that the bodily needs may be adequately met, and the parents further limit excessive drive satisfaction 'thereby initiating the child's own ego mastery of the id'. It is considered then that the parents subsequently provide patterns for identification which are necessary for the building up of an independent structure (Freud, A. 1965, p.46). The aggressive drive is to be considered chiefly in its relation to libidinal phases (*op. cit.*, p.62).

My own clinical experiences have led me to formulate the developmental conditions of early infancy with a somewhat different emphasis.

I believe that such a complete and primary narcissistic unity does not and cannot generally exist even at birth. It seems to imply a *complete* dependence on the mother, such as used to be thought of as characteristic of the prenatal period. Certainly there is a necessary and fateful dependence on the mother (or mother substitute) for certain basic needs, especially for food and warmth. The infant will not be able adequately to supply these predominantly on his own initiative for some months. The *independence* of the timing of his own needs from the rhythm offered him by the mother has in fact been the basis for the development of demand-feeding schedules, and a readjustment of ideas concerning toilet training. He may accommodate to her timing with more or less strain, or he may react with aversion as though to an intrusion if the discrepancy in timing is too great.

It appears to me, however, that the infant is partially independent of and separate from the mother at, and even before, birth. It has been pointed out (Greene 1958) that the foetus has already become somewhat independent of the mother in the first month of pregnancy, when the heart begins to beat on its own, at a rate which does not coincide with the maternal beat. The foetal motor rhythms also do not uniformly coincide with those of the mother, although the unborn infant may adapt in a considerable degree to the mother's heart beat, respiratory rhythm, and walking rhythm, even when these do not coincide with his own rhythms (Greenacre 1960*b*). It is considered that the neonate is made comfortable by being walked-with by his mother – in her arms or on her shoulder – because he has already become used to this when he was being carried *in utero*. His own spontaneous motions *in utero* however, are sometimes quite at variance with the maternal activities and more responsive directly to other external stimuli. Thus it would seem that the mother is only a part (though a very important one) of the environment and not the sole mediator of it immediately after birth. This margin of prenatal autonomy does not furnish adequate protection from the influence of certain maternal illnesses. The first three months of pregnancy when organogenesis is progressing rapidly is a time of special susceptibility. The second trimester is safer and the third trimester is again somewhat hazardous.

Already *in utero* the relation of the foetus to the mother involves other elements than are implied in a condition of narcissistic unity with her. Obviously this state cannot be considered as one of psychic activity due to psychic structuring, but it may mean that some elements in the unique organization of each unborn infant may influence his subsequent reaction to his mother and to the immediate outer world as well, very soon after birth, and may appreciably affect the psychic structuring when and as this becomes differentiated.

If we consider that the body-ego is the basic forerunner of the psychic-ego, it becomes clear that the development of the latter arises not only through the relationship to the mother, but in part from inborn organizing and balancing forces evident in the maturation of the infant himself. I can conceive of such a special fineness of balance in the foetal organization as would sometimes permit an unusually sensitive responsiveness to the mother *and* to the external environment very early in postnatal life. This would presage a possible later capacity for early gestalt perception, and an ability for synthesizing early sensory-motor experience. It might also contribute to facilitating the later synthesizing and integrating functions of the psychic ego. These might otherwise be regarded as furthered only by good maternal 'education'. The observations of Browne (1970) strongly suggest that there are considerable variations in the degree of dependence on the mother by the newborn infant. A group of children were studied consistently from birth until the age of 8 to 9 years. The one child who appeared most outstandingly gifted had shown an extraordinary independence from the mother and nurses from the very first post-natal days. I have discussed these possibilities in other terms in a paper on *The childhood of the artist* (1957) and in a discussion of infants' play (1969).

Facts regarding the disturbances in the foetus–mother relationship are now increasingly recognized, and it is clear that the old conception of the intra-uterine period as a nirvana, or state of bliss, is untenable. It rests on fantasy from a much later period rather than on fact. While unhealthy maternal conditions may produce disturbances in foetal growth and maturation, it also appears that the self-regulating organization of the individual foetus and the neonate is not as stable and efficient as the homeostatic system is to become in later life. But it is probable that the organically determined integrative function in the foetus is related to the later homeostatic principle, and exists in some degree even before and during the early development of the ego, when experience does not yet attain an appreciable degree of object relatedness.

It seems that the roots of aggression also belong to the primordial undifferentiated state and rest very largely on the early maturational pressures within the infant as a developing organism. The mother feels the kicks of an unborn child as independent of herself and interprets them subjectively, probably in accord with her emotional set toward her own pregnancy. We cannot suppose that the unborn infant has any reciprocal emotional reactivity. At most we would hypothesize some central nervous system registration of the activity as part of homeostatically-based developing patterns, representing a stage in the integration of the interweaving of the progressing functional processes.

But first let us consider the significance of the term *aggression*. This has been used in recent years with the meaning of cruelty or destructiveness (Hartmann, Kris, and Loewenstein 1949). In this sense, it implies an aim and an object – a condition which can only occur when there is already a sufficiently developed psychic ego capable of an appreciable degree of object relatedness. Aggression as an instinctual drive must arise from a primitive stage of organization of the individual organism, before this degree of object-relatedness has been reached. I speak of the *forerunners of aggression*, which I would see as arising from the undifferentiated stage of development, the stage dominated by the energetic growth of the individual. The inception of aggression is coincident with the very beginning of autonomous body-functioning, which will lead to the stage of body ego development during the early months of postnatal life. This in turn leads to hostile aggression.

An older meaning of the word *aggression* was that of *approaching*, *going at* or *toward*. This was usually associated with the idea of an especially energetic approach and merged into the meaning of an attack. Aggressive traits were on the whole considered desirable, indicating an individual's energetic attitude toward the struggles of life. The term seemed later to gain a stronger pejorative tone, implying, and almost limiting to, hostility, cruelty, and destructiveness. This was especially noticeable after the World Wars, perhaps with the emphasis on 'the aggressor nations' in contrast to supposedly peace-loving ones. At any rate this older meaning of aggression, as a *going-out-toward* or *approaching* seems to apply to the early expansive activity which may later sometimes develop into hostility and cruelty. Such unbridled expansion may injure that which it impinges upon, but destruction is not its aim or motivating force in any psychological sense. This is the background from which the capacity for hostile aggression in the interest of self-defence must develop. But tendencies to excessive hostility in its many various forms, have deep roots in extreme frustrations of whatever source, and increase from the more compli-cated struggles with hostility incident to the later libidinal-phase developments, especially the anal and oedipal periods. Such struggles result in deformations and special susceptibilities of later ego- and love-relationships.

The emergence of the fetish

It is obvious from the very character of the fetish that it defends against an unusually strong castration complex—so strong that an illusion of actual castration is easily aroused. The fetish is then the makeshift remedy. This situation indicates a weakness in the formation of the body-image. As this illusion of castration becomes too real, it is met with the use of a concretized symbol of the penis, which lends to it some strength and a semblance of adequacy. The compelling need for the fetish does not become fully evident until the young person is actually anticipating or seeking intercourse, usually in adolescence or young adulthood. Looking back through the work of analytic recon-struction in individual patients, one can see the outline, sometimes shadowy and sometimes distinct, forecasting this state of affairs at different stages throughout the early life. Such a defect in the early body ego, involving as it does the necessity for maintaining two opposite perceptions of the genitals, brings a corresponding weakness in the psychic ego. For the infarct in the developing sense of reality which is focused in the genitals, leads at the very least to uncertainty regarding the gender identity and may, in many instances, invade other elements in the psychic functioning. This disturbance occurs the more readily against a background of incomplete separation of the *me* from the other – specifically the mother.

In considering the antecedents of the fetish, I shall focus on three special periods of childhood. In all of these, severely unfavourable conditions tend to produce disturbances and imbalances in the somato-psychic development which *may* subsequently become manifest in fetishism. These three are: the *first two years*, the *fourth year*, and the *period leading up to and including puberty*. These are all critical periods, based on decisive stages of physical development, and anticipating and initiating obligatory changes in functioning, they are accompanied by shifts in the degree of independence necessary to proceed with the affairs of life.

The first two years

For most of the first year, the infant is predominantly dependent on the mother to supply sustenance and to supplement his own body warmth through her ministrations (clothing and covers, and actual body contact with her). He is largely dependent on his own autonomously directed resources to resist or eject stimulations which are pain provoking. Relief, when necessary, is largely through motoric responses cooperating with visceral discharge mechanisms – urination, defaecation, drooling, vomiting, and so on. The conditions which are most upsetting and disorganizing are those impacts which grossly exceed the infant's maturational readiness.

At this early stage, the infant is in a symbiotic relation with the mother, with development proceeding through the operation of the introjective–projective mechanism. Ideal conditions allow the infant to achieve increasing separation and independence gradually and at his own speed. Severe disturbances in the mother may result in actual deprivation of appropriate stimulation to the infant, the effect of which can be almost as disturbing as when the discomfort has arisen primarily in the infant. Generally, however, these early reactions to traumatic conditions are more diffuse and affect the quality of organization of the incipient ego, rather than laying down patterns as specific as we see sometimes in fetishists.

The second year after birth is marked by the considerable infantile achievements of walking and talking – accomplishments which indicate and implement the growing pressure for and satisfaction in independent activity. It is still a time of rapid growth as well as of change in functions and posture, which makes for significantly new and varying perceptions not only of the outer world but of the own body, both directly and in comparison to the bodies of others. The multiplicity of the perceptual variations leads to the beginning of symbol formation, at the same time that memory (not on a conditioned basis) is being established. There is a total body invigoration and responsiveness; some upsurge and awareness of genital sensations is indicated by the frequency with which infants at this time are observed touching or playing with their genitals. Castration fears and penis envy at this period have been recognized and variously interpreted by both child and adult analysts, and by research observers of infants in day-nurseries. This concurrence of increased genital awareness with the capacity for erectability of the total body in walking, may predispose to development of a persistent body-phallus equation. This is a somatic basis for later specific symbolization.

All this is part of a period of growing object-relatedness, with increasing capacity for meaningful attachments, both loving and hostile, to persons in the infant's *milieu*. There is less diffusion of rage in body states, as both rage and anger can now be directed at the real or supposed offender, rather than being spent on whatever is by chance at hand, whether it be the own body or an external object. The introjective–projective mechanism is still at work, though no longer as strong and pervasive as when individuation was less advanced.

The circumstances or events of this second year which contribute to the later development of manifest fetishism are of two general types: first, traumas which are of such a nature as directly to increase fears of castration, and secondly, those prolonged or chronic situations which more subtly promote uncertainty or confusion concerning the anatomical genital differences between the two sexes.

There is in any case some intrinsic castration fear in the male child, since his genitals are so exposed as to look as though they might readily be pulled or scraped off. But the greatest increase in castration fear is aroused by accidents to or operative interference with the genitals, or a contiguous area, or even other parts of the body. Since the sense of the own body is not yet firmly established, and the introjective–projective mechanism is still readily available, such traumas in other parts of the own body, or in bodies of others close to the infant, may be displaced to the genitals, introjected, and felt almost as though directly experienced. In this situation, vision is probably the sense through which any severe injury to 'the other' (the 'not me' in Winnicott's terms) is taken in. This visual incorporation is associated with a sympathetic responsiveness or resonance in parts of the infant's own body, which correspond to the observed injured area of the other's body. The earlier mirroring reaction of the first year is already developing into a capacity for imitativeness which may be expressed in consciously directed forms of behaviour or in less precise sympathetic body responses.

The integration of the inner representation of the own body has progressed sufficiently that the various body parts belong to each other in a fairly consistent functional way. This is evident in, and necessarily accomplished and consolidated in, the early stages of walking and talking. Widening but precise volitional-goal directness of the body activities is in process, but is still faltering and uneven. In other words the infant's separation from the mother and her substitutes and extensions, has progressed and is furthered by the increasing capacity for independent exploration of the outer world. During this period of increased outwardly-directed maturational pressure, the body is completing the process of getting itself together into a working unit, a process with which it has been so much concerned during the first year.

Further circumstances, fortuitous but unfortunate, and often present in this second year, may tend to increase confusion in the young child concerning the configuration of his genitals. This occurs when an infant at this age, and in the succeeding few years, is consistently exposed to the sight of the genitals of another child of the opposite sex, who is close to him in age and size. This situation is relatively common in families where young children, one- to three-years apart in age, are regularly bathed and dressed together, sleep together, and not infrequently play together nude.† Something akin to a twin relationship develops. Since the own-genital-area can never be seen as clearly or as easily as that of the other, the visual incorporation of the genitals of the opposite sex may be more clearly impressed on the child than that of the own-genitals. Conflicting impressions may then arise between what the infant sees repeatedly on the other child, and would suppose belonged to himself as well, and what he feels in any manual exploration or from the rising endogenously determined genital sensations. This situation obviously contributes to the pre-oedipal penis envy in the little girl and to the early fear of castration in the little boy, which have been observed and described in studies of infants in day nurseries. Although this state of affairs is not an essential antecedent of the development of fetishism as a perversion, in my own clinical experience I have found it a not uncommon contributing factor. Naturally the confusion of this period is increased if there has been a prolongation and intensification of the symbiotic relationship with the mother during a disturbed first year.

The fourth year and the period leading up to puberty

Two further periods of special vulnerability to castrative traumas are experienced by the child before he reaches adolescence. The first of these occurs in the fourth year, when there is regularly a definite rise in genital excitability. By this time the capacity for object relatedness has developed and the young child is now in the beginning of the

---

†One may also question whether it may be promoted in day-nurseries or in communes where groups of infants are cared for together, and are more liberally and consistently exposed to each other in the nude than might be true in individual families.

oedipal era. The second period of special vulnerability is in late latency or prepuberty, when the child is anticipating puberty and some body changes may have already become apparent.

These two periods resemble each other in that both occur at times of transition from a period characterized by increased body growth – assóciated with expanding physical activity with sexual interest driven largely by exploratory curiosity—to a period of intense sexual feelings involving attachment to another person. Both the phallic phase and the period of prepubescence are marked by awesome expectations of the opening of a new era, engendering both eagerness and fear.

Acute traumas such as operations on the genitals, or on body parts symbolically representing the genitals, are particularly disastrous if undertaken at these times. They seem realistically to verify the threat of castration in an explicit way and are often met with a strong and very resistant defence by denial. The tendency to deny may subsequently spread, in such a way as to distort grossly the character development. If a severe trauma occurs in the phallic–oedipal period the memory of it may be deeply repressed, and leave in its wake an amnesia for the whole period. During analysis, it reappears in dreams, night terrors, and episodes of acting-out. If it occurs in late latency or pre-puberty, it may be remembered in an isolated way but the emotion associated with it is denied and displaced on to other areas. Such traumas in prepuberty do not by themselves precipitate fetishism, but contribute to its emergence if earlier experiences of infancy have paved the way. Relatively slight traumatic experiences in prepuberty may be insistently recalled and even exaggerated, but then may be used as screens for earlier severe ones.†

†A fuller discussion of my ideas concerning developments in these periods is contained in earlier papers on fetishism published in the last twenty years. Chapters 2, 5, 12, 17, 18, 19 in *Emotional growth Vol. 1*, deal specifically with fetishism. The papers on 'Prepuberty trauma', 'Screen memories', and 'Respiratory incorporation and the phallic phase' (Chapters 9, 10, and 13 in *Trauma growth and personality*, (Greenacre 1952)) also deal with these vulnerable preoedipal periods. The latter paper concerned a case in which a definite fetishistic symptom was present in a woman. This is mentioned but not especially stressed.

The paper on 'Prepuberty trauma in girls' (Greenacre 1952) deserves a supplement as the title might imply a restriction of the significance of this trauma to the female sex. Due probably to the nature of my practice at that time, I had not observed any striking cases among males. More recently I have been greatly impressed with the extremely disturbing effects of special genital traumas in prepuberty boys, including manipulations of or operations on the genitals, undertaken ostensibly for therapeutic reasons. The post-puberty sequelae varied, but there was always a considerable distortion in the adult sexual performance, varying from overt perversion to denial through impotence. In any case, there were also marked defects in ego development. The degree of malfunction of the ego seemed to depend as well on the nature of the early mother–child relationship.

The fetish and the transitional object

In considering how the fetish is related to the transitional object, I shall lean very much on my own work. This developed largely from clinical investigations during the treatment of cases of overt fetishism appearing as part of a perversion. My study, beginning in the early 1950s, was first presented in a paper, published in 1953, concerning the relation of fetishism to the faulty development of the body image. It ended with two articles (1969, 1970) on the relationship between the fetish and the transitional object. My conception of the fetish as a perversion has developed further and been modified by additional clinical experience, not only with fetishism but with other related neurotic conditions in which pregenital disturbances clearly played a part in intensifying the oedipal problems and in undermining sound ego development in a variety of ways. During the last decade especially, there has been coincidentally a general awakening of interest in developments in the infant years, and observational data of co-workers have become increasingly available.

At the end of this discussion, I shall attempt to compare my own point of view with that of Winnicott, whose first paper (1953) concerning the transitional object was published in the same year as my first paper on fetishism. His subsequent work has stimulated and influenced me very much, although there are some points on which we are not in complete accord.

There are certain basic resemblances between the fetish and the transitional object. Both are inanimate objects selected and used by the individual in maintaining a psycho-physical balance under conditions of actual or potential strain. On the other hand, the transitional object appears in and belongs to infancy; whereas, the fetish – at least as used in a perversion – is commonly adopted as a necessary prop, or adjunct, for adequate adult sexual performance. While the perversion of fetishism becomes manifest under the demands of adult life, there are definite roots in early disturbances in infancy as well as in pre-puberty. The transitional object by contrast is almost ubiquitous and does not generally forecast abnormal neurotic development.

When we compare transitional and fetishistic phenomena, the differences are less decisive: the two conditions seem to overlap. Thus, fetishes, or less tangible substitutes for them, may be used as magic props during latency in attempts to ensure a good outcome in adventurous or competitive activities of a non-genital type. In some cases, the use of the transitional object is continued into latency, and with puberty becomes more insistent. This transitional object may then with puberty give way to a fully-fledged fetish or perversion. But this situation is the exception rather than the rule.

During latency generally there seems to be little difference between the sexes in regard to the use of benign lucky pieces, rituals, prayers, and private superstitions in the hope of success. A little girl in late latency once gave me one of her good-luck pieces. She called it a 'feeling stone', because it felt so good in her hand. It had a peculiar smoothness, which somehow suggested something satiny and softer than a stone. Irregular in shape, perhaps phallic, it had been a comfort to her when carried in her pocket. She did not use it in critical or dangerous situations, but rather to ensure good feeling and to protect against loneliness. It did not seem connected with any genital activity though it may have been a reminder of some such interest in the past. This kind of thing is extremely common. It seemed related to the transitional object and perhaps to an imaginary companion, and often becomes manifest at about eight or nine years of age. Later it may be continued in a less individualized form, as a girlish decoration, a bracelet, or whatever bit of jewellery is the current junior-miss fad. It contributes to collecting hobbies in both sexes. Here certainly the fetish and the transitional object merge. However, the use of the fetish is largely limited to men. Ritualistic performances and stereotyped fantasies as obligatory accompaniments of sexual activity may occur in women as well as in men: I would consider them as belonging in the group of fetishistic phenomena. They also occur and are intermittently acted out by transvestites.† The difference between the sexes, in the use of the fetish to secure sexual gratification may be due to the difference in the visibility of the genitals. Any failure of genital responsiveness in the male not only interferes with his sexual gratification, but is visible to both himself and his mate. Invoking an increased narcissistic wound, it requires a more drastic remedy.

Both fetishes and transitional objects are selected by the individual. In both instances the chosen object relates to the own-body as well as to that of 'the other', the not-me, basically the mother. There is a

---

†Here my experience is only with male transvestites. From the study of the records of female impostors, I have thought that the episodes of imposture in such women represent the acting-out of earlier compulsive masturbatory fantasies, which are essentially fetishistic phenomena. The acting-out may then be in response to a need to experience in actual reality rather than only in fantasy. This corresponds to the fetishist's need for a *concrete* object to bolster his uncertain potency.

greater variability and range of objects chosen by one adult fetishist than the transitional objects chosen by one infant. A great variety of objects may be chosen however by *different* infants. The infant usually selects a simple object at first, and only makes substitutions in the process of relinquishment. Thus the infant, in the process of developing, needs only time-insurance for his practical security. He is faithful but casual in his alternate use and neglect of this chosen comforter, as he progressively outgrows his need for its help. The adult fetishist, on the other hand, suffers a permanent need for this help and must accommodate to it. He may accept his use of it, make it ego-syntonic, and regard it as his own peculiarity, but he rarely gives it up spontaneously.

Both fetish and transitional object are clearly body related. They offer substitutes or additions to reinforce body parts or aspects which are seemingly inadequate. The fetish is characteristically something which suggests the male genital; but has some female attributes as well. In the perversion, the fetish is generally definitely visible and durable. If it is destroyed, it can usually be replaced. It seems clearly to be a direct body symbol which bridges the difference between male and female genitals.

The selection of the transitional object, on the other hand, occurs usually during the first year after birth, and is almost ubiquitous (Winnicott 1953). The object is clearly selected by the infant out of various objects in his intimate environment. It commonly is something soft which has been used in the infant's care, such as an old blanket, which is also impregnated with body odours, from both himself and his mother. Softness, smoothness, a suggestion of warmth, a kind of polymorphous pliability combined with relative durability seem to be the appealing qualities. The presence of body odour was thought to be almost indispensable. A freshly washed transitional object, which has previously been a favourite, will be rejected. More recent studies by Busch (1973) have indicated that texture is much more important than odour, and that after a freshly laundered object has been softened by being crumpled, it is readily accepted. Qualities of enhanced visibility such as bright colour and definiteness of outline do not count for much. In the end the specific transitional object may be gradually given up by being reduced to a mere token of its original form. For example, a piece of a blanket previously in the infant's crib may be chosen; but even a part of its satin binding may come to serve as a substitute for the blanket itself. It rarely is decisively disposed of, but its importance fades. The gradual relinquishment of the object suggests a spontaneous self-weaning.

While I have not made systematic studies of transitional objects in infancy, in those developmental situations observed at first hand, I have not generally detected as clear a connection between the specific qualities of the relinquished original transitional comforter and those of subsequently preferred toys, as is indicated by Winnicott. While a teddy bear or other stuffed animal may be used, children very soon turn to toys which are actively played with rather than embraced for comfort. Later, a live pet may succeed to the favoured position. We may understand this gradual change from an inanimate and poly-morphously pliable object, to a more clearly defined toy, and ulti-mately to a fully animate but cuddly pet as meeting the needs of the baby in successive stages of his own individuation. After this is well-advanced, he can risk establishing a friendly reliance on a pet that is capable of auto-locomotion. If he is not sufficiently separated from 'the other', unexpected motion, not corresponding to his own body rhythm, is disrupting. Several times, I have known babies of less than one-year to become terrified when an inanimate toy seemed unexpectedly to acquire independent motion. In one instance, it was a large ball which suddenly rolled toward the baby who was sprawling on the bed. In another, a usually stationary and inert toy began to perform, since its concealed mechanism was wound up and set in motion by a visitor, intending to amuse the baby, who, however, became extremely frightened. Rhythmic motion at a distance, the swaying of mobiles attached to the crib, the soft clapping of hands, or the fluttering of leaves in the breeze, may on the other hand, attract and fascinate. Such movement perceived from a distance may be simultaneously faintly stimulating and soothing, if the rhythm is relatively even and not associated with sudden changes in intensity or tempo. It is to vision what a soft lullaby is to hearing (McDonald 1970). Like the security blanket, it helps the infant to relinquish himself to sleep. An even beat may have a sustaining effect perhaps because of its resemblance to the rhythms of the heartbeat and of breathing in stages of healthy equilibrium.

The transitional object represents the infant's persistent, but less demanding, relationship to the mother during the process of separation. Periodic merging with her decreases as the autonomous urges due to maturation and growth take hold; ultimately then the mother becomes part of the environment in a different way. At first the infant is concerned with the transitional object as it conveys sensual familiarities, chiefly with the upper part of her body, (her breast, arms and face, probably with a diffuse sense of her whole body). This sense of familiarity is mediated largely through touch and kinaesthetic responses. Vision is probably not as important as it becomes when separation has progressed further. The mother who has been adequate and 'good enough' for her infant gradually and increasingly becomes part of the not-me environment, and as he propels himself forward, the infant adopts the transitional object to keep in touch with the mother as she used to be.

In contrast the fetish, destined to become part of a perversion, arises in response to a focused need, because of concern about the genitals. The demand for the concrete fetish characteristically emerges as a symptom later than is true of the transitional object, and is not always preceded by a transitional object. My clinical analytical observations have convinced me that the fetish, nonetheless, usually has roots in disturbances in the first 18 months after birth. There may be such conditions that the mother is not and cannot be good enough to fulfil the infant's needs adequately. It is the influence of *trauma* in these early months as well as in later situations which lays the ground for the development of a fetish, whether this may occur in infancy itself or only surfaces in a manifest form at a much later date.

Acute or chronic traumatic conditions involving the mother, or existing in other parts of the environment, or in the infant himself may contribute to the background for the later development of a fetish.†
For example, there may be severe deprivation of maternal contact, due to the absence of the mother or to her incapacitating illness, together with the substitution of inadequate, unreliable, and frequently changing caretakers; constant fighting and violently disruptive tensions in the household, which result in acute, overwhelming stimulation to the infant; acute or chronic physical trauma in the infant due to illness, operations, or sometimes to other unavoidable but drastic therapeutic procedures: in fact any state of unmanagable pain. Such conditions may be of an intensity for which no mother can offer

---

†It is interesting that when Freud first wrote about fetishism, in his '*Three essays on the theory of sexuality*' (1905), he considered that there might be some constitutional 'executive' weakness of the sexual apparatus which has been especially affected by some *trauma* (italics mine) of childhood, and that the specific nature of the trauma affected the special character of the fetish. I would suggest that the constitutional executive weakness may have been due to the disturbed conditions of early infancy, which may be so incorporated into later development as to appear functionally as part of the constitutional equipment.

sufficient comfort and relief. Infantile pain, as well as massive over-stimulation from external sources, inevitably arouses engulfing excitement which must be spent in and on the own body if maternal comfort is inadequate. Such experiences also are the forerunners of later states of blind rage. In such a situation, a transitional object might not be adequate either. The later clinical history is often that of a manifest or latent character disorder, with outbursts in which anxiety carries with it a panicky fear of exploding or 'going to pieces'.

My evaluation of the importance of these early traumatic conditions differs from that of Winnicott. He did not emphasize the influence of trauma; and believed that the fetish was derived from the transitional object and could be traced back to it. He cited cases of infantile fetishism as indications of this point of view. While, in my experience, there may be a transitional object preceding the fetish, this is not generally true in cases of fetishism developing in infancy or later as part of a perversion. Nonetheless the two objects are closely related. In most of the cases of the use of a fetish in infancy reported by Wulff (1946) and Sperling (1959), the chosen object certainly resembled a fetish more than a transitional object. These infants had clearly less than good maternal care. The need for a fetish had appeared after weaning and was more orally focused than is true in general with transitional objects. In any case the fetish, whether of infant or young adult, generally has a quality of hardness and concreteness in contrast to the preferred softness and plasticity of the transitional object.

In years past, thumb and finger sucking may have occupied a place intermediate between transitional object and infantile fetish. The tendency to suck the fingers or fist is frequently well-established in newborns, and has been shown to have begun before birth. But a generation or two ago, its persistence even in early infancy was so condemned that vigorous efforts to break the habit by interposing drastic physical restraints were undertaken. These undoubtedly worsened the situation by increasing the frustration developing with them. Prolonged finger sucking often showed a highly aggressive activity. Its prolongation into childhood may have resulted from this increased aggression of frustration, as well as earlier unusual or sudden oral deprivation, until it ultimately assumed the character of infantile fetishistic behaviour. In this respect, it may resemble the cases of infantile fetishism reported by Wulff (1946) and Sperling (1959). As already mentioned, the movement from oral to early genital pre-occupation is especially easy in the latter half of the first year, when the giving up of the breast and the increasing separation from the mother, occur at the same time as sitting-up and the first attempts at walking bring a new visual relationship to the own-genitals, often coincident with the beginning of toilet training. I have twice seen in consultation women who remained thumb-suckers into adult life. In both cases there were unusual disturbances and privations in the first years, and the clinical history indicated a severe degree of penis envy. The condition was clearly a form of perversion. Both women came from affluent but emotionally depriving backgrounds, with little maternal care. Later under the pressure of obligatory and burdensome social activities, these patients suffered such shame associated with the thumb-sucking, as well as with the conditions which formed its background that the development of heterosexual interests was grossly hindered.

By and large the effects of chronic untoward conditions in the first months are diffuse in character. There may be an increase in aggression, which is largely body bound since it has as yet no specific aim and object. An increase in body tension with a later predisposition to anxiety reactions may also follow. If such conditions are sustained, and so severe that the total resources of the infant are called into reaction, there is a tendency to a suffusion of excitation and an overflow of discharge with premature stimulation of zonal responses for which the infant is not maturationally ready. This may result in excretory and premature genital reactions, responses under strain which do not have a true phasic significance. Such conditions contribute to distortions in the body ego development as well as to intensification of problems of the oedipal period, which is especially burdened by persistent narcissistic elements (Greenacre 1952). These contribute to character disorders and particularly severe neuroses which are not necessarily of a perverse type.

From my own experience in analysing adult fetishists, I have concluded that specific severe traumas as well as prolonged traumatic conditions are of special significance in the determination of later fetishism. When such severe traumatic episodes occur in the first months of life, they contribute to the need for an infantile fetish, since a transitional object will not suffice. These are the situations in which the distressed infant *cannot* get any reasonable amelioration from his mother, or even from a soft representational substitute for her. No mother can then be 'good enough', and sometimes the infant's own body discharges cannot suffice to care for the amount of primitive aggression aroused. The body then requires something of extraordinary firmness to offer focus and limits to his explosiveness. It is in this state of affairs that an infantile fetish is adopted which is reassuringly hard, unyielding, unchanging in shape, and reliably durable. It seems probable that the introjection of such an object, which is indestructable, lends a necessary strength, a kind of spot of organization to meet the infant's otherwise bursting omnipotence, since this cannot now be lent him in a controlled way by maternal support.† It is this mechanism of projection and return introjection which continues to operate in the use of the fetish in perversions of adult life, which I detected clinically and described in my first paper on fetishism (1953).

I have already mentioned the fear 'of going to pieces' which may recur as a later symptom in both fetishists and other individuals with impaired ego development. Winnicott (1964) has made similar observations in regard to severe neuroses in adolescents, with a special fear of a breakdown.

He states the breakdown which is feared, has already been. What is known as the patient's illness is a system of defences organized against this past breakdown—the original breakdown ended when new defences were organized which constitute the patient's illness pattern. The patient's fear of breakdown has one of its roots in the patient's need to remember the original breakdown. Memory can only come through re-experiencing—the original breakdown took place at a stage of dependence on parental or maternal ego support. For this reason therapeutic work is often done on a later version of the breakdown—when the patient has developed ego autonomy and a capacity to be a person having an illness. Behind such a breakdown there is always a failure of defences belonging to the individual's infancy or very early childhood. Often the environmental factor is not a single trauma but a pattern of distorting influences, the opposite in fact of the facilitating environment which allows of individual maturation. [p.139]

He does not, however, mention these particular symptoms as of any special importance in the development of fetishism, whereas to me it is an important link in the genesis of the fetish.

In my differences from Winnicott there may be a semantic problem as well as some difference in the focusing on, and interpretation of, clinical observations. Winnicott sometimes mentions trauma in con-

---

†Winnicott (1964) refers to this situation as presenting the forerunner of 'unthinkable anxiety' which is kept away by the relationship to the mother who is good enough to put herself in the baby's place, not so much by adequate feeding as by adequate being. In her contact, she gives the infant a brief experience of omnipotence.

nection with the development of the transitional object, when he means a degree of discomfort and of mild frustration felt by the infant in the process of separation from the mother; a degree of frustration which is healthy and strengthening, rather than disturbing to the development of the 'young ego' (1971, pp.96–97). He seems to refer to severe trauma as 'actual' traumas and does not connect them at all with the fetish, which he regards anyway as a variant of the transitional object. I believe, on the other hand, that severe trauma has an obstructive influence on autonomous development and contributes to the later adoption of a fetish which is used at first as an emergency makeshift support. The need for this may become manifest in infancy, around puberty or in adulthood. It may be given up or used less needfully for periods, but is revived, reinstated, and incorporated into the sexual activity after puberty, when sexual feelings are more urgent. But its emergence into a condition of fetishism only recurs when additional traumata have been experienced in the phallic or pre-puberty periods, and have further intensified and focused the castration fears, the ground for which has been laid in the first two post-natal years.

This brings us to the consideration of the effect of any severe traumatic episode (as in contrast with chronic traumatic conditions) occurring at this early time. It has been repeatedly reported by reliable clinicians that even extremely severe traumas occurring to the infant or witnessed by him as occurring to someone (mother, sibling, a pet) in a warm relationship with him, seem often to result in singularly little disturbance. For example Winnicott has written 'Actual trauma, however, need have no ill effect as shown by the following case; what produces the ill-effect is the trauma that corresponds with a punishment already fantasied'. The implication is that if the trauma occurs very early, or is of so unprecedented a nature, that the infant has no remembered previous experience which can give meaning to the event; then the immediate reaction is soon over and no unfavourable symptoms will follow. He quotes the case of a girl baby of one-year-old who was attacked by her two-year-old brother with a hot poker which he stuck in the infant's neck just below the thyroid cartilage. An intelligent and generally jolly but rambunctious child, he had done this out of spite and was probably in a fit of jealousy toward this little intruder so close on his heels. Although the baby cried at the time, and spent six weeks in the infirmary, she subsequently seemed little affected by the experience. When seen by Winnicott, at 15 months, because of a cough, she seemed healthy and happy, showed no symptoms referable to the incident, and no undue axiety when the brother snatched toys from her or provoked her in other ways (1931, p.9). Winnicott then added that although having a hot poker put against her neck corresponded with nothing already in her mind and no ill effect could be noted, yet it was possible that when she reached a more advanced level of emotional development, anxiety might be referred back to this incident which conceivably could then appear to her as the cruel assault that it was.

Such cases may be of special significance in the background of the fetishist. I have seen the situation from a more expanded period of time than that granted to Winnicott, who was a paediatrician at the time he made this observation. I believe that such early severe traumas produce an extraordinary effect, which is not immediately evident for the very reason that they subject the infant to an experience of extreme stimulation for which he has no clear preparatory experience. In the analysis of some fetishists and one transvestite patient, I have found that such a severe trauma may remain as a submerged organization *impression* (I cannot think of a better word) which is not ordinarily available to memory but cannot be quite completely encapsulated and sealed off. There will always be some bit that will make a connection and be related to new experiences as they come along.

The deferred effects of these early traumas are of several types. At the very least, there is an increase in the anxiety connected with any new related experience. Most striking however, are the states in which new versions of the original traumas, sometimes only slightly modified by the accretions of later experiences and fantasies, are produced in extreme nightmares, fugue-like episodes of acting-out in a panicky state, and repetitive somnambulistic behaviour. Fragments of the original traumatic events sometimes reappear also in physical symptoms.

Such a concealed *impression* of the infantile trauma is characteristically reactivated, when, as frequently happens, new traumatic experiences occur at the age of two, as well as in the phallic and prepuberty periods. Sometimes these seem to have been produced under the influence of the continuing pressure of the disturbed earlier conditions, and sometimes they are fortuitous. But in any case, these are vulnerable sensitive periods, susceptible to the shock of accidents (either to the child himself or to other closely related individuals), and to illnesses bringing about rather radical therapeutic interferences, such as tonsillectomies, delayed circumcisions, hernia operations, mastoid operations, and other active corrective procedures of one sort or another. Even the repeated use of enemas may be definitely traumatic. Such practices contribute to the undermining of the sense of the body integrity, and interfere with the developing autonomy especially increasing the castration fear. Such 'real' or 'actual' attacks require a defence which will also be a supplement. For this purpose, a fantasy may serve temporarily, but a definite demonstration of phallic ability is soon demanded. Rising genital feelings initiate a period of masturbation which may become aggressively compulsive. It is often accompanied by sado-masochistic fantasies. Although begun in the search for relief, it results in an intensification of the castration fear and a general worsening of the sense of body and emotional integrity. When the young person reaches the stage of actually wanting and attempting intercourse, he finds his phallic ability wavering and uncertain especially when he is confronted with the sight of the female genitals. This situation in itself re-establishes his old uncertainty about his genital equipment. The fetish becomes the concretized substitute for the female phallus which has been intermittenly believed in, earlier in life, but realistically given up. The fetish is thus a reification of a fantasy which has proved inadequate for the actual test of intercourse.

A brief account of the first years of a fetishist patient may help to illustrate the significant connections between the preoedipal disturbances and the later perverse development. The nature of these disturbances came to light largely through the work of analytic reconstruction. It was possible some years later to verify, with slight modification, the validity of our reconstructive work. The progressive series of disturbances was as follows. During his first three years, the child was exposed to violent fights between the parents as well as to sexual scenes. The marriage was breaking up in an atmosphere of jealousy and recriminations. In the latter part of this time, the mother had two abortions, the first of which was done at home while the patient was thought to be asleep in the adjoining room. The situations of these abortions had been confused in the patient's memory, as he believed that he had seen instruments being boiled up in the kitchen in preparation for the second abortion. He later learned from his mother that this abortion had been done away from home while he was being cared for by a neighbour. A little later, in the period of three to five years, he suffered three important losses: the parents separated and he did not see his father for several years; the parental grandmother, who often took care of him, died suddenly in her sleep; and a close playmate about his own age, died suddenly of polio. When he was between five and six years old, he had a tonsillectomy done in the doctor's office: the scene of the instruments being boiled up, belonged to this event rather than to the abortion. During early latency he was himself hospitalized for a febrile illness involving considerable joint pain. In the prepuberty period, after his father had rejoined the family, the mother had a third abortion, again done at home. He was thoroughly cognisant of this, and the memory served as a partial screen to the earlier one.

Summary

The central core of fetishism as a perversion seems to lie in an extraordinarily severe castration complex. This ultimately results in an illusion of some actual impairment of the genitals. It has its beginning, however, in traumatically determined pregenital disturbances involving the body ego in process of formation and transition into the psychic ego. These distubances of the first years are such as to be focused in the genital area prematurely, either because of the specific nature of the trauma or because of its extreme or prolonged severity. In any case, both aggression and genital response are mobilized under strain before adequate discharge channels have matured. This may especially be the case, if the mother is unable for one reason or another to give the infant adequate comfort.

Such early disturbances may recur later in childhood, either fortuitously or derived from the original experiences in a compulsively repetitive fashion. Their effect depends on the degree and nature of the confusion regarding the genitals, the extent of the invasion of the sense of reality, and the nature of the utilization and control of the aggression. Corresponding to the lack of confidence in the integrity of the own genitals, there is a prolongation and strengthening of the ubiquitous illusion of the maternal phallus.

The actual emergence of the obligatory need for the fetish appears when the growing boy or young man is forced to recognize that the mother, or the woman who supplants her, lacks the male genitals. The fetish then is an object usually associated with the woman but capable of representing both sexes. It serves a function analogous to, but, in my estimation, not usually continuous with or derived from the transitional object. The typical transitional object is essentially part of normal development. The two objects are, however, related. Their atypical forms, the transitional and the fetishistic phenomena, may be indistinguishable, the one from the other.

References

Bak, R. (1953). Fetishism. *J. Amer. Psychoanal. Assoc.* **1**, 285.
—— (1968). The phallic woman. The ubiquitous fantasy in perversions. *Psychoanal. Study Child* **23**, 15.

Browne, J. (1970). Precursors of intelligence and creativity. *Merrill-Palmer Qu. of Behaviour and Development*, 16, part 1.

Busch, F., Nagera, H., McKnight, J., and Pezzatossi, G. (1973). Primary transitional objects. *J. Am. Acad. Child Psych.* **12**, 193.

Edgcumbe, R. and Burgner, M. (1972). Some problems in the conceptualization of early object relationships. *Psychoanal. Study Child* **27**, 283.

Escalona, S. (1953). Emotional development in the first year of life. In *Problems of infancy* (ed. M. J. E. Senn) pp.26, 31, 46. Josiah Macy Foundation., Packinack Lake, New Jersey.

Freud, A. (1965). Normality and pathology in childhood, assessments of development. *The writings of Anna Freud*, Vol. 6, 46–67. New York.

Freud, S. (1905). Three essays on sexuality. *Complete psychological works of Sigmund Freud*. Standard edition **7**, 153.
—— (1927). Fetishism. *Complete psychological works of Sigmund Freud*. Standard edition **21**, 175.
—— (1938). Splitting of the ego in the process of defence. *Complete psychological works of Sigmund Freud*. Standard edition **23**, 273.

Galenson, E. and Roiphe, H. (1971). The impact of sexual discovery on mood, defensive organization and symbolization. *Psychoanal. Study Child* **26**, 196.

Gillespie, W. (1940). A contribution to the study of fetishism. *Int. J. Psycho-Anal.* **21**, 401.
—— (1952). Sexual perversions. *Int. J. Psycho-Anal.* **33**, 397.

Glover, E. (1953). The relation of perversion formation to the development of the reality sense. In *An early development of the mind*, 216–239. New York. Reprinted 1956.

Greenacre, P. (1952). *Trauma, growth and personality*. New York.
—— (1953). Certain relations between fetishism and faulty development of the body image. *Psychoanal. Study Child* **8**, 70. Also in (1971) *Emotional growth* Vol. 1, 9–31 New York.
—— (1953). Prepuberty trauma in girls. *Trauma, growth, and personality*. London.
—— (1955). Further considerations regarding fetishism. *Psychoanal. Study Child* **16**, 187. Also in (1971) *Emotional growth* Vol. 1, 58–67 New York.

—— (1957). The childhood of the artist. *Psychoanal. Study Child* **12**, 47. Also in (1971) *Emotional growth* Vol. 2, 479–505 New York.

—— (1960*a*). Further notes on fetishism. *Psychoanal. Study Child* **15**, 191. Also in (1971) *Emotional growth* Vol. 1, 182–199 New York.

—— (1960*b*). Considerations regarding the parent–infant relationship. *Int. J. Psycho-Anal.* **41**, 571.

—— (1968). Perversions. General considerations regarding their genetic and dynamic background. *Psychoanal. Study Child* **23**, 47. Also in (1971) *Emotional growth* Vol. 1, 199–225 New York.

—— (1969). Discussion of Galenson's 'The nature of thought in childhood play'. In (1971) *Emotional growth* Vol. 1, 353–364 New York.

—— (1970). The transitional object and the fetish: with special reference to the role of illusion. *Int. J. Psychoanal.* **51**, 447. Also in (1971) *Emotional growth* Vol. 1, p.335.

Greene, W. A. (1958). Early object relations—somatic, affective and personal. An inquiry in the physiology of the mother–child unit. *J. nerv. ment. dis.* **126**, 225.

Hartmann, H. (1939). *Ego psychology and the problem of adaptation*, 101 and 151. Reprinted in translation. New York.

——, Kris, E., and Lowenstein, R. (1949). Notes on the theory of aggression. *Psychoanal. Study Child* **3-4**, 9–36.

McDonald, M. (1970). Transitional tunes and musical development. *Psychoanal. Study Child* **25**, 503.

Payne, S. (1939). Some observations of the ego development of the fetishist. *Int. J. Psycho-Anal.* **20**, 161.

Sperling, M. (1959). A study of deviate sexual behaviour in children by the method of simultaneous analysis of mother and child. In *Dynamic psychopathology* 221–242 (ed. L. Jessner and E. Pavenstedt). New York.

—— (1963). Fetishism in children. *Psychoanal. Quart.* **32**, 374.

Spiegel, N. T. (1967). An infantile fetish and its persistence into young womanhood. *Psychoanal. Study Child* **22**, 402.

Von Hug Helmuth, H. (1915). Ein Fall von Weiblichem Fussrichtiger Stiefelfetischismus. *Int. Z. f. art. Psychoanal.* **3**, 111.

Winnicott, D. (1931). *Collected papers*, 9, and 27–29. Reprinted 1958. New York.

—— (1953). Transitional objects and transitional phenomena. *Int. J. Psycho-Anal.* **34**, 89.

—— (1964). *Maturational processes and the facilitating environment*, 37, 89, 97, 139, and 141. New York.

—— (1971). *Playing and reality*, 80 and 96–97. New York.

Wulff, M. (1946). Fetishism and object choice in early childhood. *Psychoanal. Quart.* **15**, 450.

Zavitzianos, G. (1971). Fetishism and exhibitionism in the female and their relationship to psychopathy and kleptomania. *Int. J. Psycho-Anal.* **52**, 297.

5

The gender disorders

Robert J. Stoller

Introduction

Most psychoanalysts, following Freud (1953), believe all psychopathology, not just the sexual deviations, results – by such mechanisms as castration anxiety and penis envy in the oedipal conflict – from disturbances in the development of gender identity, that is of masculinity and femininity. This discussion, however, will be restricted to the gross aberrations of masculinity and femininity: primary and secondary transsexualism, transvestism, certain types of homosexuality, intersexuality, and certain aspects of psychosis.

A few introductory concepts may help. First, 'gender' (or 'gender identity'), which, in the past, was usually synonymous with 'sex' or 'sexual', is used here only to connote masculinity and femininity. The value in using a different word for behaviour previously included in the general category 'sexual' is that it permits one to separate out areas which are otherwise blurred. For instance, there is a purely biological connotation in the word 'sex': the male sex and the female sex. But that connotation might be inappropriate when considering those aspects of sexuality we call 'masculinity' and 'femininity'. For the latter, such terms as 'gender', 'gender identity', or 'gender role' have been applied (Stoller 1968). If sex and gender were in a direct relationship, if masculinity and femininity were simply the result of one's sex – that is, of biological factors – then the differentiation would be pedantic. But there need be little connection between one's sex (biological) and masculinity and femininity (psychological); the latter, in humans, is produced especially by environmental and intrapsychic effects.

The second concept is that sexual aberrations can be divided into two rather different sorts of conditions, the one 'perversion', and the other 'variant' (or 'deviation'). As used here, 'perversion' implies unconscious conflict; inability to indulge a forbidden, pregenital sexual activity is resolved by using the perversion as the conscious

109

manifestation of compromise. (An example is fetishistic cross-dressing.) Perversion, then, is a sexual erotic neurosis (cf. Gillespie 1964), requiring reparative activity in the cognitive aspects of the psyche, that is, ego and super-ego activities. 'Variant' ('deviation'), in contrast, is used to imply a statistical abnormality, but not a psychodynamically active, conflict-resolving state. Changes in sexual styles and customs from culture to culture and era to era can be examples of variance. Using these terms in this way frees one from labelling a person as perverse according to such external criteria as the sex of the object, the anatomy used, the standards of a culture, or prevalence rates, but rather according to the meaning the behaviour has for its owner. The definition is made intrapsychically, not by society. The idea of variance, in the above sense, expresses the belief that certain sexual practices or modes of gender behaviour may be acquired by such conflict-free mechanisms as are familiar to learning theorists; imprinting, classical and operant conditioning, and more complex forms of behaviour modification, especially in infancy and early childhood, play a part in shaping certain erotic and gender styles.

The third concept further defines 'perversion'. It is suggested that in perversion, to resolve the ever-present, unconscious conflict and to permit potency and the capacity for sexual gratification to persist, one's unconsciously desired sexual objects must be changed intrapsychically, reinvented. To do so requires disavowal, splitting, fetishization, de-humanization. This means, in simpler terms, that one's sexual object must be made less dangerous than it is imagined to be. Moreover, if we presume that the original sexual object was stronger than oneself, traumatizing, and the source of the original conflict that is now permanently internalized, one must, to restore one's sexual pleasure, triumph over the original object. Perversion remakes reality so that the victim – the perverse person – becomes the victor, while representatives of the original traumatizer – the original victor – are reduced in the perversion to being victims. (Rape grossly exemplifies these dynamics.) This process of changing trauma to triumph, however, reduces one's sexual object from an individual human into merely the representative of a class ('all females are the same'), or the parts of a human (breasts, penis), or an inanimate object whose relationship with the original human is only symbolic (clothing).

It is my thesis that only in the creation of perversion, not of variants, does this fetishization and dehumanization occur.

One last introductory concept. I distinguish a primeval stage in the development of gender identity, called 'core gender identity'. It starts at the beginning of life when psychic structure is first forming. The core gender identity – preverbal, rudimentary, but fixed as an unalterable conviction – manifests itself in that behaviour reflecting the belief 'I am a male' or 'I am a female'. This is a piece of identity, a sense of self. It is not the same as being a male or female which is a biological fact, though in almost all cases, this core gender identity depends on one's being a male or female. More precisely, it depends on one's being unequivocally *assigned* to the male or female sex. It need not depend on one's being in fact a member of the assigned sex, only that the infant, because of the anatomy of its external genitals, appears to be a boy or a girl and is so designated (see later section on intersexuality). It is rather well-fixed, unalterable, by age 3 (Money, Hampson, and Hampson 1957). Masculinity and femininity, however, are much more than core gender identity and are still forming for years after core gender identity is laid down. This later development is well known to us since Freud's explorations of the Oedipus complex.

Primary transsexualism

Male transsexualism

This person is an anatomically normal male, considered at birth to be unequivocally male, assigned to the male sex, and given a masculine name. Nonetheless, from the time gender behaviour first appears, usually somewhere around one year of age, the child behaves in a feminine manner. As speech, fantasy life, game playing, choice of clothes, and all other manifestations of psychic development progress, this boy acts as if he were a girl – even to saying in his first few years that he wishes to grow up a girl and to have a female body. There is no time, on into adulthood, when he shows masculine behaviour or desires. Although he may be forced by society to go to school dressed as a boy and to participate in activities with other males, he cannot do so successfully, no matter how severe the threats. In time, nowadays as early as adolescence, he may attempt to have his sex changed: castration of his testes and penis, creation of an artificial vagina, growth of breasts and softening of other body contours by use of oestrogens, and electrolysis to remove facial and body hair. Usually before this, he will have passed successfully as a female, unrecognized as a male even by close acquaintances; the 'sex change' completes the process of passing, and from then on 'she' will live unremarkably as a woman accepted by everyone, even including sexual partners, as a normal female.

In this discussion, only such a person will be called a primary transsexual. By far the greater number of males requesting 'sex change' do not fit this description, though in the literature they are classified as transsexuals because they also request sex reassignment. They will be discussed below ('Secondary transsexualism').

What causes primary transsexualism? When these people are seen in childhood, adolescence, or as adults (but only these people – not those who do not fit the above description) the following conditions are found.

First, the subject is a normal male: chromosomes are male (XY); gonads are histologically normal testes that produce normal male testosterone (unless destroyed by chronic oestrogen administration); the penis and the rest of the external genitals are unremarkably male in appearance and function; internal sexual apparatuses, such as prostate, are normal; at puberty, ordinary male secondary sex characteristics develop.

Second, such a person develops from a typical constellation, in which the mothers and fathers examined so far have had in common the following personality attributes. The transsexual's mother, in her childhood, developed a gender disorder in which a powerful masculine streak is mixed into her femininity. Her own mother is a cold, distant woman, with no respect for this little girl; the girl's mother (the transsexual's grandmother) makes the girl feel that femaleness and femininity are without value. Though her father enjoys her, he encourages her to share with him his masculine interests, and so he both promotes some sense of value in her being his little daughter and at the same time encourages her in masculine directions. But even his affection disappears, before her puberty, when he removes himself from her, either by leaving the family in a separation, divorce, or death, or by turning his attention to a new child, now ignoring this girl. When that happens, she begins to develop as if she would become a female transsexual; she will only wear boys' clothes, plays only with boys as an equal, especially in athletics, wishes she were a boy, and openly states she wants a penis on her body. As opposed to the female transsexual however, with the body changes of puberty her hopes of becoming male are crushed, and she puts on a facade of femininity. This leads in time to her getting married.

The man she marries is passive and distant, though not usually with overtly effeminate qualities. He has been dominated in his childhood by an over-aggressive mother and has not had a firm and masculine father. When these two people have chosen each other for marriage, they are able to play out their individual pathologies in a special family dynamic, in which the wife takes over the power in the household, openly scorning her husband, while he, bitter and ineffective, stays away, engrossed in his work and his hobbies.

This state of affairs is chronic, and yet transsexualism does not appear in all the children of the couple. In fact, the condition rarely occurs in more than one child; daughters, whatever neurotic problems they develop, do not become unusually masculine, and almost never are other sons in the family feminized. (When they are, it is because the aetiological conditions now being described were again present).

The third factor required for male transsexualism is the contribution the newborn son will make; if he is as described below transsexualism occurs. The necessary quality that, when added to the family's dynamics, will cause transsexualism, is the infant's appearing beautiful and graceful to his mother. When that happens, and when she finds he is a gratifying infant – happy against his mother's body – in those first days after he is born, she immediately develops an extremely intense, loving need for the infant. At that moment, the chronic sense of hopelessness and valuelessness from which she has suffered since early childhood is 'cured'. Now she has her perfect phallus, for which she yearned so long. This may well explain the puzzling fact that all these mothers give these sons very masculine names. The idea that such mothers really wanted a little girl does not hold up in these boys. This mother wants a son, that is, a male who has a penis, and she feels complete and full of rejoicing when she bears this infant and names him.

But the above factors do not *produce* the extreme femininity in the boy; they are only the necessary precursors. What is still needed is action in the three-dimensional world that will impinge on the infant's perceptions, stimuli so different from what occurs in the usual boy's experience that a rather pure form of femininity results.

The behaviour that thus influences the infant is the mother's handling of her baby; the style of which is dominated by her feeling that he is the first and only wonderful event of her life. The joy many mothers have with the infant they wanted, a joy that will be prolonged when the infant responds happily to his mother's mothering, is the normal version of the blissful symbiosis the transsexual's mother tries to establish with her beautiful son. For her, with her life-long hopelessness, the joy she receives is so gratifying that she cannot refrain from keeping her infant in her embrace – physically and psychologically – for too many hours of every day and after so many months that, in time, it is years that have passed. Her infant, by his presence, makes her finally happy, completing her former sense of anatomical and psychological incompleteness. In addition, and augmenting an already excessive closeness, she wishes to protect this beloved son from suffering at her hands even for a moment any of the unhappy feelings to which she was exposed throughout her infancy and childhood. So she does everything possible not to let her infant be frustrated by physical or emotional wants. Not surprisingly, he responds to such bliss by sensing what his mother wants and giving her more of it.

Unhappily, she needs her son to be an extension of her own body, always under her control and never separate enough to act so as to disturb her. In addition, with her envy, and therefore hatred, of males, she cannot stand behaviour that strikes her as masculine. This would be forceful, intrusive, 'dirty', 'nasty'. She is especially concerned that he should not behave in ways that reveal a desire to be emotionally separated from her. Of course, he has been self-selected already, in that he was biologically the right infant for her: he was beautiful, cuddly, graceful, and gentle. Now, as the months pass, she rewards all behaviour that holds him in this same form and discourages whatever she feels is rough or unloving, that is, masculine. So she creates this *thing* – not a separate person but a part of her own body – and we are not surprised to find that within a year or so, he, like she, does not know where his own body ends and hers begins: he believes himself to be as she is, female. He has, unfortunately, now and forever on, an insoluble problem, for although he feels female, both he and everyone else know he is unequivocally male. The rest of his life will be spent in the hopeless attempt to resolve this paradox.

Nonetheless, it is not inevitable that the boy will be totally feminized, for if the excessively close and blissful symbiosis were interrupted, however this cleavage might pain both parties, transsexualism would not result. One therefore waits to hear that the boy's father, on witnessing this feminization, will step in. He does not. He was selected long ago by this woman for his passivity and distance, for his ability to absorb endless scorn from her, and to persist nonetheless unchanged in his performance of inadequacy. And so, as his son develops, this father is not physically present. Yet he is kept forever present in the ambience of the home, for mother loses no chance to express her disgust with him and all men (precisely excluding, however, her wonderful son). But he leaves the house in the morning before his son has awakened, and busy with work, returns home after the boy is in bed. During weekends, father is still not present, spending his time at his hobbies or watching television. The rule is that at these times he is not to be interrupted by the children, and so the little boy does not see his father. As a result, his father is not there to interrupt the symbiosis. Additionally, this man is not there to serve as a model for masculine identification. In his almost complete absence and with his wife disparaging his image, the symbiotic process runs unchecked, and the femininity increases, nurtured and encouraged by a mother who thrills to its manifestations.

Male transsexualism is an oddity, then, not only because the condition is so strange – a male who tries to change into a female – but for reasons of interest to those concerned with psychodynamic theory. This is especially true of the oedipal development in the transsexual boy. How does it compare with that of masculine boys and with that of those who have gender perversions?

The oedipal situation in primary male transsexualism is different from that of other boys, for there is no oedipal *conflict*. In order for oedipal conflict to occur in a boy, he must desire to possess his mother and have that desire thwarted by his father, with the result that a conflict between the desire and the danger is established. But the transsexual boy does not want to *possess* his mother; instead, he would *be* like his mother (Greenson 1966). There is no erotic component to the relationship. This is not just a theoretical statement but can be seen in the boys: for example, the observation is confirmed when the boys are treated; as masculinity begins to appear, they finally direct behaviour at their mothers – also reflected in their games – that expresses desire for her as a separate person. And father is, of course, no threat. We have already noted that he is not there; in his absence, he has allowed, condoned, the symbiosis to be uninterrupted. The theoretical significance of the absence of an oedipal conflict in the creation of a major piece of psychopathology will become obvious when we discuss gender perversions.

The second oddity for the theoretician is that the transsexual, despite his apparent gross distortion of reality – he says he really is a female – is not psychotic. In the first place, male transsexuals simply do not show the clinical signs and symptoms of psychosis with which we are familiar. Additionally, those who might consider the condition a psychosis, do so because of the tremendous discrepancy between the patient's body and identity; this bizarre belief, they feel, can only be explained as a delusion (Stafford-Clark 1964; Kubie and Mackie 1968; Socarides 1970). Yet, though transsexuals believe they are females within, not one, child or adult, claims to have a female body; *that* would be delusional or hallucinatory, like Freud's Schreber case (1911) of a psychotic with transsexual delusions. Instead, they insist their gender-identity is what they sense psychically, regardless of their anatomy. We know, from observing the mother–child symbiosis, that the femininity was created there, was 'imprinted' on the infant and then encouraged as he grew. Such is not the aetiology of psychosis. And when one examines the patient, instead of one's theory, the absence of clinical psychosis fits what one knows of the children: infancy is not traumatic, deprived, or conflicted. For a further description of these aetiological factors and for more clinical data see Stoller 1968, 1975*a*.

Treatment. Our knowledge of treatment of transsexuals is still rudimentary, as is our knowledge of the effects of treatment. If one's goal is to achieve a person whose identity is congruous with his body, then the effects of treatment so far have been dismal. If one aims for the more modest goal of a comfortable patient, then the results are better but still leave much to be desired.

At present, there is perhaps reason for hope in the treatment of children (Greenson 1966; Stoller 1975*a*, Rekers, Yates, Willis, Rosen, and Taubman 1976). The earlier one starts, the better, for then treatment can interrupt the still-active family processes that create the femininity. In my experience, one does not get these children for treatment before 4 years of age, when society begins to impinge on them and their mothers, though as the public is told more about boyhood femininity, we shall begin seeing younger boys. The more the family situation approximates to that described above, the less likely the family will appear spontaneously for help; both mother and father somehow know that the transsexual boy is the focus for whatever mental stability they can maintain as a couple, and if he changes, they sense they will be affected. So neither usually spontaneously asks for help; they do not think they need help. But after a number of experiences in which strangers or teachers ask pointedly about the child's sex, or following a vigorous referral by a family physician, treatment may begin. It should encompass mother, father, and child, but it almost never does. The fathers do not cooperate, which is in keeping with what we already know of their personalities; those few who attend for evaluation do not carry through with the treatment.

Rekers *et al.* (1976) report a behaviour modification technique, described as simple, quick, and effective, that removes the femininity in feminine boys. The few follow-ups available so far indicate that the boys remain masculine. As yet unanswered is the question of whether the shift from feminine to masculine behaviour is superficial or whether it produces a more profound and permanent change in identity.

If one is committed to a more traditional, psychodynamically-oriented treatment, the mothers should be treated either with psychoanalysis or analytically-oriented therapy. The first goal of treatment is to help the mother through the depression that becomes manifest when she sees clearly that the treatment aims at taking from her her feminized phallus and that the bliss is to be ruined. If this issue can be managed, then she can be kept from sabotaging the treatment during the many hours of the day when she is alone with her son (Stoller 1975*a*). Beyond this goal, one can work with her toward character change of value to herself.

The boy's treatment in our hands has been more a re-learning experience than an insight treatment. Our research team attempts to change the child's environment (the family's interpersonal communications) rather than undo an intrapsychic conflict. And so only a masculine male therapist works with the child, and every effort is made during treatment hours to give the boy experiences in which behaviour defined as masculine becomes pleasurable. In addition, every effort is made to have the parents encourage masculine and discourage feminine behaviour at home. This is really, then, a behaviour-modification therapy. Perhaps it could be better done by those specifically trained in behaviour-modification techniques; that is an area for further research. Or perhaps the thesis is wrong and child analytic techniques should be used; since they have not as yet been tried, one cannot report how successful they might be.

Our results so far are meagre. One transsexual boy, now in his teens seems masculine (Greenson 1966). The rest of the half-dozen treated have become less committed to pure femininity; that is, they have some masculine interests and behaviour, but it is too early to predict the outcome in adult life for any of them (Green, Newman, and Stoller 1971).

In treating adult male-transsexuals, the general rule has been that whatever one does, it is wrong (Stoller 1968). All one can hope is to do the least harm and assuage the most pain. While the ideal would be a masculine man, it is hard to see how that can occur in a person who has never had any masculinity built into his personality from infancy. How can one create a major segment of personality *de nouveau* in the adult? A therapy based on the conviction that the transsexual can become masculine is based on the belief either that genuine pervasive masculinity can be created in adult life, or that there has been masculinity present, even if hidden, from childhood. One treatment team (Barlow, Reynolds, and Agras 1973) reports the ability to do just that. They have changed a primary transsexual male to heterosexual masculinity purely by behaviour-modification techniques. If follow-up shows the results have held and the patient is content, and if other workers can do the same with still more patients, then we shall finally have available a successful treatment for transsexualism.

Those who recommend analysis must recognize that there are no reports that anyone has ever succeeded in getting a primary trans-sexual into analysis, much less that the patient became masculine and heterosexual. There is one report of a psychoanalyst who had a patient whom he called a transsexual (in fact a paranoid effeminate homo-sexual) lie down in his office for six months, but even in this condition, which is not transsexualism, the treatment is reported to have failed (Socarides 1970). I have been unable ever to persuade a transsexual male to enter into any but superficial (sympathetic listener and reality manipulator) psychotherapy, much less psychoanalysis. These patients wish and permit only a supportive relationship, in which one helps them with life situations.

If one grants that there are a few people whose lot improves with 'sex change', the main problem in assisting the transsexual to change 'her' body is that of diagnosis; thousands of people these days request sex reassignment, and only a handful are primary transsexuals. Since the follow-up studies of surgical procedures are inadequate thus far, we do not know what happens when effeminate homosexuals, fetish-istic cross-dressers, or paranoid schizophrenics have their genitals removed. One can suspect that there will at times be severe psychiatric complications. Until adequate follow-up studies have resolved these questions, one hesitates to promote 'sex change'.

But there are problems even when one carefully selects candidates for hormones and surgery. Though, invariably, primary transsexuals are happier after 'sex change' and though, invariably, they never regret their changed body compared to the former male body as the years pass (Stoller 1975*a*), some gradually become hopeless: they can never deny that the changes in their body are not fundamental. They not only remember they were born male, but they know (perhaps better than many who treat them) that one cannot ever truly change sex.

As the years pass, they are also burdened by complications from the surgical procedures. The vagina scars and becomes shorter and narrower. Usually further operations are required to correct this, and even so, the vagina may not remain patent for life. Bouts of cystitis are also the rule for the operated transsexual, and though each bout can be controlled with antibiotics, the next infection always threatens.

To not 'change' the transsexual's body, is to leave 'her' chronically despairing, since it is known there are medical procedures to make 'her' body more acceptable to 'her'. On the other hand, to grant the request is to give short-term relief but another sort of despair which, I fear, may lead to suicide in some operated transsexuals.

Female transsexualism

I now believe female transsexualism to be a different condition from male transsexualism, not as, say in schizophrenia, the same condition in a different sex. The two states are comparable clinically, however. The female transsexual, like the male, is anatomically normal but wishes to have a male body and live permanently as a man. The condition starts in early childhood and, as I define it, runs uninterrupted by episodes of femininity. In time, the patient will request and perhaps receive 'sex change' procedures. In the female these are: bilateral mastectomy, panhysterectomy, and testosterone to produce male secondary sex-characteristics. In a few cases, with very uncertain results, the vagina has been closed and an artificial penis created by skin grafts.

The aetiology of female transsexualism is unclear, but some preliminary findings can be reported. In all the cases I have studied of these most masculine of females (those for whom the term 'transsexual' seems acceptable), the following family dynamics have been present.

Neither the mother nor the father of the little girl has a gender disorder, as is the case in the male transsexual. Instead, the baleful effect seems to originate in the mother being unable to function as a mother in the first months, or year or so, of her little girl's life. In most instances, this has been because the mother was sorely depressed, though in a few families the mother–infant relationship was disrupted by the mother's paranoid attitudes or physical illness. In any case, the constant factor has been mother's absence from her expected mothering role in a situation where the child knows her mother is there (not dead or otherwise totally removed) but beyond reach. This is the opposite of the situation in the male transsexual, whose mother is so over-whelmingly present. One would expect the father to act to ease his wife's pain, to husband her at this particular time in their relationship. He fails to do so, though at other times he has been effective. Instead of himself thus ministering to his wife, he moves this daughter into the vacuum.

Had the little girl been pretty and cuddly – that is, had she at birth and in the first weeks thereafter been perceived by the family as feminine – she might not have been so used. However, these female transsexuals are reported to be vigorous, ungraceful, and unpretty in infancy. So the infant is used to 'cure' the condition that makes mother be absent. In this process, father establishes a close, firm, and happy relationship with his daughter. Unfortunately, he does this by involving her in activities that interest him, and since he is masculine, he quickly promotes masculine behaviour in his daughter. Because she already has at birth a biological tendency toward activity, aggressivity, and other psychomotor behaviour that goes well with the masculinity, the ground is all too well laid for that development.

In brief, the masculinity is created in the child's unending labours to reach her distant and unavailing mother and in her gratifying, but not heterosexual, relationship with her father, wherein identification with him and his interests is promoted. The family situation creates a little husband out of this girl, and by the age of 4 or 5, she is already yearning to have the anatomical insignias of maleness. The situation is not the same intrapsychically, however, as in the male transsexual. The female transsexual's masculinity is born from pain and conflict, not bliss; from premature separation from mother rather than symbiosis. The female transsexual is constantly, unendingly, and hope-lessly trying to reach a mother who is beyond reach. She does this in her masculinity and in her attempt to simulate her father's maleness (i.e. to have her sex changed), but she will never quite be able to do so. This mechanism makes me look on female transsexualism as a form of homosexuality. See Khan 1964, for confirmation in a milder homo-sexual reaction. For a fuller description of these aetiological factors and for more clinical data, see Stoller 1968, 1975a.

Again, as was described for the male transsexual, the long-term results of the female transsexual's changing of her body's appearance never leads to a final, quiet success. The patients forever know they only simulate or approximate maleness, and as the years pass, they too may become despairing.

Treatment. Even fewer female transsexual children have been treated than male. So far as I know, the only ones treated are by our research team. We have had no success in four cases, if success is measured by onset of femininity. Once again the goal of treatment is to modify behaviour rather than create insight, for I believe that the masculinity is laid down so early and so permanently that insight techniques fail. Perhaps the therapist should be a feminine woman, if one wishes to create in the child a desire to be feminine. If the family can be induced to give up its need for the child as a substitute husband, then the mother and father may also come to cooperate in encouraging femininity and discouraging masculinity.

In adults, there are no reports of successful treatment that makes the female transsexual feminine. It is unknown how often this has been attempted, for there are no reports of such treatment. I have spent four years in psychotherapy with such a patient (unoperated) who, although I tried, only slightly shifted 'his' masculinity.

Following surgery and hormones, these patients are more content. Each establishes a permanent relationship with a woman and successfully holds down a job in an exclusively male profession.

Secondary transsexualism

Male secondary transsexuals

In this group are those biologically normal males, unequivocally assigned at birth to the male sex, who nonetheless develop a desire to be feminine and, in time, a desire to change their sex to female. They differ from primary transsexuals in two ways. First, the clinical picture is different. Secondary transsexuals do not appear feminine from the start of any behaviour that can be considered masculine or feminine (somewhere around one to two years of age). Instead, they develop for years in an ordinarily masculine-appearing manner. Beneath that surface – so they report in adulthood – there was, nonetheless, an impulse toward being feminine; this may or may not have been consciously experienced as a wish to be a girl. In time, usually adolescence or later, manifestations of the underlying feminine urges appear. The most obvious of these is an urge to put on women's clothes. This may be a symptom of a fetishistic perversion (transvestism), or of homosexuality. Person and Ovesey (1974*a*, 1974*b*) describe the development of these two types of secondary transsexuals, showing how the conditions develop as defensive structures from a matrix of masculinity and oedipal conflict (in contrast to the primary transsexuals).†

As different from most transvestites or effeminate homosexuals, however, the secondary transsexuals gradually experience transsexual impulses – the desire to be a woman – that grow in strength and last for longer periods – hours, days, and then indefinitely. These impulses do not, however, bring an end either to the fetishism in the one group or to the erotic homosexual urges in the other, nor are the masculine aspects of identity present from earliest life ever completely submerged. Because these earlier aspects of identity persist, the desire for sex change is less insistent, and the expressions of femininity less permanent and natural-appearing over time.

The second feature that differentiates primary from secondary transsexualism is the family dynamics in infancy and childhood. The constellation of forces just described for primary transsexuals has never been reported for any other of the gender aberrations, including secondary transsexuals.

Treatment. Because this is a mixed group with a variety of clinical pictures and aetiologies (Person and Ovesey 1974*a*, 1974*b*), there is no way to recommend one, clear-cut approach. In the last generation, the treatment most discussed in the literature has been hormonal and surgical 'sex change'. Unfortunately, because of the gross inadequacy of the reports, including follow-ups, we still do not know which patients do well and which poorly with these treatments. One can suspect, however, that the more the patient's personality is infiltrated with masculinity, the more risk he runs on subjecting his body to such radical anatomical and physiological changes. It is therefore important with secondary transsexuals that a careful and skilled – not perfunctory – evaluation of gender identity be performed before one plans the treatment. In the presence of even occasional masculine demeanour,

---

†They use a somewhat different classification from mine in that they describe these two types – the fetishist and the homosexual – as 'primary' and 'secondary' transsexualism and do not report on the state I have called primary transsexualism.

acceptance of having male genitals, gratifying relationships – heterosexual or homosexual – when living in roles typical for males, we probably should not recommend 'sex change' but instead try to engage the patient in psychotherapy. At the least, such treatment gives patients a chance to examine more closely their desire to change sex and often leads to their choosing to not do so.

Female secondary transsexuals

There are no reports that describe a group of females clinically comparable to the male secondary transsexuals. The reason may lie in the fact that classification is a device that artificially orders clinical phenomena which could as well be described in terms of continua. For instance, in reality there is no dividing line to separate primary from secondary transsexualism in males, but rather there are clusters of people who fall primarily in one group or the other. One could as well, however, place patients on continua of masculinity and femininity by criteria such as degree, naturalness, time of onset, and so on. In the case of female transsexuals, then, it may be that we are looking at a continuum of degrees and styles of masculinity, the extreme of which fits the above description for primary female transsexualism but on which fall less-marked cases of masculinity in females such as masculine homosexual women or masculine heterosexual women.

Transvestism

As used here, 'transvestism' refers only to fetishistic cross-dressing, that is, the use of clothes of the opposite sex to produce sexual excitement. The term will not refer to all cross-dressing, for this would include too many different conditions under the same rubric.

Male transvestism

Although sexual excitement caused by women's clothes may occur for the first time in boys as young as 5 or 6 years old or in men in their forties, it typically starts around puberty or in adolescence. At that first time, without prior warning, motivated, he thinks, only by curiosity, the transvestite puts on a garment of the opposite sex and immediately becomes greatly sexually excited, more than ever before in his life. He instantly recognizes this is a crucial experience and will now indulge in it either when there is opportunity or when he does not feel too guilt-laden. The condition may take three courses over time. For some men, a single garment or class of garments remains the preferred fetish; for another group, the original preference sooner or later spreads to a desire to be completely clothed in women's garments and to pretend for a period of time – minutes to hours – to be a woman; men of the third group (far fewer than in the first two), with some transsexual tendencies (the extreme being secondary transsexuals), learn to pass as women and spend extended periods living as women.

The aetiology of transvestism is not as clear as that of male primary transsexualism, but there is enough evidence to confirm that differences in the clinical picture are associated with differences in life history (Stoller 1975*a*).

No primary transsexuals are fetishistic (in this strict sense of the word, wherein fetishism means genital sexual excitement provoked by women's clothing); fetishism is the pathognomonic sign in transvestism. The primary transsexual wishes to wear women's clothes always, because he wants to be a female all his life; the transvestite wears women's clothes intermittently, usually only for a few minutes or hours but does not want to be a female. (In advanced cases, he may even wish to *pass* as a female, but he does not wish to *be* a female.) Women's clothes for the primary transsexual are no more symbolically significant than for a feminine woman; for the transvestite, the clothes have powerful unconscious meaning – as mother's embrace, skin, or phallus; as transitional object; as evidence to the transvestite he is not castrated; and so on (Fenichel 1953). The primary transsexual has been feminine since early childhood and is unremarkably feminine all the time, every moment of the day and night, awake or dreaming regardless of garments worn; the transvestite is masculine, except when cross-dressed. The primary transsexual is sexually excited exclusively by people of the same anatomical sex, but opposite gender-identity; the transvestite almost exclusively chooses women for his sexual partners. The primary transsexual wishes to become a normal female, to approximate which requires hormonal and surgical procedures; the transvestite has a male core gender-identity and wishes to be a male, and so he does not submit to 'sex change' surgery. The crucial difference between the two is revealed in the attitude of each toward his penis: the transsexual feels the organ is a cruel mistake that blights his life, while the transvestite's life is focused on his penis, for he is a fetishist. The transsexual wishes to be a female; the transvestite wishes to be a male. The primary transsexual's aberration is (in keeping with my definitions earlier) a sexual variant; the transvestite's aberration is a perversion.

The transsexual was created in a blissful symbiosis; what are the aetiological factors in the transvestite's early life?

Let us first mark this finding: in no case of transvestism reported in the literature, and in no case seen by myself or my colleagues, has the history of the family dynamics of the male transsexual been given. Instead, something crucially different occurs in all cases where there are reports given of early childhood and in all cases investigated by our research team: rather than a lengthy period of blissful symbiosis, the transvestite-to-be is allowed to develop a male core gender-identity; he accepts himself as belonging to the male sex in the manner as do other boys. Following that stage, he also develops masculinity. In other words, whatever flaws there are in the mother–son relationship of transvestites, the boy separates from his mother's body and individuates into someone who believes himself to be a male (sex) and a boy (gender-identity and -role). This indicates that something in the range of a typical oedipal situation exists; at least the stage for an oedipal conflict has been set by the creation of a boy who values his maleness and masculinity (and therefore can be threatened by its loss). In addition, the boy, in separating psychologically from his mother, has her before him as a separate, desired, opposite-sexed object. In his childhood, therefore, he is exposed, more or less, to the temptations and threats of the oedipal conflict, essential for the development of masculinity, whether comfortable or perverse-ridden. Transvestites' mothers, from reports in the literature and from working with transvestites, their mothers, and wives, are a hetero-geneous group of women (Stoller 1968). Transvestites' fathers, about whom I know less, are also mixed: some seem distant and passive, as are fathers of male primary transsexuals, while others are frightening, angry, punishing men who, though all too present, are about as unreachable as an object for love and identification, as would be a distant and passive father.

In many cases, what seems to set off the process that leads to fetishistic cross-dressing is an attack on the boy's masculinity. Frequently (but not invariably) this will be a precise event: an older woman or girl – mother, sister, other female relative, or neighbour – puts women's clothes on the little boy *in order to humiliate him*. This act induces castration anxiety, or, as I prefer to look at it, a threat to one's identity: it is not just the fear of losing his genitals that frightens the boy but the significance of his genitals in fixing him as a member of the sex to which he has long since committed himself in his core gender-identity. In certain cultures and in certain eras boys may be dressed in girls' clothes. This in itself does not cause transvestism, for the purpose is not to humiliate the child. It is not the cut of the clothes but the intent of those who clothe the boy that makes the difference.

Other humiliations or other severe threats to the integrity of one's maleness and masculinity may also predispose a boy to fetishism; the work of Greenacre (1953, 1955, 1960, 1969) and Bak (1953, 1968) indicate as much.

But this, so far, is only trauma; yet perversion is pleasure. How is the latter accomplished? And where lies the conflict supposedly essential for the definition of perversion? One conflict lies, I believe, in the oedipal situation. The issue for the boy who is to become a transvestite is how he can protect his maleness, preserve his masculinity, permit his genital eroticism to develop, and to succeed in growing up to be an intact male, a man, a lover of women (who will substitute for his original desired object, mother), and a person with identity still intact – more or less. Since those are the problems confronting every growing boy (except the transsexual or maximally disrupted children such as the severely mental deficient, brain damaged, or autistic), we need to find other conflicts, specific for the transvestite.

The route *via* the oedipal conflict to a desired woman is additionally blocked for the transvestite by that first cross-dressing episode, a sharp, focal attack square upon his masculinity. It augments his fear of women (produced by their power to humiliate) and his hatred and envy of them (that they can be so strong and so effortlessly do so much harm), and results in a need for revenge on them (to bring the pleasure of victory to what had been traumatic). The conflicts here are between desire to harm females and fear of their strength, between wanting to have them (heterosexuality) and wanting to be one of them (identification with the aggressor), between preserving one's maleness, masculinity, and sexual potency and giving in to women's castrating attack by becoming a woman. Each of these conflicts is solved by the perversion: beneath the women's clothes and the *appearance* of being a female (no penis), the transvestite has secretly triumphed. His penis is still there and functioning. More, it is *really* there, triumphantly erect, victoriously male. By the expedient of seeming castration ('see me looking like a woman'), he escapes with his penis intact ('but I secretly still have my penis'). For a fuller description of these mechanisms, see Stoller 1975*a*, 1975*b*.

Treatment. So far, no children who are transvestites are reported to have been treated. Although there are not, as yet, published reports on adolescents, a few have been treated by my colleagues at our medical centre. All have been seen in psychotherapy but none in analysis. Three have stopped the behaviour; the fourth stops intermittently. We are hopeful, but it is too early to presume these are cures and not just intermittent episodes of non-perverse activity as are so often found in untreated transvestites. If one judges from the literature on adults, the prognosis for giving up the behaviour is perhaps nil. At any rate, there are no reports, with careful follow-ups, of any fetishistic cross-dresser who has stopped (including not fantasizing it during intercourse and masturbation) for years, if the treatment is psychoanalysis or other psychotherapy. There are no cases in the analytic literature of a permanent shift in psychodynamics in such a patient, so that one might be assured that the underlying forces have changed enough to permit the perversion to disappear.

More optimistic is the work of behaviour therapists. In brief, they state – though with adequate follow-ups so far – that the more fetishistic the transvestism, the more likely is it that the symptom can be suppressed by behaviouristic techniques. The more the transsexual elements in the patient's identity, the poorer is the prognosis; that is, the more the patient wishes to pass, the longer the episodes of passing, the more fantasies the patient has of having a female body, or the more the patient wonders whether to have transsexual surgery, the less effective is behaviour modification (Gelder and Marks 1969).

Female transvestism

Fetishistic cross-dressing is essentially unheard of in women. While women cross-dress, they do not do so because the clothes excite them erotically. In all the literature (in English), there is only one report of a woman so excited (Gutheil 1964). I have had two others as patients and a third known only through letters. In all these, genital excitement came from putting on men's clothes and feeling as if a man for the moment. The individual garments were not exciting, however, until the woman anticipated wearing them. None was compelled by erotic need to cross-dress; for none was it the preferred or most intense sexual behaviour; none was fascinated by men's clothes; none lingered over the texture, style, or smell of the clothes.

Homosexuality

Because homosexuality is taken up elsewhere in this volume, it will only be discussed briefly here and only as concerns its gender aspects.

Male homosexuality

We consider here only effeminate homosexuality, but at the start I place a caution that this is probably not a unitary condition with a relatively organized aetiology, consistent from case to case. Rather there are many homosexualities with varied aetiologies, dynamics, and clinical pictures. In the following discussion, I only emphasize features frequently found in effeminate homosexuals and leave out a present-ation of variation existing in this 'condition'.

As in differentiating primary transsexualism from transvestism, I use the theoretical framework touched on in the beginning of this chapter in order to distinguish dynamics found in these different conditions. Again it will be helpful to separate out the dynamics of perversion – which I believe are generally present in the homosexualities – from those of more simple deviation (a matter of autonomous character structure, non-conflicting from the start).

Our first clue is in the clinical appearance of the effeminate homo-sexual as compared to the primary transsexual or transvestite. The transsexual is feminine. 'Feminine' implies a clinical picture in which the person appears, behaves, and fantasies in a manner falling within the range of what is considered 'feminine' for that culture; most of all, the implication is that this appearance is unremarkable, normal, easy-going, natural, not an act or an effort, not a performance that would bring applause or admiration from onlookers. It is habitual and permanent. Such is not the picture in the effeminate homosexual. The term 'effeminate', in contrast to 'feminine', implies caricature, mimicry, the secret revelation of masculinity and maleness. There is something exaggerated or unnatural, a display, a sarcasm. And that is what underlies the behaviour. The effeminate homosexual does not wish to be a woman or have a female's body. Although his admiration for women may have led to considerable identification with them from childhood on, the admiration is mixed with envy, anger, a clear, even if subtle, underlining in one's behaviour that one is not a woman but a man making fun of a woman.

The source of this anger and envy is typically found in the childhood of effeminate homosexuals. It has become folklore by now, the observations having been made by so many people – one need not be an expert – that the mothers of such boys or men are overprotective (Bieber *et al.* 1962). When one observes closely the mother–child relationship described as 'overprotective', one finds that the closeness between mother and son, and the great gratifications granted by mother, come only when the boy does what she wishes. As long as he does not stir her envy and anger toward males, she will gratify him. For she is a woman who hates males. So he learns, by the system of reward and punishment she has set up, that behaviour she considers masculine will be punished but that soft, graceful, passive, 'sweet' behaviour will please her. In order to avoid her punishment – her withdrawal of love – the boy must suppress evidence of masculinity, and he can do so only with effort, pain, frustration. His feelings about his mother's 'love' are mixed. Yet to express the anger directly would be to bring her wrath down on him, and so it must go under cover. The disguise is in the effeminacy, where, in his mimicry, he subtly adds anger to his gentle, unmasculine appearance. In that way, though seeming to comply with his mother, he is secretly hostile and, in fantasy, victorious over her.

But why does he suffer when she wishes him unmanly? – the transsexual does not. The answer can be found in the histories as given by the parents and in the analyses of such homosexuals, when childhood memories are recovered. As different from the transsexual, the effeminate homosexual, like the transvestite, has had the opportunity to develop *some* masculinity during early childhood. He has a male core gender-identity on which he has built some masculinity, and especially, some capacity to see his mother as an external, heterosexually desired object. It is his masculinity, his need to reach for his mother, his entry into an oedipal situation, that sets off his mother's punishing reaction. She forces down expressions of his masculinity, but she would not do so had they not had the chance to develop. In passing, it is worth noting that severe attacks on his masculinity by his father may also push him toward the defence of homosexuality. Perhaps these attacks will not succeed in making him homosexual unless mother fails to protect the boy from father's attack.

If, then, we look again at the clinical picture of the effeminate homosexual, we find, as with the transvestite and in contrast to the transsexual, that the behaviour is the result of trauma, conflict, and conflict resolution. The homosexual does not wish to be a female; quite the opposite. He loves his penis and the gratifications it brings. The problem for him is that the way has been barred to gratification provided with a female.

These homosexualities, in summary, are perversions, not simply variants. The difference, as Freud has long since indicated (1953), is found in the oedipal conflict and focuses on the importance of the penis (important not only for sexual gratification but, at a more primitive level, for preservation of identity).

Female homosexuality

Rather than discussing female homosexuality, which is taken up in more detail elsewhere in this volume, and about which I know too little, I wish to discuss briefly very masculine women. There are several types I can separate off in a preliminary manner: 'butch'† homosexuals, mothers of male transsexuals, 'unrealized' transsexuals, transsexuals, and 'penis' women. The clinical differences between these groups are not sharp enough to make this a true classification; all, I believe, are points on a homosexual continuum.

The 'butch' homosexual believes she is a female, and while envying and identifying with males (comparably to the way effeminate male homosexuals react to females), she is militantly proud of being a female and insistes hers is a superior state to any male. She believes she understands women better than do men and can make a better lover and friend for a feminine woman. She believes herself homosexual and states she would not have it any other way.

The mother of the male primary transsexual, strongly identifying with males, has had a period in her life when she wished to become a male. Having some femininity implanted in her in childhood, she consciously gives up her desire to be a male with the onset of puberty. Unable to make a homosexual adjustment, she disguises herself as a heterosexual and lives permanently as a married woman, yet a hater of masculinity.

The 'unrealized' transsexual (secondary transsexual?) is a female who at the start believes herself a homosexual and lives as a homosexual

---

†There is no non-slang word for indicating an exaggerated masculinity compared to (natural appearing) masculinity, which is the equivalent of 'effeminate' *vis à vis* 'feminine'.

in the homosexual community. Because she is exclusively masculine, she gradually finds herself revealing her marked masculinity; in time, she comes to feel she should be a male and fairly late in life makes mild moves toward 'sex change'. The intensity of her transsexual drive, however, is less than in the transsexual and the length of time she needs to find her full masculinity is far greater.

The female transsexual need not be considered again, except to recall the notion above that female transsexualism may simply be the most advanced degree of the masculine female homosexual. Because in all these females, the masculinity is probably forced on the girl by painfully applied conditions in her family during childhood (balanced by undue encouragement to identify with father), these character disorders are not comparable psychodynamically to male transsexualism.

By 'penis' women I mean an extremely small group of biologically normal females (I have only seen three) who hallucinate a penis as a permanent, three dimensional, intrapelvic structure. They do not hallucinate this as a symptom of a psychotic episode but rather *feel* a penis within themselves all the time, at any time of the day or month, undiminished with the passage of years, even in the absence of any other signs of clinical psychosis. Extensive study of one such patient revealed this to be, as one would expect, a homosexual defence (Stoller 1973). This condition is the extreme version of the often-heard fantasy of women that they wish they had a penis or dreamed they were a man.

Intersexuality

'Intersexuality' is used here in the sense it generally has nowadays – to indicate that one or more of the major criteria for defining sex (chromosomes, gonads, external genitals, internal sexual apparatuses, and hormonal state and secondary sex characteristics) are abnormal. This is not the place for a careful discussion of the biological features or classificatory systems possible in intersexuality. It is enough here to indicate rules and hypotheses that touch on behaviour influenced by the physical abnormality. See Chapter 14.

Intersexuality was a fundamental concept for Freud's general theory of psychology, where he called it 'bisexuality'. Reviewing what was known from embryology and animal research in his day, he became familiar with findings that revealed aspects of both sexes in all humans (1905). This biological bisexuality he considered the 'bedrock' on which all normal and abnormal psychology is built (1937).

Time has borne out these important findings, although significantly modifying them. At present the evidence indicates that, except for the chromosomes, in all mammals including humans, all cells, tissues, and organs begin in a state of femaleness. Only if androgens are added (their production apparently controlled in the foetus by the Y chromosome) will a normal male result. In many ways, the male is an androgenized female; for instance, the penis is an androgenized clitoris, for without androgens a clitoris results in both sexes, and with enough androgens (but only at a precise stage of foetal development) a penis results in both sexes. Especially interesting are the recent studies revealing clearly in mammals that a male's masculine behaviour requires perinatal priming of the brain (hypothalamus) by androgens during a critical period specific for each species. In the absence of masculinizing hormones, masculine behaviour does not occur, and instead the adult animal acts feminine. This rule of the primacy of femaleness is less biologically imperative, and post-natal learning more influential, the higher the species' position on an evolutionary scale. To what extent this rule holds in humans is still unclear, since one cannot perform the testing experiments on the human foetus or infant. Studies of chromosomal/endocrine disorders in man tend, however, to bear out the fundamental rule: the absence of androgens in the foetus produces varying degrees of anatomical femaleness, absence of anatomical maleness, and a tendency toward behavioural femininity in the patient, whether chromosomally female or male. On the other hand, large amounts of circulating foetal androgens produce varying degrees of somatic masculinization (maleness) and masculine behaviour in the child and adult, whether chromosomally male or female. The literature elaborating these findings is reviewed in Galpaille 1972; Stoller 1975*a*. What makes the matter still unclear is the question of how much do post-natal, environmental (that is, interpersonal), and intrapsychic effects override these biological tendencies in man. In my opinion the rule in humans is that in gender behaviour, psychological effects *can* almost always overpower the biological. The transsexual would seem a good test of this: in the absence of any demonstrated biological abnormality in pre or post-natal life and under the influence of a specific set of family dynamics playing on an infant male selected for his beauty, extreme femininity results. At the other extreme, there seem to be rare cases in which the biological is the overpowering influence (Money and Pollitt 1968; Stoller 1968); an unusually large number of males, hypogonadal during foetal life, have disturbances in masculinity even to the point of feeling themselves to be girls in childhood and adult life.

Hermaphrodites – those whose external genitals do not have the appearance normal for their sex – present a 'natural experiment' testing the hypothesis that in humans, the interpersonal, rather than the biological, is the greater influence in the development of masculinity and femininity (Money, Hampson, and Hampson 1955, 1956; Stoller 1968). In such situations, once again, family attitudes primarily determine the child's gender-identity. Regardless of the rest of the criteria for establishing sex (chromosomes, gonads, and so on), if the infant's genitals at birth look appropriately female and the infant is unequivocally assigned to the female sex, the core gender-identity will be 'I am a female', and the equivalent with males and maleness. Then, as with the completely normal female or male, on being assigned to the appropriate sex, one develops a core gender-identity consonant with the *assignment*, not the biology of one's sex. For instance, the otherwise normal female or male, but with external genitals appearing like those of the opposite sex, will be assigned to the wrong sex; if unequivocally thus reared, the child develops a clear-cut gender-identity in keeping with the assignment, not the biology. Or, a different example, when the genitals look hermaphroditic, that is, have attributes of both sexes, if the parents are uncertain of the child's sex (as, for instance, when a physician tells them that the sex is not yet determined or is unclear), then a hermaphroditic core gender-identity results (Stoller 1968). In this situation, the child grows up with an unalterable sense of either being a member of both sexes or of neither.

Treatment. We need not discuss the hormonal or surgical management of the intersexed patient; more important, anyway, are the rules of identity formation that should underlie the decisions of the surgeon or endocrinologist.

The key concept in treatment is the core gender-identity. We have noted that once the sense of belonging to a sex is established (around 3 years of age) it is very difficult to modify this fundament of identity. Everyone has a permanent sense of belonging to one sex or the other, except in the unhappy situation of those with a hermaphroditic identity; these people feel they belong to a sex to which no one else belongs; they feel they are freaks.

After early childhood, then, the established core gender-identity probably cannot be changed. One should recommend that treatment in the intersexed patient who unequivocally believes himself a male or herself a female be planned around this established identity; there should be no treatment the success of which would require that the core gender-identity change (Money, *et al.* 1955; Stoller, 1968). Therefore, even though the anatomical and physiological condition will require more hormonal or surgical management, the body should be modified so as to best approximate to the identity. The patient, saddened by his inadequate physical state, will still be less traumatized than the boy or man suddenly told he is in fact female; or similarly in the case of a girl. For example, there is a common hermaphroditic state in otherwise biologically normal males, in which the penis is the size of a clitoris and the rest of the external genitals may also at birth have a female look. If the child is brought up a female, she may suffer from the knowledge she is sterile and needs oestrogens to maintain a feminine figure, but to tell her at age 6, or 16, or 26 that she is a male may be catastrophic. Even if the diagnosis of maleness is properly made at birth, because there is no present-day surgical technique to build a functioning penis, the child can be brought up as a girl. The surgical and hormonal problems are manageable: remove the testes (usually cryptorchid), surgically create an artificial vagina, and administer oestrogens at puberty. The result is a normal-looking female.

The case of the patient with a hermaphroditic identity confirms the rule that core gender-identity should determine mode of treatment. This is the person so often noted in the literature who can change sex with minimal distress at any time in life. For such a patient, after years of uncertainty and feeling unhuman, it is most supportive to be told by a medical authority that the uncertainty will be resolved and that he really is a male (she really is a female). The patient then gladly submits to the change of sex. Although the core gender-identity does not change, one's adjustment in the world often does. But when an intersexed patient, believing without suspicion he or she belongs to the assigned sex, is suddenly authoritatively told this was a mistake, the consequence may be the onset of psychosis (Stoller 1968) or the start of life-long despair and withdrawal from others. See also Chapter 14.

Psychosis

Gender disorders are commonly seen in psychoses. Freud used this finding as the keystone for his theory of the aetiology of paranoia. He said that the homosexuality (perhaps better termed transsexualism, for the symptom usually takes the form of ideas about one's sex changing), latent and unacceptable in the patient, becomes the core of a conflict that can only be solved by a delusion (Freud 1911).

Although ideas about sex change are present in transsexuals and in paranoids, the two conditions need not be confused. The paranoid has the other manifestations of psychosis (such as remaking of reality other than that related to changing sex, or a thinking disorder); the transsexual does not. The paranoid is clinically paranoid (suspicious, irritable, self-referent, subject to supernatural forces), the transsexual is not. The paranoid man is not feminine nor is the paranoid woman like a man; the male transsexual's behaviour is unremarkably feminine, and, if one were not specifically told that 'her' body was male, the patient could scarcely be distinguished from another woman in regard to femininity; or comparably for the female transsexual. The paranoid feels threatened by the possibility his body might change its sex, the idea of sex change being alien, ego-dystonic; the transsexual yearns for the body to change. The paranoid believes his sex is fundamentally changing; the transsexual does not believe his sex changes but only that the external appearance of it has changed. The paranoid believes his sex change will occur because of supernatural forces; the transsexual believes he can accomplish 'sex change' only by his dealing with the real world. The paranoid's transsexual fantasies emerge only during the psychosis and disappear from consciousness if it ends; the transsexual's desire to be a member of the opposite sex has been conscious since the earliest childhood and has never changed, regardless of treatment or other life circumstances.† The paranoid states are a defence; male primary transsexualism is not.

In short, the paranoid states clinically do not look like primary transsexualism, their psychodynamics are grossly different, and they develop from aetiological factors unlike those in transsexualism.

Conclusions

Underlying the above descriptions of clinical states are rules and hypotheses that may help clarify issues of diagnosis, dynamics, and treatment.

†I trust that no one will think, because beneath the paranoid's conscious rejection of transsexual impulses are unconscious desires, that therefore the dynamics are actually the same in the paranoid and the transsexual. That style of theorizing would throw away the gains ego psychology has brought to theory and practice.

(a) The earliest stage in the development of gender-identity (masculinity and femininity) is the core gender-identity, a taken-for-granted, usually unfelt (but not dynamically unconscious) state of acceptance of oneself as a member of one's assigned sex.

(b) In almost all humans, regardless of biological state, unequivocal assignment to one sex or the other and the continuing adherence to that assignment by parents in their behaviour toward their child creates core gender-identity; in humans, the biological state, to the extent it contributes, is a silent undercurrent rarely powerful enough to overcome parental influences in the opposite direction.

(c) Core gender-identity, once formed, cannot be displaced.

(d) Two different classes of dynamics may underlie the aberrations; the first is that of neurosis production – perversion – in which conflict, defence, and compromise formation in order to resolve conflict produce a psychodynamically unendingly active state. The other – variant – creates an aberration in which the above dynamics are not at work. The difference between the two is especially in the dynamics of hostility; in the perversion, hostility is directed to one's sexual objects, who must be demeaned, fetishized, dehumanized, before they can be found safe enough to be approached erotically. In the variants, this dynamic of hostility is not an issue.

(e) Careful observation of the patient in the present, plus careful history-taking, allows one to separate out as different conditions primary transsexualism, secondary transsexualism, transvestism, homosexuality, intersexuality, and psychosis.

(f) What Freud often called 'homosexuality' and put at the centre of psychological development, both normal and pathological, might nowadays more accurately be called 'transsexual tendencies'. This adds the connotation of an impulse toward sex change to the connotation of 'homosexuality', which focuses only on the more superficial aspect: object choice.

(g) The most profound aberration of gender – the earliest to form, the least likely to change by life-experiences or treatment – is primary transsexualism, and yet, at odds with commonsense expectation, the condition is caused by atraumatic, non-conflictual learning experiences, accomplished primarily within a timeless, excessively close physical and emotional intimacy with mother.

(h) If core gender-identity is so difficult to modify after childhood, then the more its presence makes up the gender disorder being considered, the poorer the prognosis for change. This suggests that we should either develop new treatment techniques for modifying core gender-identity (psychoanalysis does not), or we should design our treatments recognizing they will be limited to the extent that the pathology is a reflection of core gender-identity.

References

Bak, R. C. (1953). Fetishism. *J. Amer. Psychoanal. Assoc.* **1**, 285.

—— (1968). The phallic woman: the ubiquitous fantasy in perversions. *Psychoanal. Study Child* **23**, 15.

Barlow, D. H., Reynolds, E. J., and Agras, W. S. (1973). Gender identity changes in a transsexual. *Arch. Gen. Psychiat.* **28**, 569.

Bieber, I., Dain, H. J., Dince, P. R., Drellich, M. G., Grand, H. G., Gundlach, R. H., Kremer, M. W., Rifkin, A. H., Wilbur, C. B., and Bieber, T. B. (1962). *Homosexuality*. New York.

Fenichel, O. (1953). The psychology of transvestitism. *Collected papers*, New York.

Freud, S. (1905). Three essays on the theory of sexuality. *Complete psychological works of Sigmund Freud*. Standard edition, **7**, London.

—— (1911). Psychoanalytic notes on an autobiographical account of a case of paranoia (dementia paranoides). *Complete psychological works of Sigmund Freud*. Standard edition, **12**, London.

—— (1937). Analysis terminable and interminable. *Complete psychological works of Sigmund Freud*. Standard edition, **23**, London.

Gadpaille, W. J. (1972). Research into the physiology of maleness and femaleness. *Arch. Gen. Psychiat.* **26**, 193.

Gelder, M. G. and Marks, I. M. (1969). Aversion treatment in transvestism and transsexualism. In *Transsexualism and sex reassignment* (eds. R. Green and J. Money). New York.

Gillespie, W. H. (1964). The psycho-analytic theory of sexual deviation with special reference to fetishism. In *The pathology and treatment of sexual deviation* (ed. I. Rosen). London.

Green, R., Newman, L. E., and Stoller, R. J. (1971). Treatment of boyhood 'transsexualism'. *Arch. Gen. Psychiat.* **26**, 213.

Greenacre, P. (1953). Certain relationships between fetishism and the faulty development of the body image. *Psychoanal. Study Child* **8**, 79.

—— (1955). Further considerations regarding fetishism. *Psychoanal. Study Child* **10**, 187.

—— (1960). Further notes on fetishism. *Psychoanal. Study Child* **15**, 191.

—— (1969). The fetish and the transitional object. *Psychoanal. Study Child* **24**, 144.

Greenson, R. R. (1966). A transvestite boy and a hypothesis. *Int. J. Psycho-Anal.* **47**, 396.

—— (1968). Disidentifying from mother. *Int. J. Psycho-Anal.* **49**, 370. ·

Gutheil, E. A. (1964). Quoted in *Sexual aberration*, Vol. 1 by W. Stekel. New York.

Khan, M. M. R. (1964). The role of infantile sexuality and early object relations in female homosexuality. In *The pathology and treatment of sexual deviation* (ed. I. Rosen). London.

Kubie, L. S. and Mackie, J. B. (1968). Critical issues raised by operations for gender transmutation. *J. nerv. ment. Dis.* **147**, 431.

Money, J., Hampson, J. G., and Hampson, J. L. (1955). Hermaphroditism: recommendations concerning assignment of sex, change of sex and psychologic management. *Bull. Johns Hopkins Hosp.* **97**, 284.

——, ——, ——, (1956). Sexual incongruities and psychopathology: the evidence of human hermaphroditism. *Bull. Johns Hopkins Hosp.* **98**, 43.

——, ——, ——, (1957). Imprinting and the establishment of gender role. *Arch. Neurol. Psychiat.* **77**, 333.

—— and Pollitt, E. (1964). Psychogenetic and psychosexual ambiguities: Klinefelter's Syndrome and transvestism compared. *Arch. Gen. Psychiat.* **11**, 589.

Person, E. and Ovesey, L. (1974a). The transsexual in males. I. Primary transsexualism. *Amer. J. Psychotherap.* **28**, 4.

—— and —— (1974b). The transsexual syndrome in males. II. Secondary transsexualism. *Amer. J. Psychotherap.* **28**, 174.

Rekers, G. A., Yates, C. E., Willis, T. J., Rosen, A. C., and Taubman, M. (1976). Childhood gender identity change: operant control over sex-typed play and mannerisms. *J. Behav. Therapy Exper. Psychiat.* **7**, 51.

Socarides, C. W. (1970). A psychoanalytic study of the desire for sexual transformation ('transsexualism'): the plaster-of-paris man. *Int. J. Psycho-Anal.* **51**, 341.

Stafford-Clark, D. (1964). Essentials of the clinical approach, In *The pathology and treatment of sexual deviation* (ed. I. Rosen). London.

Stoller, R. J. (1968). *Sex and gender Volume I: On the development of masculinity and femininity*. New York.

—— (1973). *Splitting*, New York.

—— (1975a). *Sex and gender Volume II: The Transsexual experiment*. London.

—— (1975b). *Perversion*. New York.

6 Exhibitionism, scopophilia, and voyeurism

Ismond Rosen

Exhibitionism

Definition

An exhibitionist may be defined as a man who exposes his genitals to someone of the opposite sex outside the context of the sexual act. When it serves as the major source of sexual pleasure, or is compulsive or repetitious, exhibitionism is regarded as a perversion. Genital exhibitions occur normally in both sexes in childhood, and in adults as a prelude to sexual intercourse where they can be a source of added pleasure. Homosexual acts of this nature will not be considered here. In the adult these belong properly to the category of homosexuality, whilst among boys and young adolescents exhibitionism often forms part of normal exploratory behaviour (Kinsey, Pomeroy, and Martin 1948).

The perversion of genital exhibitionism does not occur in women. Ford and Beach (1952) in their study of 190 communities found no peoples who generally allowed women to expose their genitals under any but the most restricted circumstances. Even the wearing of clothes had as its function the prevention of accidental exposure which might provoke sexual advances by men. In those few societies where women deliberately exposed their genitals, the Lesu, Dahomeans, and the Kurtatchi, this was apparently done as an advance for intercourse with a particular man. Exhibitionism could thus be characterized as an arrest at the stage of courting behaviour, which was one view Havelock Ellis held of the condition. Fenichel (1945) noted that women who had a preference for genital exhibitionism in fore-pleasure, revealed in analysis that they had retained to a high degree the illusion of possessing a penis. What relationship this has to the infrahuman primate series is hard to say. In these animals the receptive female exposes her genitals to provoke sexual advances. Zuckermann (1932) and others regard the large size of the clitoris in anthropoid apes as phylogenetically a primitive character. The absence of the perversion of genital exposure in women has been explained by the difference in development in the two sexes with regard to the castration complex. Absence of the penis in the woman is felt as a narcissistic injury; the exhibitionism is displaced on to the whole of the rest of the body, especially the breasts, and on to a show of attractiveness. Therefore the showing of the genitals cannot have the reassuring effect it has in men. It has however been observed historically in the Balkans among peasants, and also in prostitutes in London, where these women expose themselves as an affront. See also Zavitzianos (1977).

Generally speaking, it is the woman, or girl as she is in 60 per cent of cases, who, on being exposed to by a man, feels insulted and who retaliates by calling the police. In Britain, exhibitionism is an offence known as Indecent Exposure, legal details of which are to be found in Chapter 13.

Historical

The literature dealing with exhibitionism is still rather meagre and has been well reviewed by both Karpman (1925, 1948) up to 1926, Rickles (1950), Mohr, Turner & Jerry (1964), Gebhard (1965), and Rooth (1976). Excellent clinical descriptions occur in the early psychiatric writings (Lasègue 1877; Garnier 1900; Maeder 1909; Strasser 1917). Later authors of mainly psychoanalytical persuasion have provided extended case histories and further understanding of the psychological mechanisms (Freud 1905; Stekel 1912, 1920–21; Sadger 1921; Sperling 1947; Christoffel 1936, 1956). However, certain basic problems still require further elucidation.

Many authors have drawn attention to the archaic quality of such an act and the inherent expression of primitive phallic worship. Lasègue, who rendered the first clinical description and coined the term exhibitionist in 1877, and Garnier (1900), both described cases where there was habitual exposure in churches. The latter's oft-quoted case held the act in great veneration. This patient felt that when women were in an attitude of devotion, they would realize the seriousness of the exposure and gratify him by showing profound joy on their faces and by exclaiming 'how impressive Nature was when one sees it in these circumstances.' At that time, and until recently, sexually aberrant behaviour was regarded as part of a neuropathic taint (Krafft-Ebing 1906; Hirschfeld 1936). Havelock Ellis (1935) equated exhibitionism with a pseudo-atavism. This he qualified as 'there being no true emergence of an ancestrally inherited instinct, but by the paralysis or inhibition of the finer and higher feelings current in civilization, the exhibitionist is placed on the same mental level as the man of a more primitive age.'

The difficult question of sexual symbolism is raised in this connexion by authors such as Rickles and Karpman who feel that the exhibitionist expresses in his act the ancient rituals associated with phallic worship. This is part of the ontogeny recapitulates phylogeny theory; certain forms of primitive physical development assumed to have been passed through by the human species are repeated during the development of the individual human embryo. Similarly the emergence of psychological states, such as the appearance of the Oedipus complex and the super-ego or conscience in the child, is thought of as a repetition in the individual of earlier experiences in human social life. With great advances in the fields of genetics, early infant development and ethology, more detailed knowledge is required of the factors affecting both the transmission of acquired social and psychological behaviour, and the effect of the environment on its final form in the new generation. One cannot equate actions in primitive peoples, which had come to have a highly specific complex symbolic content, with behaviour that is normally found in childhood, although the form of the act is similar. Repetition of species behaviour (which Jung called the collective unconscious, and which followers of Freud accepted as factual without the need for special terminology) properly belongs to the phase of childhood where it appears only as a tendency, and gains its specific symbolic content from social experience. This social situation is the relationship the child has with its parents in the earliest years and is expressed by the terms Oedipus complex during the phallic phase, and by pre-oedipal relationships during the earlier oral and anal phases. Thus in the exhibitionist all the instinctual urges are transmuted and coloured by the prism of these early family ties.

Exhibitionism is usually regarded as reinforced by constitutional disposition. Two cases of this series had fathers who were known exhibitionists. The literature has many examples of the syndrome occurring in several members of the same family. However, the term 'constitutional' remains unsatisfactory, and too general in explaining what portions of a behaviour pattern or tendency are inherited on a genetic basis, and what is acquired through intra-uterine and later developmental influences.

Incidence

Exhibitionism is one of the commonest sexual deviations in this country as witnessed by criminal statistics and treatment figures. The offence of indecent exposure formed one quarter (490) of Radzinowicz and Turner's total of 1985 sexual offenders in their 1957 study. This represented approximately one third (2279) of the 6161 sexual offenders found guilty in 1959. Taylor (1947) found that indecent exposure formed nearly a third of all sexual offences. Other studies published in America show this to range from 20 to 35 per cent of all sex offenders. Arieff and Rotman (1942) found that their 100 unselected cases constituted 35 per cent of the sex offenders seen at the Psychiatric Institute of the Municipal Court of Chicago. Hirning (1947) reported 60 exhibitionists and 105 cases of other sex offences in a 10-year study of cases referred by the courts to the psychiatric Division of Grasslands Hospital, Westchester County, New York. Rickles (1950) found 48 exhibitionists out of 152 sex cases (35 per cent) at the Behaviour Clinic at King County, Washington. In Radzinowicz' study 80 per cent of indecent exposures were first offenders. The other 20 per cent formed the largest recidivist group of all sexual offenders and were also amongst the most difficult to treat. Only 24 per cent of the cases charged with indecent exposure were referred by the courts for medical reports in 1954. The number of cases referred seems to be rather low compared with the high proportion of frank psychiatric illness, and serious personality disorder amenable to therapy, reported in the literature.

The factor of age was elicited from the Mohr, Turner, and Jerry (1964) study in Toronto, where the majority of exhibitionists were in their twenties. In England and Wales, the figures between 1958 and 1970 show that the incidence for adults remains steady, but doubles for offenders under the age of twenty-one years; the total annual convictions for indecent exposure were approximately 3000 for this period, making it the most common sexual offence.

Where there is exposure to young children, the prognosis worsens, both for repetitions and for the incidence of later paedophilia. The link between exhibitionism and violence is discussed at length in the literature. Gebhard (1965), showed that one-fifth of his exhibitionists' previous sexual offences, which contained no exposures, involved the use of force. Bauer (1970) quoted by Rooth (1976) reported findings in Germany indicating an increasing sadism in exhibitionism which reflected a general rise in violence in all sexual crimes. Petri (1969) attempted to predict which exhibitionists might become violent later, because of the relatively high incidence of offenders, 12 per cent in one series of rape, arson, or robbery with murder, who had previously presented as exhibitionists. Further cases are mentioned where eleven rapists were previously exhibitionists. Petri's classification for predicting future violence is given in order of increasing seriousness:

(a) Simple exposure.

(b) Simple exposure with masturbation.

(c) As for (b), but where communication is attempted, such as speaking, shouting, or whistling.

(d) Exposure which includes touching or handling the victim.

Rooth (1973) found a low incidence of sexual offences involving force in his series of thirty persistent exhibitionists. He concluded that the exhibitionist act might actually protect against violence in the persistent offender, and suggested the exhibitionists could not be regarded as a homogeneous group of offenders. The typical, confirmed exhibitionist may well not be a danger, but forensic series tend to be dominated by single-offence exposers, who need not necessarily share the same characteristics; and it may be that the violent minority will prove to come predominantly from the ranks of the incidental as opposed to the habitual offender.

In a diagnostic series, the numbers and types of cases found often reflect the attitudes of the referring sources. Thus clinics attached to courts or prisons refer the more severely disturbed patients. In the Portman Clinic 1964 series, cases were sent from many different courts, prisons, and other clinics, a high proportion of which were referred with a view to possible treatment. For the preceding 5 years the Portman Clinic had seen an average of 154 sexual offenders annually out of a total average number of 536 new cases referred. Sixty per cent of these cases were referred by the courts. Of this 154, 50 cases or approximately one-third, were exhibitionists. These proportions accurately represent the national distribution, and are in keeping with the incidence reported in the literature.

Although the series of cases to be reported here is statistically significant only in that it represents a high proportion of those cases taken on for treatment at the clinic, nevertheless the results of such treatment which are later reported would seem to have some general validity.

The clinical material in this chapter is based on personal observations made at the Portman Clinic over a 2-year period on eighteen cases treated with group therapy in three separate groups, and six others treated with individual psychotherapy. Both treatments were on a weekly out-patient basis on psychoanalytically orientated lines. There were two adult groups which ran for 9 months and 1 year respectively and an adolescent group with boys aged 15–17, meeting for nearly 6 months. This presentation will deal with phenomenology from a dynamic psychoanalytic point of view, with special reference to two aspects. Firstly, character formation and its links with the Oedipus complex and early object relationships; secondly, the exhibitionist's handling of his instinctual drives with particular reference to his aggression, narcissism, and depression. Emphasis will be placed on the importance of early pregenital experiences for later phallic levels of fixation. These processes will be illuminated by the progress made in the therapeutic groups, which will also be described. The results of treatment and a follow-up study will be found at the end of the chapter.

Classification

Exhibitionists can be usefully classified into main groups, with gradations in between. The first is the *simple* or *regressive* type, where the exhibitionist act follows as the result of some rather obvious social or sexual trauma, disappointment or loss, or as an accompaniment to a severe mental or physical illness, including the vicissitudes of old age and alcoholism. These people tend to be rather reserved and shy with social and sexual inhibitions and fears, but their personalities are on the whole relatively good ones, as seen in their intimate associations and work records. Maclay (1952) has given an excellent account of what he calls 'compensatory types' where 'the exposure is an act of more or less normal individuals, and is in the nature of an anomalous form of the ordinary sexual advance'. These cases would fit into this group.

Personality disturbance is much more intense in the second group which is the *phobic–impulsive* type. The quality of the personality defects is usually dependent on the pattern and intensity of the infantile level of fixation and the defence mechanisms employed. Examples are given below. In this group one finds persons who regularly exhibit and become recidivists. Where the impulsive aspect predominates they are often of an amoral cast of mind, prone to other forms of character disorder and actual perversion such as transvestism and voyeurism, as well as the commission of crimes of stealing. Thus Richard, exhibiting his feminine attire, wandered on to the wrong beat and was picked up with the other girls and driven in the Black Maria to prison, where his true sex was discovered. Several of the patients were voluble sea-lawyers, two of whom gravitated towards the office of shop-steward, where they exercised a capable irresponsibility combined with a constant shiftlessness of employment. This need for frequent change of object, whether job, possessions or interests, was typical of many patients and revealed their pre-oedipal character fixations. Even in their arguments they usually ended up identifying and agreeing with the other side. In this group, too, could be found well-developed phobic disorders of both hysterical and obsessional type. For example, Peter, a highly intelligent patient, had constant recurring fantasies that his genitals would be bitten off by sharks in the swimming pool, bath water, and bed, which was evidence of his severe phallic castration anxiety expressed in phobic terms; while a part-time musician, of whom we had three, had to pick up all the papers in the street prior to exposing himself. This obsessional symptom was an intensification of the reaction formation of tidiness as a defence against the anal component of 'dirtiness' in the act of exposure.

From an examination of the literature and the observations made on The Portman Clinic 1964 series of patients, it seems clear that this phobic-impulsive group exists as a syndrome or entity, separate from cases where exhibitionism occurs symptomatically in the presence of other specific causes. Some controversy exists about the diagnostic classification of this syndrome; whether it belongs to the psycho-neurotic compulsive group, or to the impulse neuroses or perversions, which some classify among the psychopathic personalities. Apart from the question of nomenclature, treatment is dependent on the diagnosis preferred; diagnosis should be based on the psychopathology.

Phenomenology and psychopathology

The phenomenology of the exhibitionist act is a complex and fascinating one, the full understanding of which would give the clue to many processes hitherto unexplained. The pre-conditions and liability for such responses exist in childhood where desires and acts of exhibitionism are normal in both sexes and undergo a process of repression.

In the exhibitionist the normal process of repression is either exaggerated, leading to severe inhibitions, both sexual and social, or is incomplete, where there has been either intense prohibition or stimulation of interest in the boy's body and his genital functions by mother. Both Rickles (1950) and Karpman blame the heightened sense of narcissism on mother's excessive attention to the boy's body and his genitals. The unrepressed exhibitionist urges serve to hold deeper sexual wishes towards the mother in unconscious control. The age of subsequent onset of exposure is highly variable and dependent on chance environmental stimuli. Two patients described games of 'look and show' with girls, many years before puberty. Thus in these two persons the normal latency phase was seriously interfered with, or with regard to exhibitionist tendencies, failed to occur. The latency period, following the oedipal stage and lasting until just before puberty, is characterized by strong reaction formations against infantile sexuality, plus the growing sublimatory interests in boyhood pursuits. Several adolescents exposed themselves due to the intensity of sexual feeling during puberty and the teens. It is quite often the case that the youth is already in a state of sexual excitement when the sudden presence of a female causes him to objectify the experience through her. For example, boys masturbating alone in their rooms, or urinating in the country in apparent solitude, may see passers-by from a window or other vantage point, and believing themselves to be unnoticed, complete an act, or succumb to sudden impulse. Two men started in their late teens and early twenties following their only intercourse experiences, which were with prostitutes while on service, and which were profoundly shocking and disappointing. It was as if all their fears of inadequacy and of the damaging effect of intercourse with a woman thereby gained material proof. Commencement at later decades was usually a result of loss or frustration, which although not manifestly sexual, nevertheless symbolized a blow to their self-esteem and masculine pride, and was associated with feelings of depression. The circumstances of the first exposure experiences contribute to an habitual pattern which is set up. This template is made use of by the police to apprehend such unfortunates. The conditioning varies proportionately and is stronger in youth, although new additional patterns may be later established. Ford and Beach (1952) state that males who have mated with females in a particular place often show signs of sexual arousal the next time they are taken to the same enclosure. There soon develops a strong tendency to approach and remain within the setting previously associated with sexual satisfaction, and to respond sexually to any other individual met there.

This capacity for conditioning seems to stem from the high degree of fused aggression and libido which, having been withdrawn from previous objects, is freely available when the penis, highly charged with narcissistic libido, is exhibited. This has significance for treatment, because where such specific habits exist, each major pattern and element of the situation, for example, the age of the victim, the place, time of day, general mood, and so on, must be worked through in therapy; otherwise a trigger mechanism may still be set off by the presence of some of these stimulus elements. Thus one patient, aged 40, in individual psychotherapy had analysed his need to exhibit to young schoolgirls on the road walking home from the station. His desire and fantasies of exposure no longer existed in that situation. He then required to work through urges to expose himself while travelling on trains, wishes not yet under full control. This man had an unresolved oedipal conflict of high intensity and had been forced from the age of 8 by schoolgirls into exposing himself. The difficulties with his father were mirrored in his reacting badly to any superiors or masculine authority. This led to a feeling of suppressed resentment at work demands, and a sense of injustice at the failure to secure promotion. Exhibitionism was a release for these feelings. Prior to psychotherapy he was treated with stilboestrol which succeeded in banishing all his sexual fantasies. On stopping this drug the urges and fantasies of exposing himself returned immediately. By means of psychotherapy he was able to have a normal sexual life with his wife and he lost the urge to expose himself. But he was still advised to avoid those situations which previously presented a source of stimulation, which it was felt could still be dangerous if he regressed when he became depressed or angry. One feature of this patient's illness was the severe social ostracism and active anonymous hostility vented on him and his family, as a result of his court appearances being reported in the newspapers. While freedom of the Press must be earnestly upheld, the publication of details of sexual offences may result in exaggerated social sanctions, or as sometimes happens in certain much publicized cases, in a false sense of heightened esteem in the offender. The wisdom of or justification for such publication should be further examined in the light of modern knowledge.

The precipitating event may therefore be primarily one of two types. The first is that of internal sexual excitement arising spontaneously as in the adolescent, or aroused in him by sexually stimulating sights. The patient, Peter, first exposed himself at his window in response to a little girl doing handstands next door. He could never resist the sight of a girl's knickers after that. In the second type, exposures occur as a result of a non-sexual tension situation which nevertheless has the symbolic meaning of loss of security or castration. Thus a young artist exposed himself in his car on two occasions when going home from the dentist. The unconscious awareness of a dental attack as symbolizing castration was quite clear. Depressions following loss of work or status were common causes. Often there was a mixture of the two in a complex way. The act itself, however, is usually an impulsive affair, which, when the urge arises, is beyond the capacity of the individual to control. A feeling of inner tension prevails which seems similar to that described by Freud (1905) for an infantile sexual aim; it is felt as unpleasure, is centrally conditioned and then projected on to a peripheral erotogenic zone, in this case, the genitals. On exposure the exhibitionist becomes aware of intense genital sensations and a sense of inner pleasure, in excess of anything else he has experienced, including heterosexual orgasm. There may or may not be an erection and masturbation may or may not be indulged in. The fact that neither erection nor ejaculation is necessary for the experience of specific pleasure is evidence of the hyper-libidinization of the genital area. The sexual pleasure may be short-lived or endure for a long time. Usually, however, there is a return of self-critical faculties and many, overcome by their guilt and remorse, are easily apprehended and form the bulk of the first offenders. Many patients pride themselves on their self-control and high moral standards in other spheres. Those who plan their exposures may go undetected for years. The picture is therefore one of a temporary suspension of super-ego control as far as these unconscious instinctual desires are concerned, the ego being forced to participate in the performance of an organized act, but powerless to control the timing of it. Like the infant, the exhibitionist can neither tolerate tensions, nor wait for his needs to be satisfied. Both must be dealt with immediately. Instead of thinking they pass directly into action.

The recognition that the adult exhibitionist acts out a partial aspect of instinctual behaviour normally expressed in childhood and subsequently repressed, was first adumbrated by Freud in the *Interpretation of Dreams* (1900) and later fully described in his classical *Three Essays on Sexuality* (1905). This position was maintained with little change by Fenichel, who regarded exhibitionism as the 'simple overcathexis of a partial instinct' which was a denial of or reassurance against castration anxiety and the Oedipus complex. The Oedipus complex in its positive aspect may be said to be dominated by the boy's aggressive feelings against his father and his tender wishes towards his mother. Its negative side, which is present in varying degrees in exhibitionists, is that of a wish to take mother's place with father by identifying with her. Castration anxiety is the unconscious fear of the boy's own aggressive feelings plus the fear of the father's retaliation. While Freud felt strongly about the specificity of castration anxiety as fear of loss of the genitals, he nevertheless saw it as part of a sequence of bodily loss starting with the birth process and followed by weaning and the loss of faeces.

In its intensity, castration anxiety represents all the anxieties of loss ever experienced, while the aggression felt towards the father and expected in retaliation seems to be the sum of all previous aggression, from whatever stage and source.

In animals, reaction to fear takes one of two pathways. Either there is action, in the form of fight or flight, or there is complete immobility as if transfixed. These two patterns of behaviour are seen extremely well in the exhibitionist. In Freud's description of exhibitionist dreams, the factor of sudden physical immobility is shown to be a characteristic feature; lesser degrees of inhibition are extremely common, and are discussed in detail by him, the association between the wish to exhibit sexually and inhibitions to activity of any sort are clearly linked in these dreams, much as one finds it in the everyday life of the exhibitionist. During the time of greater fear or tension, there is the sudden impulse to exposure as an aggressive act. But this act is also a safeguard against still more dangerous fighting. One patient called Bill had several previous convictions for indecent exposure, voyeurism, and stealing. He only attended the first meeting of the first group, but returned a year later having lost his wife and job, and desperately seeking help. Having stopped exposing himself, he was afraid that if he lost his temper he would murder someone. He was taken into the second group, and described his enormous powers of control which suddenly gave way if his self-esteem was threatened, or if a superior was unfair. An ex-boxer, he was a potential murderer and everyone recognized it. The group was quite subdued for two sessions when he talked at length about his difficulties. He then found a new job and social interests and became calmer. Later some members began to assail him in a subtle way, and he left the group, unable to tolerate this aggression and what he regarded as the therapist's unfairness to a particular member.

We must now try to understand what loss of love and self-esteem means, in terms of early object relationships. This is because there is a fundamental relation between the mechanism of depression and impulse neurosis. Both depressives and impulse neurotics are greedy people, dependent on narcissistic supplies from outside. Freud laid down a timetable of libidinal development in the infant, which progresses from auto-erotism, to narcissism, to true object relationships. Thus in the stage of narcissism, loss of an object or a reduction in the amount of love shown, leads to a withdrawal of libido from the object and its re-direction back on to the infant's own body. The part of the body participating in this narcissistic regression is dependent on the degree to which earlier fixations have occurred in the genital and pregenital phases of development. An examination of the total personality characteristics and mental associations reveals the amount and quality of these fixations; derivatives thereof colour the exhibitionist act itself. The exhibitionist regresses to the sadistic phase of childhood, where any loss of object, self-esteem or threat of rejection results in a withdrawal of libido from the object or external reality, and a subsequent investment of this libido as secondary narcissism in the infant's own body via a specific organ, his penis.

Certain exhibitionists seem to be fixated at the oral level. Thus loquacious Dick described himself as a 'mouth in trousers'. The hostility of the oral phase, seen as biting and devouring, is projected on to the outside world and a similar retaliation is expected. It is the strength of this fixation which gives to later objects such as the female genitalia their hostile oral character. Christoffel (1936) postulated colpophobia, fear of the female genitals, as the basic fear in exhibitionism. Melitta Sperling (1947) reported the analysis of a single case of exhibitionism in which an oral fixation was the most important determinant of the condition. This operated through the unconscious equation of breast with penis. The patient could not overcome the trauma of weaning and early separation from mother.

At the stage of object relationship, the libido is similarly withdrawn from the object, but then a mental image of the lost object is taken into the self by the process of introjection and represented therein. This leads to an identification with the lost object and is one of the mechanisms of character formation. The time sequence of these developmental phases is important and the stage of object relationship takes place about the time biting and anal interests are becoming prominent, at about the eighth–ninth month. Winnicott (1958) has described certain phenomena of the transitional phase between oral erotism and true object relationship. One of these transitional phenomena is the infant putting his thumb into his mouth, while the fingers of that hand caress the nose or face. Exactly similar behaviour occurred as a regressive phenomenon in Roger, a youth of 17. His sullenness and silence during the adolescent group mirrored his relationships generally. He treated his parents at home as complete strangers and never spoke to them. With gentle handling and time he evinced a pleasant if rough demeanour in the group and settled down to work at a new job extremely well. When the group ended, he continued in individual psychotherapy. Each session commenced with a cheery account of the week's successful happenings, then he would lapse into silence. This withdrawal became more profound in later sessions, when the thumbsucking and face caressing would occur in a hypnoidal state from which he was hardly rousable. He lost his exhibitionist urges, but the underlying object losses which were exposed resulted in his being sent away, as he had a kleptomaniac episode of stealing from a garage he was passing. A similar hypnoidal phenomenon was seen to affect the whole second adult group on one occasion as a response to inconsequential compulsive talking by one member. Winnicott (1958) has described both pseudologia fantastica and thieving in terms of 'an individual's unconscious urge to bridge a gap in continuity of experience in respect of a transitional object.' Some exhibitionists appear to react to loss with mechanisms from this transitional phase.

When the stage of object relationship is reached with its sadistic biting and anal aspects, the individual becomes aware of himself and others as hostile and threatening. He has great difficulty in dealing with the objects he introjects. The complex mechanisms of this phase belong to the study of depressions and super-ego development. Exhibitionists tolerate loss very badly and expose themselves as a defence against the accompanying depression. One patient out of this series exposed himself one week after the death of his father. Another adult group member showed only few signs of depression when reporting a still-birth to the group eagerly awaiting news of the delivery. As a group they could become more depressed over this, than he could as an individual.

Greenacre (1952) has examined the resultants of childhood stimulation which is either premature, too intense, or too frustrating. She believes that these, if early lead to an increased somatization of memories and symptoms; if severe and massive, to the utilization of all possible channels of discharge; and in states of frustration or over-stimulation, that genital arousal occurs from an early time. Also, that genital performance may be used very largely in the service of pregenital aims, yet retaining genital form and even a modicum of genital pleasure.

In many exhibitionists, although the organ involved is the genitals, the mechanisms employed from an economic point of view is that set up by the oral-sadistic phase. The importance of oral factors as components of the castration complex has been discussed by Stärcke (1921), Fenichel (1931), and de Monchy (1952).

The problem may therefore be stated as follows. Does the exhibitionist regress to the oral sadistic phase of childhood when he meets the difficulties aroused by the Oedipus complex in the genital phase, when castration anxiety is at its height? Or are there fixations and components from the pregenital phases (oral and anal) which influence both the castration complex and the Oedipus complex? The exhibitionist's relationships with his parents (and his wife) are difficult to understand in the light of the classically described Oedipus complex. Towards both parents there is an ambivalent love–hate relationship, which in its heightened state is characteristic of the pregenital pre-oedipal phase. This was clearly revealed in many patients during their treatment. Thus towards the mother there was love expressed in a pre-oedipal way via a strong feminine identification. This feminine identification was found to be present in all the patients, even in the unlikeliest member John, who was a shop manager and who, though inhibited, appeared a virile family man. It was discovered that he prided himself on being able to handle ladies' dainties better than any of his female staff. The feminine identification was also an aspect of the negative Oedipus complex, where the son is desirous of replacing mother in father's affections. This provides an obvious stimulus to a homosexual attachment and inclination, and the act of exposure to a woman is also a defence against this homosexual component and full feminine identification. The difficulties of dealing with the latter in treatment are discussed in the section on group therapy.

The erogenous pleasure gained in the act of exposure leads to a heightened self-esteem or narcissism. Freud postulated that exhibitionism remained more narcissistic than any other partial instinct because it originated in the precursor of looking at oneself. This provided the connection with another partial instinct, that of scopophilia, the sexualization of the sensations of looking. Scopophilia and exhibitionism usually exist as instinctual counterparts in the same way as sadism–masochism, active–passive wishes, and masculine–feminine strivings.

Allen (1974) examined scopophilic–exhibitionistic conflicts as factors in the formation of neuroses, in everyday life, and the treatment situation, and the implications of providing cathexes for creativity. Perversions based on these conflicts were not studied. The conclusions reached were that 'the partial instincts of scopophilia and exhibitionism were present in everyone, tending to form defensive polarities in the psychological economy'. 'Looking–showing defences affected learning, life-style and functioning: traumatic scopophilic and exhibitionistic incidents of early life can become the basis for later screen memories and acting out. Dreams occur in which the patient is primarily an observer.' 'Looking and showing factors constantly influence the psychoanalytic process for both analysand and analyst: every correct interpretation indicates to the patient that he has been perceived accurately and that the analyst is able to observe and exhibit his findings.'

Scopophilia and voyeurism

Scopophilia, the pleasure in looking, can also become a perversion, which is known as voyeurism. Freud (1905) defined it as a perversion if '(a) it is restricted exclusively to the genitals or (b) if it is connected with the overriding of disgust (as in the case of *voyeurs* or people who look on at excretory functions), or (c) if, instead of being *preparatory* to the sexual aim, it supplants it. This last is markedly true of exhibitionists, who, if I may trust the findings of several analyses, exhibit their own genitals in order to obtain a reciprocal view of the genitals of the other person.' In the perversions, the presence of exhibitionism always means an associated voyeurism and vice versa, even if only present unconsciously.

Scopophilia is thus the taking in of impressions visually, and during the first year of life may be linked with the way objects are taken in via the mouth, or sensations experienced by touch; looking and touching are intimately associated. If, however, the oral incorporative experiences are unsatisfactory and come to be characterized by greed, hunger, and insatiety, with fears of the ensuing hostile aspects, then the visual functions may come to have a similar quality and be felt as devouring, compulsive, and later be defended against by complex inhibitory systems of lack of interest or learning difficulties. The visual component of castration anxiety is exemplified in the classical myth where Oedipus blinds himself as a retribution for his incestuous crimes. These visual–oral–phallic aspects are described in detail in Fenichel's paper 'The scoptophilic instinct and identification' (1954).†

It seems that the excess of aggressive energies and their lack of fusion with libidinal elements require other bodily systems to be more highly charged as a way of dealing with them. Thus other ectodermal structures such as the skin participate in and express the 'unpleasure' or tensions. Several of the patients reported the active existence of skin complaints of the nature of eczema and allergy, this being a rather frequent finding in the literature. Exhibitionism however is mainly linked with the phallic stage of experience; the greatest investment of narcissistic libido being concentrated on this organ due to its significance for procreation. The scopophilic instinct becomes prominent again in the phallic stage when curiosity and research about sexual matters becomes intensified. Thus from an economic point of view libido from both the oral and phallic stages finds a common pathway for expression and, later, repression. The reaction formation against scopophilia is shyness. The earliest intimation of shyness seems to have its origins at the time in the infant's life when it is learning to distinguish between familiar figures and strangers. Work reported by Ambrose (1961) on the smiling response in infants, shows that following a peak of smiling responses to both mother and strangers, which occurs at 20 weeks with institution infants and 13 weeks with home infants, there is a decline in response-strength towards the strangers, so that by the age of 5–6 months the child seems able to discriminate well between mother-figure and strangers. Other observers attributed this falling off in smiling response to a fear of strangers; Ambrose records it as also being due to factors of curiosity and exploration. This development coincides with both the oral-sadistic phase and the important time when the child comes to see its mother more as a whole person or object. She may be incorporated as a source of pleasure; the stranger however leads only to further tensions. The reaction formation of shyness occurs at the early oedipal phase at the age of 3 or 4 years, when curiosity, concept formation and the thirst for knowledge are aroused strongly. As Freud (1905) has stated, 'in scopophilia and exhibitionism the eye corresponds to an erotogenic zone.'

Thus, disturbances in these stages of development are likely to be

†Fenichel is one of the authors who prefer the term scoptophilia to scopophilia. The latter has been used here because it is better in keeping with the original Greek, *skopein*, to look.

reflected later in specific disorders which are found in varying degrees in all exhibitionists. The difficulty in object relationships is seen in the exhibitionist act itself, where the woman exposed to does not have the characteristics of a whole person for the exhibitionist. She is merely there to provide a narcissistic gratification and proof against castration. Most patients readily agreed that they 'would run a mile' if the woman to whom they exposed themselves were to respond. Even for those who claim the act as means of sexual stimulation, doing it to a *complete stranger* robs it of the quality of fore-pleasure as exposure before normal intercourse my be, and turns it into an aggressive act. The exhibitionist therefore reverses the childhood formula of avoiding strangers in order to perceive mother more wholly. Exposure to the stranger is still dangerous but preferable to exposing to the familiar woman who stands for mother because of the greater danger inherent in the castration complex. Many patients were extremely prudish with their wives; they took care never to let each other be seen in the nude, and their pattern of sexual behaviour in intercourse was rigidly conventional. There is general agreement in the literature on the puritanical attitude towards sex in the families of exhibitionists as well as in themselves. The highly inhibited and shy exhibitionists are therefore a result of the excessive reaction formations against scopophilia. In the group they could not talk, as everyone was strange, and in a few cases months passed before they could be induced into making spontaneous comments. One of the commonest complaints was of having nothing to talk about. It was well known that individuals with such complaints are usually poor readers due to their difficulties in taking in visual impressions. The importance of good reading ability as expounded by Mortimer Adler in *How to read a book* is most instructive here. He points out the philological connexion between the words 'to read' and oral behaviour. Previously 'read' was the term given to the ruminant's fourth stomach. Oral terms are also used to denote understanding, such as the 'digestion' of a passage.

One of the commonest inhibitions observed in the group was that of inability to initiate any activity. When the talkative members were absent, one was able to analyse the fears of commencement as mechanisms for controlling instinctual drives. At least two talkative persons should be in the group to balance the shy silent ones, as lengthy silences are absolutely intolerable to the latter and should be avoided. Richard left the group never to return, during a silence near the end of the first group when attendances were low. Further, there is little to talk about if there are learning difficulties and facts cannot be taken in due to a repression of curiosity. The ideas underlying their silences were a mixture of castration fear and narcissistic inferiority, namely that what they had to say had already been said, or would be a paltry contribution, and that they would be laughed at by others. Thinking, as a mental function, was extremely difficult and no thoughts were present. This was in marked contra-distinction to the compulsive talking felt by two disinhibited members, one of whom was Dick, the 'mouth in trousers'.

Glasser (1978) discusses the conflict between the ego and the super-ego in the exhibitionist. He agrees with Rooth (1976) that exhibitionists are under-achievers, and posits that the failure to reach adequate goals may be due to the passive resistance of the ego against the sadistic demands of the super-ego. Some secondary gain accrues to the ego as a result. The exhibitionistic act is a manifestation of active, compelling defiance against the super-ego; this attitude manifests itself in all spheres of psychic activity, especially those imposing moral and ethical restraints.

Treatment

The treatment of exhibitionists and voyeurs must always be made on the basis of an individual assessment. In general the therapy of choice is some form of psychoanalytical treatment, individual or group psychotherapy, though counselling in simple inhibited adolescents may suffice. The more pronounced the accompanying personality disorder and the tendency to repeat, the greater the need for intensive transference therapy.

All patients appearing in court should have a medical report. It is to be preferred that the psychiatrist making the report should be responsible for the subsequent treatment advised either by undertaking to give the treatment personally or under his supervision, or making suitable prior arrangements elsewhere.

Some patients of the simple regressive type may respond to the shock of the court appearance, fines or imprisonment, but these have a minimal effect on the phobic-impulsive group.

Stilboestrol was useful in controlling intensive urges for a time while psychotherapy was being arranged or started, but was otherwise purely palliative, carried its own risks of feminization and was temporarily castrating. It is non-curative. For further details of antiandrogen therapy, which is preferable to the oestrogens, see Chapter 1 p.21.

Surgical castration would seem to be completely uncalled for in this condition.

Exhibitionists have been treated successfully by a variety of behaviour therapy techniques – systematic desensitization, Bond and Hutchinson (1960), Rognant (1965); electric aversion therapy, Fookes (1969), Evans (1970). See Chapter 12.

McGuire, Carlisle, and Young (1965) put forward the hypothesis that masturbatory fantasy entrenches deviant sexual behaviour. Evans (1968), finding that exhibitionists who masturbated with deviant fantasy responded poorly to deconditioning therapy, cautioned the subjects against such practices. Stephenson and Jones (1972), and Jones and Frei (1977) treated exhibitionists, who were previously resistant to change, successfuly using provoked anxiety in special settings. The latter experimenters induced their subjects to undress before a mixed audience, and to relate verbally their feelings, events, expectations and attitudes, including those attributed to the victim. The experience aroused tension, hostility, shame, and disgust. Severe anxiety was the predominant feature, partly based on the variable proximity of the audience, which could move closer to within four or five feet of the subject, and which produced anxiety because the distance from the victim or audience was no longer in the control of the subject. The high anxiety was thought to facilitate the re-examination of previously held attitudes, which were then corrected by a kind of aversive conditioning. At the fifth weekly session, video tapes were taken and played back to the subject the next week. Video-taping was repeated and played back again. The results were that exhibitionism was eliminated entirely in ten out of fifteen subjects, with partial successes in two. Six subjects refused to participate or failed to complete, making a 30 per cent failure apart from those who did not improve. This method of treatment, which induces a high level of anxiety, was also used to treat exhibitionists by Serber (1970) and Wickramasekera (1972). These authors pay great attention to the behavioural aspects of their treatments, but do not appear to understand in any depth the nature of the symptom, or the interpersonal relationship problems of their subjects, including the changes which are induced. Rooth (1976) expresses the view that behaviour therapy 'holds out the promise of bringing his exposure more rapidly under control' ... 'but the possibility remains that group therapy might in the long term be more beneficial because of other, less definable changes, such as an improvement in interpersonal relationships'.

Voyeurism – a clinical case study

Details of a case of voyeurism will now be presented. Apart from the significant psychopathology, the difficulties in dealing with this recidivist patient from a social and therapeutic point of view are salutary and reveal areas of interaction that deserve of public and professional notice.

Noel was in his middle twenties, and had eight previous convictions for 'peeping Tom' offences. These were mainly for watching women in public lavatories, the last one being combined with that of stealing for which he was sentenced to 6 months' imprisonment. He was first sent by the court for psychiatric opinion aged twenty, and his progression both medically and criminally was briefly as follows. At first he was given a conditional discharge and he commenced treatment which was hypnosis. He appeared to respond, but after 2 months failed to attend. Later he was arrested for a similar offence, was put on 2 years' probation and treatment was continued in irregular unco-operative fashion. Several other court appearances soon followed, he being bound over and then being fined £25 for breach of recognizance. His attitude was one of great resentment to his parents and indifference towards the court. The diagnosis was that of immature psychopathic personality. Diagnoses by later psychiatrists who saw him aged 23 were that of immature and unstable personality with psychopathic traits, and compulsive abnormal sexual behaviour. By this time he had had a course of psychotherapy lasting a year, the results of which he was pleased with, and also a course of hormone treatment to diminish his sexual desires. He had married during this period and no further hormones were prescribed so as not to interfere with his marital sexual life. A year later the psychiatrist referring him from one of H.M. Prisons to The Portman Clinic thought that he was suffering from a psycho-neurotic illness with obsessive compulsive features, stemming back to childhood or adolescence, and was in need of further treatment.

Noel was then treated with weekly analytic psychotherapy when the following picture slowly emerged. His problems stemmed directly from a very disturbed early family background, characterized by his subjection to intense stimulation of an aggressive and sexual kind, together with deprivation of understanding and affection, at times alternatively, at others concurrently. As a child of 8–10, he would get resentful with his mother and express this in cruelty to animals. He had to show off to the other boys, or be silly to gain their attention. He craved his father's attention and admiration, but the latter took all his exploits and excellent sporting abilities quite coolly.

He reported satisfaction during sexual intercourse with his wife, but disgust on completion, and was compelled to think of millions of others having intercourse at the same time, like animals. When it was interpreted to him that he then became conscious of his parents' intercourse, he associated to his first ever awareness of primal scene activities at the age of 4, and ever since then, because of the paper thin walls. He was terrified, prayed they would stop, and later lay awake waiting for a repetition of the event, feeling left out and resentful. He had a similar set of fantasies about the toilet where the sounds fascinated and disgusted him. The similarity of his feelings concerning his wish to see women in lavatories and his mother in intercourse was revealed. He felt that seeing women in the toilets was a way of degrading them. By his offences and court appearances he was able to hurt his mother. Not only was his feeling of being left out by his parents a cause of intolerable loneliness, but he also had to defend himself against the wish to become like mother. Thus artistic sensitivity to poetry and music was a source of fear as this aroused a feeling of feminine identification, and was checked by his daring exploits. But he would imitate women's toilet behaviour he had seen, by squatting and arranging his clothes. Thus he came to do actively what was done to him passively when young. He felt humiliated at being bathed by mother up to the age of 11 and humiliated women in return. As an adult, he thought mother was oversexed as she came into the bathroom at inopportune moments, and when he became angry, she would say 'You've got nothing to look at', which led to his first voyeuristic acts in public. He then admitted to conscious thoughts of intercourse with mother. He said that this was the worst kind of incest and he found such ideas quite intolerable, but that going into toilets was the next best thing to intercourse with mother. The importance of his voyeuristic acts as a defence against his intense incestuous desires for his mother, as well as an expression of them, became clear. In his teens he would try and see mother without any clothes on and was given a hiding by her for observing her at her toilet. This also linked up with memories of discovering mother's soiled sanitary towels as an adolescent and as a small child, which aroused his disgust and the thought that if father only knew about these things what he would say; the sexually arousing effect of all this was clear, and the anal-sadistic aspects emphasized. His voyeurism was therefore a compromise mechanism which prevented and yet satisfied his wish for intercourse with mother and led to severe punishments, for he would frequently be caught, as it were, on purpose. The punishments had different significant aspects; through them he could show his masculinity to mother, make up for his sense of genital inferiority, further humiliate his parents, and counter his fears of a feminine identification. He felt his parents wanted a girl instead of him, and as a child he had fantasies of being a girl. He said he would hate to be a woman, because of chaps like him frightening them in toilets, afraid of being raped or murdered. The sado-masochistic elements in this case are quite striking; one source of such satisfaction was always the publication of his name or misdemeanour in the newspapers. The merits in Press publication of details of sexual misdemeanours remain debatable, and in many countries are disallowed. Though social sanctions such as losing jobs and friends followed, the narcissistic satisfaction was enormous.

Noel gave evidence of oral sadism as well as the anal sadism described above. His boyhood cruelties were prolific. He dug tunnels in ponds and filled them with frogs, newts, eels and adders, watched them tangling together, then would cut them to bits with a knife, or pour on oil and set them on fire. Games of torture were frequent and included fantastic 'dares'. But this sadistic approach was contradictory; he would never hurt a bird under any circumstances and was a keen ornithologist. Birds were thought of as tender; amphibians could be tortured or burned, and mammals killed. He once killed his own pet rabbit, but could not put an injured bird out of its misery. Once at school he spoiled a prize cabbage the children were growing by poking his finger through it – and when later an interpretation about his wish to damage mother's breast was given on different material, he associated back to the cabbage and said that it had to be holed exactly in the centre. This was interpreted as representing the nipple and he then talked of his fantasies which were similar to a recent murder case where the woman was bodily mutilated. He had thoughts of cutting a woman's breasts right off where they joined the rib cage, and added that he also had fantasies of cutting women's nipples out. He continued to describe how, when he was younger and was served mince meat and mash, he would mix it all up and make the food into a square, then make a ploughed field out of it with a fork, then cut the centre square and eat it, then a square on the left, right, north and south, then other squares, but could not finish it like this and had to gobble it all up. The interpretation was made that the squares were to take the breast shape away. He replied that it was very significant when people drew doodles. He drew triangles, a large one which he then bisected, added other triangles and suddenly had to do figures of eight and then put circles into the centres of the triangles.

What needs to be emphasized here is that despite his nuisance value to women in toilets, the moral suffering inflicted on his family, and a single physical altercation with his father and fights with his brother, none of these oral sadistic fantasies were acted out with women. The perversion of voyeurism and his complex defensive mechanisms were able to keep them all at bay. This is in marked contrast to one of Hyatt Williams' (1964) cases, where almost the precise sexual fantasies were acted upon in reality. During treatment, with increasing insight his aberrant impulses were able to be resisted, and his relationships and his work level improved.

The picture of family life seen through Noel's emotions and fantasy was certainly not visible even to the trained observer. His parents were eminently respected in their neighbourhood, and presented to legal and medical authorities as well adjusted, responsible persons who had made great personal sacrifices in order to advance their son's education. They were completely at a loss to understand his behaviour, and were responding to advice to be as tolerant as they could towards his misdemeanours.

During treatment at the clinic the patient re-lived much of the original feelings associated with the experiences described. He became extremely sensitive to loneliness and acted out his voyeurism when he became depressed, for example, when a social engagement with his wife suddenly could not be kept. His treatment could not be carried to a successful conclusion although he was making excellent progress, as he had to be transferred to a new therapist after 6 months. Although the changeover was carefully handled by all concerned with his full knowledge and agreement, and he liked his new female therapist, stating he preferred her to a male doctor, this provoked a fresh burst of voyeuristic activities for which he was sentenced to prison. Although it was suggested to the magistrates that treatment as an in-patient was infinitely preferable to imprisonment in view of his excellent progress and co-operation in treatment, his record was against him. The view was taken that he was morally degraded and had brought great shame on his wife and had further failed to benefit from the opportunity for treatment; he deserved punishment and could have treatment again after his prison sentence; in the meantime, society should be protected from such as him. Although he was originally referred to The Portman Clinic for out-patient treatment from prison, an earlier psychiatrist had recommended in-patient psychotherapy. In fact he really required much more intensive therapy such as psychoanalysis from the start, prescribed early on in his history, but the number of trained psycho-analysts working in the field of delinquency is extremely limited; their skill has to be technically diminished by having to give analytic psycho-therapy instead of full analysis to make help available to a greater number of National Health Service patients.

The diagnostic differences noted above are due to varying aspects of his psychopathology being presented at different times. The psycho-pathic quality refers to the early oral elements with their impulsiveness and denial, while after a certain amount of treatment, the more com-pulsive anal-obsessional mechanisms were observed with their better control and improved prognosis. Magistrates have usually been found to be extremely co-operative over allowing patients who have repeated their misdemeanours during the early stages of therapy to continue with their treatment. It is clearly impossible to alter the compulsive psychological mechanisms quickly and so prevent recurrences and further legal proceedings. The emphasis should be on prescribing correct medical treatment early on, even though it may seem more intensive than warranted by the offence, but lack of facilities prompts a legal progression of discharge, probation, fine and prison, with a corresponding psychiatric scale of medical report, superficial talks, drugs, and intensive analytic psychotherapy. Perhaps an ideal as des-cribed long ago by Silverman (1941) is still too remote in this country. He described a situation in an American city, where the police gave a sexual exhibitionist the opportunity to consult a psychiatrist before charges were preferred. If treatment was found to be possible and was embarked upon, the charge was dropped, and no unwelcome court appearance and newspaper publicity followed.

Prevention of recidivism is important. It should be possible to detect the potential repeater by the type of character structure found at the time for the first medical report, so that these cases can be referred for intensive therapy from the outset, instead of going through a process of hardening and inner despair.

Group therapy

Due to the vast amount of data and the complexity in reporting clinical material available from three different therapeutic groups, the follow-ing presentation will be made.

1. A clinical account of some treatment sessions in sequence from the first adult group, followed by the details of one session as an example.
2. A general survey of some of the technical problems and transference phenomena.

Clinical report of group therapy sessions

The following is a clinical report on sessions of the first adult group of sexual exhibitionists which met weekly for 75 minutes. It is based on the sequences of the first half of the group therapy, followed by a report of one whole session in detail. The group started with two meetings in July, before the break for the summer holidays, and met regularly thereafter until March of the following year. The members were originally eight in number. No rigid selection of criteria were used, and those awaiting psychotherapy were offered group therapy. It was extremely difficult to keep patients waiting who were in urgent need of treatment for perverse sexual impulses, and the one patient who never attended the group was seen just prior to the summer holidays, but required admission to Horton Hospital soon after, for depression and his concern about his psychic urges. He never replied when treatment was offered after his discharge.

Seven persons attended the group at any time, two of them subsequently lapsing. One, Bill, only attended the first meeting. He was over 40, an exhibitionist, voyeur, and thief, who had over a dozen convictions to his credit and was pessimistic about treatment. He returned later and was a member of the second group for a while.

To acquaint the reader with the lives and work of these patients in the group, I shall start with a thumbnail sketch of each one, referring to them by assumed Christian names. They were Tom, Peter, David, John, Richard, Michael. Patients were addressed formally in the sessions.

TOM was 25, tall, dark, and usually in working clothes. He was married with children, and was employed in a large works. His first offence for indecent exposure was at the age of 16, and a year later he was put on probation for minor stealing offences and sent to a hostel. He disliked the hostel, ran away, was sent to prison and from there to borstal. He escaped, was caught and sent to prison. He decided to become a model prisoner, behaved perfectly and after a few months sought special privileges on these grounds. In a meeting before the Prison Governor he was told he had shown no improvement in behaviour.

He retorted that he had been so good he had no room to improve and was perfect. The need for improvement was insisted upon, so, losing his temper, he flung a bottle of ink at them, overturned the table, and walked out. Now he could improve, and he did so, with an early release.

He had no difficulty with the law again until 7 years later when he exhibited himself publicly, but for 2 years there had been sexual difficulties with his wife, leading to abstinence. During group treatment, and through the probation officer's valuable talks with his wife, full normal intercourse was re-established. Tom's relationship to his parents gave the key to his attitude to life. His father was an obsessional personality who was a moral coward, especially during air raids, while his mother was strong and dependable. Tom identified with her and at the age of 16 he chased his father out of the house – it was at this age that his exposures started. All his life he had been looking for a hiding. He was a very angry young man indeed, especially in the group at times. His I.Q. was 126.

PETER, aged 26, was an intellectual, and the brains of the group. His manner was that of an impartial pedant, always ready to lead discussion, argue in theoretical terms about psychology, and take over the role of leader in the group. He appeared to have a good deal of insight until one realized that he expressed no affect and that this was all part of an intellectual defence and that he had a similar split between a loving relationship with a woman and a sexual life. For him the ills of society could be healed by a return to an unhibited biological sexual existence. In his family life he regarded his father as a failure, his mother as a model of perfection, and he had successful brothers several years older, one of whom seduced him into masturbating him when he was 8 and chagrined him by not returning the compliment. He had a fairly free sexual life, essentially got on poorly with people and was married to a girl his intellectual inferior. They parted when his compulsive revelations about his inner fantasy disgusted her. His exhibitionism apparently started aged 19 when he watched a girl of 11 doing handstands in the garden next door, and he exposed himself in his upstairs bedroom. This subtle surreptitious game continued for a year, after which he openly showed and masturbated in parks. He was excited by the sight of little girls' knickers and was an intense voyeur. He had never been caught. His avowed intention was to excite women for masturbation or intercourse.

DAVID was aged 24, a well-turned-out, pleasant, gentle-looking sales-man. He was quiet, maintained his individuality in the group and was referred for masturbating at open toilet windows in office blocks to female staff. His father, a regular soldier, was killed on D-day. He lived with his aged, ailing mother. He had been in the army and his only experience of intercourse was during a drunken Geisha week-end, in Tokyo, and was highly unsatisfactory. David had a steady girl-friend whom he had known for years and planned to marry later. He treated her with utmost respect. He suffered with asthma and nervous dermatitis. He was absent for a quarter of the meetings with dermatitis and away another quarter due to work demands. He felt his troubles would be over if he could have intercourse, which he was too gentlemanly to perform. His I.Q. was 108.

JOHN was aged 40, and the oldest member. He was on probation with a condition of treatment. Pleasantly middle aged, dressed in a neat sports coat, with a row of pens in his top pocket. He too was quiet, most attentive, and weighed his words ponderously. For some time all statements were prefaced by 'If I can put it this way', or 'How shall I say?', or 'May I say?', the following statement usually being a generalization, or a detraction to pour oil on a group difficulty, or to come to the therapist's aid if attacked. John's demeanour was blandly enthusiastic – 'we're all nice chaps'. He was a manager, happily married with children, and said he came from a happy home and had none of the difficulties the others reported, especially about homo-sexuality. He had courted his wife during the war, by leaving camp without permission and riding to see her on his motor bike. John would exhibit himself alighting from his car on his way home to any passing women, but dreaded any contact with them. This had happened two to three times weekly for 8 months. He was upset by a manager being appointed over him. However, he lost his position due to newspaper publication of the offence, but luckily secured a better post in the same trade. His I.Q. was 117.

RICHARD was aged 37, a mechanic was was married, with one child. He was the nattiest, flashiest, dresser of all, with a grey suit, blue suede shoes, and dark blue tie with glass sparklers on it. He was good-looking in an effeminate way. He had three previous convictions, although his present attendance was voluntary. The first was aged 28 for exhibitionism. The second aged 30 was most astounding; he was picked up by the police as a prostitute as he had happened to wander into the wrong area while indulging his transvestite bent. He was only discovered when he had to undress. Ever since the age of 10 he had wanted to be a girl. He was the middle of seven children, three boys and four girls, and his father, an engineer, brutally knocked the family about, in one case breaking his brother's arm by hurling a chair at him in an argument. Although his father died 25 years ago, he seemed to have left his mark. Richard had also been induced into passive homosexual practices for the last 5 years. His last court appearance, aged 37 was for indecent exposure. He exhibited to any female in the street or parks, without erection or ejaculation, and described an 'exhilarated feeling inside' which lasted for a long time; he had regular sexual intercourse but this did not satisfy him as much. He was variable in the group, reticent about his pervert proclivities which were only just held in check by his attendances, but he would argue and expostulate if he was sure there would be no real counterattack. He enjoyed berating other social groups such as 'bank-clerks'. His I.Q. was just over 100.

MICHAEL, aged 29, who lapsed after the eighth meeting, was the most uncontrolled member of the group, like a chunk of primary process. His parents separated when he was three and he shuffled thereafter between relatives and boarding schools. He was taken into care and sent to an approved school aged 14, because of passive homosexuality. He exposed himself and masturbated to girls in the dark, in cinemas and on beaches, and was excited by the sight of girls' knickers. He was convicted for indecent exposure aged 24 and 27 and was on probation with a condition of treatment. He claimed his trouble was due to his never having had sexual intercourse, though he compared himself to his father who, he said, had even made another girl pregnant when he was born. He moved around constantly, although apparently he was a good worker as a fitter, and a shop-steward. Michael sat through the first meeting sprawled out in his raincoat and hat. He would burst into meetings late, argue firmly and inconsequentially about wage rates and hold the group's attention by his imperturbable vigour even when attacked. He settled down remarkably, came neatly dressed and showed flashes of helpful insight. He claimed to be able to control his proclivities by willpower, and later reported that he had had intercourse with a young lady he had been seeing for some time, and seemed to be improved. His I.Q. was 96.

BILL has been described on p.149.

The first two meetings were concerned with problems of control of their perverse sexual drives. Michael said he could control his by willpower, and Bill said this was not so; he had willpower beyond the average and could not. He said further that even marriage made no difference, and John and Richard confirmed this, which shattered David, who saw marriage as the end to his problem. The question of punishment was raised, Michael supporting prison as a useful deterrent. But Tom and Richard disagreed from personal experience, and John said even a police caution initially had not helped. They went on to talk of the social implications of their acts. John and Tom had both lost their jobs and their families had suffered. John brought up the question of newspaper publication of their misdemeanours and its effect on their lives. (This topic was raised on many occasions and there were newspaper cuttings later on reporting subsequent offences by Tom. Although harmed by such reports, Tom nevertheless upheld the freedom of the Press. He was getting his punishment.)

The main interpretations at this stage were that they were all different individuals united through suffering the same complaint; that exhibitionism was normal in childhood and that we needed to try and explore earlier memories as a pattern for present behaviour; that their offences were serious in so far as they offended society. The group were intrigued by the fact that women did not suffer from this complaint and it was interpreted that they exhibited themselves in other ways. Michael said he wouldn't exhibit again because he would think of what it was like for the woman, especially if she were his daughter. But he decried the way women dressed to excite men, and how he wanted to touch them.

After the summer break Peter joined the group. John asked if there was place for further members, and on being questioned related how a man had exposed himself to his (John's) daughter of 10. She had told her mother, who telephoned the police. John felt pity for the man, was prepared for him to come into the group, as he was with the same probation officer, and the group agreed. He did not think his daughter had been harmed, but all reference to his feelings about his wife's action was avoided and the therapist purposely refrained from interpreting this.

The talk ranged on the attitude of workmates, who in reality seemed to forget about the incident after a short while. One amusing aspect however was that to be a successful exhibitionist one seemed to need a good memory for faces. Tom did not have one, and apparently actually exposed himself to a woman working in his own, though admittedly large, department. He said he had no idea who she was, and the group laughingly suggested he approach and ask her. Sessions later Peter reported how on his prowls he tried to pick up two young women in the street, launching forth with 'Haven't we met somewhere before?', whereupon they said 'Aren't you the chap down by the river, but you had a beard then!' These disturbances of visual memory were a result of repression of scopophilic tendencies.

Tom talked about his strong sense of morality and how it would be impossible for him to have extra-marital relations. Incidentally his probation officer was co-operating well in dealing with his wife, and helping her to overcome her sexual difficulties. Richard then talked of how prison made one more perverted although it was supposed to be helpful, and exhibitionism was only one of his difficulties. Sex could take thousands of different forms. Peter questioned whether he was afraid of homosexual difficulties and Richard said yes. Peter then said he had never had any experiences like that, then checked himself and said yes, there was one, and that he had thoughts that he might be homosexual too. Then he said something about 'all of us coming here and exposing ourselves before you, a beautiful girl', looking at the therapist and adding 'I wonder why I said that?' The transference aspect of this remark was noted and reserved for future use. The group were taken aback and led away from this to females exhibiting themselves. It was interpreted that the group was not confined to talking about exhibitionism, but that this was only one of the types of early sexual behaviour levels one could be stuck on. The purpose here was to try and liberate their fantasy, and also to discover the extent of their difficulties; while not frightening them away with interpretations one had to try and hold their urges in check.

At the end of the meeting Tom reported privately that he had in fact exhibited himself again. He was encouraged to discuss it at the next meeting. This he did 2 weeks later, describing how his bicycle had turned into his usual haunt, 'as if of its own accord', and he had partially exhibited himself to two girls. He felt very ashamed but a new feature had appeared; he wanted to apologize and made to do so, but they ran away. This need for apology was accepted as a hopeful sign, attributed to the work of the group. Peter resented having to be interrupted in a lengthy intellectual argument about lowering the age of consent which would solve everything. Still it was felt we had to come to Tom's aid and discuss his problems further. But Michael interposed and described his compulsive feature of having to pick up all the papers in the street before he could expose himself. This animated the group to discuss tidiness and Tom interjected aggressively, looking at the therapist, 'You seem to have rather a nice suit on but your underwear is probably filthy underneath.' He then talked about his drawers at home being untidy and Michael shouted out 'drawers' significantly, to mean underclothes. It was interpreted that being tidy or dirty were mechanisms for the discharge of tensions and were opposites such as looking and exhibiting were, both belonging to a more immature phase.

Meetings at this time tended to be dominated by Peter, either in argument with Michael or in discussion with John or the therapist. Members generally talked to the therapist or into the group as a whole, unless actually arguing with one another. But then discussion turned more and more on their relationships with each other. They decried the odd times of arrival of members, asked for more group time, and complained of the warming up period of each session which was stressful. This was linked with their difficulties in making relationships with people, and how they denied the need for relationship in their acts of exhibitionism, which took place with complete strangers. This led to a discussion on the defiance of authority, with Tom relating his stormy past; Peter telling how he had been punished for purposeful misdemeanours at school; and Richard describing how he told lies to his wife in the evening when he wanted to go and commit an offence, but 'did not knock her about to get out'. Although Richard became very angry, she didn't let him out, and he cooled off and then felt all right. This seemed a typical adolescent rebellion, and the 'not knocking his wife about' was in relation to his own father's behaviour. These were interpreted, and the description of the vicious father then emerged from him. Peter talked of his failed father and Tom angrily despised his father at length for his weakness. The therapist interpreted Tom's defiance of authority as stemming from this and he seemed thunderstruck. John talked of his happy home life and though generally silent, nodded in assent to all the proceedings. Michael said how his father went round 'giving everyone babies' and said 'I must take after him.' It was interpreted that he was really rather afraid of the opposite sex, and had little to do with them, and everyone laughed. Perhaps this fantasy indicated his fear of identification with his father. Michael left the group when it was explained that although it was a condition of treatment for him to attend, he could have individual therapy instead; the group was purely voluntary. He much later applied to come back but could not attend regularly. Much resentment was voiced against him after he left, especially by Richard.

Richard talked of how he could not show his affectionate feelings to his wife, but could to his son, and the interpretation was given that if he let his feelings go, he might beat his wife as Tom did, as all his feelings had to be kept in check. Peter said, 'If one is stopped, the other is stopped too', and went on to describe how he couldn't achieve having the ideal mother, although his wife's hair was black like his mother's. In fact his wife was the very opposite of an intellectual. The therapist interpreted that it was not permissible to achieve one's mother in reality. Wherever possible, the therapist tried to make interpretations that would have general group validity. Subsequent interpretations of aggressive behaviour in the group, especially to the therapist, as reliving old angers about father, were most helpful. On one occasion the therapist was asked why similar interpretations were not made about John. It was replied that he had given no such material, having always maintained that his parents were happily married. But this brought up a repressed memory of how at the age of seventeen he had bought a motor bike and expected to be severely chastised by his father. The latter, however, merely said how grieved he was with his actions, and John, disappointed in his father's weakness, described how he suffered a shock, and ascribed this own passive relationships with superiors to this. Later he became very active in the group, especially after his use of phrases such as 'May I say ...?', etc., had been interpreted. Peter noted that these phrases were always addressed to him and he interpreted his wish to treat all problems in the group as things to be overlooked, or as avoidances. John reported how he was active in public speaking at parent–teacher meetings now, and quite recently he had been challenged by an employee to a fight and had gone outside and lightly returned the first blow, which so humiliated the other fellow that he himself roared with laughter and felt triumphant. Previously he would have mediated a middle path to avoid any disturbance. How John later took over the leadership of the group by actively dislodging Peter is shown below in the description of the complete session.

Peter finally told the group about his homosexual relationship with his brother and made his feelings overt for the therapist, as the one from whom he sought a similar experience. However, he insisted that his relationship with the therapist excluded the rest of the group, and there followed discussions over many sessions about whether one came for an individual relationship with the therapist or fitted into the group. Peter would purposely use psychological jargon which the group could not understand, question others, make tentative interpretations to them, and so play the role of assistant psychiatrist. This was always interpreted as his resistance to fitting in as a member of the group, his difficulty in expressing his feelings, and his need to split feelings and intellect. He described himself as a compulsive talker and slowly began to evince his real feelings and fears; his feelings of physical inadequacy which Richard echoed. He described his castration fantasies; of sharks being in the swimming pool and around his bed, which would bite off his genitals, and he brought up early memories of seeing little girls' genitals which had been, as it were, cut off. However, the rest of the group weren't up to this level of fantasy, and their reaction to him generally was one of growing antipathy because of the social difference and his intellectual hostilities, while they always granted him his right of leadership because of his superior education. Peter, while losing no opportunities to attack others under interpretation from the therapist, nevertheless openly started to admire Tom's moustache, and tried hard to get Richard to discuss his homosexuality and transvestism; but Richard had had a series of arguments with Tom about their respective jobs and their merits as workers. Tom seemed to come off best in these, and Richard, retiring into passivity, stated that 'he wasn't going to argue, as you never knew how far you could go with some people', meaning his fear of Tom losing control of himself in the group.

We must return to Tom because he fell deeply into trouble with the law. While on his way to the eighth session, he was arrested a block away from the clinic for exposing himself. Apparently a woman had been exposed to and a policeman had jumped into a taxi, ridden down the road and seen Tom. He denied the charge and was brought face to face with the woman who made it. She said she was not sure if he was the man, but at the police station they told her that he had been up for this charge before, and this seemed to have confirmed her opinion. He was charged and subsequently fined, his attendance at the group probably having been instrumental in preventing his being sent to prison. Nevertheless, from his evidence it was extremely doubtful whether he actually committed this offence. He maintained his innocence throughout and on the strength of his previous truthfulness it was hard for anyone in the group to disbelieve him.

Adult exhibitionist group session

Present: Peter, Tom, John, Richard

The group started late with only Peter and John. Peter commented that this evening it was rather like some committees at work. Other members of staff could go to these committees and on occasions there were more staff than committee. It seemed that here there were 'two of us, two of you' (two patients, therapist and observer). The therapist commented that perhaps Peter felt out-numbered. Peter went on that during this last week he had felt independent of the group, that he did not need the group. The therapist suggested that this was how he felt in any group, even in a twosome with a woman, and Peter agreed. The therapist commented that Peter needed to lead in the group or else he could not belong to it; there was no halfway house for him.

Richard arrived later at 7 o'clock and commented 'You started sharp tonight', and Tom came bustling in shortly after. Peter made his 'Good evening' deliberately stand out from the rest. Peter, who had again been the group leader, or had tried to be, now relapsed into the background a little. Tom was brought up to date with the evening's proceedings but he ignored this and proceeded to tell a weak joke which he had heard at work and which he felt compelled to tell: 'A man had gone into a pub for a drink and there had been only one other person in the bar, a girl in the corner. He asked what she would like to drink and she said "A pint of beer, please." Seeing the man's surprise she said, "Don't be put off by the dress, it's only for show." ' There was scarcely a murmur from the group. Peter did not understand and made this plain to Tom in a very castrating sort of way. He then forced a laugh and Tom explained that 'she' had been a 'he'. (In addition to this condescension towards Tom, Peter was once later in a similar attitude towards John, and on one occasion stood up to open the window for him.)

Apropos of the story, Peter asked Richard whether this was not his problem; would he not like to talk about it now? Richard shook his head, Peter went on to say, by way of reparation towards Tom, that he (Tom) also wanted to bring up this topic tonight and he thought this was Tom's way of doing it. Peter thought if they got on with the discussion of homosexuality they could then move on to other things, and he thus began to lead the group. It seemed to the observer that Peter's attitude was to curry favour with the therapist.

Tom broke in with seemingly little relevance that he had been aggressive that week. Last Friday he had gone to the pictures with his wife and their enjoyment had been spoilt by a group of Teddy-boys in front. He had gone down to ask them to be quiet and was surprised to find that they were all girls. None the less, there were some boys there who were making a noise in the gangway by the wall. They were calling across to their friends on the other side of the audience. Tom asked them if they would mind being quiet; he had paid to see the film and wanted to see it. One of the boys replied 'I've met your sort before', and Tom said 'Oh no you haven't. If you had, you'd never be saying that'. The boys were quiet for a while after that. This little bit was completely by-passed by the group and John, picking up again the reference to homosexuality, asked Peter about masturbation. They agreed that mutual masturbation was homosexual but were not clear about self-masturbation. Peter described what he thought was normal sexual development, from self-masturbation through mutual masturbation to heterosexual mutual masturbation and finally to a normal sexual relationship. John observed that Richard and Tom did not recognize this homosexual factor.

There was a silence, broken by John saying he wanted to bring up the discussion which had taken place last week when the group had officially ended and the therapist had gone. Tom had complained then of his frustration in the group and that he was afraid of bringing this topic up because he thought he would 'blow his top' if he did, but he gave permission for anyone else to bring it up. The therapist commented that there was tension all round this evening (this was really an understatement) and he interpreted Tom's 'joke' as an attack upon Richard, a provocation of him. But the group did not pursue this point either, and John now proceeded to attack Peter most forcefully. He drew attention to the fact that talking was difficult for him (he had a very bad attack of laryngitis that evening). He said that Peter did not lead the group because the group did not follow, and anyway, said John, wagging his finger at Peter, 'you can't ruddy well lead the group', because Peter was a patient in the group. He, John, could not lead the group for the same reason. The therapist pointed out that he *was* leading the group, and that in a sense whoever was talking at a particular time was leading the group at that point. Nevertheless, John denied his leadership role in his usual terms of 'circumstances' and by use of the word 'naturally'. He thought that Peter, by virtue of his intellect, was perhaps the one most fitted to lead the group. He reminded the group that he would have to leave soon (at the end of last week he said he would have to leave at 7.35 this evening). It seemed rather as though he were stirring things up and then leaving them. He got agitated and talked about blowing his top at work. If people were making a mess of their jobs and realized that he knew this and mended their ways he was satisfied; but what he could not stand (at this stage he was standing up and putting his coat on, very red in the face) were the apprentices who, after he had spent 3 weeks showing them their job and had in all spent 130 hours on each of them, still became slipshod the moment his back was turned; he had had enough of this. And he went.

There was a long silence broken by Peter, who had been considerably taken aback by this onslaught. He said it was the first time anybody had left the group except once when he had gone at 7.55, and he had wondered then what had gone on after his departure. The therapist said he wanted to bring up what happens when he goes. There were spontaneous comments from the three. Richard spoke of relaxation and Peter said things went back to man-in-the-street level and they became ordinary people. Richard said that he was sick of the word 'intellectual', which he had heard so often in the last few weeks.

Tom began talking about the conscious restraint he put upon himself in the group. He was afraid that if he did not, in spite of the frustration, he would blow his top. This was related to his incident in the cinema and in previous sessions when similar interpretations had been given that he wanted to beat Peter up, and that 'the only time you can be like father is when you are beaten up by father like a man'. Tom referred to a row which had taken place between his parents when he was young. Mother had finally blown her top and thrown a plate on the floor or at father, who had gone out to the garden and stayed there. The therapist commented that mother had in fact behaved like the lad. She had become angry and aggressive and father had taken a passive role in going out and staying out. Tom went on to say that men who fight each other sometimes have the greatest respect for each other afterwards and become the greatest of friends, even though it may have been a 'blood bath'. The therapist interpreted the homosexuality in this and at this point Peter was under great stress, although by and large he enjoyed this session in which Tom was, so to speak, put in his place. Tom went on that his father, he felt, was a cissy, and Peter took up the point that 'the only person we could justifiably, and I use the word justifiably in inverted commas, call cissy in the group is Mr. ——' (Richard). Richard did not rise to this at all and the therapist commented to the effect that Tom and Richard were father figures to each other, that Tom provoked Richard because he wanted Richard to attack him, because Richard's passivity was the passivity of his father who had not beaten him, and this was what Tom wanted; but that Tom also stood for Richard's father in personality in that he was a man who was violent and who could, for example, break a chair over his son's arm, and hence Richard, having had experience of this sort of father, was reluctant to say anything in the group. This defence of Richard was appreciated by him and having remained silent for most of the evening he joined in a little later for almost the first time. Tom went on that he had 'got to respect' the therapist because he had done so much for him, and Peter took up this point, particularly the word 'got', and interpreted it. Tom retreated behind a plea of a poor education but the therapist pointed out that the word 'got' was used and that in fact was what Tom meant. Tom became angry and said that the therapist's interpretations angered him, that they were wrong, he had often only half finished, the words were twisted, and so on; what were they getting at in the group on this occasion? The therapist replied, 'We are trying to get at what you mean by blowing your top.' Tom's complaining that he was getting angry with the doctor, was interpreted as his being angry as a boy with his father for being inadequate. The interpretations, though nominally rejected, were obviously in fact going home; Peter complained and attacked Tom that he (Peter) had in fact interpreted the word 'got' before the therapist, but actually the attack had been directed upon the therapist and not himself (Peter). The implication was that he wanted Tom to attack him, as part of a homosexual attack from his brother and father.

Tom went on to talk about discipline and the virtues and values of it, and how he admired the German army for this while the Japanese were pretty terrible. Richard would not have this and said the German army was bad itself, witness Buchenwald and Belsen, both of which he had seen shortly after the war ended. Tom would not allow that this was in fact a general standard of the behaviour of the German army in the last war. Tom extolled the virtues of discipline, which was interpreted by the therapist as his need for a strong father to control his aggression, and he was reminded also of an incident to which he had referred in a previous session when, as a result of this discipline in the

Guards, fifteen men had been unnecessarily drowned. But in his plea for greater humanity, Richard had the best of the exchange, and this marked the beginning of a change in his submissive, complementary role towards Tom (and his own father) and the establishment of a relationship in reality of equality, or even superiority, which previously existed only unconsciously in his ego-ideal.

General comments. Peter started off trying to lead the group and later made a second attempt but finally had to give up. An enormous amount of hostility and aggression was released this evening, particularly by John but also by Tom, and it may well be that this has gone as far as it safely can and that perhaps a switch to a more sexual topic rather than an aggressive topic would be in the interests of the group. Peter this evening deliberately re-introduced the use of Christian names in an attempt to lead the group.

Technical problems and transference phenomena

As will be seen in the following reports of group sessions, initial remarks in the group were usually addressed to the therapist. From the outset all these approaches were carefully directed by the therapist to the group as a whole. In this way, social relationships were encouraged rather than narcissistic gratifications. Patients were made to regard each other as possible sources of narcissistic supply, though a low estimation of their colleagues' ability to satisfy their needs for help and understanding was openly voiced. The first few sessions were devoted to a discussion of personal theories of why they exposed themselves, and how they should be punished or treated. The question of self-control was paramount and via these topics the patients described their backgrounds, personalities and pathological behaviour. In the main, whatever topic was discussed there were always two fairly distinct poles of opinion. This polarity functioned on all topics, and interpretations were made in such a way as to include all the members of the group depending on their position along a dimension between the two poles. Thus the introduction of Bill into the second group appeared to be a successful move. He could be presented to the others as an example of pure activity and aggression, in contrast to their passivity. Much of the talk relating to aggression was applicable directly to their sexual fantasy and behaviour.

A mechanism that was operative when one had representatives of opposite poles on the same dimension, was the tendency to identify with the opposite type of behaviour – 'I wish I could take a leaf out of your book'. However, the identification and envy was only partial, leading to a limited growth along the dimension rather than a complete switch from passivity to activity, such as may occur with the return of the repressed during impulsive behaviour. Further, they experienced the permissiveness of both types of behaviour in the group, with the accent on control of extremes. There was the verbalization of affect for both types; a reduction of inhibition for the repressed and a new mode of expression for the impulsive.

Talking about a 'dimension of personality', along which all members could feel suitably placed, gave them an objective correlate in the group which provided a framework for the description of dynamic past behaviour and its reliving in the group. In this sense, the transference relationship was not to the leader of the group, but to the group as a whole, where the affective reactions to any one member were described on the dimension of either communication or aggression. This led one to determine which dimensions were suitable for exposition. Those used were activity–passivity, aggression–love, control–lack of control, masculine–feminine, infantile regressive behaviour versus mature reality directed responses. Actually, the 'love' aspects were not made much of because, in an all male group, the homo-erotic element was excessively stimulated early on. The view members took instead was that of identification or support against attack in argument.

Attendance at the group was intensely discussed and in one patient absence came to symbolize exposure. An intellectual process was set up in place of impulsive action but the patient regarded the punitive aspects of the results of exposure greater than that accruing from one absent session. Thus a more socially accepted way of acting out was provided, which could subsequently be dealt with by the group.

The next phase of the group was that of patients finding interest in other members as individual personalities rather than in their behaviour. This led to further identifications, and, more important, to differences, of a polar kind among themselves. Not only were these perceived as existing between two individuals but clear divisions among all the members occurred. This was especially notable in both adult groups with regard to the degree of inhibition and reserve felt by some members and the almost total freedom of instinctual expression in others. Members expressed the wish that the inhibited could be more liberated and that the impulsive could gain control. Thus the group set its own therapeutic aims as a social norm against which their own personalities were mirrored, and any progress assessed.

Members were encouraged to talk about their experiences of exposure and the active wishes to repeat this. Controlling these desires was vital as nearly all of them were on probation and a breach meant possible detention. It took quite some time before the urges could be brought under control and several members of all three groups exposed themselves during treatment. In three cases the magistrates in their wisdom imposed fines, and allowed them to continue treatment, but two adolescents were sent away after further repetitions.

Acting out of exhibitionist urges appeared to cease when the patient had reached a certain level of ability to verbalize his instinctual urges and had some feelings of security in the therapeutic relationship which was set up. In the group, numerous minor symbolic exhibitionist acts occurred all the time and became interpreted by the members themselves as such. The energies released became cathected to the group situation. Patients reported how they found themselves thinking more and more about the group between sessions; some could use thoughts of the group to control urges to expose themselves.

At a later stage a group transference phenomenon called complementation was displayed. This term has been used by Foulkes and Antony (1957) in their description of their own groups and of Kreitman's work with 'murderous mothers' at the Maudsley Hospital, and refers to the way in which members reacted in a lock and key fashion with each other's psychopathology. Tom for instance would have lengthy provocative arguments with Richard, who was also a transvestite, and whose father had been so actively hostile as to break his brother's arm in an altercation. Richard had retreated into a feminine identification on these grounds. In the group Richard was afraid of Tom possibly losing control of himself and becoming violent, in the way that Richard's father had behaved. He would withdraw and act passively when he felt threatened, but in time learned to stand up to Tom verbally. Simultaneously, Tom could feel chastened and controlled by interpretations which revealed that he was goading Richard in much the same way as he had acted towards his own father, whom he regarded as a moral coward. Tom stopped exhibiting but acted out his wish to be beaten. He reported how he stood up in a local cinema full of cat-calling Teddy-boys and told them to shut up. To his surprise and disappointment, they did. The operation of these dimensions of activity–passivity, masculinity–femininity, aggression–love and control–lack of control, acting through the Oedipus complex, was instructive.

One of the effects of the complementation was an intensification of the transference towards the therapist, thus incidentally allowing for further interpretation of the transference relationship and for increased therapeutic potentialities. An excellent example of this is given in the report of the full session above, where Tom, having expressed the sort of resentment already described, turned his hostility on to the therapist, allowing the same interpretations to be made in the group situation.

There are certain advantages in treating groups composed of patients with a single shared diagnosis or instinctual proclivity such as exhibitionism. These are the greater ease with which polarities of identification and difference in personality traits can be delineated; the reciprocal facilitation between this delineation and complementation phenomena; an increased intensity of group transference in affective or feeling terms; and the establishment of clear group ideals of behaviour as attainable norms.

Much of the aggressive behaviour and actual exposure was also a defence against the feminine identification with mother and thus also against homosexuality. Overt homosexual feelings became prominent and were interpreted in the first group. This seemed to contribute materially to the dissolution of the group as too great anxieties were aroused. Interpretation of these feelings, although present, were studiously avoided in the second group. Both Slavson (1954, 1956) and Hadden (1958) found that homosexuals tended to create either too much disruption and anxiety in groups, or dropped out themselves because of difficulties in discussing their problems. Litman (1961) found that one or two sexual deviants could be successfully treated in a neurotic group provided that there were women present; the feminine reactions served to buffer the rest of the group against excessive anxiety about male homosexuality. In the first group, the need for women to be introduced was specifically requested by one member, Peter, at the time when homosexual anxieties were mounting, and he was openly expressing homosexual advances to the therapist in the transference based on experiences with his brother. Unfortunately the group could not be reconstituted with female members as this would have broken the conditions of the research setting. In any case, in the group transference, feminine roles were projected on to the therapist, so that the request for female members was a resistance to the analysis of the homosexuality aroused. Thus Peter, who was highly intelligent, used defences of intellectualization and rationalized his exhibitionism as sexual advances made in a sexually inhibited abnormal society. His condition would disappear, he argued, if free love were instituted. He was a well-controlled voyeur and exhibitionist who had never been caught and came voluntarily for treatment. He used his considerable powers of argument aggressively in the group in a subtle way to maintain his superiority, leadership and narcissism. When this was analysed by the group, he lost the leadership of the group, showed immature dependency reactions and threatened to leave. This was a repetition of his emotional relationships which had always been superficial, and which had led to an estrangement with his wife to whom he verbally exhibited his sexual difficulties in a sado-masochistic way. He gained considerable maturity, and ability to feel, through the group, and at follow-up two years later reported no overt exposures, some sexual difficulties of an immature kind, and a working towards greater maturity in relationship with women (see follow-up letter).

Strange as it may seem, it was possible to deal indirectly with their sexuality a great deal of the time by discussing the patients' aggression. *This functional equivalence of exhibitionism for the expression of aggression is noteworthy.* John attended both groups, and from being quiet and retiring in the first group later became the dominant personality. The rivalry for leadership in the group was a transference of oedipal and sibling relationships, and was analysed as such, first by the therapist and then actively by the members themselves.

The role of the therapist was emulated in patients' active attempts to help and understand each other. Thus in the second adult group Harry, aged 21, who had never known his father and was brought up in a completely feminine environment with his mother and several aunts, formed a strong attachment to the therapist. His exposures were deliberate and the source of great pleasure. He travelled 40 miles to the group, and after treating all the members with disdain began to take an interest in helping the most inhibited members and being actively hostile to John, the family man. Both these affectionate and aggressive impulses were worked through and he became a charming and sympathetic person, who married during the course of treatment and lost all his wishes to expose himself. In his case the therapist provided an ideal male figure on whom he could model himself and with whom he could identify, thus filling the gap of the absent father in his childhood; while John the family man was used to express his hostility towards the absent father. In his follow-up letter he described a return of urges to expose during a severe depression, but no exposures resulted.

Perhaps the greatest technical problem of an out-patient group of sexual deviates is how to keep the group alive from the point of view of membership. Immature, impulsive, pleasure-seeking individuals are notoriously irregular in any social behaviour. That the groups survived as long as they did was gratifying; and due to unceasing interpretations by the therapist, efforts on the part of the psychiatric social worker, who sat in as an observer, and due to the close contacts with the respective probation officers, and the patients' families. If a patient missed two sessions without apology, a letter was sent to him; if he missed three, a letter went to his probation officer. (For further information on the role of the probation officer in the treatment of sexual deviants, see below.) It was thought wiser to have a closed group, even though members were down to two on occasion, than a continuous open group with regular newcomers, in order to gain a sense of personality definition among the members. Further, certain patients would not continue treatment after their 1-year condition of treatment was over; others had to move out of London or found it difficult to attend for a variety of reasons. Thus towards the end of both groups the numbers had dwindled. This put a great strain on those present, and was reflected in Richard's leaving the group. It was generally felt that many of the patients would have benefited from further group treatment; hence John was included in the second group, although it made for some technical difficulties. This raises the question of whether a pre-scribed period of 1 year as a condition of treatment is wise; in all groups voluntary attendance was stressed in that even if patients were on a probation order with a condition of treatment, if they did not want to attend for group therapy voluntarily, other treatment would be found for them. These issues were amongst the earliest faced in the group. What can better determine growth towards maturity than the issues of free choice in a social setting or an interpersonal relationship?

The adolescents presented the greatest difficulties, both with regard to regularity of attendance and their extremes of shyness, inhibition, or acting out of instinctual drives. In general, when there was a good attendance for any regular period, say a few weeks, they would find the session enjoyable, talk amiably about their interests and girl-friends and gain a feeling of support from the group solidarity. But due to the small numbers of available cases, it was not possible to constitute a good regular out-patient group. It was impossible with these means for certain members under strong emotional stress to maintain control of their sexual urges, and although they were offered individual treatment two were finally sent to borstal. Acting out of exhibitionist and aggressive anti-authoritarian wishes through dangerous driving, especially on motor bikes, was noted and required interpretation to avoid serious personal injuries resulting. Certain inhibited members did extremely well, but nevertheless one is forced to conclude that out-patient group treatment for adolescent sexual offenders requires very special conditions and that individual therapy is preferable.

Many of the inhibited adolescents gained great benefit from regular personal contact with their probation officers. This would be a treatment of choice in certain cases where there is immaturity, a need for identification with a strong but helpful male figure, and relatively minor sexual behaviour of an exploratory kind in a first offender.

Results

The results of treatment and follow-up in individual cases are listed together with other details of the history in Table 6.1.

Most psychiatric follow-up studies utilize either the morbidity figures of hospital re-admissions or responses to postal enquiries. In dealing with criminal cases, assessments are usually made on a basis of subsequent convictions. In this study wherever possible letters were sent to both the patient and the probation officer. The follow-up date denotes responses to the last communications sent.

Some of the difficulties in completing accurate follow-up studies with out-patient delinquents are as follows.

Patients who have been placed on a probation order, or treated as a condition of probation laid down by the court, often cease treatment once these terms have been complied with, and wish to put the whole experience behind them. Efforts to communicate with patients by letter or personal visits are then resented as intrusions into their personal privacy. A letter enquiring for follow-up details may be socially disastrous as it reveals past problems which may have been successfully hidden from intimates.

At the end of treatment, all patients were instructed that if they felt the danger of exhibitionistic lapses they should report for further help. In court referred cases, with subsequent offences, the probation officer is usually made aware of this fact, or the Clinic is asked for a report of previous treatment if the case comes up in a new court. Thus where no further communications were received from patients and probation officers were unaware of further difficulties, it was presumed that the patient had not been convicted of a further offence; though it must be admitted that in some cases urges to exhibit and even occasional acts of exhibitionism might occur in a 'satisfactory' case where supervision had ceased. Usually, however, lapses were brought to the notice of some authority.

Differences in the quality of improvement are hard to assess in a statistical manner. Thus in some cases, real personality improvements had taken place although occasional lapses in response to severe situational stress had occurred. Two patients married, and eight showed greatly improved relationships at home and at work.

The letters that follow, written by four patients and edited to preserve anonymity, are examples of the quality of improvement.

1. Your letter has just been forwarded to me, and I will answer it in the form of a report on the case with which we were concerned. I expect you will agree that this is quite appropriate as we are dealing with the matter by correspondence. You will understand that the subject's feelings about the case, and many of the details, will not come across in a report of this kind.

The subject now feels that the complex of behaviour and desires with which you are familiar has become integrated into his personality in a somewhat matured form, and no longer has the dissociated compulsive character that it had before. It is matured in the sense that, (i) he no longer feels these desires towards girls of pre-adolescent age, (ii) he initiates a friendly relationship with girls from this age onward, whereas previously the behaviour manifested itself in a 'social vacuum', and (iii) the specific behaviour characteristic of the case now occurs, if at all, after several weeks during which the subject plays with the young girl – and her friends if she is with them – and takes the opportunity, while for example helping them climb trees, etc. – of fondling her in an affectionate but discreet manner. In fact, on only one occasion in the last six months, has there been anything more than this fondling, and that took the form of 'wanting to go to the toilet' in some bushes after telling the girls so that she could keep away. In fact the subject reports that the 14-year-old girl on this occasion looked covertly at him while he was semi-concealed behind a bush, and this excited him to the point of ejaculation with very little manual stimulation. The subject and the girl went on picking berries, as before, without the situation having apparently proved traumatic. After that occasion the girl was always with friends on the few occasions when the subject met her, and circumstances effectively terminated the relationship.

At present, the subject has no similar involvement, but reports that he has seen a very well-developed girl of 14 or thereabouts with whom he would like to establish the same sort of relationship.

Table 6.1 Results of treatment and follow-up of cases of exhibitionism treated with individual group therapy

Name and age	Marital status	I.Q.	Exhibitionism				Treatment		
			Frequency	Offences	Other symptom manifestations	Previous treatments	Portman Clinic Psychotherapy Sessions		
							Individual	Group
John (41)	M.	115	3 times	Indecent exposure	Nil	Nil	Nil	64
Donald (28)	M.		Frequently for years	Indecent behaviour	Psychopathic personality Chronic masturbation	Nil	Nil	22
Tom (25)	M.	126		Enclosed premises Stealing. Indecent exposure × 2		Nil	Nil	24
Peter (30)	M.	125 +	Frequently		Character disorder	Nil	Nil	27
David (24)	S.	108	Frequently	Indecent exposure 8 previous offences	Nil	Nil	Nil	10
Richard (37)	M.	100	Frequently	Masquerading as female prostitute Indecent exposure × 2	Transvestite. Passive homosexual	Nil	Nil	25
Bill (36)	M.	93	Frequently	13 previous convictions 2 × indecent exposure, voyeurism 3 × stealing, assault	Uncontrolled aggression	Nil	Nil	5
Michael (29)	S.	100	Frequently	Care and Protection Indecent exposure × 2	Immature personality	Nil	Nil	6
James (29)	M.	104	Occasionally	Indecent exposure. Insulting behaviour	Nil	Nil	Nil	18
Eric (23)	S.	119	3 times	Indecent exposure × 2	Nil	Nil	Nil	11
George (23)	S.	122	Very frequently	Indecent exposure	Immature personality	Nil	Nil	32

| Results | Follow-up | | | Final result |
	Duration after treatment	Patient	Probation officer	
Recovered	18 months	No reply	Satisfactory work and home conditions. No repetitions	Symptom free. Personality improvement
Improved +	6 months	No reply		Improved
Improved + +	16 months			Improved
Improved + +	18 months	Greatly improved		Improved
Improved +	36 months	Married, recovered		Recovered
Improved	24 months	No reply		Improved (slightly)
Unchanged	18 months	No reply	Personality difficulties a great handicap. No further sexual exposures	Personality unchanged. Improved
Improved	36 months	Greatly improved. Stable at work. No repetitions		Recovered
Improved + Discontinued treatment	18 months	No reply	No further contact after 1 year condition of probation and treatment	Improved
Improved + +	18 months	No reply	Improved	Improved
Married. Improved + +	12 months	?	Satisfactory	Improved

Table 6.1 *(continued)*

Name and age	Marital status	I.Q.	Exhibitionism		Other Symptom manifestations	Treatment		
			Frequency	Offences		Previous treatments	Portman Clinic Psychotherapy Sessions	
							Individual	Group
Harry (26)	S.	119	Frequently	Larceny Indecent exposure	Nil	Nil	Nil	20
Roger (26)	M.	99	Frequently	Indecent exposure	Nil	Sedatives	Nil	39
Stephen (15)	S.	124	12 times in 6 months	Indecent exposure × 2	Enuresis	Nil	Nil	6
Dennis (15)	S.	108	Frequently	Breaking and entering Indecent exposure larceny	Immature personality	Nil	Nil	34
Jack (16)	S.	103	Once	Indecent exposure	Immature personality	Nil	Nil	23
Keith (15)	S.	116	Frequently	Indecent exposure. Care Committee	Behaviour disorder	Psychotherapy	Nil	10
Don (16)	S.	115	Frequently	Larceny × 3	Enuresis	Nil	Nil	24
Rupert (19)	S.	109	9 times	Indecent exposure	Immature personality	Nil	11	Nil
Max (38)	W.	116	Frequently	Indecent exposure × 4	Severely emotionally disturbed	Psychotherapy	8	Nil
Robert (53)	M.	108	Twice	Indecent exposure	Nil	Nil	5	Nil
Leonard (16)	S.	106	Frequently	Indecent exposure	Immature personality	Nil	18	Nil
Joe (49)	M.		Frequently	Indecent exposure × 2	Uncontrollable aggression	Nil	11	Nil
Ralph (46)	M.		Frequently	Indecent exposure	Nil	Stilboestrol	23	Nil

| Results | Follow-up | | | Final result |
	Duration after treatment	Patient	Probation Officer	
Improved +	18 months	No reply		Improved
Improved + +	18 months	No reply	Satisfactory	Improved
Improved	24 months		'Completely adjusted'	Greatly improved
Improved	24 months	Continued treatment at another clinic. Further minor traffic offences. Personality greatly improved	Two further episodes of masturbation in public, and, in a state of depression	Greatly improved personality. Better sexual adjustment, two offences of exposure
Greatly improved	24 months		Personality developed considerably, Satisfactory	Greatly improved
Committed to Approved School	36 months		Indecent exposure Shopbreaking Still in need of treatment	Unchanged
Personality Improved Larceny committed to Borstal	24 months		Made good progress at Borstal. Released	Borstal. Improved
Greatly improved	24 months	Nil	Nil	Improved
Remarried. Improved				Improved
Greatly improved	24 months	Nil	Highly satisfactory	Greatly improved
Greatly improved	24 months	Nil	Satisfactory	Greatly improved
I.S.Q. Indecent exposure		Admitted to hospital for in-patient psychotherapy	Improved by stay in hospital	Relapsed. In-patient treatment with improvement
Greatly improved				Greatly improved

The subject feels that this sort of emotional involvement grades into his (by social standards) 'normal' sexual desire for older females, being only modified at the lower age-levels by social sanctions against more complete physical inter-course with young girls, and by the natural and learned restraint of girls of this age, which only force or psychological compulsion on the part of the subject would overcome. As you know, neither of these expedients has the slightest appeal to this particular subject.

From economic reasons, the subject is living a rather limited social life at present, and has not yet found a woman of what he would regard as a suitable age for the kind of intimate friendship he most enjoys – a woman of about 25 years. He reports that he had just such a relationship before going abroad, though it was unfortunately brief because of that. In the past few weeks there has been an unsatisfactory affair with an 18-year-old girl: unsatisfactory because of the extreme difference of interests and the refusal of the girl to allow the natural process of foreplay leading to sexual intercourse to proceed very far. Again, before going abroad, the subject met and had coitus on one occasion with a 17-year-old girl, who was unable to respond or experience pleasure in the act because of frigidity which she said was habitual. The subject wonders whether there is some objective characteristic of the, shall we say, 15–20 age group, perhaps connected with the war, which accounts for the difficulty he has in establishing satisfactory social or sexual contact with them. He contrasts this with the rather parental, though strongly sexual, affectionate feeling he has for girls up to about 15 from puberty, and with the egalitarian affection he can feel for women over about 20, again with a sexual component, of course.

As regards his marriage, the subject reports that his wife has hardened towards him after the long separation, and there is no feeling of love or affection between them. Perhaps a divorce will be arranged eventually.

In summary, the subject feels that he is now at least a whole personality, even though social sanctions make it necessary to be discreet about one aspect of it.

2. I have received your letter and felt that I should like to write back, first I am feeling quite well at present, I have not had any treatment since my last attendance at the clinic, as regards to being any better, let's say I am not any worse, although in all fairness, I must say that in my wife's opinion she thinks I was better for the treatment, myself I would not like to say. I feel that I was not getting anywhere, at the time I was attending the group was breaking up fast. There was only two of us there, I felt very awkward to say the least, and if you remember at the time, I did not stay, and left early. At first I was not fully aware of what the treatment entailed, but I am willing to try anything, if I thought it would be to my advantage. At the time I do feel that I was not getting anywhere, but that of course is only my opinion, you people know more about these things than I do. At least I am grateful for all you

have done for me, I know it must mean a lot of work. I think the best thing I can do is to leave it to you to decide which you think is best for me, I am willing to try anything. I have not had any further trouble with the basic problem, but I know myself that I am far from cured shall we say. I still have these urges, although my wish to be feminine is far greater, I notice this in all the things I do, this seems to be my greatest problem at present. I am wondering if any of the others are still attending. However, I will leave things as they are at the moment, hoping that this will be some guide to you.

3. I'm sorry to have kept you waiting for a reply to your letter, as you know it was always one of my faults to keep postponing things and, as you can see, I haven't changed much.

I have been debating whether to write you, as about a month ago I had been going through a rather depressing period and I had the old feeling coming back. Although I never exposed myself, I thought about it several times, and only fear of the consequences saved me.

This depression was due to my wife and I having a rather upsetting period. Being rather young, she misses her work and freedom, and what with now having a baby to care for, she gets very irritable and I'm on the receiving end.

I find it very hard not to give up, and if it weren't for the baby I think I would. I am still looking for the unobtainable in life, work and women. All pretty women still attract me, and if I had the chance to be unfaithful I would. When I am out on my own I still get that wonderful sense of freedom, and its times like these when the desire to expose myself is greatest.

I think what I miss most of all is the chance to discuss these things and if there was the opportunity of joining another group, I would, willingly.

4. Many thanks for your letter dated 17th of this month.

I will answer it the best way I can, because I am no authority on the matter in question.

Incidently, did you get my phone message last Wednesday evening? If you didn't it was to inform you that all letters are answered by me on Sunday mornings only, as I am fully engaged during the week.

Now to answer your letter. You say, you hope I am feeling well, thanks a lot. I am in great form at the moment, only wish there were more than 24 hours in a day, then I could get some more of my private work attended to. But my Sect. thinks otherwise.

The treatments you are giving are causing some anxiety, so I gather from your letter, as to whether it is doing any good to people and if it has, to what extent. Well as far as I am concerned, it had little value, that is why I stopped coming along and what is more I am glad I did, because I wanted to and I succeeded in doing, conquering this whole problem on my own, I started doing it, I stopped it, and I will tell you how. When I stopped coming along to the meetings, I did so because I wanted to spend more time at music and forget the past, but build up a future, which I am still doing. Coupled with this, I have grown up mentally and act more like a man than a child. I have become hard in many ways, mixed with people (except those not connected with music) gone out with one or two girls.

If I felt like relieving myself, I lie on my bed and do so, with the aid of a picture of a half naked girl. I don't let it bother me. If I started doing it in front of girls again it most certainly would. That's all there is I can say. I am going out with my girl friend at the moment, I have never touched her because we hope to get engaged at Christmas, not only that, we are always talking about Modern Jazz.

Group treatment

Thirteen adult patients attended two groups with an average attendance of twenty-three sessions each. All except two patients had been before the courts. Eight could be classified as recidivists, four of whom had been convicted of additional non-sexual offences such as stealing or assault. All thirteen cases were of the phobic-impulsive type, seven were mainly phobic and six mainly impulsive.

Follow-up studies on these thirteen cases revealed that there was an average follow-up period of 20 months after cessation of treatment, at which date no known convictions had occurred. Fitch (1962) examined men convicted of sexual offences against children. Fifty per cent of reconvictions (30 cases out of 59) for sexual and other offences took place within 19 months over a 79-month survey period. The ability of patients to remain without indictment for 20 months or more, therefore has some prognostic significance. It was thought that urges to perform exhibitionistic or other indictable acts were possibly still present in four patients, but under control. In the others, these had apparently ceased.

There is no doubt that analytical group psychotherapy is efficacious in the treatment of the adult severe phobic-compulsive exhibitionist. It was generally felt that treatment for a longer average period than 6 months was required.

Mathis and Collins (1970) and Truax (1970) emphasize the importance of treating sexual deviants in a group consisting of people with similar problems, where the shared needs and experiences can be utilized to dissolve the defence mechanisms of rationalization, isolation, and denial. A similar group approach with serious sex offenders in Broadmoor is described by Cox in Chapter 12.

Adolescent group

Five patients aged 15–16 attended the group. Attendances were irregular and the results on the whole were uneven and unsatisfactory. Two boys with inhibited personalities obtained great benefit, while the three remaining were compulsive in type and had committed other offences, although two of them showed great personality improvement as a result of later individual psychotherapy. In these three boys, there was a change in the type of offence to that of a compulsive non-sexual kind, in two of stealing, and in the other of reckless motor cycling.

One must therefore conclude that whereas group psychotherapy can help the inhibited shy adolescent, it is of little benefit to the compulsive instinct-ridden patient. For these, intensive analytic psychotherapy and close supervision would be required. Reality difficulties with the parents are often great obstacles to treatment in these boys.

Individual analytical psychotherapy

Six patients were treated with weekly analytical psychotherapy for an average attendance of twenty-one sessions. All were referred by the courts and except for one patient they had exposed themselves frequently.

In all but one case they lost all urges for exposure and there have been no notifications of relapse after a 2-year follow-up period. In the single case who relapsed, in-patient psychotherapy was later given with improvement.

An attempt has been made in this chapter to correlate the psychiatric and psychoanalytic approaches to this problem. Although the call is always for more research into pathology and treatment, society must keep up with the advances in knowledge that have already been made. There is now much evidence that with skilled psychotherapeutic care, many exhibitionists and voyeurs can be relieved of the torture of compulsion and avoid the shame of social sanctions and imprisonment. The costs of providing such skilled help as against the costs of custodial care and suffering to others are difficult to evalute, but as exhibitionism has one of the highest recidivist rates of all sexual offences, medical opinion and possible therapy should be sought early. Unfortunately not all eclectic treatment which passes for psychotherapy is of the same order, or of a level to help such persons.

References

Allen, D. W. (1974). *The fear of looking*. Bristol.

Ambrose, J. A. (1961). The development of the smiling response in early infancy. In *Determinants of infant behaviour* (ed. B. M. Foss). London.

Arieff, A. J., and Rotman, D. B. (1942). 100 cases of indecent exposure, *J. nerv. ment. Dis.* **96**, 523.

Bauer, G. (1970). *Kriminalistik* **24**, 145.

Bond, I. K., and Hutchison, H. C. (1960). Application of reciprocal inhibition therapy for exhibitionism. *Canad. med. Ass. J.* **83**, 23.

Christoffel, H. (1936). Exhibitionism and exhibitionists. *Int. J. Psycho-Anal.* **17**, 321.
—— (1956). Male genital exhibitionism. In *Perversions: Psychodynamics and Therapy* (ed. S. Lorand and M. Balint). New York.

de Monchy, R. (1952). Oral components of the castration complex. *Int. J. Psycho-Anal.* **33**, 450.

Ellis, H. (1935). *Psychology of sex*. New York.

Evans, D. R. (1968). Masturbatory fantasy and sexual deviation. *Behav. Res. Ther.* **6**, 17.
—— (1970). Subjective variables and treatment effects in aversion therapy. *Behav. Res. Ther.* **8**, 147.

Fenichel, O. (1931). Antecedents of the Oedipus complex. In *Collected Papers*. London.
—— (1945). *The psychoanalytical theory of neurosis*. New York.
—— (1954). The scoptophilic instinct and identification. In *Collected Papers*. London.

Fitch, J. H. (1962). Men convicted of sexual offences against children. *Brit. J. Crim.* **3**, 18.

Fookes, B. H. (1969). Some experiences in the use of aversion therapy in male homosexuality, exhibitionism and fetishism-transvestism. *Brit. J. Psychiat.* **115**, 339.

Ford, C. S., and Beach, F. A. (1952). *Patterns of sexual behaviour*. London.

Foulkes, S. H., and Anthony, E. J. (1957). *Group psychotherapy*. London.

Freud, S. (1900). The interpretation of dreams. *Complete psychological works of Sigmund Freud*, Standard edition **4**. London.
—— (1905). Three essays on sexuality, *Complete psychological works of Sigmund Freud*, Standard edition **7**. London.

Garnier, P. (1900). Perversion sexuelles, comptes rendus. *Congrès International de Médecine.*

Gebhard, P. H. (1965). *Sex offenders*. New York.

Glasser, M. (1978). The role of the super-ego in exhibitionism. *Int. J. Psychoanal. Psychother.* In press.

Greenacre, P. (1952). Pre-genital patterning. *Int. J. Psycho-Anal.* **33**, 410.

Hadden, S. B. (1958). Treatment of homosexuality by individual and group psychotherapy. *Amer. J. Psychiat.*, **114**, 810.

Hirning, L. C. (1947). Genital exhibitionism: an interpretive study. *J. clin. Psychopath.* **8**, 557.

Hirschfield, M. (1936). *Sexual anomalies and perversions.* London.

Jones, I. H. and Frei, D. (1977). Provoked anxiety as a treatment of exhibitionism. *Brit. J. Psychiat.* **131**, 295.

Karpman, B. (1925). The sexual offender. *Psychoanal. Rev.* **12**, 151.
—— (1948). The psychopathology of exhibitionism; review of the literature. *J. clin. Psychopath.* **9**, 179.

Kinsey, A. C., Pomeroy, W. B., and Martin, C. E. (1948). *Sexual behaviour in the human male.* Philadelphia and London.

Krafft-Ebing, R. v. (1906). *Psychopathia sexualis.* New York and London.

Lasègue, C. (1877). Les exhibitionnistes. *L'Union Mèdicale, troisième série* **23**, 709.

Litman, R. E. (1961). Psychotherapy of a homosexual man in a heterosexual group. *Int. J. Gr. Psychother.* **11**, 440.

MacLay, D. T. (1952). The diagnosis and treatment of compensatory types of indecent exposures. *Brit. J. Delinq.* **3**, 34.

Maeder, A. (1909). Sexualitat und epilepsy (exhibitionismus). *Jb. Psychoanal. Psychopath.* Vol. I.

Mathis, J. L. and Collins, M. (1970). Mandatory group therapy for exhibitionists. *Amer. J. Psychiat.* **126**, 1162.

Maguire, R. J., Carlisle, J. H., and Young, B. G. (1965). Sexual deviation as conditioned behaviour: a hypothesis. *Behav. Res. Ther.* **2**, 185.

Mohr, J. W., Turner, R. E., and Jerry, M. B. (1964). *Paedophilia and exhibitionism.* Toronto.

Petri, H. (1969). Exhibitionismus: Theoretische und soziale Aspekte und die Behandlungs mit Antiandrogen. *Nervenarzt* **40**, 220.

Radzinowicz, L. and Turner, J. W. C. (1957). *English studies in criminal science,* Vol. 9, *Sexual Offences.* London.

Rickles, N. K. (1950). *Exhibitionism.* London.

Rognant, J. (1965). Exhibitionnisme et deconditionnement. *Ann. méd-psychol.* **123**, 169.

Rooth, F. G. (1973). Exhibitionism, sexual violence and paedophilia. *Brit. J. Psychiat.* **122**, 705.
—— (1976). Indecent exposure and exhibitionism. In *Contemporary psychiatry.* Selected reviews from the *British Journal of Hospital Medicine.* (ed. T. Silverstone and B. Barraclough).

Sadger, J. (1921). *Die Lehre von den Geschlechts Verurrungen.* Wien.

Serber, M. (1970). Shame aversion therapy. *J. Behav. Ther. exptl Psychiat.* **1**, 213.

Silverman, D. (1941). Treatment of exhibitionism. *Bull. Menninger Clin.* **5**, 85.

Slavson, S. R. (1954). *Re-educating the delinquent, through group and Community participation.* London.

—— (1956). *Fields of group psychotherapy.* New York.

Sperling, M. (1947). The analysis of an exhibitionist. *Int. J. Psycho-Anal.* **28**, 32.

Stärcke, A. (1921). The castration complex. *Int. J. Psycho-Anal.* **2**, 179.

Stekel, W. (1912). Zur psychologie des exhibitionismus. *Zbl. Psychanal.* **1**, 494.

—— (1920–21). On the psychology of exhibitionism. *Z. Sexualwissenshaft* **7**, 241.

Stephenson, J. and Jones, I. H. (1972). Behaviour therapy technique for exhibitionism. *Archiv. Gen. Psychiat.* **27**, 839.

Strasser, C. (1917). The psychology and forensic consideration of exhibitionism. *Alienist and Neurologist* **38**, 239.

Taylor, F. H. (1947). Observations on some cases of exhibitionism. *J. ment. Sci.* **93**, 631.

Truax, R. A. (1970). Discussion of Mathis and Collins (above). *Am. J. Psychiat.* **126**, 1166.

Wickramasekera, I. (1972). A technique for controlling a certain type of sexual exhibitionism. *Psychother. Theory Res. Pract.* **9**, 207.

Williams, A. H. (1964). The psychopathology and treatment of sexual murderers. In *The pathology and treatment of sexual deviation.* (ed. I. Rosen). London.

Winnicott, D. W. (1958). Transitional objects and transitional phenomena. Chapter in *Collected Papers.* London.

Zavitzianos, G. (1977). More on exhibitionism in women. *Am. J. Psychiat.* **134** (7), 820.

Zuckerman, S. (1932). *Social life of monkeys and apes.* London.

7 Clinical types of homosexuality

A.Limentani

Introduction

In recent years there has become apparent an increasingly marked division in the attitude to homosexuality: at a time when there is a growing tendency for people in all walks of life to regard homosexuality as normal, there remain many who use the term in a derogatory and insulting manner, quite often with an implication of social menace. The view presented in this chapter is that homosexuality is a syndrome, and that it is not sufficient to regard it only as an adjustive process, as was proposed by Sullivan (1955).

With the abolition of the more restrictive of the laws touching on relationships between individuals of the same sex, and the increased permissiveness in contemporary society, it has become apparent that homosexuality remains a condition which may in certain specific instances require treatment.

When treatment is discussed among psychotherapists, opinion is sharply divided; quite apart from doubts and divergent theoretical considerations as to what constitutes homosexuality, views appear to range from unreasonable pessimism to excessive optimism. This state of affairs is particularly unwelcome in a field which demands both co-operation and a multilateral approach to the patient's problem, taking into account that where one form of treatment may fail, another may succeed.

Generally, psychiatrists and psychotherapists are in no position to ignore homosexuality as a syndrome, as it may quite unexpectedly appear as a complicating feature in almost any form of mental illness. For instance, it may be part of the individual's personality and character, and not in the least responsible for behavioural disorders requiring psychiatric assessment; it may be the basic underlying cause of such a condition as alcoholism, or drug addiction; or it may be a complicating factor in a case of neurotic sexual impotence, when psychotherapy will fail to make a real impact unless the homosexual elements have been thoroughly covered.

It must be appreciated, however, that clumsy and tactless attempts to bring into the light less conscious aspects of a patient's sexual orientation may prove quite damaging to the course of any form of psychiatric intervention. The nature and depth of homosexual elements, whether conscious or unconscious, should be of more than passing interest both to the psychiatrist and the psychotherapist. A thorough assessment is imperative in the case of the homosexual who wishes to be rid of the deviation.

It is entirely understandable that any diagnostic attempt in relation to so varied a condition as homosexuality may be met by considerable scepticism or frank disbelief. How could we expect to make sense of a situation where an interest in a person of the same sex (commonly referred to as *homosexuality*) is the only common feature in the cases of the paedophiliac (where the central force is likely to be a narcissistic disturbance), and the man who is pathologically jealous of his wife (who might easily be the victim of unresolved oedipal conflicts)? The psychopathology of sexual deviation is, as has been pointed out in previous chapters, extremely complex, and the aetiology of the homosexual syndrome is unquestionably multifactorial. Readers of the relevant literature, not necessarily psychoanalytical, will be impressed by the fact that each writer tends to have a definite view, and in the end the impression is created of an almost limitless number of clinical conditions. In this presentation, an attempt is made to individuate the more recognizable of such clinical types by using both the psychoanalytic and psychiatric models.

Some clinical types of homosexuality and their specific psychopathology

In purely descriptive terms homosexuality can be repressed, sublimated, fantasied, or manifest. Each sub-division carries its own specific symtomatology, capable of influencing the individual's state of mind, his interpersonal relationships, and his role in society. Repression plays an extremely important role. For instance, repressed homosexual impulses and conflicts may represent the main aetiological factor in sexual impotence and frigidity. When repression is excessive, sublimatory activities will be impaired. When it is ineffective, the deviation may still not be manifest, but derivative patterns of behaviour will appear. Pathological jealousy is a classical example of this, and is well matched by the opposite attitude, that is the wish to share or exchange partners.

The relation of the ineffective repression of homosexual impulses to paranoia was first described by Freud (1911), linking it with the turning of love into hate. It is important to emphasize that Freud indicated that the whole process is latent (unconscious). A criticism of this important psychoanalytic finding disregards its unconscious nature by adducing evidence that a great many persons are paranoid without becoming homosexually orientated (Friedman, Kaplan, and Sadock 1972). This criticism also emphasizes that the majority of homosexuals do not develop paranoid delusions. It is, however, the central point of the thesis put forward in this chapter that the development of homosexual impulses and attitudes can be and often are used as a defence against neurotic and psychotic processes.

Little needs to be said about those cases where homosexual fantasies have broken into consciousness with much suffering and discomfort, but it should never be assumed that this is an indication of confirmed sexual deviation. On the contrary, such fantasies are often a last line of defence against heterosexuality which appears dangerous owing to its association with strong aggressive impulses, and particularly incestuous wishes. The patient's fantasies are a good indication of the effectiveness or failure in all methods of treatment (Marks, Gelder, and Bancroft 1970). Studies which ignore fantasies (Randell 1959) will give an entirely different exposition of the psychopathology of transsexuals, as compared with those studies which have taken them into account (Hoenig, Kerna, and Youd 1970), when they will show the importance of the homosexual element.

In manifest homosexuality, all defensive barriers against the acting-out of deviant impulses have broken down. It is in these cases that accurate assessment becomes a matter of the utmost urgency and importance, as it will guide us towards appropriate treatment or masterly inactivity, as the case may be. The innumerable types of deviation met in the literature, and in clinical practice, can be divided into three ill-defined, yet clearly recognizable groups.

Group I

In this group, manifest deviant behaviour, often associated with compulsive related day-dreaming, aims at preventing the emergence of heterosexuality, and is the presenting symptom in a large number of individuals who are basically latent heterosexuals. Some writers refer to these as pseudo-homosexuals, an unsatisfactory term as it implies a falseness in their state of mind which is not reflected by their feelings. Attachment to members of the same sex is linked with the flight from the opposite sex, which is perceived as being dangerous, threatening, and domineering. Oddly enough, the attempt to deny the very existence of the opposite sex is frequently a sign that one is dealing with latent heterosexuality rather than true deviation. A guideline in differentiating them further from 'true' deviants is guilt, which is almost always present, particularly in those who seek guidance or help. It is necessary to distinguish the guilt derived from external circumstances, social or moral influences, from that derived from unconscious psychopathology, whether it is related to the residual heterosexual conflicts at the root of the deviation, or to the homosexual activity itself.

In early papers, Freud (1905a) recognized that psychoneuroses could exist side by side with manifest perversions, and suggested that heterosexuality had been totally repressed in such cases. The psychopathology will be that of a psychoneurosis; the homosexuality indicates the persistence of a particularly severe oedipal conflict and castration anxiety. The dangers related to the expression of heterosexual impulses are obviously of such a nature that it is not sufficient to rely on the usual neurotic defence mechanisms to ward off fears rooted in the subject's internal world and object relations; the deviation is there to create a citadel, which in practice becomes a prison which affords a degree of security.

Anxious, hysterical or obsessional personalities are common in this clinical type. It is particularly the association of homosexuality and obsessional traits which is likely to produce a picture of shallowness of affect, ruthlessness, and compulsive behaviour, consisting of a constant search for a partner, and rare engagement in sustained or deep relationships. Any attempt at controlling or curtailing the sexual acting-out is followed by an outbreak of anxiety and depression. The depth of character and personality disturbance needs to be assessed carefully as it may affect the outcome of the treatment. The presence of serious obsessive–compulsive traits may defeat all therapeutic efforts.

The following case is fairly representative of a clinical picture with a good prognosis encountered in this group. An intelligent young man with mildly obsessional personality traits had become seriously depressed and suicidal whilst still at university, following disappointment in a homosexual love affair. At the age of $3\frac{1}{2}$, he had been separated from his parents, when he was sent to a war-time nursery in England. This was a severe traumatic incident which coloured all his subsequent relationships, as all human beings were regarded as unfaithful and untrustworthy. He was totally impotent when he first approached a girl, and soon after he became involved with a male homosexual friend. He felt extremely guilty about his sexual activities and agonized over them, but he relentlessly continued to importune his friend who eventually showed little interest in and no affection for him. He responded well to psychoanalysis and after it was ended he married, had children, and had a very successful career. After ten years there has been no recurrence of homosexual interests. It is worth noting here that once the homosexual attachment could be analysed and understood within the transference relationship, his condition did not differ from that of a classical straightforward psychoneurosis capable of responding well to psychotherapy.

The occurrence of homosexual behaviour as a substitute symptom has been described in the literature (Thorner 1949), and is of considerable clinical interest when the possibility of removing it is a real one. This writer reports that in the course of treatment, and concurrent with a period of sexual abstinence, a young patient developed a status asthmaticus. This symptom was linked with conflicts over aggression and was quite troublesome, until he convinced himself that he was homosexual and acted on that belief. The relationship between sexual deviation and certain psychomatic states, such as ulcerative colitis, is very obscure. Many observers have reported on the occurrence of haemorrhoids quite suddenly in the midst of a homosexual conflict.

Group II

This group includes all cases of 'true' perversion when the disturbance is deep, and the defence against heterosexuality seems almost of secondary importance. Depression is a common presenting symptom with or without periodicity, but conscious guilt is generally absent. Careful investigation will readily show that the homosexuality is employed as a massive defence mechanism, aimed at warding off overwhelming separation and psychotic anxieties, a dread of mutilation and even disintegration. Bizarre acting-out, marked identification with the opposite sex, promiscuity, and a preference for very brief contacts with partners, associated with a tendency to congregate in public lavatories, is sometimes suggestive of a prepsychotic condition or even psychosis. 'True' deviants seek treatment for reasons such as difficulties arising at work or in personal relationships, and occasionaly because of some offence which has involved them in court proceedings. They specifically ask that nothing be done to change their sexual orientation. Focal therapy may appear indicated, but in practice it is difficult to carry out because of the interaction between the sexual maladjustment and other ego disturbances. It is therefore essential that, before under-taking any form of treatment, due notice be taken of the value attached by the patient to the deviation in fighting off loneliness, isolation, alienation, and aggressiveness.

There are three identifiable clinical types:

Narcissistic disorders of character and personality are very commonly found in homosexuals of both sexes included in this group, where paedo-philiacs are largely represented. The history will often show the pre-sence of psychological disturbance in the parents, severe deprivation, and traumatic experiences. There is a tendency to seek partners, younger or of a similar age, but frequently the need to protect and to be protected, to nurse and to be nursed is the primal force in these associations (Freud 1910). The search for a narcissistic love object may even induce a man to look for a partner who is overtly antagonistic to homosexuality, as he may also be (Khan 1970). Phallic over-valuation is the rule, with loss of self-esteem and a readiness to feel hurt and injured. A double deviation is present when a man is both homosexual and paedophiliac.

Homosexuality as a defence against severe depressive states is probably much more common than is generally recognized. The diagnosis is difficult as the presence of reactive depression, which responds to superficial intervention,. hides the true nature of the problem. Early traumas, sudden deaths in the family, or separation and divorce of parents in infancy are valuable diagnostic pointers. Some writers see the behaviour of homosexuals who struggle with the threat of severe depression as a solution of the past conflict over weaning, which is felt as not only a narcissistic injury, but also a blow to the infantile omnipotence (Bergler 1951).

In the male, unbearable depressive thoughts and feelings, probably originating in very early infancy, make it possible for him to have physical contact with any woman as the penis is experienced as a thoroughly bad part of his body (Rosenfeld 1949). Marked passivity in sexual relations serves the purpose of recovering the lost potency and acquiring something good. At times, the only safeguard against psychotic depression, apathy and despair is to become and act the part of the good mother to the partner (Khan 1970).

The serious consequence arising from the sudden failure of the homosexual solution aimed at alleviating depressive feelings can be seen in the following case history. A young woman was referred because of violent rages, in the course of which she was dangerous both to herself and a woman companion. The destructive outbursts of violence had begun after the breakdown of a long-standing lesbian relationship. She had suffered from recurrent depressive attacks for many years and had been very promiscuous. In the course of extended assessment interviews she recognized that she had used her compulsive lesbian activities as the 'cure' for her unbearable depression, as she could rely on sliding into a state of mild euphoria after successful sexual exploits. At the time of the referral she longed for the woman who had jilted her to come back, and her woman companion (a non-practising lesbian) was gradually becoming the object of her hatred and murderous feelings. Admission to hospital was the only solution.

Homosexuality as a defence against paranoid anxieties and related states. The turning of hatred into love can be found in early and late psycho-analytic writings (Freud 1920, 1923; Nunberg 1938). Glover (1938) has also noted that a perversion will involve the use of libidinization and idealization of the object as a defence against aggression and anxiety, whilst Freeman (1955) has drawn attention to the psychotic quality of the fears and the castration anxiety experienced by the true homosexual in relation to men and women alike. Projection dominates the emotional life of a certain type of homosexual, bringing some relief but much confusion. This defence mechanism implies the throwing out of unwanted or dangerous parts of oneself, which will fill the environment with a host of threatening and persecutory objects to be dealt with by the appeasement implicit in homosexual acts and relationships (Klein 1932; Rosenfield 1949). In certain cases, it is clear that behind the phallic preoccupation and castration anxiety there is a marked fear of the loss of individual identity and of total disintegration. In cases where severe paranoid anxiety is hidden beneath a manifest homosexuality, hostile and greedy oral impulses are directed against authority figures and partners, turning them into retaliatory figures. On the other hand, these men will appease by submitting to anal intercourse and reassure themselves by fellatio about the destructiveness of their biting and devouring impulses.

Not infrequently, the deviation which presents as a simple neurosis or as a sexual disorder attributable to biological forces, conceals a fully fledged paranoid schizophrenia (Socarides 1970). Even when paranoid anxieties have erupted into florid schizophrenia, in spite of manifest homosexual activities, the perversion acts as a brake on the threatened acting out of murderous impulses. This was seen very clearly in the following case. A 24-year-old man had been a compulsive homosexual for as long as he could remember. He would roam the streets at night looking for a 'victim', someone who could tolerate his castrating anus. He came for treatment because of his uncontrollable rages at work, where he would break furniture or get involved in violent fights with fellow workers. At intervals he would experience vivid auditory hallucinations associated with his homosexual 'victims'. During the hallucinatory episodes, he would seek hospital care voluntarily, as he would no longer trust his homosexual acting-out to protect him against killing someone. It is difficult not to believe that this might well have happened in the absence of such an outlet.

Group III

This group includes all those cases of actual (as opposed to fantasied) bisexual behaviour which occur in situations of stress, prisons, and special social and cultural surroundings. Psychiatrists are often under pressure to regard this abnormal behaviour as merely the result of contingency, which is hardly the case. However, in recent times, cases of 'false' actual bisexuality have become fairly prevalent amongst some young or even middle-aged persons, who are searching for new experiences; there will be no difficulty in distinguishing these from the genuine cases, as the feelings associated with the acting-out are wholly egodystonic.

Psychopathic disturbances are prevalent in the male whilst immaturity is a dominant feature in the female. Both sexes will exhibit a profound tendency towards dependency in relation to mother or her substitutes; as a rule, there is a severe dissociation between the female and male parts of the personality, aggravated by very active projections, splitting processes, and multiple identifications. Many studies tend to concentrate on the examination of the perversion, taking the heterosexuality for granted, in spite of the obvious lack of gratification and serious disturbances present in this particular area.

Actively bisexual individuals can of course create a very striking impression of being unable to choose between a heterosexual and a homosexual object. However, a careful analysis of all that is involved will reveal that whilst longing for an idealized father to rescue them from an impossible predicament, in their dealings with their love attachments, these men and women seek to re-enact an anaclitic and narcissistic type of object relating (Limentani 1976). The sudden removal or unavailability of either sexual outlet is known to cause severe depression and to have precipitated suicidal acts.

Discussion

There is considerable danger in attempting to classify clinical types by forcing them into diagnostic categories. Provided, however, that the classification is not applied rigidly, it may prove of value in deciding the most suitable treatment, bearing in mind a number of eventualities. For instance, some neurotic patients included in the latent hetero-sexual group will occasionally show the familiar picture of phobic anxiety or of a compulsive symptom covering up a psychotic illness. Equally the homosexuality linked with a depressive illness might turn out to be an excellent psychotherapeutic proposition.

In general, all those cases which can be considered as belonging to the latent heterosexual group should be offered whatever type of psychotherapy is available over an extended period. Behaviour therapy may be indicated as a preliminary step. Careful selection may be rewarded by considerable therapeutic success. The deviation in the true homosexual is very unlikely to be influenced; in this case all forms of psychotherapy regularly prove disappointing. A complete and satis-factory change in this type of homosexual interests and behaviour is unknown to the present writer. It should also be stressed that with the increased knowledge of the problems linked with narcissistic disorders, the psychotherapy of homosexuality associated with such conditions carries a more favourable prognosis than hitherto.

The homosexual syndrome, as it has been described in relation to certain clinical types, is seen as part of a defensive movement directed at lessening anxiety or at creating barriers against the eruption of unbearable conflicts, and quite often simply at ensuring survival. In this context, the defence includes all the techniques used by the ego to dominate, control, and channel forces which might lead to neurosis or psychosis. It follows that the homosexual solution is a defence which when encountered should be treated with the utmost caution, especially in those cases where its removal is under consideration. It is necessary also to stress that whenever homosexual inclinations are predominant, treatment of any psychological disturbance may disturb a delicate balance within the sexual sphere.

Attempts to treat all kinds of homosexual behaviour indiscriminately, without reference to personality, character, and associated psychological disorders must be held responsible for the excessive and unnecessary gloom shared by psychiatrists and the public at large with regard to the likelihood of influencing the course of this condition.

References

Bergler, E. (1951). *Neurotic counterfeit sex*. New York.

Freeman, T. (1955). Clinical and theoretical observation on male homosexuality. *Int. J. Psycho-Anal.* **36**, 235.

Friedman, A. M., Kaplan, H. I., and Sadock, B. J. (1972). *Modern synopsis of psychiatry*, Chapter 14 p.250. Baltimore.

Freud, S. (1905a). Three essays on the theory of sexuality. *Complete psychological works of Sigmund Freud*. Standard edition **7**, 125. London.

—— (1905b). Footnote p.146.

—— (1910). Leonardo da Vinci and a memory of his childhood. *Complete psychological works of Sigmund Freud*. Standard edition **11**, 59.

—— (1911). Psychoanalytic notes on an autobiographical account of a case of paranoia. *Complete psychological works of Sigmund Freud*. Standard edition **12**, 3. London.

—— (1920). The ego and the id. *Complete psychological works of Sigmund Freud*. Standard edition **19**, 3. London.

Glover, E. (1938). The relation of perversion formation to the development of reality sense. *Int. J. Psycho-Anal.* **14**, 486.

Hoenig, J., Kerna, J., and Youd, A. (1970). Social and economic aspects of transsexualism. *Br. J. Psychol.* **117**, 163.

Khan, M. M. R. (1970). Le fetichisme comme negation du soi—Fetichisme du prepuce chez un homosexual: notes cliniques. *Nouv. Rev. Psychoanal.* **11**, 77.

Klein, M. (1975). The psychoanalysis of children. In *The writings of M. Klein* Vol. II, Chapter 12. London.

Limentani, A. (1976). Object choice and actual bisexuality. *Int. J. Psychoanal. Psychother.* **v**, 205.

Marks, I., Gelder, M., and Bancroft, J. (1970). Sexual deviants two years after electrical aversion. *Br. J. Psychol.* **117**, 137.

Nunberg, H. (1938). Homosexuality, magic and aggression. *Int. J. Psycho-Anal.* **19**, 1.

Randell, J. B. (1959). Tranvestism and transsexualism. *Br. Med. J.* (**ii**), 1448.

Rosenfeld, R. (1949). Remarks on the relation of male homosexuality in paranoia, paranoid anxiety and narcissism. *Int. J. Psycho-Anal.* **30**, 36.

Socarides, C. W. (1970). A psychoanalytic study of the desire for sexual transformation. (Transsexualism: the plaster of Paris man). *Int. J. Psycho-Anal.* **51**, 341.

Sullivan, H. S. (1955). *Conceptions of modern psychiatry*, p.85. London.

Thorner, H. A. (1949). Notes on a case of male homosexuality. *Int. J. Psycho-Anal.* **30**, 31.

8
The homosexual dilemma: a clinical and theoretical study of female homosexuality

Joyce McDougall

Introduction

I hope to show in this chapter that female homosexuality is an attempt to resolve conflict concerning the two poles of psychic identity; one's identity as a separate individual and one's sexual identity. The manifold desires and conflicts which face every girl with regard to her father have, in women who become homosexual, been dealt with by giving him up as an object of love and desire, and by identifying with him instead. The result is that the mother becomes once more the only object worthy of love. Thus the daughter acquires a somewhat fictitious *sexual identity*; however, the unconscious identification with the father aids her in achieving a stronger sense of *subjective identity*. She uses this identification to achieve a certain detachment from the maternal imago in its more dangerous and forbidding aspects. As far as the idealized aspects of the mother-image are concerned, these now seek satisfaction in a substitute relationship with a homosexual partner. This over-simplified statement of the 'homosexual solution' to oedipal distress, as well as to preoedipal conflict and narcissistic integrity, raises many questions. I hope to offer partial answers to some of them.

What are the reasons that might force a small girl to give up her love for her father? And by what means does she arrive at an identification with him instead? Why is the mother felt to be so dangerous? What factors have hindered identification with the genital mother who has sexual relations with a man? What lies behind the frantic idealization of women? And what does she have to offer to her idealized women partners?

Over and beyond these questions which relate to the inner object world and the oedipal structure, are others which concern female sexuality in general. What is the role of 'penis envy' and of 'castration anxiety' in homosexuality? And what of the body image itself? How is it possible to maintain the illusion of being the true sexual partner to another woman? When we have some tentative answers to these questions, we shall be better equipped to broach the investigation of the homosexual relationship and all that it unconsciously represents. But let us first glance back some forty years to the earliest psychoanalytical paper ever published on the subject.

'No prohibitions and no supervision hindered the girl from seizing every one of her rare opportunities of being together with her beloved, of ascertaining all her habits, of waiting for her for hours outside her door or at a tramhalt, of sending her gifts of flowers, and so on. It was evident that this one interest had swallowed up all others in the girl's mind'. Thus in 1920, did Freud describe the passion of a young homosexual patient for an older woman. In reconstructing the genesis of his patient's homosexuality Freud reveals that the daughter, having reached a 'normal oedipal attachment' to her father, renounced all love for him at a period when she unconsciously desired a child from him. This period coincided with the mother's pregnancy. Thus it was the mother – unconsciously hated rival for the father's love – who gave birth to the child longed-for by the daughter. The traumatic effect of this event appears to have led the young girl to a bitter rejection of all men, while she herself 'changed into a man, and took her mother in place of her father as her love-object' (Freud, 1920). From this time onwards, she pursued with amorous devotion women slightly older than herself. At the time of her consultations with Freud, she was enamoured of a lady of doubtful morality, albeit of distinguished family; and of whom her father particularly disapproved. The young woman nevertheless arranged to be seen by her father in the company of her beloved. He turned upon her with a look of hatred which she construed to mean: 'You are forbidden to love this woman'. But to her unconscious mind the silent message read: 'and you shall not have me either'. Following the exchange of angry glances between father and daughter, the woman friend was enraged at finding herself to be an object of disapproval, and ordered the girl to leave her and to refrain from ever addressing her again. In the girl's mind, both man and woman refuse her the right to sexual possession of a woman but unconsciously, as Freud's paper shows, the daughter takes this interdict to mean that she has no right to take her mother's place and to desire her father's love for herself. Faced with rejection by both father and mother, she makes a final symbolic gesture in an attempt to possess and punish the two objects of her desire – she throws herself into the railway cutting with the intention of committing suicide. In this tragic fashion she hurls a protest against the double abandonment, along with her feeling of utter helplessness, and her belief that there is nothing left to live for.

Freud elicits from this fragment of an analysis an insight into the young girl's secret sexual wishes towards her father and her symbolic attempt, through her suicidal gesture, to compel him to give her a child. It is an oedipal drama. Freud's conclusions might lead us to suppose that narcissistic mortification alone explains the young woman's suicidal leap. However, oedipal rage and pain in the face of the fact that one is barred forever from the fulfilment of incestuous childhood wishes is a universal sexual trauma. Why is this young patient, and many others like her, so specially marked by the traumatic nature of human sexuality and oedipal disillusionment? Why such a desperate solution? Although her suicide is mobilized by oedipal distress, we are witnesses at the same time to a *preoedipal* drama which Freud does not explore. This paper predates by some ten years Freud's startling discovery of the little girl's preoedipal conflicts in her struggle for sexual identification (Freud 1931, 1933). Long before the classical oedipal phase, she must come to terms with her love–hate relationship with her mother; she must achieve an identification with her as an individual and separate being, as well as identifying with her on a sexual plane. It is evident that her chances of achieving psychic independence, without undue guilt and depression, depend to a large extent on the mother's willingness to allow her girl-child to become independent of her, as well as her willingness to help her daughter in her sexual-identifications. These in turn require the mother to acknowledge her daughter as a rival with feminine aims and desires, and to accept the daughter's love for the father. Clearly this also involves the father's attitude to his little girl, and the extent to which he is willing to offer her his strength and love, and thus to help her disengage herself from her mother. If the parents suffer from unconscious conflicts, which *interfere* with the girl's attempts to come to terms with her narcissistic and erotic wishes, and with the necessity to face sexual realities and accept her own sexual-identity, then she runs the risk of receiving confusing messages. These will jeopardize her growing feeling of identity and of outer reality, and affect the structuring of her libidinal and aggressive impulses. Furthermore, it is on this basis that she must face, and eventually work through, the conflicts of the classical oedipal crisis. It is perhaps justifiable to propose that it requires two problem parents to produce homosexual offspring.

Freud's paper states clearly his thesis that his young patient's suicidal attempt was an unconscious acting-out of a phallic union with her father. But we must add to this symbolic reconstruction that she was, at the same time, enacting the dissolution of her infantile relationship to her mother. She is, at last, a woman asserting her right to sexuality and motherhood, no longer in need of another woman in order to complete her own femininity. She had assigned to her woman friend the role of an idealized mother. Endowed with beauty, surrounded by lovers, she was, to the eyes of the ardent young girl, a perfect portrait of femininity, and thus possessed of manifold gifts which the girl considered were denied to herself and which, in childhood, she had believed were uniquely reserved for her mother. Her conscious wish to be an object of erotic desire for the other woman and to take sexual possession of her masks not only her desire 'to be a man' as Freud put it, but also her child-like wish to obtain all the hidden treasure the woman is felt to hold – the right to the man and his penis, as well as to the child he will give her. When her homosexual quest is thwarted, she seeks to punish both the man and the women, for she demands something from each of them. In her suicidal leap, she attempts an ultimate and secret fulfilment of these wishes and, as Freud points out, at the same time obtains punishment.

An alternative solution to her conflict might have been the establishment of overt homosexual relations, and in fact Freud's paper leads us to suppose that such was the case with his young patient. Her homosexual activity would then carry the same unconscious significance as her suicide attempt. Namely a symbolic fulfilment of wishes, both loving and destructive, originally directed towards the parents. I am not maintaining that a homosexual solution to oedipal and narcissistic problems is the equivalent of suicide but on the contrary that such an outcome may serve to ward off states of depression or depersonalization and thus act as a bulwark against suicide or psychic death.

I first became interested in the unconscious significance of homosexual relationships when I had several homosexual patients in analysis, within a relatively short period of time. Three of these were women and, before their long analyses were terminated, I had two more such patients. In spite of their individual differences, these women showed striking similarities in their ego-structure and in their oedipal background. Their violence was particularly evident, as was the complicated defensive struggle against it, especially when these violent feelings were directed to the sexual partner. Equally striking was the fragility of their sense of identity as expressed in periods of depersonalization, bizarre bodily states, and so on; particularly if the relation to the love-partner was felt to be threatened, whether by external circumstances or from within. One patient, for example, on learning that her lover was to leave her unexpectedly for three days, exclaimed: 'I felt the room swimming around me when I read her letter; I couldn't think where I was and I had to bang my head against the wall until I came to my senses'. On a similar occasion, she stubbed burning cigarettes out on her hands in order to bring to an end the painful sensation of loss of body-ego boundaries (Federn 1953). Another patient cut her hands with a sharp knife and burned pieces of her skin when deserted by her lover of the moment. These patients were expressing not only their almost symbiotic dependence upon their partners, but also the terror and violent rage which the experience of separation and loss aroused. All these patients manifested equally intense reactions to men – but from men violent attack was anticipated. One of my patients kept a stiletto in her pocket; another hid a large kitchen knife in her purse. Both claimed to be protecting themselves from attacks by taxi-drivers and passers-by. In addition to isolated episodes of confusion and depersonalization, all suffered from periods of intense depression connected with failure in their relationships, or with failure in their creative and professional activities. Work-failure was frequently the conscious reason for coming to analysis. In my work with them, I came to understand that their sexual and love relationships were often used as a manic screen against depressive feelings and persecutory fears, a magic shield against fantasied attacks or threatened loss of identity.

The oedipal story and the oedipal structure

I make distinction here between the personal family history which emerges through childhood memories, conscious assessments and what we might call the parental imagos, and the unconscious symbolic structures to which the childhood experiences, plus the inner fantasy world of the individual, have given rise. These structures affect not only the ego, its defensive system, and the internalized objects of love and hate, but also relations with external objects. If we give to the concept of *structure* the significance assigned to it by Levi-Strauss (1949), we may readily accept that the *oedipal structure* is a nuclear one in the unconscious basis of the personality. Not only does it determine ego-identity in its narcissistic and sexual aspects, it also imprints a pattern on instinctual aims and eventually will structure interpersonal as well as intrapersonal relationships. The profound symbolic significance of the 'Oedipus complex' cannot be reduced simply to the story of the child and his parents. Nevertheless, it is only through piecing together this 'story' that we can arrive at any understanding of the symbolic structure of the ego and its objects of desire.

In homosexual men and women, we find a family romance of a specific kind, and one which needs to be carefully analysed, if we are to understand both the personality structure which results, and the role of homosexual objects in the psychic economy. In addition therefore to corresponding factors in ego-structure and in the defence mechanisms used to maintain its precarious equilibrium, there is a striking similarity in the way in which these patients present their parents. My female homosexual patients might all have been of the same family, so much did the parental portraits resemble one another. My own clinical observations have been amply confirmed by the findings of other analytic writers on this subject, in particular Deutsch (1932, 1944–5), Socarides (1968) and Rosen (1964). The descriptions which follow continue, to a large extent, an article on the unconscious significance of the object relationship in female homosexuality (McDougall 1970). If I quote rather extensively from this earlier paper it is because I have very little to add to this particular aspect of homosexuality.

The father-image

As we shall see, the father is neither idealized nor desired. If not totally absent from the analytic discourse, he is despised, detested, or denigrated in other ways. Intense preoccupation with the noises he makes, his brutality, insensitivity, lack of refinement, and so on, all contribute to giving an anal-sadistic colouring to the portrait. Furthermore his phallic-genital qualities are contested, since he is often presented as ineffectual and impotent; there is no feeling of a strong, loving father nor of a man whose character might be considered as essentially virile. In the daughter's inner psychic world, the once phallic father has regressed to being an anal-sadistic one.

Olivia, a pretty young woman in her twenties, who in the first years of her analysis lived with an older woman to whom, she said, she was 'married', came one day to her session looking physically ill and brandishing a letter from her father. 'I have to go back to Florence for the holidays, to be with the family! It makes me sick. I couldn't sleep all night. Thought I was going to vomit...I can't bear the sound of my father with his horrible throat noises and coughing. He only does it to drive me mad. I can't stand looking at him. He makes little twitching movements with his face. Disgusting.' In earlier sessions, she had recalled that his beard used to scratch her when she was little, that his voice was sharp and frightening; in fact every memory connected with him portrayed his presence as an intrusion of a violent kind; warmer and more tender memories did not appear till some two years later. As far as Olivia knew at this point in her analysis, she had always hated him and believed he hated her, too. She continued: 'I'm so afraid that I shall have an "attack" when I get back to Florence—and my father hates me more than ever when I'm ill and can't leave the house'. Olivia here refers to a phobia of vomiting, which was sufficiently severe to cripple most of her social relations and was one of her principal reasons for coming to analysis. Olivia continued to 'vomit up' her distressed and hateful feelings about her father. 'I'm sure he is responsible for my attacks. He tries to make me ill. You probably don't believe it but I know he would like to kill me.' Olivia had passed through periods when she even imagined her father's plotting with his employees to liquidate her. In her third year of analysis, she amended this belief to: 'My father is not aware of it, but *unconsciously* he would like to kill me'. At this point Olivia was no longer compelled to go out armed with a knife against the men who might attack her.

Karen, a talented actress, came to analysis because of severe anxiety attacks which stultified her work when she was in front of an audience. As her analysis progressed, she was able to give a fantasy content to her phobic attacks; it was as though she might suddenly defaecate or vomit on stage. 'When I think of my father I hear him clearing his throat of mucous, blowing his nose, horrible noises seemed to spread over the dinner table and envelop us all [herself and her sisters]. I used to think I would faint when he spoke to me, as though he were going to spit at me. I'd like to tear his guts out, filthy pig! Makes you want to vomit'. On another occasion she said: 'As a child I was always afraid of losing control of myself. I used to faint a lot. Every morning before going to school I would pray "Please God, don't let me vomit today"'. At other times she recalled a frightening fantasy, that has persisted for some twenty years, in which her father would creep up behind her to cut off her head. 'I think he must have *threatened* to kill me when I was little. I would jump whenever he came up behind me. I always kept a safe distance from him, would never sit beside him in the car'.

Eva says: 'I can't describe the terrible look on my father's face. Even though I've done nothing I'm always afraid he will shout at me . . . and he's so rude at the table. My heart races as though he's going to kill me. When he's there I'm paralysed with fright and can't eat or talk'.

Sophie, a gynaecologist, living with a woman colleague, paints in slightly different colours the same basic portrait of the denigrated father: 'He's a rich and successful businessman, but basically he's just a peasant; retarded ideals, no sensitivity. No one could make a move in the household if he were not in agreement. He would throw violent tantrums like a child. He hates women; he would tell with pride of the time he slapped his sister publicly because she was out walking with a boy. No one can look up to such a father'.

We see from these examples, which could be multiplied, that the paternal imago is strong and dangerous. Physical closeness to the father gives rise to feelings of fear or disgust. The daughter thus presents a childhood situation in which the father is kept at arm's length and there follows a fantasy struggle against being invaded by his tics, mucous, angry voice, and similar intrusions. The anal quality of the descriptions is evident, as is the idea of a sadistic attack. The very concentration on the father, his gestures, noises, words, and attitudes gives some indication of the uneasy excitement attached to this image. One has the impression of a little girl in terror of being attacked or penetrated by her father. The emphasis on his dirty, noisy, or unrefined qualities, and the intensity of her repudiation of him as a person, gives us an inkling of the way she has used regression and repression to deal with any phallic-sexual interest he might have aroused. In addition, there is much evidence to point to the fact that the girl-child has been obliged to find psychic defences to deal with the *unconscious problems of the father* regarding femininity.

These suppositions are further corroborated by the observation that in the early stages of analysis there is rarely any reference to the father's genital sexuality, or even to his masculine activity in the outside world. His sexual relation to the mother is totally blotted out, and his achievements in the professional world are despised or minimized. The defensive value of this impotent image is clear: if he is castrated there is little fear of desiring him as a love object. The reason for this destroyed and denigrated introject, and the manner in which it becomes deprived of all phallic-genital quality remains to be explored. Important at this point, is some insight into the unconscious *identification with the father* which these patients had constructed.

At the beginning of her analysis, Olivia always dressed in stained jeans and vast thick sweaters. She complained of the women in her environment who criticized her appearance, refusing to accept her for what she was. 'I'm scruffy; I look like a grubby boy. I'm convinced you aren't interested in me either; I don't suppose you even want to go on with my analysis!'. She then asked if many attractively dressed women came to consult me, then dissolved into tears saying she was 'dirty, clumsy, and disgusting'. At the same time she asserted that it would be impossible for her to be otherwise. 'I'd feel ridiculous dressed up like a *woman*. Besides I can't bear to hear them cackling about fashions and make-up. All my life my mother made me get dressed up to go to receptions. I always felt angry and ill'.

Olivia here applies to herself the identical terms with which she castigated her father. Largely lost to her as an object, except for her passionate hatred of him, she is now identified with him in the form of a regressed image, possessed of disagreeable and dangerous anal qualities. She also wore a thick leather wristband for a time, believing it gave her 'an appearance of strength and cruelty', but the extent of her identification was unknown to her, since she projected a large part of this dangerous strength and cruelty onto the world of men in general. She went outside protected by her knife against sadistic attack; the fact that it was she who wielded the knife and might therefore be considered as dangerous did not occur to her. Anticipating our discussion of the mother's role in this curious oedipal tangle, we might point out that the partial identification with the father imago is felt to be forbidden by the mother and to be criticized and despised by other women. Olivia also fears in this session – and indeed for some two years of our analytic work together – that the analyst too will cast her out for those traits in which she unconsciously identifies with her father's strength. These elements clearly represent a vital part of her identity, and one which she feels she must struggle to preserve. Although her narcissistic identification with a father conceived of in anal-sadistic terms is highly conflictual, it is of cardinal importance to Olivia's self-image, and indeed forms an important dimension in her homosexual attachments.

Karen, in her own inimitable style, revealed the same self-portrait.

'I'm just a piece of shit, and that's exactly how everyone treats me. But my friend, Paula, saw me quite differently. And that's how I knew she really loved me. She liked my craziness and she didn't treat me like shit!' She then added defensively, no doubt wondering if the analyst could love her and accept her as she was: 'I haven't had a bath for weeks and I don't give a damn. I smell like a skunk and I love it. Can you smell it?' Clinging narcissistically to her body products and odours, Karen added a style of dress which carried out the same idea. When obliged to wear 'feminine' clothing she felt anxious and uncomfortable. The sadistic intentions imputed to her father were also important elements in her own fantasy life. She often imagined herself killing men. 'I'd like to kill some man – any man – and drive a knife right through his belly.' She frequently dreamed of chopping men up, and at these times was afraid to go out in the street, unless accompanied by her lover, for fear that men were plotting murder against her.

It is interesting to note that Sophie, who considered her father to be a woman-hater, told me in her first interview that *she* was a misogynist, although exclusively homosexual in her love-relationships. She too felt 'like a castrate' (her own term) if she wore dresses instead of her well-tailored trouser suits. Sophie was more aware than any of my other homosexual patients of the underlying hatred and general ambivalence attached to her homosexual loves, although her identification with an anal-sadistic father was entirely unconscious.

I come now to another essential aspect of the father-image, and one which has considerable importance for any understanding of the symbolic oedipal structure and its particular fragility. This in turn has momentous consequences for the structure of the ego and the maintenance of ego-identity. Behind the 'castrated' image, behind the regressive libidinal involvement with an exciting and frightening anal-sadistic father, lies the image of the father who has *failed in his specific parental role*, leaving his small daughter a prey to a devouring or controlling, omnipotent maternal image. The mother, usually represented, as we shall see, as the essence of femininity and in no way a masculine-phallic personality is nevertheless felt to have secretly destroyed the father's value as an authority figure, and to have aided the child in denying his phallic-genital qualities. The primal scene, if acknowledged at all, is conceived of in sadistic terms, and is usually attributed to the mother's stories of the sexual brutality, and so forth, to be expected of men. The mother's apparent complicity in the quasi-total destruction of the masculine image of the father is a constant theme. One mother plotted with her children to steal small sums of money from the father; another aided her child to conceal poor school marks. One patient claimed that her mother refused to allow the father to come near her when she was young, on the grounds that he was disturbing to her because she was 'nervous and delicate'. Karen's mother frequently discussed with her daughter the eventuality of a divorce from the father, the underlying idea being that she and the mother would be better off alone; another constantly decried the father's family background. In spite of a childlike delight in believing that they were more important to mother than was the father, these children nevertheless bitterly resented the father's exclusion and blamed him for not having played a parental role to help them become independent of the mother. The extent of the threat, which this destruction of the parental-image represented, was only slowly brought to light in analysis, although detectable in certain anxiety symptoms from the outset.

Karen described a dream thus: 'There was a little boy running in front of a car. A woman driver rides right over him and leaves him paralysed. My father just stands there saying he doesn't know where to go for help. I scream "You're a doctor aren't you? You could be hanged for refusing to help someone in mortal danger". Then I take the baby to a woman doctor myself. She sprays it with ether but I keep on calling my father to come and help me'.

Karen's associations lead to angry rantings against the father and to details which identify the damaged baby boy as a representation of herself, and the woman doctor as the analyst. Let us reconstruct the latent meaning of the dream insofar as it pertains to the present discussion. The little boy's accident symbolizes castration in a global sense – he is paralysed as Karen feels herself to be most of the time. The damage is caused by a woman driver – Karen says: 'My mother's a terrible driver. Never looks where she's going!' But it is also a woman (analyst–mother) who is supposed to repair the grave damage to which the father is indifferent – homosexual relationships will 'repair' her and end her own feeling of being paralysed, as well as the longed for completion of herself. However, the dangers which lurk in the latter solution, when lived out in the analytic situation, are revealed in Karen's associations to the woman doctor's 'treatment'. 'Ether' says Karen, 'will either lull you into insensibility so you feel no more pain – or else it kills you outright': the analyst–mother, like the homosexual partners, may lull the damaged baby back into the fantasied bliss of the mother-nursling fusion, but this quest may also kill the baby. The rejecting father abandons his child to the overpowering, seductive mother who, in return, only offers psychic death. What was once a phallic-libidinal demand has now regressed to a cry for help; but the father does not heed her appeal.

A dream of Olivia's reveals a similar unconscious picture of the father. In her dream, she watches a mother-cat delivering kittens. The kittens are born with their eyes open and this means they are going to die. She makes desperate attempts to save these babies, first putting them into a box to small for them, where they suffocate. Then she puts them out with the mother-cat in the snow, where they continue to fare badly. Her father is there with the mother-cat and she begs him for help. He replies that he is too busy, he has a business meeting. She turns back to the kittens and finds they are all dead. In recounting her dream, Olivia burst into tears saying the dream was like real-life in that her father would not care if *she* died. The kittens doomed to die *because their eyes are open* was a reference, in primary process thinking, to an early primal-scene memory. Olivia had once observed her parents making-love when they believed she was asleep, and she had described her mother, when recounting this screen-memory, as 'the cat who got the cream'. She was three years old at the time; one can detect in the dream story her wish that her mother's babies would die, but what had eventually died in the tiny girl's mind was the hope that she might one day identify with the mother-cat, and have access to a genital father-image and the right to live kittens all of her own. Her associations to this dream all led to a feeling that she was 'destroyed' on the inside. At the time of this dream she had suffered for several months from amenorrhoea; although we were able to understand later that this symptom also signified her desire to have a child, in her fantasy at this point in time she was empty and finished as a woman; the dead kittens represented herself and her unborn children doomed to extinction. In the dream, it is to her father that she turns to save her from the situation in which her femininity is at stake. He does nothing and the end result is death.

Behind the conscious wish to eliminate or denigrate the father, all of my homosexual patients revealed narcissistic wounds linked to this image of the *indifferent* father. Strengthened by the conviction that the mother forbade any loving relationship between father and daughter, these women tended to feel that any desire for the father, his love or his penis, was dangerous. Such a wish could only entail the loss of the mother's love and bring castration to the father. Thus the daughter's consciously avowed dislike of the father was experienced as a gift made to the mother. In turn it gave rise to many fantasies of a revengeful and persecuting father, and subsequently to the fear of men in general.

What light do these brief clinical examples shed on the relation of the homosexual to her father? There is practically no trace of the normal-neurotic solutions to oedipal wishes. The father has become lost as a love-object, and equally lost as a representative of security and strength, which bars the way to future genital relations. In addition, in her attempts to deal with her primitive libidinal and aggressive wishes, the small girl's ego has undergone profound modifications. The discarded paternal object has been incorporated into her ego-structure never to be given up. No other man ever takes the father's place in the homosexual girl's psychic universe. The renunciation of the father as an object of libidinal investment, does not correspond to the relinquishing of the oedipal object which we find in heterosexual women; nor, in consequence, does it lead to the formation of symptoms to deal with frustrated oedipal wishes and castration anxiety which we find in most neurotic structures. Instead there is identification with the father, but this identification, while it might be said to prevent further ego-disintegration, itself has crippling consequences for the ego, for it is an identification with a mutilated image, possessed of disagreeable and dangerous qualities. The ambivalence inherent in any process of identification is here immeasureably heightened; the ego runs the risk of suffering merciless attacks from the super-ego for these identifications which nevertheless form an essential part of the individual's identity. The depressive reproaches which the homosexual so frequently heaps upon herself bear the stamp of the classic reproaches of the melancholic (Freud 1917). They represent an attack upon the internalized father, yet this narcissistically-important, and zealously-guarded, object of identification is a bulwark against psychotic dissolution. The pregenital super-ego results in ego-fragility, and in impoverishment or paralysis of much of the ego's functioning.

We are still faced with the question as to why the little girl, in her attempt to internalize something as vitally important to her ego and to her instinctual development as the phallic representation of her father, is able to do so only at the expense of object loss, ego impairment, and considerable suffering. A fuller understanding of her inner psychic reality requires us to turn now to an investigation of the relationship with the maternal imago.

The mother-image

The complicity with the mother has already been noted; however, there is little identification with her. Invariably these mothers are described in idealized terms – beautiful, gifted, charming, and so on. The mother is felt to be possessed of all the qualities which the daughter lacks. What is striking in this unequal situation is that it is taken for granted. There is no conscious envy of the mother. Furthermore she emerges as the sole safeguard against the dangers of living, dangers coming from the father as well as the outside world. At the same time the mother is frequently felt to be in danger herself; fears of her imminent death are quite common. In fantasy, she is the victim of fatal accidents, or illnesses, or the prey of would-be attackers. Coming closer to the source, she is threatened with abandonment or excessive domination by the father. He is believed to make unfair demands upon her sexually or otherwise.

Identification with such an imago presents two main difficulties. Any aspiration towards narcissistic identification is doomed to failure because of its excessively idealized qualities; these in turn are maintained in order to repress a fund of hostile and destructive wishes directed towards the internalized mother. She must remain an unattainable ideal at the price of a continuing narcissistic haemorrage in the daughter's self-image. Secondly, this attitude is reinforced by the destructive nature of the primal-scene fantasies. There is no trace of an idea that the parents might be complementary to each other sexually, or that the mother is enhanced in any way by her relation to the father. Frequently the parents' sexual relationship is totally disavowed on a conscious plane; analysis reveals that, behind this denial of sexual realities, there are sadistic and frightening images of the sexual relationships and of the father's penis. Thus there is no wish to identify with the mother in her genital role. The wishful fantasy of all these patients might be summed-up as a desire for total elimination of the father and the creation of an exclusive and enduring mother–daughter relationship. This latter fantasy is lived out in the sexual relationship with women partners, who thus become mother substitutes, frequently with alternating roles, each being at times the mother, at times the child. Elaborations of this wish are often reiterated in the early transference situation. Its aggressive elements usually are strongly repressed.

Again, I draw on examples from my experiences in analysis. Olivia described her mother as 'talented and beautiful; she was a public figure and everyone adored her ... I always wanted to be near her, like they did. Whenever she went out I was haunted by the idea that she would get run over ... She's pure and innocent, can't imagine that anyone can have evil thoughts ... the only trouble is that she can't understand what it is to be ill. She was never sick. ... Somehow she was never there when I needed her. I wonder if all my stomach troubles wern't a way of keeping her near me'.

Eva would say: 'I loved her so much; and she looked so pretty. She had lots of beauty treatments and still looks very young for her age. I used to save up all my pennies to buy flowers for her when I was little'. (Later she stole money from her father to give flowers to the girls she was in love with at college). 'When she was caring for my little sister I was almost ill with longing for her. Sometimes I would try to be ill so that she would keep me at home with her'. Later, she added: 'But somehow it was as though you couldn't get close to her. She wasn't mean but she gave things instead of love'.

Before exploring the many layers of the maternal imago, let us briefly recapitulate the parental images as revealed in the early stages of analysis. Father is the repository of all that is bad, dirty, or dangerous, while mother is pure, beautiful and clean. Above all, she is maintained as a *non-conflictual* object. She is the fountainhead of all security—a security later sought in other women who become objects of sexual desire. She is thought to possess highly valuable feminine attributes, but these evoke no conscious jealousy. The daughter hopes to have access to some of these qualities later by loving another woman. The one sour note in the lovely-mother theme is the impression that she is narcissistically involved with herself, and is lacking in understanding. However, these traits are in no way resented by the daughter in her attempt to keep intact the idealized image: indeed they regarded themselves as unworthy, unlovable children, who had been a disappointment to their mothers. All my patients, as the analysis proceeded, began to reveal and explore quite different aspects of the mother-image of which two seemed particularly important; the first concerning their own ambivalent feelings towards her, and the second giving some indication of the mother's ambivalence. The first, already hinted at, was a constant concern for the mother's health and safety. Obsessive images of her falling fatally ill, of finding her dead, or cut to pieces were frequent. This was often expressed through a compulsive need to phone her constantly when separated, or rush back to her during vacations. Often these identical fears were transferred globally onto female partners. The need to stay very close, to control the mother's movements to the best of their abilities, and to smother her with solicitude, thinly veiled the underlying aggressive content. The emphasis was on mother's indispensibility to the child, and it was only much later that the patients were able to discover that this was felt to be a demand *stemming from the mother*; to be independent of her would have been both disloyal and dangerous. The fantasies that the mother, or the sexual partner, might fall victim to a fatal catastrophe were consciously considered a total threat to the patient's personal safety and her object world, but as time went on she could not avoid becoming aware that these were magical means of preventing dangerous impulses in herself from *destroying the maternal object*.

The second theme which turned up with unfailing regularity was that of a rigidly-controlling mother wielding omnipotent power over the body of her child, meticulously preoccupied with order, health, and cleanliness. The underlying feelings to which this particular relationship to the mother gave rise are typified in a remark of Karen's: 'My mother hated everything to do with my body. She used to smell my clothes all the time to see if they were dirty. When I defaecated she treated it like poison. For many years I believed my mother did not defaecate. In fact I still find it hard to believe!' The examples are legion. One patient was forbidden to mention her excretory needs. She was taught at an early age to cough politely to draw attention to such things. She always felt dirty and ashamed because of her body functions. Another mother referred to constipation as 'back trouble' and forbade her daughter to look at her faeces. These aspects of the 'anal' mother who rejected all that may be attached to the concept of anal eroticism had a markedly inhibiting effect upon the integration of the anal components of the libido as we have seen. The displacement of these components onto the phallic image of the father have also been noted.

The controlling and physically rejecting aspects of the maternal imago came slowly to consciousness and stirred-up considerable resistance, since this was felt to be an attack upon the internalized mother, and involved the risk of being separated from an almost symbiotic relationship in the inner object world (Mahler and Gosliner 1955). The feeling that their bodies, and their whole physical selves, had been severely rejected by the mother was most painfully brought to light by these patients, although their own often violent rejection of their bodies was conscious from the beginning. 'My body is repugnant to me, especially my breasts. Everything about me that is flabby is disgusting. I have always tried to have hard strong hands. My hands resemble my father's and help to cover up all that is moist or wrong with my body. I still get terribly anxious concerning urine or shit – I cannot accept these functions; they are somehow disgustingly femin- ine'. Thus did Sophie express her feelings towards her despised bodily self. When younger she used to torture herself with a razor blade in order to 'purify' herself, but this compulsive behaviour was no longer necessary after her first homosexual experiences. The reverse side of this maternal rejection and hatred of their physical-selves was expressed by all these patients through fantasies of loving *another woman's body*. They would lavish on a female partner caresses, minute explorations, tenderness, and all the loving that they unconsciously demanded for their own bodies – believed to be ugly and deformed, physically weak, or unhealthy. One patient described the 'recovery' of her own body through her female partner in these terms: 'Until I met Sarah I had no body, only a head. I always worked well at school to please my mother. Going into the street was a nightmare; I felt awkward, unstable and monstrous, yet I was not aware of any individual parts of my body. Sarah brought my hands and feet, and my skin to life. But I still don't have much. I cannot bear to have my breasts touched. I love her genitals but cannot let her touch mine.' Similar intense bodily conflict was manifested by another patient, in that the dangerous fantasies attached to her own body and genitals were projected onto her partner as well. This patient proclaimed a total lack of both clitoral and vaginal sensation, and indeed was confused about where her vagina was located. She would imagine it constricting or cutting like a knife. She had a recurrent fantasy in which she gave birth to a child in broken segments; it later became evident that she attributed to her vagina both oral-devouring and anal-constricting functions. In her first homosexual experience, when she was eighteen years old, she became excited when her partner demanded clitoral stimulation and was happy to administer these caresses to her friend. But when the friend asked her one day to put her fingers into her vagina she drew back in horror, 'I was sure my fingers would get stuck inside her and that it would require the services of a surgeon to separate us. I was so terrified. I just could not comply with her request'. This fear of 'getting stuck' was connected to an unconscious aspect of her relation with her mother. Her mother's vagina would demand that she remained perpetually attached, like a phallic organ, and nothing short of a surgeon's knife could separate them. That this patient's father was a noted Parisian surgeon made her reflection pertinent and rich in symbolic meaning. Only an effective father could protect her from the maternal wish to make her into a permanent phallus.

These fragments from sessions shed further light upon the tenacious, yet frightening, tie to the negative aspects of the internalized mother. The patients all unconsciously regarded themselves as an indispensable part or function of the mother (Lichtenstein 1961). The feeling of being mother's 'phallus' was a narcissistically enhancing aspect, but it was inevitably accompanied by the idea that one was a faecal object, despised yet omnipotently controlled by her. The daughter invariably came to feel that she existed to enhance the maternal ego; one is tempted to believe that these patients served as counter-phobic objects with regard to deep anxieties on the mother's part (Winnicott 1948, 1960). Two further remarks express vividly the complex and primitive tie to the mother, and the danger involved in wishing to dissolve it, terrifying and crippling though its maintenance might be. 'The feelings I have about you [the analyst, at a moment of intense maternal transference] are insupportable. I have never loved nor hated anyone so much in my life. If I love you you will destroy me; if I hate you you will cast me out forever.' Loving meant devouring; for long periods of time it was important to this patient to believe that I hated her. This made her feel safer and also enabled her better to support her strongly sadistic and hateful feelings towards me. 'If you love me I am lost, for then you will destroy me and throw me out like shit – or else you will tie me up to you forever – like my mother did.'

Another patient expresses the same ideas in the following fantasy: 'My mother and I are fused together. At one end we are sealed by our mouths and at the other by our vaginas. We make up a circle bound by cold steel bands. If it breaks we shall both be torn'. This fantasy, which continued through several sessions underwent the following trans-formation: 'I broke that circle when I first loved another woman. But there was only one vagina – and my mother got it! With her icy fingers she closed mine up forever'. The same patient often felt that if anything worked well in her life (she was an artist), or if she had success or pleasure with her work, her mother was liable to fall dangerously ill and die. Identical terror in the symbiotic relationship is vividly expressed by Mary Barnes whose account in *Two accounts of a journey through madness* (Barnes and Berke 1971) lays strikingly bare the force of an attachment to this kind of internalized mother-image. Mary writes: 'It was difficult for my mother to be loved and she didn't understand about unconscious motives....Once I told her, "Mother, it seemed to me that I caused all Peter's illness and all your sickness!"...Feeling happy, enjoying myself, instinctively I would wonder, is mother ill?...It's only safe to be dead, in a false state, or hidden away, shut up somewhere, mad Mary'. The patients I am discussing chose other solutions (which we will examine in detail later) than that chosen by Mary Barnes; for them it was heterosexuality and the world of men which had to be 'kept dead, hidden away, shut up somewhere', while mother was constantly repaired and reassured. The fear of becoming separate and independent led, in many of my patients, to an inability to work or to create. If ambitions of this kind were pursued with success, it was invariably at the price of considerable anxiety and fantasies of the mother becoming ill or dying. It was perhaps no accident that two of the mothers of my patients did actually fall gravely ill, at times when their daughters were beginning to create successful careers for themselves; another suffered from inexplicable haemorrhages when her daughter married. The latter patient, during this upheaval, dreamed that her mother had lost her legs and that she was condemned to walk underneath her mother, taking the place of legs. How can a leg separate from its body? And what sort of independent existence could it hope for? And again how can the mother-body function if its legs decide to leave it? Such are the dilemmas facing the homosexual patient when she begins to desire a loosening of the bonds which tie her to the internalized mother. Either she will become nothing more than an amputated limb, or her mother will seek revenge or die. In most cases these desperate feelings are transferred onto the sexual partner. Said Sophie: 'Since my friend has come to live with me I feel sure I exist. It was like that when I was a child. I only existed in my mother's eyes; without her I was never quite sure who I really was'.

To sum up the salient features of the maternal imago we might say that, *first, the mother is felt to have destroyed the public image of the father and to act as a forbidding barrier between father and daughter; behind this image stands the mother-with-the-enema who took possession of the child's body and its contents. This usually resulted in very early control over bodily functions which, far from liberating a small child, renders her ever more dependent upon the mother; finally, there is the fantasy that the daughter is part of mother's very essence and vice versa – a symbiotic fantasy in which each keeps the other alive; there can never be two women; to separate from the mother (or later substitutes) means to lose one's identity.*

Apart from the homosexual object-choice, one other outcome of this particularly-lopsided family constellation is a nexus of character traits which affected most of my patients, and which I have also noted in clinical writings by other analysts. Unless compensated by meticulous reaction-formations these patients tend to display an inability to organize their lives in even the smallest details. Some of them seemed to live in the midst of disorder and confusion to a punitive degree. The inability to work constructively, or even in some cases to arrange papers, to pack a suitcase, to make a decision, exemplified the fear that independent ego-activity is dangerous. The feeling of being an incomplete entity, ill-defined, incapable, vulnerable, is the inevitable result of the unconscious symbiotic relationship. The non-integration of the anal components of the libido, in such a way as to be useful to the ego, weakens further the personality structure. Nothing can be achieved, or, if achieved, retained. One had the feeling that these patients were forced to prove that nothing could be accomplished without the constant aid of the mother or mother-substitute. The mother who fosters precocious bodily and ego controls of all kinds in her child, with the desire that the child should *perform for her*, deprives the child of the right to perform for her own pleasure.

Penis envy and the phallus concept

Before summarizing the oedipal constellation and the specific type of unconscious structure it gives rise to, we should first examine the role of 'penis envy' in homosexually, as compared with heterosexually, oriented women. I should like to recall the elements of this concept in Freudian theory, and the theoretical distinction between 'penis' and 'phallus' since it is important to any understanding of the symbolic structure which contributes to the formation of sexual deviation.

Freud regarded *penis envy* as a fundamental element in the organization of feminine sexuality; this envy is considered to arise as a result of the discovery of the difference between the sexes, the little girl feeling deprived as a consequence (Freud 1925). This feeling of deprivation involving as it does ignorance of the existence of the vagina leads to the feminine castration complex (Freud 1908). During the oedipal phase, penis envy is expected to give way to two transformations of the basic wish to have a penis of one's own: the wish to acquire a 'penis' inside the body, usually in the form of the wish for a child, and the desire to receive pleasure from the man's penis in the sexual relationship (Freud 1920, 1933). Failure to achieve these transformations may result in neurotic symptoms and character problems. The same wishes may also find sublimatory expression.

The term *phallus* has a symbolic significance. As his researches progressed Freud became increasingly interested in what he designated as 'the phallic phase' of libidinal development, in children of both sexes. The term *penis* came to be reserved for the male organ in its anatomical reality, while the *phallus* referred to all that the penis might symbolise in psychic reality – power, plenitude, fertility, and so on. A phallic significance may thus be conferred on any part-object such as breast, faeces, urine, child, or an adult person used as a part-object. In recent analytic writings (Grunberger 1971), the phallus is taken to be the symbol of narcissistic integrity; or again as the fundamental significant of desire (Lacan 1966) for either sex. Most analysts would agree today that the penis-envy concept, with its symbolic phallic overtones, applies to both sexes; if the little girl is envious of her brother's sexual organ, the little boy equally as envious of the large paternal penis. But over and beyond these envious attitudes to the penis, interest is centred on its symbolic significance: the importance of the phallic organization in the libidinal development of boy and girl, and its structuring effect in the oedipal situation (Kurth and Patterson 1968). This phase of development marks a turning point in psychic life, with lasting consequences on the acquisition of sexual-identity and the unconscious structuring of sexual desire. The *phallus*, as the psychic representative of desire and narcissistic completion, plays the same role for both sexes, but the attitude to the *anatomical penis* is necessarily different. The fact that the penis is a visible sexual organ, and that in our phallocentric society the male is regarded as the more privileged, gives woman specific problems to overcome, and it is less than likely that these are simply resolved, as Freud claimed, by her eventually having a child. Indeed should she regard her child as the equivalent of a penis, or even as her *phallus*, that is the object of her desire and the means of being sexually and narcissistically complete, she has resolved little of her basic sexual and relational problems, and can scarcely avoid creating graver ones for her child. To understand the girl's specific conflicts in regard to phallic wishes, we must add that these have their prototypes in the earliest mother–child relationship. The first phallic object, in the symbolic sense, the earliest object of narcissistic completion and libidinal desire, is the breast. This particular connotation of the 'phallic mother' as the omnipotent mother of the nursing situation, object not only of the baby's needs but primordial object of erotic desire was first noted by Brunswick (1940). 'The term "phallic mother"...is best designated as the all-powerful mother, the mother who is capable of everything and who possesses every valuable attribute'.

With regard then to phallic envy and its specific development in the little girl, we may trace its origins to the desire to possess for oneself the breast-mother, object of desire, of pleasure, and of need, and thus trace 'penis envy' from oral sadistic 'breast-envy' through its various anal representations to its investment in the penis. From this point of view 'penis envy', in the form of wishing to have a penis and envy of those who possess one, is only one manifestation, in a continuum, of possible objects of desire in their manifold pregenital, genital, and sublimated forms. Either sex, in the attempt to find a solution to infantile sexual and narcissistic longings, might come to the erroneous conclusion that the secret to all fulfilment is to be possessed of a penis but, for the reasons already stated, this is more likely to be the little girl's fantasy. Clinical findings and observations of children, all confirm the importance of penis envy in women but rarely explore the many roots of this complex wish. It cannot be explained by the simple megalomanic wish to possess everything one does not have. Reference has been made to the fact that it conceals early oral longings. We must add to these important dimensions all the thoughts that the little girl has about her father's penis. Father usually comes to represent authority, order, and the outside world; and his penis comes to symbolize these qualities in the unconscious. But over and beyond this, he is also seen as the object of mother's interest and sexual desire. Thus the penis may signify a narcissistic enhancement to be desired as such; a symbol of power and protection; the object of mother's desire. It is evident that this powerfully-cathected, phallic symbol will inevitably represent, in the eyes of the little girl, the principal object needed to guarantee mother's love and sexual interest, as well as an important possession with which to earn respect from the world in general. In consequence boys are considered to hold an extremely favoured position.

There is yet another dimension to the little girl's phallic envy. For both sexes, the wish to be the exclusive object of the mother's love and desire is coupled with a fear of the pregenital mother-image: the controlling and demanding mother of the anal-sadistic phase of development, and the equalling terrifying mother of oral fantasy; the little girl tends to feel that the possession of a *penis* would protect her from enthralment and submission to these omnipotent aspects of the mother-imago; the boy would not only have more to offer but also runs no risk of being a rival to the mother.

It is understandable therefore that an overwhelming majority of women find difficulty in resolving the problems of 'penis envy', the more so since on attaining motherhood they tend to transmit their neurotic solutions to their daughters; for woman must be held responsible in large part for the 'solutions' to the problems of penis envy and castration anxiety, since she herself plays a considerable role in the idealization of the penis and the depreciation of femininity.

In her contribution to a book on female homosexuality, Torok (1970) writes:

We are right when we suppose that this age-old inequality requires woman's complicity, in spite of her apparent protest shown by penis envy. Men and women must be exposed to specific, complementary affective conflicts to have established a *modus vivendi* which could last through many civilizations.... At the end of the anal stage the little girls should be able to achieve in masturbatory fantasy a simultaneous identification with both parents in terms of their genital functioning. But there are two obstacles: first, the one originating in the anal period, namely that autonomy in masturbatory satisfaction necessarily means a sadistic dispossession of the mother and her prerogatives; second, the Oedipal obstacle, according to which the re-creation of the primal scene, by identification with both parents, also implies supplanting the Mother, an exacting, jealous and castrated Mother, and an envied, depreciated, and at the same time overvalued Father. The only way out of this impasse to identification is the establishment of an inaccessible phallic ideal.... When women holding such imagoes have to deal with married life, they suddenly find themselves confronted with their latent genital desires, even though their affective life is immature for want of heterosexual identification, as they are still dominated by problems of the anal stage. Thus the fleeting Oedipal hopes will soon give way to a repetition, this time with the husbands, of the anal relationship to the Mother, a relation which is then confirmed by penis envy. The advantage of this situation consists in avoiding a frontal attack on the maternal imago and also in avoiding the feeling of deep anxiety at the idea of detaching oneself from her domination and superiority.

The homosexual woman and the penis

The above passage delineates subtly the background to a *neurotic* solution to the problems of the sexual difference, the frustrations of the oedipal situation, and the ideals of present day society. What of the homosexual woman and her particular solution? To begin with, her wish for a penis of her own and all it represents is not, as with the heterosexually orientated, totally unconscious. The homosexual's desire for a personal penis is frequently conscious, intense, and detached from the man. Many homosexual women recount dreams in which they have a penis, and devise sexual games with a fabricated penis. One of my patients refused to go out of her home during adolescence unless she first tied around her genital area a fictitious penis. Although terrified that this might be discovered she was equally terrified to leave the house without it. A colleague discussed with me a similar patient, who binds her breasts and ties on a false penis in order to face the world. This patient took hormones which she hoped would produce male secondary sexual characteristics, and was investigating the possibility of having her breasts removed. 'My breasts have been bound for two years now ... everybody thinks I am a man. I shave every second day. When I flirt with girls I satisfy them sexually, but I always remain dressed. I cannot bear to be touched'. The wish to have an anatomical penis sometimes reaches hallucinatory dimensions. Certain of my patients described the impression of really being possessed of a male genital. One referred to this 'penis' as her 'phantom organ' and likened it to the illusions of amputated patients who can still 'feel' the missing limb. This patient also thought of having her breasts removed and, like the patient who took hormones, she could not bear to be touched by her partners. As with many of these women, her sexual pleasure was to procure pleasure for the partner. The penis wish is therefore extremely complicated in homosexual women; not only does it exist to repair a fantasied castration but it is also intended *to keep dormant any feminine sexual desires*. The patient who always wore a fabricated penis in adolescence reached a point in her analysis where she began to explore her overwhelming guilt about this behaviour. She suddenly wished to make herself a penis once more; it no longer seemed such a hideous crime. 'Last night I made myself a penis out of some bits of material. I tried it on and caressed it, and I felt flushed and excited. Then suddenly I had a strange urge to push it inside my body. It nearly frightened me to death.' The vaginal sensations and feeling of desire filled her with anxiety, and the thought came to mind that if she were to give in to such feelings she would go crazy, explode, or die. That night she dreamed that her mother was dying. In fact the cruel and prohibiting part of the internalized imago was about to die as the daughter became sexually alive. We were later to discover that this play-penis had also served to block clitoral as well as vaginal sensation, and thus contributed to reinforce the blocking of genital desire.

As we have seen, the deep sense of prohibition and of being threatened by the mother is not the only reason for the wish for a personal penis. The father's penis has been divested of its symbolic phallic function and significance. To the extent to which the penis is a penis-attached-to-a-man, it is a dangerous image, endowed with violent and destructive qualities. Since at the same time the primal-scene is envisaged in anal-sadistic terms, men are believed to harbour sadistic or humiliating desires towards women. There is no image of a 'good penis'; the penis is never envisioned as a pleasure-giving, healing, or narcissistically enhancing possession when offered to the woman in a heterosexual relationship. In addition, since the father's penis was denied by these patients, much of their own sexual activity was a protest designed to prove that the mother had never desired the father nor his penis, and that in fact a penis was quite unnecessary to the sexual act with a woman.

Behind the 'bad penis' images, analysis reveals equally dangerous breast fantasies in which the breast is felt to be a poisoning and persecutory object. The equation of breast and penis in the unconscious is inevitably linked to oral-sadistic fears of a paranoid or schizoid kind, and, of course, is not limited to a homosexual organization. The tragedy of the homosexual girl's psychosexual development is rooted in the fact that the penis has become detached from the father, the part-object taking the place of the total-object: it is introjected as such, to prevent further regression to the traumatic prephallic era, in which the mother is felt to contain the phallus – not only the father's penis but the power of life and death over her child. According to the possible variations in the unconscious family constellation, the penis-image and its phallic symbolic meaning will vary for different homosexual women. Briefly speaking, we might say that there are two main poles, one in which depressive anxiety is uppermost, and the other in which per-secutory anxiety dominates. In the first case the aim of *repairing* the partner is uppermost and may include a measure of self-reparation, the split in the self-image being repaired narcissistically through a sexual object who is *like oneself*. At the other end of the scale the *fear of the homosexual object* leads, because of paranoid projection, to an over-whelming need to dominate the object erotically, the orgasm of the partner carrying the meaning both of possession and castration. Such women frequently seek no orgastic pleasure for themselves and, if their terror of total loss-of-self is strong, they will assume a male identity with somewhat delusional conviction, leading in certain cases to operations intended to 'transsexualize' their bodies. The women dominated by such deep anxiety frequently claim that they are *not homosexual*. Their unconscious identity-image would tend to uphold that they are really men imprisoned in female forms. In practice, they avoid any personal orgastic pleasure while seeking to procure sexual pleasure for their partners. Desire centred only on the climax of the partner characterizes a number of homosexual women. To seek direct erotic pleasure jeopardizes the deep feeling of masculine identity. This in turn is vitally necessary to ward-off anxiety of psychotic dimensions concerning the body-image and the feeling of identity, both being felt to be threatened by the internalized mother and to carry a danger of fusion with her.

This brings us to the crucial role of castration anxiety in homo-sexual women: it is perhaps evident from the clinical fragments quoted here that the fantasy of being castrated is more profound, more globally disturbing, than is the case with women who have developed neurotic symptoms or neurotic character traits to cope with castration anxiety at its different levels. It is clear that castration anxiety is not limited solely to phallic anxiety, stemming from the phase in which the sexual difference becomes significant; nor is it limited to the 'narcissistic castration' resulting from the oedipal crises, when the small child discovers that he is forever outside the sexual bond of the parents, and that his incestuous longings will never reach fulfilment. The anxiety felt by these patients concerns *not only their sexuality but their feeling of subjective identity as separate beings*. This might well be named 'primary castration', the prototype of later 'castration anxiety'. If unresolved, that is, if the small girl fails to accept and compensate adequately for the recognition of otherness, then she risks the loss of her ego-boundaries, of aphanisis and psychic death.

Castration in this global sense is actually the equivalent of accepting reality, and has to be symbolised in the same way that phallic-castration anxiety has to be elaborated psychically for the establishment of sexual reality and gender identity. Homosexual relations avoid the many-sided problem of classical phallic-castration anxiety by the simple exclusion of one of the sexes; but homosexual activity and its ensuing relationships also aid the ego in dealing with the more

overwhelming anxiety concerning separateness and fear of disintegration. However, the homosexual way of life is inadequate to cope with
all of these problems. Much anxiety is left over and thus we find in
these patients many poorly structured neurotic symptoms – phobic
formations concerning oral anxiety (anorexia, bulimia, addictions,
and vomiting phobias are frequent), phobic–obsessional symptoms
concerning anal and urinary functions, masochistic body rituals, and
persecutory fears. Hypochondriacal anxiety and somatizations are also
common (Sperling 1956). All of these syptoms are deeply rooted in
the early mother–child relationship, at which time the stage is set for
many of the 'acting-out neuroses', including a homosexual resolution
of oedipal stress at a later period. The latter solution is more apt to
arise when the father has unresolved homosexual problems and feelings
of envy, and hatred for women.

The homosexual relationship

In his comprehensive book *The overt homosexual* (1968), Socarides
writes:

Most overtly homosexual women will in treatment acknowledge the mother–
child relationship which they have with the love object.... The homosexual
woman is in flight from the man. The source of this flight is her childhood
feeling of guilt toward her mother, the fear of merging with her and the fear of
disappointment and rejection at the hands of the father if she dared to turn to
him for love and support. If she expected that her father would fulfil her
infantile sexual wishes there is a masochistic danger present, too. Or she may
feel that her father would refuse her and then she would suffer the danger of
narcissistic injury. The end result is to turn to the earlier love object again – the
mother – more ardently than before. However, she cannot return to the real
mother due to her fear of merging and being engulfed.

My own clinical experience confirms the extensive researches of this
author. But I would like to add to his summary a brief examination of
the dynamic changes in the psychic economy consequent upon the
establishment of overt homosexual relationships. Most of my patients
were conscious of an intense feeling of having triumphed over the
mother, and a wish that she would feel abandoned and punished. This
was usually covered by a thin veneer of concern about her feelings,
and a fear that she might take revenge of some kind. 'Somehow I
deliberately let my mother find out about my love affair with Susan.
She was absolutely furious, of course – and I was secretly glad, as though

I wanted to punish her for something. When she learns I'm in analysis with a *woman*, it'll just kill her!', remarked one of my patients pointedly. There is a large measure of triumph over the father also, since the homosexual solution implies the denial of the father's phallic role and genital existence, and the proof that a woman does not need either a man or a penis for sexual completion. The homosexual triumphs finally over the primal-scene and sexual reality.

A further source of gratification lies in the fact that the new relationship is an overtly erotic one. Masturbation and sexual desire, always felt to have been forbidden by the mother, are welcomed by the partner and guilt feelings are thus diminished. Many old conflicts between mother and daughter are also eclipsed in the relation with the mother-substitute. In general the real mother has always complained about the unfeminine daughter who refused to dress in pretty clothes, was not interested in boys or parties, behaved in ways which seemed irresponsible, unusual, disorderly and secretive. Now all these same character traits are accepted and even highly valued by the homosexual partner. The unconscious significance of this acceptance is far-reaching, for hidden under the surface of the ruthless, non-conforming, anal-erotic child, is the internalized father, and in consequence an anguished fear of losing the identification with him which guarantees ego-identity. This the mother has never accepted, while the father has frequently reinforced this outcome by his own conflict with femininity.

One of my patients recounted a poignant moment with her lover which epitomizes the 'reparative' dimension of the homosexual love-relation. She lived with an older woman, upon whom she was extremely dependent. Although she had many proofs of her friend's devotion to her, she always feared that one day she might vomit and that her friend would then throw her out. She suffered in fact from a severe vomiting phobia. One evening she had a genuine digestive upset and, knowing that she was about to vomit, she called to her friend to do something to stop it happening. In answer to her plea, the friend held out her hands so that the young woman might vomit into them. She did so, exclaiming 'Now you will never love me again!' But her lover deposited a kiss on the regurgitated meal as a sign of total acceptance. This unusual exchange had a profound meaning, and an equally profound effect on the young woman. She was able to analyse, in the months which followed, the unconscious significance of her phobia, and to understand that her friend's gesture meant acceptance of, and forgiveness for, all her forbidden erotic fantasies concerning the father's penis as well as repressed sadistic wishes. Her body-image, always experienced until then as a faecal object which should be discarded, became an object of value.

The many sided importance and structuring aspects of anal-erotic and anal-sadistic fantasy has already been stressed; the patient just quoted is a crystalline example of a fantasy common to most homosexual women, namely that being a women is equivalent to being a pile of faeces. 'She imagined herself as a very aggressive unattractive, destructive and "smelly" object. She "gave off smells" and was filled with bad things. She had deep feelings of guilt for her aggression towards both her father and her mother. "If I show my evilness everyone will abandon me . . . . This aggression was turned against the self in dreams and made her feel bad as if she were "a piece of smeared faeces."' (Socarides, 1968). Such deeply destructive feelings, along with the damaged self-image, are partially healed by the homosexual relationship, where each partner may play the 'holding function' of the 'good enough mother' of Winnicott's writings (1960). 'She is less cruel to me than I am to myself', said Sophie one day talking of her lover. These women are often incapable of being 'good mothers' to themselves, and can only bestow love on another woman. Something which is missing in the inner-object world is thus sought in the partner: through identification with her, instinctual satisfactions as well as certain lost parts of the self are recovered.

The aggressive wishes which seek to be contained in the homosexual act and object relation go further back than the phallic-genital frustrations of the oedipal situation, further back than the anal phase of integration, back, as we have seen, to archaic sexual objects, long before the conscious differentiation of the sexes (Klein 1950, 1954). If the homosexual girl's secret desire at the phallic-genital level is to obtain the sexual emblems of the other sex – the symbolic unattainable phallus, with which to attract the mother's desire – the underlying wishes are those of the baby, all that the infant-self unconsciously still demands. This might be summarized as the wish to obtain for oneself, and forever remain in possession of, the breast-mother. Not only is the difference between the sexes disavowed, but also the difference between one person and another, one body and another, the baby and the breast. Such satisfactions and gratifications are hoped for within the erotic homosexual bond. But since this is built upon the greedy oral-love of the earliest relationship, it includes the aim of possessing the object to its own destruction. The underlying fantasy, not only of having castrated but also of having lost or destroyed the object, gives rise to intense depressive feeling.

We have up till now been examining the positive aspects of the homosexual relationship; however, it is evident that few of the basic conflicts are resolved and that the new relationship contains the seeds of its own destruction. Analysis invariably reveals the greedy and destructive, as well as the manipulatory, anal-controlling aspects of the relationship. The need to idealize the partner, the sexual act, and the relationship as a whole is present in order to protect the love-object from the fantasied attacks that the individual would like to make upon it. The homosexual needs to believe that her relationship to her partner is reparative and healing. While it is true that concern for the object mitigates greedy oral destructiveness, this unconscious content contributes to the evanescent quality of many homosexual affairs. 'I realize more and more that I am crazy to go on caring for her so much. I admit I grabbed at her to live with me because my last friend left me so suddenly and I just can't live alone. Nor can she [the present friend]; but where I really care a lot about her – her failures, her insomnia – she doesn't even know who I really am! My professional problems bore her to tears. I'm sure if I suddenly stopped bringing home money she would leave me immediately for another woman.' This remark from one of my patients is one I have heard in different versions from other homosexuals.

Such insights are extremely painful to the individuals concerned, and in fact they are only uncovered in analysis when the patient discovers to her astonishment that history is repeating itself; not only does she perceive this with respect to her various lovers, she also comes to realize that a piece of infantile history is being re-enacted: she is once again the little girl performing solely for the narcissistic enhancement and the emotional security of the mother. Thus the tendency to reduce the love-partner to a part-object, to victimize her, and to control her every movement is only equalled in intensity by the fear of becoming, oneself, the part-object, magnetically fixed upon the partner. Such patients seek therefore to play an essential and irreplaceable role to the partner, and sometimes end-up doing many things for the other woman to the detriment of their own interests or of their work. Here the wheel has come full circle to the childhood relation with the mother; the ego thus continues to pursue its instinctual aims and to maintain its fragile identity along the lines traced out in childhood.

The oedipal structure and the ego defences

The oedipal organization as an unconscious nuclear and structural model of the personality should serve as a starting point for our summary of the findings in this paper. As we have seen, the homosexual girl has regressed in face of the oedipal situation and restructured her sexual desires in terms of the dyadic mother-relationship; thus the father's penis no longer symbolizes the phallus and she herself embodies the phallic object. Through unconscious identification with the father, and by investing her whole body with the significance of the penis, she is now able in fantasy to fulfil a woman sexually. Instinctual regression from phallic-genital, to anal-erotic and anal-sadistic expression, has left its mark on the object-relationship and has also been invested in character-traits. Oral-erotic and oral-sadistic wishes, because of their frightening nature, are kept in check in large part by the homosexual relationship and the sexual act itself. Addictions and compulsions (such as kleptomania) (McDougall 1970; Schmideberg 1956) are frequent secondary symptoms to deal with these primitive, repressed impulses. There is no dissolution of the oedipal conflict: with regard to the heterosexual object, narcissistic mortification has led to complete conscious withdrawal from the father; insofar as homosexual oedipal wishes are concerned, the homosexual woman has also failed in the integration of these into her personality structure for their normal resolution would have led to identification with the genital-mother. Instead, the primal-scene is denied, and then reinvented with the exclusion of the male and the penis. Following Bion (1970) we might say that these children have refuted the oedipal myth and created a private one instead. The homosexual 'solution' to id wishes and relational problems has its counterpart in the ego structure. From the standpoint of clinical categories we are dealing with an unconscious organization which is neither a classical neurotic nor a psychotic one. There are neurotic defence mechanisms at work, but they are not sufficiently organized to protect sexual-identity; in addition, there are a number of psychotic defences which have gone into the homosexual solution and the maintenance of its basic illusions. In fact we find here the splitting of the ego's defensive shield, as described by Freud in his 1938 paper on this subject. This would seem to provide the nodal point for the conception of a 'third structure'. Although this identical oedipal and ego structure is found to underlie all sexual deviations (Rosen 1964; McDougall 1972) it seems to me inaccurate to refer to this as a 'perverse' structure since it is not limited to the sexual perversions. The defensive splitting and the continual acting-out to compensate for what is missing in the inner psychic world can also be found in many severe character neuroses, in patients with addictions and anti-social symptoms, as well as in psychosomatic patients (Sperling 1968; McDougall 1974). What is more specific for homosexual women is the pathological introjection of the father figure, and the erotization of defences against the depressive and persecutory anxieties which result from these distorted structures.

Splitting mechanisms play a particularly important role in the ego organization. Not only is there a split in the defensive mechanisms but there is also a split in the inner object world (Gillespie 1956a and b). The image of womanhood held by these patients is divided into a highly idealized and a totally castrated one – so idealized that it is felt to be inaccessible, and so castrated that they must disguise their femininity by all the psychic means at their disposal. As long as this type of splitting process can be maintained – and it requires constant projection and disavowal of reality to do so – the ego can protect its identity. Further extension to the splitting tendencies is to be seen in the redistribution of the split-off fragments. Although the failure of early splitting into good and bad (which if unhealed leads to a psychotic resolution) has been avoided there is nevertheless a specific splitting along sexual lines – a 'good' sex and a 'bad' sex. This is similar to the 'false splitting' described by Meltzer (1967). 'Bad parts' of the self along with bad feelings attached to the internalized mother are projected onto the father, and subsequently onto men in general, and may lead to a paranoid attitude towards men. But this ensures the 'good' which is invested in fantasies of reparation of self and partner, and hopes for recovering lost parts of the self. However, if the female object, which unconsciously contains so much hatred and so many 'bad' parts of the infantile-self, comes too dangerously close to being a *conscious* container of hatred then the fear of the partner may triumph over the eroticized defences, and this would lead – outside of an analytic situation – to the risk of psychotic episodes of a paranoid type. At this point the loved and the hated person coalesce; not only sexual desire, but all desire, the desire to live, is threatened. Mary Barnes (1971) described the feeling that all instinctual movement on her part was forbidden: 'The "right" thing had always been what someone else wanted of me.... Not separate, my desire had to go through someone else. As if I was a tiny baby, I could only be satisfied through 'Mother' gauging my needs.

In her womb, the food of blood from her, to me. The trouble with me had been my real *Mother* hadn't really wanted me to have it, food. She had never had any milk in her breasts. She couldn't; she hated me. Yet she told me she loved me, and wanted me to eat.... I had to starve to death to satisfy my Mother'. Mary Barnes had found no protective halt, such as the creation of homosexual relations to live out sexual desire and to protect her, as she 'went down' in the depths of her tortured relation to her inner objects. The harsh pregenitalized super-ego of the homosexual is quadrupled in psychotic dissolution. If the neurotic may be said to fight for his sexuality and the psychotic for his very life, the homosexual (along with all 'third structure' people) might be said to have found a half-way station between these two aims, in which psychic death is avoided and only one's sexual-self is denied. The homosexual girl's unconscious identification with the father gives her a separate identity and enables her to enact the reparative role, in the guise of sexual partner, repairing thus all the fantasied attacks contained in her intense demand for possession of the sexual- and autonomous-self of her partner. This of course is not genuine repar-ation, and comes within the scope of all that is included in the term manic defence as defined by Klein, Heimann, Isaacs, and Riviere (1952) and Winnicott (1935). It is nevertheless a powerful and protective structure within the ego.

Reference has already been made to the fantasies of the maternal breast as a bad and poisoning object, and to the way in which the homosexual act may keep fears of being destroyed (because of one's incorporative desires) at bay. But to the extent to which such fears dominate the picture and come close to consciousness, we are moving nearer to a psychotic structure than to a deviant sexual one. The same basic fears may also be elaborated through other forms of compulsive behaviour such as alcoholism, bulimia, and so on. Since the father symbolically embodies the acute paranoid fears, and since persecutory anxiety arises from contact with him, this psychic split gives the homo-sexual girl the chance to preserve her ego from dissolution; but if such fears return to the *maternal image* there is little chance of a satisfactory homosexual solution. She is also compelled to maintain her ego-identity on another front, by keeping her distance from men, for any close affective contact with them will make her lose the 'internalized penis', the fantasy on which her identity is built. She is constantly and compulsively driven, in her dilemma, to endless repetition in her erotic relationships. Over and beyond the masochistic danger of self-surrender, she is equally menaced by the potential upsurge of her violently ambivalent feelings towards her partners. Homosexual relationships move continually between two poles: the fear of losing the other, which results in a catastrophic loss of self-esteem – leading to loss-of-identity feelings or suicidal impulses; and the arousal of cruel and aggressive feelings to the partner which give rise to intolerable anguish. As a consequence of excessive idealization of the partner, homosexual relations contain, to a greater extent than heterosexual ones, a hidden dimension of envy. Thus, in spite of its reparative aspects, the homosexual situation is inevitably precarious. A sexual identity that disavows sexual reality and masks inner feelings of dead-ness can only be maintained at a costly premium. The homosexual pays dearly for this fragile identity, heavily weighted as it is with frustrated libidinal, sadistic, and narcissistic significance. But the alternative is the death of the ego.

What may psychoanalysis hope to achieve for the homosexual woman? The analyst, whatever his personal wishes may be, can only dedicate himself to leading his patient as far as possible on the road to self-discovery, which may or may not lead to her giving up her homosexual life. The important aim is to bring to her consciousness the varied aspects of her internal drama which until now have escaped her, along with the conflictual roles played by the internalized parents, and the intense feelings of love and hate attached to them. She will then be in a position to retrace what she understood to be her place and role in the family constellation. Only in this way may she come to recognize her own conflicts and contradictory pursuits, along with the intricate network of defences constructed since infancy to deal with confusion and mental pain.

Among other factors, the analytic harvest includes a transformation of the body image. Where she once conceived of herself as ill-made, disorganized, dirty, or sick, she now is able to make a truer appreci-ation of her physical self. The old hypochondriacal anxieties become less, and often disappear entirely. More solidly 'embodied', the patient comes to a different appreciation of herself and her capacities in professional and other social fields.

For many, there is an equally important change in the feeling of sexual identity. In spite of the fact that these patients rarely come into analysis in order to become heterosexual, many do in fact give up their homosexual pursuits and become wives and mothers. Others are not drawn to the heterosexual arena. In spite of its pitfalls, the homosexual solution offers a certain security. However the conviction of having chosen and consciously assumed one's homosexuality is in itself a positive factor in comparison with the former feeling of compulsion. Thus these patients are often able to create more stable, less ambivalent, relationships with their partners, and find themselves better armed to face homosexual conflict.

References

Arlow, J. (1954). Perversions: theoretic and therapeutic aspects *J. Amer. Psychoanal. Assoc.*, **2**, 336.

Bak, R. (1956). Aggression and perversion. In *Perversions: Psychodynamics and Therapy* (ed. S. Lorand and M. Balint). New York.

Barnes, M. and Berke, J. (1971). *Two accounts of a journey through madness*, London.

Bion, W. (1962). *Learning from experience*. London.
—— (1970). *Attention and Interpretation*. London.

Brierley, M. (1932). Some problems of integration in women, *Int. J. Psycho-Anal.* **13**, 433.
—— (1936). Specific determinants in feminine development. *Int. J. Psycho-Anal.* **17**, 163.

Brunswick, R. M. (1940). The pre-oedipal phase of libido development. *Psychoanal. Quart.* **9**, 293.

Deutsch, H. (1932). On female homosexuality. *Psychoanal. Quart.* **1**,
—— (1944–5). *Psychology of women, Vols. 1 & 2*. New York.

Federn, P. (1953). *Ego psychology and the psychoses*. London.

Freud, A. (1951). Homosexuality. *Bull. Amer. Psychoanal. Assoc.* **7**, 117.

Freud, S. (1908). On the sexual theories of children. *Complete psychological works of Sigmund Freud*. Standard edition **9**. London.
—— (1915). A case of paranoia running counter to the psychoanalytic theory of the disease. *Complete psychological works of Sigmund Freud*. Standard edition **14**. London.
—— (1917). On transformations of instinct in anal erotism. *Complete psychological works of Sigmund Freud*. Standard edition **17**.
—— (1917). Mourning and melancholia. *Complete psychological works of Sigmund Freud*. Standard edition **14**. London.
—— (1920). The psychogenesis of a case of homosexuality in a woman. *Complete psychological works of Sigmund Freud*. Standard edition **18**. London.
—— (1922). Some neurotic mechanisms in jealousy, paranoia and homosexuality. *Complete psychological works of Sigmund Freud*. Standard edition **19**. London.
—— (1924). The loss of reality in neurosis and psychosis. *Complete psychological works of Sigmund Freud*. Standard edition **19**. London.

—— (1925). Some psychical consequences of the anatomical distinction between the sexes. *Complete psychological works of Sigmund Freud*. Standard edition **19**. London.

—— (1931). Female sexuality. *Complete psychological works of Sigmund Freud*. Standard edition **21**. London.

—— (1933). Femininity. *Complete psychological works of Sigmund Freud*. Standard edition **22**. London.

—— (1938). On the splitting of the ego in the defensive process. *Complete psychological works of Sigmund Freud*. Standard edition **23**. London.

Gillespie, W. (1956a). The general theory of sexual perversions. *Int. J. Psycho-Anal*. **37**, 396.

—— (1956b). The structure and aetiology of sexual perversion. In *Perversions: Psychodynamics and Therapy* (ed. S. Lorand and M. Balint). New York.

Glover, E. (1933). The relation of perversion-formation to the development of reality-sense. *Int. J. Psycho-Anal*. **14**, 486.

—— (1960). *The roots of crime*. London.

Grunberger, B. (1971). *Essais sur le narcissisme*. Paris.

Jones, E. (1927). The early development of female sexuality. *Int. J. Psycho-Anal*. **8**, 459.

—— (1934). The phallic phase. *Int. J. Psycho-Anal*. **13**, 1.

Klein, M. (1950). *Contributions to psychoanalysis*. London.

—— (1954). *The psychoanalysis of children*. London.

—— (1957). *Envy and gratitude*. London.

——, Heimann, P., Isaacs, S. and Rivière J. (1952). *Developments in psycho-analysis*. London.

Kurth, F. and Patterson, A. (1968). Structuring aspects of the penis. *Int. J. Psycho-Anal*. **49**, 620.

Lacan, J. (1966). *Ecrits*. Paris.

Levi-Strauss, C. (1949). *Les structures elementaires de la parenté*. Paris.

Lichtenstein, H. (1961). Sexuality and identity. *J. Amer. Psychoanal. Assoc*. **9**.

McDougall, J. (1970). Homosexuality in women. In *Female sexuality* (ed. J. Chasseguet-Smirgel). Michigan.

Mahler, M. and Gosliner, B. (1955). On symbiotic child psychosis. *Psychoanal. Study Child*. **10**, 195.

Meltzer, D. (1967). *The psychoanalytical process*. London.

Nunberg, H. (1938). Homosexuality, magic and aggression. *Int. J. Psycho-Anal*. **19**, 1.

Rosen, I., (ed.) (1964). *The pathology and treatment of sexual deviation*. London.

Rosenfeld, H. (1949). Remarks on the relation of male homosexuality to paranoid anxiety and narcissism. In *Psychotic states*. (ed.) London.

Schmideberg, M. (1956). Delinquent acts as perversions and fetishes. *Int. J. Psychoanal*. **37**, 422.

Socarides, C. (1968). *The overt homosexual*. New York.

Sperling, M. (1968). Acting-out behaviour and psychosomatic symptoms. *Int. J. Psycho-Anal.* **49**, 250.

Torok, M. (1970). The significance of penis envy in women. In *Female Sexuality*. (ed. J. Chasseguet-Smirgel). Michigan.

Winnicott, D. (1935). The manic defence. In *Collected Papers*. London.
—— (1948). Reparation in respect of mother's organized defence against depression. In *Collected Papers*. London.
—— (1951). Transitional objects and transitional phenomena. In *Collected Papers*. London.
—— (1960). The theory of the parent-infant relationship. *Int. J. Psycho-Anal.* **41**, 585.

9 The psychoanalytic theory of homosexuality
with special reference to therapy

Charles W. Socarides

Introduction

In the early years of psychoanalysis, Freud (1905), Sadger (1909), and Ferenczi (1909) had perceived the interconnection between infantile sexuality, perversions, and neurosis, and arrived at the conclusion that a neurosis represents the negative of a perversion. A formulation of the essential psychological developmental factors in homosexuality was described by these foremost psychoanalytic investigators of their time around 1910. For example, they stated that in the earliest stage of development, the homosexual-to-be experiences a very strong mother fixation. Upon leaving this attachment, he continues to identify with the mother, taking himself narcissistically as the sexual object. Consequently he searches for a man resembling himself, whom he attempts to love as he wishes his mother had loved him. Clinical investigations of the genesis of the constellations responsible for this developmental inhibition uncovered an unresolvable oedipal conflict.

Freud saw that the determinants toward homosexuality came during adolescence, when a 'revolution of the mental economy' takes place. The adolescent, in exchanging his mother for some other sexual object, may make a choice of an object of the same sex. In addition, the presence of an unloving cruel father increased the difficulties in the formation of male identification (Freud 1921).

The clinical papers of that era focused almost exclusively on the failure to resolve the oedipus complex, as the causative factor in homosexuality. Freud himself was not content with this application of the oedipal theory as the definitive answer, and stressed the necessity to seek out other determinants, namely, the psychic mechanism responsible for homosexuality, and an explanation of what determines this particular outcome rather than another. He concluded that homosexuality represents an inhibition and dissociation of the psychosexual development, one of the pathological outcomes of the oedipal period.

243

Analytic investigation, at that time, had not disclosed any single genetic or structural pattern that would apply to all, or even a major proportion of, the cases of sexual inversion. It would be the task of future investigators, Freud wrote, to determine what genetic developmental factors were essential for the production of homosexuality, to elucidate a structural theory for understanding homosexuality, to examine therapeutic problems inherent in the treatment of homosexuals, and to shed light on the connection between the sexual instinct and the choice of object in homosexual behaviour.

Freud found difficulty in drawing a sharp line between normal and pathological behaviour. He stated that, in cases where exclusiveness of fixation (obligatoriness) was present, we are justified in calling homosexuality a pathological symptom (Freud 1905). He maintained that constitutional factors played a part in sexual perversions, but they played a similar role in all mental disorders. This in no way indicated any repudiation of the role of psychological factors in a predisposition to homosexuality: in fact, he was emphasizing precisely these developmental factors.

From the outset, therefore, homosexuality was considered to be a recognized form of perversion along with fetishism, voyeurism, paedophilia, transvestism, and so on. Subsequent psychoanalytic investigations have more than amply substantiated this position. Most psychoanalysts define perversion as an habitual deviation from the prevailing sexual norm. A homosexual may be defined an an individual who engages repetitively, or episodically, in sexual relations with a partner of the same sex, or experiences the recurrent desire to do so. If required to function sexually with a partner of the opposite sex, he can do so, if at all, only with very little or no pleasure. In homosexuality as in other perversions, genital sexuality is replaced by one component of infantile sexuality. Perverse acts are distorted exaggerations, and have a quality of uniqueness and stereotypy which does not appear in normal persons, except as introductory activities prior to intercourse. The true homosexual has only one way of gaining pleasure, and his energies are concentrated in this direction. His capacity is blocked for other pleasures by some obstacle, which is more or less overcome by the perverse act. The gratification of the perverse instinctual drive actually constitutes the end-product of a defensive compromise, in which elements of inhibition as well as gratification are present. The component instinct itself has undergone excessive transformation and disguise to be gratified in the perverse act.

The perverted homosexual action, like the neurotic symptom, results from the conflict between the ego and the id (a concept developed in 1923), and represents a compromise formation, which at the same time must be acceptable to the demands of the super-ego. As in the case of neurotic symptoms, the instinctual gratification takes place in disguised form, while its real content remains unconscious. However, a perversion differs from a neurotic symptom, first by the form of gratification of the impulse, namely, orgasm; and secondly, in the fact that the ego's wishes for omnipotence are satisfied by the arbitrary egosyntonic action. It has been discovered that the defensive aspects of homosexuality are crucial for promoting object relations and sustaining identifications. In homosexuality, the fusion of aggressive and libidinal impulses, the presence of guilt, and the need for punishment, play important roles. Homosexuality differs from neurosis in that the symptom is desexualized in neurosis; discharge is painful in neurosis, but brings genital orgasm in the perversion.

Gillespie's (1956) important paper on perversions in general represented the state of psychoanalytic theory and understanding of homosexuality at that time. His work was remarkably comprehensive, taking into account infantile sexuality, and affirming that the problem of homosexuality lies in the defences against oedipal difficulties. It underlined the concept that in homosexuality there is a regression of libido and aggression to preoedipal levels, rather than a primary fixation at those levels; it stressed the importance of ego behaviour and ego defensive manoeuvres, as well as the importance of the Sachs mechanism; it delineated the characteristics of the ego, which make it possible for the ego to adopt a certain aspect of infantile sexuality thereby enabling it to ward off other aspects. The super-ego has a special relationship to the ego, which makes the latter tolerant of this particular form of sexuality. A split in the ego often coexists with a split in the sexual object so that the object becomes idealized, 'relatively anxiety-free and relatively guilt-free in part'.

In the past two decades, increasing emphasis has been placed on preoedipal phase difficulties as causative of homosexuality (Arlow 1952; Socarides 1960, 1962). This can be seen in psychoanalytic studies, such as those of Bychowski (1945), van der Leeuw (1958), Fleischmann (1960), and Socarides (1968a, 1968b, 1974). The last edition of this book (Rosen 1964) includes numerous statements on the aetiological significance of preoedipal developmental pathology in homosexuality, as well as other perversions. In 1967, in a paper entitled 'A unitary theory of sexual perversions: theoretical considerations' presented before the American Psychoanalytic Association, I proposed that the genesis of homosexuality and perhaps all of the sexual perversions may well be the result of common core disturbances which occur earlier than has been generally assumed and accepted, namely, in the preoedipal phase of human development (Socarides 1978).

Aetiology

Several psychoanalytic hypotheses attempt an explanation of the basis for sexual object choice in homosexuality. The first, originally suggested by Freud (1905), was that of constitutional bisexuality; this assumed in essence that in addition to an innate constitutional sexual predisposition to opposite-sex partners, there exists a similar unconscious and innate predisposition to same-sex partners. Freud felt that man's bisexuality, in interaction with experiential factors in childhood, was responsible for the expression of one choice or the other. He later placed less emphasis on the constitutional factor, suggesting that 'the connection between the sexual instincts and the sexual object' is not as 'intimate' as one would surmise – both are merely 'soldered together'. He warned that we must loosen the conceptual bonds which exist between instinct and object: 'It seems probable that the sexual instinct is in the first instance independent of its object nor is its origin likely to be due to the object's attraction'.

Bieber (1959) holds that, where reproduction depends on heterosexual mating, there are built-in mechanisms to guarantee heterosexual arousal and behaviour. In mammals, the built-in mechanisms are largely mediated through olfaction. Evidence is accumulating that olfaction is operant in human sexual development (Bieber 1959; Kalogerakis 1963). Neurologica and humoral mechanisms in concert with experiential factors under normal childhood conditions, according to these authors, guarantees heterosexual object choice. In my opinion, such primitive neurological guarantees are unlikely. Similarly, the theory of constitutional bisexuality, as an aetiological factor in the development of the homosexual perversion, can be viewed as having outlived its scientific usefulness for man does not 'inherit any organized component mechanisms that would – or could – direct him to such goals as mating or choice of mate' (Rado 1955). In man, due to the tremendous development of the cerebral cortex, motivation – both conscious and unconscious – plays the crucial role in the selection of individuals and/or objects that will produce sexual arousal and orgastic release. Where massive childhood fears have damaged and disrupted the standard male–female design, the roundabout method of achieving orgastic release is through instituting male–male or female–female patterns. Such early unconscious fears are responsible not only for the later development of homosexuality, but for all modified sexual patterns (perversions) of the obligatory type.

In all homosexuals, according to the preoedipal theory of causation, there has been an inability to make the progression from the mother–child unity of earliest infancy to individuation (Socarides 1968*b*). One of the consequences of this inability to traverse the separation-individuation phase successfully is a deficient and distorted sense of sexual identity. This becomes a source for future disturbances in sexual object choice and aim. The background of homosexuals studied (Bieber *et al.* 1962) commonly reveals a pathological family constellation† in which there is a domineering, psychologically-crushing mother, who will not allow the child to achieve autonomy from her, and an absent, weak, or rejecting father, who is unable to aid the son to overcome the block in maturation. As a result there exists in homosexuals a partial fixation with the concomitant tendency to regression to the earliest mother–child relationship.

Preoedipal theory of causation

The preoedipal theory rests on two pillars: the first is the presence of a fixation in the preoedipal phase of development; the second is the Hans Sachs (1923) mechanism of sexual perversion. According to my observations, the genesis of homosexuality may well be the result of disturbances which occur earlier than has been generally assumed. These early phases are not truly undifferentiated, and they are already manifesting important beginnings of structure formation (Arlow and Brenner 1964; Hartmann, Kris, and Loewenstein 1946). Fixation to the mother, and the characteristically narcissistic object choice of the homosexual may be traced back to the earliest preoedipal phase of the mother–child unity.

It may be assumed that relations, as they develop out of the original unity in the undifferentiated phase, are the forerunners of later object relations. Qualitative and quantitative factors, specifically the diver-

---

†It should be noted that Freud, with remarkable prescience, had predicted such a family constellation in 1905.

gent tendencies in the separation processes beginning at birth – one leading to separateness and differentiation, and the other toward retaining the primitive state of the original unity – leave their imprint on the developing modes of instinctual manifestations and on ego formation. They exercise a determining influence in the structuring of the introjects and their subsequent projective dramatization in the external world.

The fantasies and latent dream thoughts of the adult about his earliest experiences are representative of what once was the earliest reality. Thus external situations become internalized in the structure of the ego. Introjection and projection are ego-building mechanisms of the infant, becoming, through change of function, defensive devices of the child's developing ego.

The normal child must find his own identity as a prerequisite to the onset of both true object relations and partial identifications with his parents (Jacobson 1964). To the homosexual, the mother, during infancy, was dangerous and frightening, forcing separation, and threatening the infant with loss of love and care on the one hand; while on the other, the mother's conscious and unconscious tendencies were felt as working against separation. Anxiety and frustration press for withdrawal of libidinal cathexis from the mother, and result in a shift of libido economy toward increased aggression. This image of the introjected mother leads to a split in the ego. In his narcissistic object choice, the homosexual not only loves his partner as he himself wished to be loved by the mother, but reacts to him with sadistic aggression, as once experienced toward the hostile mother for forcing separation.

The unconscious hostility reinforces the denial of any loving and giving aspects of the mother. The homosexual seeks to rediscover in his object choice – in the most distorted ways – the primary reality of his narcissistic relationship with the different images of the mother (and later of the father) as they were first experienced. The first introjection of the mother image predisposes the pattern of later introjections.

Homosexuality, therefore, can be seen as a resolution of the separation from the mother by running away from all women. In fantasies and actions, in reality, in the compulsive hunting for partners, the homosexual is unconsciously searching for the lost objects, seeking to find the narcissistic relationships he once experienced in the mother–child symbiosis. The homosexual is trying to undo the separation and remain close to his mother in a substitutive way, by using the male. He is trying to be one with her, and to seek out the reduplication of himself as an object.

In 1923, Sachs provided psychoanalysis with a most important explanation of the mechanism of sexual perversion. This discovery has not been widely applied to clinical material and the paper has remained untranslated until recently. He noted that, in homosexuality, a particularly suitable portion of the infantile experience or fantasy is preserved through the vicissitudes of childhood and puberty, and remains in the conscious mind. The rest of the representatives of the instinctual drives have succumbed to repression, instigated by their all-too-strong need for gratification or stimulation. The pleasurable sensations belonging to infantile sexuality in general are now displaced onto the conscious 'suitable portion of infantile experience'. This conscious suitable portion is now supported and endowed with a high pleasure reward – so high, indeed, that it competes successfully with the primacy of the genitals. What makes this fragment particularly suitable? The pregenital stage of development upon which the homosexual is especially strongly fixated must be included in it; and it must have some special relationship to the ego which allows this particular fragment to escape repression. In this connection, one must remember that in the ego itself unconscious elements are present, for instance, guilt and resistance. Instinctual drives are themselves in a continual struggle through the developmental stages of life. The complete subjugation of one which grants much pleasure may not be completely possible. Very often what we have to resign ourselves to is a compromise, allowing pleasure to remain in a partial complex to be taken up into the ego and to be sanctioned, while the remaining components are detached and repressed more easily. This separation or split '...in which the one piece [of infantile sexuality] enters into the service of the repression and thus carries over into the ego the pleasure of a pregenital stage of development, while the rest falls a victim to repression, appears to be the mechanism of perversion' (Sachs 1923).

We know that the most difficult work of repression is almost always the detachment from the infantile object choice, the oedipus complex, and the castration complex. The partial drive does not continue directly into homosexuality, but only after it has passed through the permutations of the oedipal conflict. This is a kind of working-over that wipes out traces of the oedipus complex, eliminates, for example, the important individuals involved, eliminates one's own self-involvement, and the product becomes the perverse fantasy. It can then enter consciousness and can yield pleasure.

It would follow that fantasies which lie outside the circle of infantile sexual gratification present themselves as a 'way out'. For instance, in male homosexuality there is an extremely strong fixation on the mother which cannot be dealt with. The end result becomes a fixation on the homosexual's own sex, as a result of narcissism and in the retreat from later castration anxiety. This is incorporated into the ego and is acceptable to it. In essence, there has been taken over into the ego a portion of what would otherwise be repressed. Nonetheless, the rest of the repressed portion may still remain strong enough to threaten a breakthrough during later life, and the homosexual may, at any time, develop neurotic symptoms.

In homosexuality, the instinctual gratification takes place in a disguised form while its real content remains unconscious. We must constantly re-emphasize that we are not dealing with an aspect of infantile sexuality, which was allowed into consciousness and which the ego could somehow tolerate; the homosexual symptom does not come about simply because the boy, once disturbed in his sexuality by castration fear, regressed to that component of his infantile sexuality which once in childhood gave him security, or at least reassurance against his fears, and at the same time obtained orgastic relief. The over-emphasis on the infantile expression of his sexuality simultaneously serves to reassure him, and to maintain a repression of his oedipal conflicts and other warded-off remnants of infantile sexuality. This is a partial repression of infantile sexuality wherein other parts are exaggerated. Repression itself is facilitated in homosexuality, through the added dividend of some other aspect of infantile sexuality being consciously stressed (Sachs 1923).

Homosexuality, therefore, is a living relic of the past, testifying to the fact that there was once a conflict, involving an especially strongly developed component instinct, in which complete victory for the ego was impossible and repression was only partially successful. The ego had to be content with the compromise of repressing the greater part of infantile libidinal strivings (primary identification with the mother, intense unneutralized aggression toward her, dread of separation), at the expense of sanctioning and taking into itself the smaller part. As an illustration one might consider the repression of wishes to penetrate the mother's body, or the wish to suck and incorporate and injure the mother's breast. In these instances, a piece of infantile libidinal striving has entered the service of repression, through dis-placement and substitution. Instead of the mother's body being pene-trated, sucked, injured, incorporated, it is the male partner's body which undergoes this fate; instead of the mother's breast, it is the penis with which the patient interacts. Perversion thus becomes the choice of the lesser evil.

Two defence mechanisms, identification and substitution, play a crucial part in the framework of the above structure. The homosexual makes an identification with the masculinity of his partner in the sexual act. In order to defend himself against the positive oedipus complex, that is, his love for his mother, hatred for his father, and punitive aggressive drives toward the body of his mother, the homosexual substitutes the partner's body and penis for the mother's breast.

In every homosexual encounter, there is a hidden continuation of the close tie to the mother through the breast–penis equation. The reassuring presence of the penis in place of the breast allows the homo-sexual to feel that he is faithful, loyal to, and simultaneously main-taining the tie to the mother, but at a safe distance from her. He divests himself of oedipal guilt by demonstrating to her that he could have no possible interest in other females. Furthermore, he is protecting the mother against the onslaught of other men's penises, allowing penetration into himself instead.

Homosexuals desperately need and seek a contact whenever they feel weakened, frightened, depleted, guilty, ashamed, or in any way helpless or powerless. The male partners whom they pursue are representatives of their own self in relation to an active phallic mother. They achieve masculinity through identification with the partner's body and penis. The men chosen as partners represent their forfeited masculinity regained. In the patients' words, they want their 'shot' of masculinity. They then feel miraculously well and strengthened, and thereby avoid regressive and even disintegrative phenomena. They instantaneously feel reintegrated upon achieving orgasm with a male partner. All their pain, fear, and weakness disappears; they feel 'well' and whole again. Marked improvement in therapy is seen subsequent to the patient's recognition of these primitive mechanisms.

The homosexual comes to realize in later phases of treatment that he is engaged in an act of major self-deception, having been victimized into sexual activity with individuals of the same sex by certain intricate psychic transformations. He has not given up his maleness at all; he urgently and desperately wants to be a man but is able to do this only by transiently identifying with the masculinity and penis of a partner in the sexual act.

Homosexuality thus serves to protect the personality against regression. In the most severe cases, if homosexual behaviour did not occur, the patient would proceed to severe regression experienced as a threat of loss of ego boundaries and dissolution of self. Overt homosexuality is crucial for the survival of the ego, when it is faced with the catastrophic situation of imminent merging with the mother and pull toward the earlier phases of development.

In the threatened reunion with the mother one can discern:

(a) a wish for and fear of incorporation;

(b) a threatened loss of personal identity and personal dissolution;

(c) guilt feelings, because of a desire to invade the body of the mother;

(d) an intense desire to cling to the mother, which later develops into a fear of and wish for incestuous relations with her;

(e) intense aggression of a primitive nature toward the mother.

At a conscious level, the patient attempts to compensate for this primary nuclear conflict by certain activities designed to enclose, ward off, and encyst the isolated affective state of the mother–child unity. Therefore, he does not approach any other woman, especially sexually, as this will activate the fear of the mother–child unity. He does not attempt to leave mother, because this would only provoke engulfing, incorporative tendencies on her part. Any attempt by him to separate produces an exacerbation of his unconscious ties. He therefore strives to keep the optimal distance/closeness ('safest closeness') to her, while remaining asexual to other females. All sexual satisfactions are carried out through substitution, displacement, and other defence mechanisms. Having already made a female identification, he restores strength through transitory male identification with his male partner. However, while substituting a man for sexual intercourse, he is unconsciously enjoying sexual closeness to both mother and father simultaneously.

One cannot leave this section on aetiology without acknowledging the author's indebtedness to the monumental contributions of Mahler and her co-workers in elucidating separation-individuation processes (Mahler 1967; Mahler, Perl, and Bergman 1975). For the homosexual has failed to make the intra-psychic separation from the mother at the proper stage of development, and as a result there remains a chronic intra-psychic stimulation to which he remains fixed despite the fact that he may have in part successfully passed other developmental and maturational phases. Because of the infantile deficiency, compensating deviant structures will have been formed in other maturational phases, such as impaired gender (sexual) identity, and ego deficiencies.

Classification

Over seventy years ago, Freud (1905) proposed a classification based on both conscious and unconscious motivation. He divided homosexuals into absolute inverts, whose sexual objects are exclusively of their own sex, and who are incapable of carrying out the sexual act with a person of the opposite sex or deriving any enjoyment from it; amphigenic inverts, whose sexual objects may equally well be of their own sex or of the opposite sex, because this type of inversion lacks the characteristic of exclusiveness; and contingent inverts who, when circumstances preclude accessibility to partners of the opposite sex, may take, as their sexual objects, those of their own sex.

Current research leads me to define five major types of homosexuality.

Preoedipal type

This type of homosexuality originates from a fixation to the preoedipal stage of development (from birth to three years of age). It is unconsciously motivated and arises from anxiety. Because non-engagement in homosexual practices results in intolerable anxiety, and because the partner must be of the same sex, it may be termed obligatory homosexuality. This sexual pattern is inflexible and stereotyped.

Severe gender-identity disturbance is present: in the male, a faulty and weak masculine-identity; in the female, a faulty, distorted, and unacceptable feminine-identity, derived from the mother who is felt to be hateful and hated. This disturbance is due to a persistence of the primary feminine identification. In the female, there persists an identification with the hated mother which she must reject. It is essential here to differentiate between primary and secondary feminine identification. Following the birth of the child, the biological oneness with the mother is replaced by a primitive identification with her. The child must proceed from the security of identification and oneness with the mother to active component separateness – in the boy toward active male (phallic) strivings, and in the female to active feminine strivings. If this task proves too difficult, pathological defences, especially an increased aggressiveness, may result. These developments are of the greatest importance for the solution of conflicts appearing in the oedipal phase and in later life. In the boy's oedipal phase, under the pressure of the castration fear, an additional type of identification, secondary identification with the mother, in a form of passive feminine wishes for the father is likely to take place. However, beneath this feminine position in relation to the father, one may often uncover the original passive relation with the mother. In the oedipal phase of the girl, fear induced by both parents – a conviction of rejection by the father because she is female, and by the mother because the latter is hateful and hated – leads to a secondary identification. This results in passive feminine wishes for the mother, and a masculine identification superimposed on the girl's deeper hated feminine identification, in order to secure the 'good' mother (the female homosexual partner later in life).

The anxieties which beset persons of this type are of an insistent and intractable nature, leading to an overriding, almost continual search for sexual partners. The homosexual act is needed to ensure ego survival, and transiently stabilize the sense of self. Consequently, the act must be repeated frequently out of inner necessity, to ward off paranoidal and incorporative fears. There are rare exceptions in this type, who cannot consciously accept the homosexual act and struggle against it and in whom, therefore, the symptom remains latent. The homosexual symptom is egosyntonic as the nuclear conflicts have undergone a transformation and disguise. The aim of the homosexual act is ego survival and a reconstruction of a sense of sexual identity in accordance with anatomy. The male achieves 'masculinity' through identification with the male sexual partner, and receives reassurance against lessening of castration fear. The female achieves 'resonance' identification and anxiety relief, but she also creates the 'good' mother–child relationship.

There is a predominance of pregenital characteristics of the ego in these patients, for example, remembering is often replaced by acting-out, and there is a persistence of primitive and archaic mental mechanisms (Freud 1905).

Oedipal type

This type of homosexuality stems from a failure of resolution of the

Oedipus complex; castration fears lead to the adoption of a negative oedipal position, and a regression in part to anal and oral conflicts. The male assumes the role of the female with the father (other men); the female takes the role of the male to the mother (other women). Homosexual wishes in this type are unconsciously motivated, and dreaded; engagement in homosexual practices is not obligatory. The sexual pattern is flexible in that heterosexuality can be carried out and is usually the conscious choice.

Gender-identity disturbances of masculine sexual identity in the male, or deficient feminine sexual identity in the female, are due to a secondary identification with a person (parent) of the opposite sex in this type. This is simply a reversal of normal sexual identification in the direction of the same-sex parent.

The anxiety which develops in the male is due to fears of penetration by the more powerful male (father); the female fears rejection by the more powerful female (mother). Common to both are shame and guilt arising from super-ego and ego conflicts, conscious and unconscious, attendant to engaging in homosexual acts in dreams and fantasies, and, occasionally, in actuality under special circumstances of stress. Homosexual acts in this type are attempts to ensure dependency and attain power through the seduction of the more powerful partner.

Primitive and archaic psychic mechanisms may appear due to regression. These are intermittent, often absent, and do not lend a stamp of pregenitality to the character of the individual as in the preoedipal types. A careful developmental history and longitudinal study of a patient's life will indicate preoedipal or oedipal type of character structure. The homosexual symptom is ego-alien. Although unconsciously determined, it is not the outcome of the repressive compromise (Sachs mechanism) as described in preoedipal homosexuality above. The symptom may remain at the level of unconscious thoughts, dreams, and fantasies, as it is not a disguised acceptable representation of a deeper conflict. When it threatens to break into awareness, anxiety develops. However, under certain conditions, for example defiant rage overriding the restraining mechanism of conscience, periods of intense depression secondary to loss, with resultant need for love, or need for admiration and strength from a person of the same sex, homosexual acts may take place. Such acts, however, do not achieve the magical symbolic restitution of the preoedipal type. They may indeed exacerbate the situation through loss of pride and self-esteem.

The aim of the homosexual act is to experience dependency on and security from 'powerful' figures of the same sex. The sexual pattern of the negative oedipal type is not as inflexible or stereotyped as in the preoedipal type. There are exacerbations and remissions in the sense of masculine identity (in the female, in the sense of pride and achievement in feminine identity) secondary to successful performance in other (non-sexual) areas of life. Such feelings of success diminish, or even cause a disappearance of, any fantasied or actual need for sexual relations with persons of the same sex. This symptom picture described above is often seen in obsessional character neuroses, secondary to experiencing a defeat in their external lives with resultant regression.

Situational type†

Homosexual acts may take place when there is an environmental inaccessibility to partners of the opposite sex. The behaviour is consciously motivated. The acts are not fear-induced, but arise out of conscious deliberation and choice. The person is able to function with a partner of the opposite sex. The sexual pattern is flexible and these individuals return to opposite-sex partners when they are available.

In connection with the situational type, Bieber (1972) reported that men who had not been homosexual prior to military service, were found, with rare exceptions, to have refrained from homosexual activity throughout their tour of duty despite the absence of female partners. This finding suggests a possible revision of the concept of situational homosexuality in instances where the coercive factor is absent. Much of the so-called 'situational factor' in prisons is an outcome of the struggle for dominance and is, in fact, rape.

Variational type†

The motivations underlying this form of homosexual behaviour are as varied as the motivations which drive men and women to pursue power, gain protection, assure dependency, seek security, wreak vengeance, or experience specialized sensations. In some cultures, such surplus activity is a part of the established social order; in others, entirely a product of individual enterprise contrary to the general social order. The homosexuality practiced in ancient Greece was in all probability variational in type: there were strict laws against it, except for its practice during a brief period in late adolesence and penalties included disenfranchisement of those engaged in catamite

†The terms situational and variational were introduced by Rado (1949).

activities (anal intercourse) (Lacey 1968). Sentiments expressing admiration and affection for youth (so-called homosexual sentiments) short of homosexual relations in ancient Greece were allowed. In ancient Sparta homosexuality could be punished by death.

The behaviour is consciously motivated. Homosexual acts are not fear-induced but arise out of conscious deliberation and choice. The person is able to function with a partner of the opposite sex. The sexual pattern is flexible and these individuals do return to opposite-sex partners when they so prefer.

Variational homosexuality may occur in individuals who seek to gratify the desire for an alteration of sexual excitation, often for reasons of impotence or near-impotence in the male partner of the heterosexual pair. Much of the heterosexual group-sex activity currently reported includes homosexual behaviour between male and female participants and is of this type. In some instances, individuals with unconsciously derived homosexual conflicts take part in such group activities, in order to act our their homosexual wishes and simultaneously to deny their homosexual problem. Variational homosexuality may also be seen in the neurotic, psychotic, and sociopath. It frequently occurs in those suffering from alcoholism as well as in depressive states.

Latent type

There is much confusion in the use of the term 'latent homosexuality', due to the misleading concept of constitutional bisexuality, which implies that, side-by-side with an innate desire for opposite-sex partners, there exists an inborn desire for same-sex partners. Correctly, latent homosexuality means the presence in an individual of the underlying psychic structure of either the preoedipal or oedipal type without overt orgastic activity with a person of the same sex. The shift from latent to overt, and the reverse, is dependent on several factors:

(a) the strength of the fixation at the preoedipal level (quantitative factor), severity of anxiety, and the intensity of regression from the later oedipal conflict.

(b) the acceptability of the homosexuality to the ego (self), the superego (conscience mechanism), and the ego ideal.

(c) the strength of the instinctual drives, that is libido and aggression.

The latent homosexual may not have any conscious knowledge of his preference for individuals of the same sex for orgastic fulfilment. On the other hand, there may be a high degree of elaboration of unconscious homosexual fantasies and homosexual dream material, with or without conscious denial of its significance. They may live an entire lifetime without realizing their homosexual propensities, managing to function marginally on a heterosexual level, sometimes married and having children. Another pattern is that of the individual who, fully aware of his homosexual preference, abstains from all homosexual acts. Others, as a result of severe intolerable stress, infrequently and transiently do engage in overt homosexual acts, living the major portion of their lives, however, as latent homosexuals. In the latent phase, they may maintain a limited heterosexual functioning, albeit unrewarding, meagre, and usually based on homosexual fantasies. Or they may utilize homosexual fantasy for masturbatory practices, or may abstain from sexual activity altogether. These individuals are, of course, truly homosexual at all times; the shift between latent and overt, and the reverse, constitutes an alternating form of latent homosexuality.

All forms of latent homosexuality are potentially overt. Social imbalance – where severe inequities exist between one's survival needs, due to the failure of society to ensure their adequate satisfaction – has a precipitating effect on some borderline and/or latent cases of both preoedipal and oedipal homosexuality. Such imbalance also brings a flight from all aspects of masculine endeavour and a retreat to a less demanding role. This is a possible explanation of the apparent rise in the incidence of male homosexuality during periods of social turbulence, when many traditional roles, privileges, and responsibilities are overturned. The same factors may cause an increase in female homosexuality.

Clinical picture

The clinical symptoms in the history of the fully-developed preoedipal homosexual have an almost classic, unvarying pattern, although the symptoms themselves may vary quantitatively from patient to patient. In adulthood, he constantly yearns and searches for masculinity, and by engaging in homosexual acts incorporates the male partner and his penis, thus 'strengthening' himself. Almost every homosexual en-counter first concerns itself with disarming the partner, through one's seductiveness, appeal, power, prestige, effeminacy, or 'masculinity'. This simulation of the male-female pattern (active versus passive, the one who penetrates versus the one who is penetrated) should not lead to the conclusion that the motivation of either partner is to achieve femininity; both partners are intent upon acquiring masculinity from each other. Despite surface manifestations of the degree of apparent affection, beneath such tender affectivity is the homosexual's motivation to disarm and defeat, conquer and control, the sexual object. While feelings of love and affection may be present, these are highly charged with neurotic fears and inhibitions. Premature attempts at sexual relations with women on the part of these men may result in severe anxiety from fears of engulfment, a sense of bodily disintegration or other regressive symptomatology. It must be remembered that the homosexual act 'magically' produces a psychic equilibrium, which temporarily withstands the multiple anxieties which beset the homosexual.

As a result of this faulty gender-identity, there are pronounced feelings of femininity which are a result of the persistence of the primary feminine identification with the mother. Corresponding feelings of a deficit in masculinity engender anxiety when he attempts performance in the appropriate gender-role.

The homosexual attempts to maintain a similar position of optimal distance to women as he did to his mother. Fear of the sudden approach of women results in the sensation that he will be engulfed, incorporated, or devoured. This reflects the original fear of his mother's engulfment and control, and in part reflects his wish for, and dread of domination. It is then generalized to a fear of all women and fear of engulfment by them, especially by the female genitalia and the pubic hair. The patient continues in a life-long intense oral-sadistic relationship with the mother and other women. This intense sadism towards women is disguised by its opposite, a masochistic attitude towards them. Mixed with active homosexual feelings toward men, there are passive homosexual feelings towards men as there were towards his father. The latter are often repressed. There is in the unconscious a wish to take the place of the mother in sexual intercourse, both to protect and supplant her and to wreak vengeance on the father through appropriating his penis. This pattern can be seen to arise from the early wish and/or dread of extreme closeness to the mother, the intense dependency on her for a feeling of well-being and survival and the intense identification with her.

Incorporative anxiety, such as fears of swallowing parts of one's own body, fears of internalized harmful objects, and projective anxieties, as indicated by fears of poisoning, bodily attack, and mild fears of persecution, arise from the predominance of archaic primitive psychic mechanisms derived from an earlier period of life.

The anamnestic material continually reveals the striking theme of his existence, namely: an inability to make the intrapsychic separation from the mother and as a consequence severe anxiety upon attempting separation (in the psychic sense) from her. This can be noticeable from the earliest childhood and continuing throughout life.

Psychoanalytic theory

For many years, the lack of a systematic study of ego-psychology, and the absence of a concept of ego-development comparable to the phases of libidinal development, presented difficulties in the application of structural concepts to homosexuality, as well as to other perversions. Furthermore, the development of a comprehensive systematized work on the principles and techniques of psychoanalytic therapy of homosexual individuals has been slowed by questions as to the exact psychic aetiology (including misunderstandings surrounding the issue of contitutional bisexuality). Other contributing factors are suggested by the following observations:

(a) psychoanalysis has shown that patients who experienced mostly pain and suffering from their condition are motivated to change; others very often are not;

(b) the intolerance of these patients to experiencing anxiety, and the relief from anxiety while acting-out has previously led to therapeutic nihilism and counter-transference reactions;

(c) the neutralization of conflict allows for the growth of certain ego-adaptive elements of the personality, so that some homosexuals may appear on the surface not 'ill' at all, except for a severe deficiency in functioning in their sexual life;

(d) of all the symptoms of emotional origin which serve simultaneously as defences, homosexuality is successful in its capacity to provide, for limited intervals, not only a neutralization of profound psychic conflicts and struggles, thereby promoting a pseudo-adequate equilibrium, but also a high pleasure reward (orgasm).

Our present, more optimistic, outlook for the alleviation of this disorder has been enhanced by researches in ego-psychology; advances in analytic technique, which deepen our understanding of both the transference relationship and the analytic situation, thereby making it possible to define more clearly the nature of ego-pathology in the narcissistic neuroses; and research findings derived from psycho-analytic observational studies on the mother–infant relationship which illuminate aetiological processes.

Reports of results and therapy

In 1905, Freud wrote that the only possibility of helping homosexual patients was by commanding a suppression of their symptoms through hypnotic suggestion. By 1920, he believed that psychoanalysis itself was applicable to the treatment of sexual deviations, including homo-sexuality. His criterion of care was not only a detachment of cathexis from the homosexual object, but the ability to cathect the opposite sex with libido (that is, become emotionally involved).

In 1950, Anna Freud stated that many of her patients lost their per-version as a result of psychoanalytic treatment. This occurred even in those who insisted they wished to remain homosexual, having sought therapy only to obtain relief from their associated symptoms.

Several sources have reported a significant proportion of cases with successful outcome. An unpublished informal report of the Central Fact Gathering Committee of the American Psychoanalytic Associ-ation (1956) was one of the first surveys with 66 cases. Of the group of 32 cases which completed treatment, eight were described as cured, thirteen as improved, and one as unimproved. This constituted one-third of all cases reported. Of the group of 34 cases that did not complete treatment, sixteen were described as improved, three as untreatable, five as transferred. In all such reported cases, follow-up communication verified assumption of full heterosexual role and function.

In 1953 the Portman Clinic survey in England reached the following conclusions. 'Psychotherapy appears to be unsuccessful in only a small number of patients of any age in whom a long habit is combined with . . . lack of desire to change' (Glover 1960). The Portman Clinic, under the direction of Glover, divided the degrees of improvement into three categories:

(a) cure – abolition of conscious homosexual impulse and development of full extension of heterosexual impulse;

(b) much improved – the abolition of conscious homosexual impulse without development of full heterosexual impulse;

(c) improved – increased ego integration and capacity to control the homosexual impulse.

In conducting focal treatment (brief therapy aimed at the relief of the homosexual symptom), Glover states that the degree of social anxiety which prevails, particularly among patients seen in private, is based on a projected form of unconscious guilt. He is of the opinion that the punitive attitude of the law and society enables the patient to project concealed super-ego reactions onto society or the law. A therapist must decide whether to treat homosexuality through the regular course of depth therapy, or whether he and the patient will be satisfied with focal relief. In any case, the therapist must deal with both conscious and unconscious guilt, severe anxiety upon the patient's attempting heterosexual relations and, of course, oedipal conflict and castration anxiety. It was deemed necessary to demonstrate to the patient the defensive aspects of homosexual relationships. Only by uncovering the positive aspects of his original relationships to women (mother, sister) and revealing their associated anxieties or guilts (real or fantasied), derived from the hostile aspects of these early experiences can heterosexuality be attained.

While statements of therapeutic effectiveness and cure of homosexual patients are frequently encountered in the publications of individual psychoanalysts, detailed individual case reports of successful resolutions of overt homosexuality of the obligatory type are relatively scarce, only seven being known to this author: Flournoy (1953), Lagache (1949), Poe (1952), Vinchon and Nacht (1931), Wulff (1940), and Socarides (1968b, 1969). In addition, important insights into a successful resolution have been proposed by Bergler (1956, 1958), Bychowski (1945, 1954), Anna Freud (1951), Freud (1905, 1920), Glover (1933, 1960), Lorand and Balint (1956), Nunberg (1938), Rosenfeld (1949), and many others.

In 1962, Bieber *et al.* presented a systematic study of 106 male homosexuals. Their results did much to clarify the progress in therapeutic knowledge and effectiveness. Out of the 106 homosexuals, who undertook psychoanalysis with members of the Society of Medical Psychoanalysts (New York City), twenty-nine (27 per cent) became exclusively heterosexual.

My own clinical experience with homosexual patients in private practice may well be (with the exception of Bergler) one of the most extensive. During a ten-year period, from 1967 to 1977 I have treated psychoanalytically 55 overt homosexuals. Of these patients, 44 were in long-term psychoanalytic therapy of over a year's duration (average 3.5 years): the number of sessions ranged from three to five per week. In this group, there were only three females.

The remainder (11) were in short-term analytic therapy (average 6-7 months) at two to three sessions per week. Three were female.

In addition, full-scale analysis was performed on 18 latent homosexuals, in whom the symptoms never became overt, except in the most transitory form. Thus the total treated in short- and long-term analysis, whether overt or latent, was 73.

Finally, over 350 overt homosexuals were seen in consultation (averaging one to three sessions) during this ten-year period.

A definitive breakdown and analysis of the therapeutic results in these various groups is currently being written. I can report, however, that of the 44 overt homosexuals who have undergone psychoanalytic therapy, 20 patients, nearly 50 per cent, developed full heterosexual functioning and were able to develop feelings of love for their heterosexual partners. This included one female patient. These patients of whom two-thirds were of the preoedipal type and one-third of the oedipal type, were all strongly motivated for therapy.

General problems

My remarks are restricted to the psychoanalytic therapy of overt male homosexuality of the obligatory type. This type of homosexuality is exclusive, arises from unconscious conflicts, and is not due to situational or variational motivations. In these individuals non-engagement in homosexual practices would induce severe if not intolerable anxiety. Oedipal homosexuality see p.254 is a different form of homosexuality which may be treated similarly to a neurosis.

We are confronted at the outset with apparently formidable difficulties in the psychoanalysis of those with a full-developed homosexual perversion. Homosexuals bear and carry with them characteristics that are present in most individuals who suffer from impulse neuroses; addiction, delinquency, and narcissistic personality disorders. Because of their pathological narcissism, they seem to be unable to maintain a continuity of analysable transference relationships. Their relationship to the therapist therefore often abounds with fusion of self- and object-images, primitive forerunners of identification. They often suffer from poor object relationships and/or lack of object constancy. The symptom is egosyntonic and there is a great deal of acting-out. Furthermore, they appear at times intolerant of postponement of impulses. From clinical experience, I believe these formidable issues can be met and resolved, as they have been in many instances of borderline conditions, narcissistic personality disorders, and impulse neuroses.

For example, the need for homosexual activity is often of extreme intensity and is carried out often in states of utmost necessity. This requires a modification of technique which requires understanding of the individual underlying structure and meaning of the homosexual act (A. Freud 1954). With most homosexuals, it is wise neither to encourage nor prohibit homosexual activity. The patient, through the analysis of the unconscious motivation and fantasy leading to the homosexual act, will thus at a suitable point in therapy be able to decide on a course of action. Also the patient must not engage in what may be experienced as a 'self-castration', through self-prohibition of homosexual acts, until this facet of the unconscious problem has been understood and thoroughly analysed. Nor will the patient flee the therapy as a result of unwise prohibitions against homosexual activity.

One basic concern is that the resisting forces, which may be necessary for the ego not to collapse, should not be suddenly overwhelmed. We do not intend a sudden, unopposed breakthrough of id derivatives (as seen in pre-psychotic cases). Variations of technique are necessary, therefore when manifestations of transference or resistance exceed in force, or malignancy, the amount with which we are able to cope. In order to adequately control transference and resistance, there may be an increase or diminution of sessions, or the patient may occasionally not lie on the analytic couch but engage in face-to-face therapy for shorter or longer periods of time. Often, anxiety is thereby lessened, distortions or an appearance of negative transference can be kept at a manageable intensity, regressive episodes can be more easily managed, and face-to-face discussions may dissipate distrust and lessen the severity of projective anxieties. Against this backdrop, the analysis of dreams, fantasies, transference, and resistance proceeds as in any other psychoanalytic therapy.

One of the major resistances continues to be the patient's misconception that his disorder may be in some strange way of hereditary or biological origin or, in modern parlance, a matter of sexual 'preference' or 'orientation', that is, a normal form of sexuality. These views must be dealt with from the very beginning. They often stem from the fear that destruction of homosexual pleasure will leave the individual without any pleasure.

During the course of therapy there is a revival and working-through of the following psychodynamic issues.

(a). *Persistent stimulation of the child's aggression by the mother*, throughout early and late childhood, has resulted in an unalleviated guilt binding the child to her; any attempt at separation induces severe anxiety. The increase in both primary and secondary aggression, due to frustration, leads to fears of violent destructiveness aimed at all love objects. While these feelings undergo reaction-formation into their opposite, they are rediscovered during the course of therapy. As an illustration, after two-and-a-half years of analysis one patient, Paul, a 23-year-old accountant, discovered that his homosexual feelings were filled with violent impulses. 'When I get a sexual feeling, the man must be extremely submissive, as I say this I get a dizzy feeling as though I'd like to punch these men, or strangle them, or strangle their genitals by pulling them off, tearing them off, and causing them pain and enjoying the pain. I'd like to see the pain on their faces. I'd get a real charge out of this. I have many angry feelings within me and all this facade of being nice to people, it's all an act.... And I hate my mother so. I hate her for all that she did to me, her selfishness and everything being for her. I feel like crying, and I feel awful, and the hate is getting more and more about all the things that have happened to me, and I guess I've wanted to kill her for a long time. Then I wouldn't be weak and helpless.'

(b) *The presence of a distorted body ego.* Paul noted: 'You know, I don't feel I have my own body. I want someone else's body. My body is flat. I guess because the penis is flat, or never gets erect with girls. I keep looking for a body in another man, and that's one of the reasons for choosing a man, especially if he's clothed and looks very masculine. It seems I'm reaching for that when I want a man. It has to do with the muscles. I want more muscles. I was never allowed to do anything that would make muscles for me, such as sports. My mother would laugh at me and say to me, "What are you trying to be? A killer?" She would make fun of my penis. She used to say, "You'll hurt yourself if you ever have sex." She said if I ever exercised strenuously or lifted heavy things I might hurt my penis.'

As he improved (during the second year of analysis), he experienced a stabilization of his body ego. 'What I don't like now is if I go out and I want a man to look at me, to like me, I don't like that feeling. I don't know myself when I do that anymore. I can't feel my body or my face when I do that. It takes me a while to get over it.' He did not wish to experience these feelings as he had begun to feel full-bodied, having reconstructed his body-ego; he felt pride, in his movements, in his new identity. 'There's a lot more independence in me now. I don't even try to force my heterosexual feelings any more.'

(*c*) *The substitution of the male partner for the mother* as a love object to avoid both oedipal (incest) and preoedipal conflicts.

(*d*) *The imperative need for homosexual relief* and the conditions under which this occurs.

(*e*) *The homosexual's characteristic demeaning and degrading of the father*, often quite openly. He identifies with the aggressor (mother). This, however, produces guilt in therapy, and is an impediment to his feeling of being entitled to be a man.

(*f*) *The homosexual makes an identification with his partner* in the sexual act. Homosexual contact promotes a transient, pseudo-strengthening of his own masculinity and identity, which must constantly be repeated or a psychic 'decompensation' occurs. The homosexual seeks masculinity, not femininity, and knowledge of this unconscious motivation becomes a potent source of strength, reassurance, and determination for change in the direction of heterosexual functioning. The important discovery that the interpretation of the patient's actions which most achieves relaxation of resistance is his attempt to acquire masculinity through identification with the partner and his penis in the homosexual act was made by Anna Freud in 1949. After this interpretation is worked-through, the patient may be able to function heterosexually, going through a strong narcissistic-phallic phase, when women serve only the 'grandeur' of his penis. The unconscious fearful fantasy of homosexuals, that they would dissolve in a woman at the height of the sexual act (fear of engulfment) is another important interpretation.

(*g*) *The nuclear preoedipal anxieties.* While the analysis of oedipal fears of incest and aggression is of paramount importance in the analytic work, it is vital to the understanding and termination of homosexuality that the nuclear preoedipal anxieties, for example, the primitive fears of incorporation, threatened loss of personal identity, engulfment by the mother, and personal dissolution which accompany any attempt to separate from the mother, be revealed.

(*h*) *Breast–penis equation*. The penis of the partner is revealed to be a substitute for the feeding breast of the sought-after 'good' mother. The homosexual therapy escapes the frustrating cruel mother, and makes up for the oral deprivation suffered at her hands.

(*i*) *An intense yearning for the father's love* and protection exists at unconscious levels, a further frustration of the need for masculine identification. The homosexual act dramatizes the aggression and yearning toward all men as a consequence.

Our current state of knowledge of the course of psychoanalytic treatment of the homosexual, as well as our increasing ability to deal with the vicissitudes to be encountered, owes much to Glover's earlier observations summarized in *The roots of crime* (1960). He noted that in the early stages of analysis there are, of course, many indications of spontaneous transference, some of which can be recognized as essentially maternal in origin. There exists in particular a passive receptive attitude to interpretation, which alternates with disappointment when this is not forthcoming. But as is only to be expected from the first, open expressions of active analytic rapport take the form of father transferences in which the positive elements at first predominate.

It is essential, however, to uncover any negative elements of the father transference; only when these have been fully ventilated is it possible for the deeper mother transferences, both positive and negative, to appear. Many analytic failures, in the sense that the patient retains his homosexual system even if only in a less marked form, are due to the failure to uncover and analyze these potential mother transferences, which at first are almost exclusively saturated with pregenital sadistic fantasy. With the successful overcoming of these deeper regressive phases, the prospects of a successful outcome are greatly improved. As a rule, the first sign of fundamental improvement is the appearance of anxieties which would ordinarily set up neurotic defences. These differ from the earlier manifestations of social anxiety, which are encountered at the beginning of the analysis of most homosexuals. The deeper anxieties gradually give place to guilt reactions, and it is at this point that super-ego analysis can be made effective. This calls for persistent ventilation of the projection systems by means of which the patient covers his guilt. During this period the patient may manifest a number of transitory symptom formations of a conversion type, and his inhibitions in work and in social contact may be exacerbated.

Once these have been worked-through, the way is open to analyze the genital kernel of the repressed oedipus complex which the homosexual has used every unconscious mechanism to conceal.

Glover correctly concluded that under present conditions of selection, success in treatment depends upon the following factors:

(a) the effectiveness with which the purely psychological disposition to homosexual object choice can be uncovered;

(b) the degree to which current ego difficulties and frustrations can be offset;

(c) the degree of transference rapport that can be established.

The first of these factors depends on the amount of primary gain secured through the perversion; the second, on the amount of secondary gain obtained in current life; and the third, on the degree of potential accessibility of each case. As in all other forms of treatment of mental disorder, the third factor is by far the most important.

Selection of cases

It must be remembered that the treatment of any perversion threatens to rekindle the very conflicts from which the patient has fled by means of his perversion, and 'to destroy a pleasure ... the only sexual pleasure the patient knows' (Fenichel 1945). However, even individuals who are 'at peace' with their perversion may have a determination to get well. Central to the issue of prognosis and selection of cases is to what extent this determination can be awakened. The determination itself may have multiple motivations, and in every case a trial analysis will have as one of its aims the evaluation of the will to recover.

The best cases are those in which the patient feels 'worse', not only from the point of view that his perversion may be accompanied by neurotic symptoms, but that he can no longer tolerate his homosexual adaption. Such a patient seeks analysis because he is unable to achieve any form of true ego-satisfaction in his perversion. The instinctual discharge via homosexuality has led to a sense of depletion, exhaustion, and a wish to turn away from the homosexual object. This reduces his satisfaction and expectations in life, and leads ultimately to despair and a need to undergo treatment.

Even the most serious of cases of homosexuality will yield to therapy, if the patient seeks therapy, when he feels severely distressed about being homosexual, not only because of guilt or shame, but because he finds his homosexual life meaningless and extra-territorial to the biological realities of life around him. Hopefully, he may have more that a vague awareness that he is the victim of internal psychic disturbances, which have left him no choice but to engage in homosexual activities.

An important criterion is that the patient experiences inner feelings of guilt capable of being used analytically. This strong inner feeling of guilt derives from the unconscious wishes of an aggressive and libidinal nature, experienced under the disguise of homosexuality. The absence of conscious guilt usually does not mean that the patient does not suffer from guilt, but instead that it is experienced by him as a need for punishment. Once the patient sees that his guilt arises from internal conflict, and not simply from the mores of a condemning society, he is at last on a path towards the beginning of the resolution of his homosexuality.

Ideally, homosexual patients should voluntarily seek therapy and not be under duress from parents, or other authority figures. For they are beset by savage unconscious drives against their parents, a hatred that is in direct proportion to their wild, self-damaging tendencies which their aggressive homosexuality camouflages.

Beneath an apparent willingness to get well, the real intent of some patients may be to prove that homosexuality is as 'rational' as heterosexuality. It is obvious that, as long as the patient remains committed to the idea that his interest in same-sex partners represents the expression of an inherent biological choice, the benefits of therapeutic help are limited. It must be made clear to the patient that neither homosexuality nor heterosexuality are innate behaviour patterns, but are learned.

Another criterion is the degree of self-damaging tendencies in the patient. Hopefully, if the patient views this damage socially, personally, and in the work area, as somehow arising from or being due to his homosexuality, there may be strong motivation toward change.

The therapist must also consider the strong preference for homosexual reality rather than homosexual fantasy. The homosexual is suffering from irresistible impulses, in which the striving for security and the striving for instinctual gratification are intimately commingled. He begins to perceive that this tension is like a dangerous trauma, and his aim is to get rid of tension and in addition achieve sexual gratification. Gradually he becomes aware that these drives are not experienced in the way his other normal instinctual drives are experienced, and he wishes to change them. With therapy he ultimately moves in the opposite direction; first preferring homosexual fantasy instead of acting-out the irresistible impulse, and finally attempting heterosexual fantasy, and then heterosexual reality.

The problem of narcissism

In some homosexual patients, the sexualization of pathological narcissism through homosexuality may appear to be the central clinical problem. Careful scrutiny will reveal whether we are dealing with an eroticized statement of what is basically a narcissistic personality disorder (many narcissists may fleetingly engage in homosexual activities without suffering from the true perversion), or whether the pathological narcissism is but one aspect of the homosexuality. My comments here are directed toward the latter situation.

In homosexuals a weak ego-structure is further burdened by narcissistic and pre-narcissistic dispositions. This type of ego-structure makes the ego particularly vulnerable to the impact of libidinal stimulation, and renunciation of primitive gratification becomes difficult if not seemingly impossible. In place of object cathexis, the ego seeks gratification in a short-circuited act between the self and pseudo-objects, for instance, between various susbstitutes for the ego and for parental images (Bychowski 1945). In his repetition compulsion, the homosexual dramatizes a repeatedly unsuccessful attempt of the ego to achieve mastery of libidinal and aggressive impulses, and of the originally archaically cathected objects. The ego, when faced with the task of object cathexis, experiences a threat of further impoverishment. Concomitantly we find a lack of neutralized energy indispensible for control, postponement, and anticipation of gratification.

The homosexual, alongside those with narcissistic personality disorders, has specific assets which differentiate him from the psychotic or borderline individual. Unlike the latter, homosexuals have 'attained a cohesive self, and have constructed cohesive, idealized, archaic objects'. They are not seriously threatened by the possibility of an 'irreversible disintegration of the archaic self, or of the narcissistically-cathected, archaic objects' (Kohut 1974). Furthermore, they are able to establish specific, stable, narcissistic transferences, which allow the therapeutic reactivation of the archaic structures, without the danger of their fragmentation despite regressive episodes. In two earlier papers, *A provisional theory of etiology in male homosexuality* (1968a) and *Sexual perversion and the fear of engulfment* (1973), I described, utilizing case material, the homosexual's tendency to severe regressive episodes during therapy which proved to be not only reversible, but of extreme value therapeutically. Thus like narcissistic personality-disorders, homosexuals are analyzable. The spontaneous establishment of one of the stable, narcissistic transferences is one of the best and most reliable signs which differentiate these patients from psychotic or borderline cases, on the one hand, and from ordinary transference neuroses, on the other. Therefore, a trial analysis is of greater diagnostic and prognostic value than overt behaviour.

The homosexual, like those with purely narcissistic personality disorders, suffers from 'specific disturbances, in the realm of the self and those of archaic objects cathected with narcissistic libido [self objects]' (Kohut 1974). Archaic, over-estimated configurations have not become integrated with the rest of the personality and result in the adult personality becoming impoverished.

Kohut warns that it is unwise to prematurely confront the undisguised narcissistic manifestations of the split-off sector 'with reality in the form of educational persuasion, admonition and the like...' The exception is when a 'chronic defensive grandiosity' has secondarily become surrounded by a system of rationalizations analogous to the disguise in a phobia. Thus, the homosexual with a severe narcissistic conflict poses special problems in that therapy produces severe depression, feelings of emptiness, worthlessness, and attacks of narcissistic rage. See also pages 70–3.

Findings from a recent panel on the psychoanalytic treatment of male homosexuality

The structure of homosexuality consists of neurotic conflicts involving both anal and genital stages of sexual development, and the oedipal phase. These are superimposed on a substratum of deeper preoedipal nuclear conflicts. The vicissitudes of the preoedipal conflict pass through later developmental periods and complicate, add to, and give a particular configuration to the later conflict. All oedipal conflicts have an admixture of the preoedipal danger. Therefore, psychoanalysis is the treatment of choice for this disorder. Both preoedipal and oedipal anxieties can be relieved, through the revival of infantile memories and traumatic states, and the reintegration of the individual achieved. Treatment of preoedipal damage requires, in addition to the uncovering techniques of psychoanalysis, educational and retraining measures, more intensive support and intervention and modification of the handling of transference, resistance, and regression. These, and other important considerations were both reviewed and elaborated upon by panelists at a 1976 meeting of the American Psychoanalytic Association, as reported by Payne (1977).

Stoller proposed that the more feminine a boy is, the more likely will he be to desire someone of the same sex, and the earlier will his overt homosexuality begin. Furthermore, in his opinion, the less likely is it that either the femininity or homosexuality can be reversed by psychoanalysis. He believed that hope of changing homosexual behaviour also decreases with the patient's age. 'Malignant femininity' must be distinguished from the more 'benign' kind, and treatment should be instituted as soon as possible for the latter.

In a similar vein, Person opined that 'psychoanalytic intervention is usually indicated only for those homosexuals who are within the range of normal masculine gender behaviour. [However, even in such cases there may be an unconscious primary feminine identification beneath this outward appearance.] Within this range there are differences in terms of ego-integration, object relations, defence mechanisms, and predominant psychodynamic constellations' (Payne 1977). The treatment approach is determined more by ego-strength than by the intensity of the homosexuality. The homosexual patient typically struggles between fears of abandonment and fears of engulfment at the hands of the mother. From her own clinical experiences, she noted that these fears emerge strikingly in the transference, especially with a woman analyst. In the transference, the patient needs to control the relationship through putting 'distance' between himself and the therapist, to prove to himself that he is not at the mercy of a malevolent mother figure. He may, therefore, interrupt the treatment at various times. Person spoke of a variety of secondary factors which considerably complicate the clinical picture. For example, she defines two subgroups of homosexuals who although falling within the normal range of masculine gender, show differing degrees of involvement in the homosexual world – 'sexual homosexuals' and 'socio-sexual homosexuals'. Social treatment problems emerge, particularly when undertaking the treatment of the 'socio-sexual homosexual'. The prognosis for the 'sexual homosexual' is not necessarily better than that for the homosexual who is immersed in the homosexual world. It is guarded in those in whom homosexuality emerges late in life, after a family has been established, 'because of the capacity for denial and lack of insight, which has previously virtually sealed off the homosexual's conflict from awareness' (Payne 1977). The special problems in the treatment of the 'socio-sexual homosexual' are due to the 'easy gratification of the neurotic and narcissistic wishes, gratifications that tend to consolidate a patient's identity as a homosexual and tip the balance towards homosexuality' (Payne 1977, pp.109–190). She notes that such homosexuals feel that they reap 'benefits characteristically open only to a woman.' Such a homosexual feels 'glamorous', avoids the demands of financial responsibility, experiences an excitement due to the ease of access to sexual partners. These are antidotes to depression and act collectively as a hypomanic defence. Thus, any move towards giving up homosexuality, even when self-imposed, may be seen as a serious imposition 'restricting instinctual freedom as well as threatening the loss of homosexual identity' (Payne 1977).

Socarides noted that the nature of the spontaneously developing transference is more crucial to the analysability of homosexual patients than is the presenting symptomatology or the life history. This is true even in very effeminate homosexuals. He found that most homosexuals have achieved sufficient self-object differentiation and internalization of object-representations to be able to form a transference neurosis. They have adequate capacity to circumscribe regressions that occur in the transference, and a reliable-enough observing-ego to permit those transference neuroses to be analysed. The maintenance of the working alliance is of the greatest importance in the analysis of homosexual patients. The therapist may be reacting too negatively, since he may be viewed as a threat to the presenting symptom that is ego-syntonic, affords orgastic release, and creates a temporary equilibrium in the patient. The new attachment to the analyst permits the patient to reduce homosexual practices by protecting him against his dangerous, destructive masculine impulses. Regressions may serve as resistances, but they enrich the transference. During severe regressive states, childhood events may be relived in the transference with dramatic impact and vividness, permitting strong abreaction and furthering the patient's understanding of his earliest nuclear conflicts which were causative of his condition. It is vitally important that these regressive states do not lead the analyst to abandon the analysis, or to modify the basic analytic approach beyond what is necessary, although some supportive measures may be given.

Concluding remarks

Given the appropriate selection of cases, the ultimate success or failure of psychoanalysis of homosexuality lies in the thoroughness with which the analyst explores not only the unconscious libidinal phases of the negative oedipal complex and the reactive aggression with which these are associated, but also the effect on ego and super-ego structure of those identifications and introjections that are laid down during the preoedipal phase of development. The meaning of the preoedipal factors can be obtained from a study of the fantasy systems both conscious and unconscious.

Of paramount importance is the degree of transference rapport which can be established. Hopefully, an active analytic rapport of a positive nature may take place, in the form of a father transference in which the positive element predominates. It is essential to uncover the negative elements of the father transference so that the patient may be enabled to delve into the deeper mother transferences and the preoedipal material.

It will be noted that the social anxiety and social guilt, which the patient complains about, enables him to project concealed super-ego reactions onto the law or society. Having worked-through this material, the patient will begin to strike against a core of sexual anxiety and guilt pertaining to his oedipal-period aggression.

A process of sexual re-education may be necessary at certain favourable points in the analysis. This may consist of systematic sexual instruction, particularly since the unconscious fantasies of homosexuals tend to promote a number of conscious myths of a phobic nature which inhibit any attempt to put into action heterosexual impulses. However, as in the basis of all education, the best means of accelerating the education or re-education of homosexuals is to uncover and decrease inhibiting anxieties and, where possible, also to uncover the sources of infantile anxiety and guilt. Lastly, it can be stated that, hopefully, a development of greater tolerance among sections of the community for the homosexual, who has previously been treated as a scapegoat and criminal will lead homosexuals who are amenable to treatment to attempt such therapy. However, to accomplish this end, homo-sexuality of the obligatory type must be acknowledged as a psycho-sexual disorder, for which therapy is not only possible but necessary since the condition requires careful psychoanalytic attention. One's compassion for the plight of the homosexual, his responsiveness as a patient, and his value as a human being in interaction with the scientific challenge and fulfilment posed by his intrapsychic conflicts, leads to a mutuality of gratitude and satisfaction between patient and psycho-analyst, which well justifies the commitment to the attempted alleviation of this important and serious disorder.

References

American Psychoanalytic Association (1956). *Report of the central fact gathering committee.* New York (unpublished).

Arlow, J. A. (1952). Psychodynamics and treatment of perversions. *Bulletin Am. Psychoanal. Assoc.* (Panel Report) **8**, 315.

—— and Brenner, C. (1964). *Psychoanalytic concepts and the structural theory.* New York.

Bergler, E. (1956). *Homosexuality: disease, or a way of life?* New York.

—— (1958). *Counterfeit sex.* New York.

Bieber, I. (1959). Olfaction in sexual development and adult sexual organiz-ation. *Amer. J. Psychother.* **13**, 851.

—— (1972). Personal communication to the author.

——, Dain, H. J., Dince, P. R., Drellich, M. G., Grand, H. G., Gundlach, R. H., Kremer, M. W., Rifkin, A. H., Wilbur, C. B., and Bieber, T. B. (1962). *Homosexuality: a psychoanalytic study of male homosexuals.* New York.

Bychowski, G. (1945). The ego of homosexuals. *Int. J. of Psycho-Anal.* **26**, 114.

—— (1954). The structure of homosexual acting-out. *Psychoanal. Quart.*, **23**.

Fenichel, O. (1945). *The psychoanalytic theory of neurosis.* New York.

Ferenzi, S. (1909). More about homosexuality. In *Final contributions to the problems and methods of psychoanalysis.* New York.

Fleischmann, O. (1960). Choice of homosexuality in males. In panel report on theoretical and clinical aspects of overt male homosexuality, *J. Am. Psychoanal. Assoc.* **8**, 552.

Flournoy, H. (1953). An analytic session in a case of male homosexuality. In *Drives, affects, behaviour* (ed. R. M. Lowenstein). New York.

Freud, A. (1949). Some clinical remarks concerning the treatment of male homosexuality. (Abstract) *Int. J. Psycho-Anal.* **30**.

—— (1951). Homosexuality, *Bull. Amer. Psychoanal. Assoc.* **7**, 117.

—— (1954). Problems of technique in adult analysis. In *Bulletin of the Philadelphia Association of Psychoanalysis,* **4**.

Freud, S. (1905). Three essays on the theory of sexuality. *Complete psychological works of Sigmund Freud.* Standard edition **7**, 125. London.

—— (1920). Psychogenesis of a case of homosexuality in a woman. *Complete psychological works of Sigmund Freud.* Standard edition **18**, 145. London.

—— (1921). Group psychology and the analysis of the ego. *Complete psycho-logical works of Sigmund Freud.* Standard edition **18**, 67. London.

Gillespie, W. H. (1956). The general theory of sexual perversion. *Int. J. Psycho-Anal.* **37**, 396.

Glover, E. (1933). The relation of perversion formation to the development of reality sense. *Int. J. Psycho-Anal.* **14**, 486.

—— (1960). *The roots of crime*. London.

Hartmann, H., Kris, E., and Lowenstein, R. M. (1946). Comments on the formation of psychic structure. In *Papers on psychoanalytic psychology*. New York.

Jacobson, E. (1964). *The self and the object world*. New York.

Kalogerakis, M. G. (1963). The role of olfaction in sexual development. *Psychosom. Med.* **25**, 420.

Kohut, H. (1974). *The analysis of the self: a systematic approach to the psychoanalytic treatment of narcissistic personality disorders*. New York.

Lacey, W. K. (1968). *The family in classical Greece*. New York.

Lagache, D. (1949). De l'homosexualité à la jalousie. *Revue Francaise de Psychoanalyse* **13**, 351.

Lorand, S. and Balint, M. (1956). *Perversions: psychodynamics and therapy*. New York.

Mahler, M. S. (1967). On human symbiosis and the vicissitudes of individuation. *J. Amer. Psychoanal. Assoc.* **15**, 740.

——, Perl, F., and Bergman, A. (1975). *The psychological birth of the human infant: symbiosis and individuation*. New York.

Nunberg, H. (1938). Homosexuality, magic and aggression. *Int. J. Psycho-Anal.* **19**, 1.

Payne, E. C. (1977). Psychoanalytic treatment of male homosexuality. (Panel Report). *J. Amer. Psychoanal. Assoc.* **25**, 183.

Poe, J. S. (1952). The successful treatment of a forty-year-old passive homosexual based on an adaptional view of sexual behaviour. *Psychoanal. Rev.* **39**, 23.

Rado, S. (1949). An adaptional view of sexual behaviour. In *Psychosexual development in health and disease* (ed. P. H. Hoch and J. Zubin). New York.

—— (1955). Evolutionary basis of sexual adaptation. *J. Nerv. Ment. Dis.* **121**, 389.

Rosenfeld, H. A. (1949). Remarks on the relation of male homosexuality to paranoia, paranoid anxiety and narcissism, *Int. J. Psycho-Anal.* **30**, 36.

Sachs, H. (1923). On the genesis of sexual perversion. *Int. Psychoanal.*, 172. (Translated by Hella Freud Bernays, 1964; New York Psychoanalytic Institute Library).

Sadger, J. (1909). Zur Aetiologie der contraren Sexualempfindungen. *Med. Klinik*.

Socarides, C. W. (1960). Theoretical and clinical aspects of overt male homosexuality. (Panel Report). *J. Amer. Psychoanal. Assoc.* **8**, 552.

—— (1962). Theoretical and clinical aspects of overt female homosexuality. (Panel Report). *J. Amer. Psychoanal. Assoc.* **10**, 579.

—— (1968a). A provisional theory of etiology in male homosexuality: a case of preoedipal origin. *Int. J. Psycho-Anal.* **49**, 27.

—— (1968b). *The overt homosexual*. New York. (Reissued 1977).

—— (1969). The psychoanalytic therapy of a male homosexual. *Psychoanal. Quart.* **38**, 173.

—— (1973). Sexual perversion and the fear of engulfment. *Int. J. Psychoanal. Psychother.* **2**, 432.

—— (1974). Homosexuality. In *American handbook of psychiatry Vol. III.* (2nd edn.) (ed. S. Arieti.) New York.

—— (1978). A unitary theory of sexual perversion. In *The new sexuality and contemporary psychiatry.* (ed. T. B. Karasu and C. W. Socarides). New York.

van der Leeuw, P. J. (1958). The preoedipal phase of the male. *Psychoanal. Study Child.* **13**, 352. (New York).

Vinchon, J. and Nacht, S. (1931). Considerations sur la cure psychanalytique d'une nevrose homosexuelle. *Revue Francaise de Psychanalyse* **4**, 677.

Wulff, M. (1941). Ueber einen Fall von männlicher Homosexualität. *Int. Z. F. Psychoanal.* **26**, 105.

10 Some aspects of the role of aggression in the perversions

Mervin Glasser

Introduction

Anyone considering sexual deviance should keep in mind the distinction between a true perversion and the perverse elements which may feature in the sexual life of normal people or people suffering from various forms of disturbance. The vast majority of people may, from time to time, indulge in sexual fantasies which deviate from the culturally accepted norms, and many people may even put such fantasies into occasional practice, particularly as foreplay. But when the sexual deviance is a persistent, constantly preferred, form of sexual behaviour which reflects a global structure involving the individual's whole personality, I consider it appropriate to use the term 'perversion', despite its pejorative overtones, as a diagnostic designation like 'obsessional neurosis' or 'paranoid schizophrenia'. In this chapter, then, I shall be limiting my discussion to some of the critical contributions aggression makes to the aetiology, development, and nature of the perversions.

The 'core complex'

When we treat perversions, we invariably come to recognize a particularly important complex of inter-related feelings, ideas, and attitudes. I refer to it as a *'core* complex' because the various elements that go to make it up are at the centre of the pervert's psychopathology and fundamental to it. Aggression is a major and integral element of this complex but for the sake of clarity of exposition, I shall discuss the part it plays separately in the next section.

A major component of the core complex is a deep-seated and pervasive longing for an intense and most intimate closeness to another person, amounting to a 'merging', a 'state of oneness', a 'blissful union'. The specific versions of this longing are as varied as the individuals who express them. For example, a transvestite patient in the course of his treatment once spoke of imagining himself crawling up the birth passage and curling up snugly inside the womb; while on another occasion, when talking about the coldness and hardness of the city, he expressed his longing to be back in the country, 'at one with the earth and the grass and the trees, part of Mother Nature'. This longed-for state implies complete gratification with absolute security against any dangers of deprivation or obliteration and, as will be seen later, a totally reliable containment of any destructive feelings towards the object.

Such longings are, of course, by no means indicative of pathology; on the contrary, they are a component of the most normal of loving desires. However, in the pervert it persists pervasively in this most primitive form even when later developmental stages modify its manifest appearance. Such 'merging' for him does not have the character of a temporary state from which he will emerge: he feels it carries with it a *permanent* loss of self, a disappearance of his existence as a separate, independent individual into the object, like being drawn into a 'black hole' of space. There are individual variations depending on the particular vicissitudes of the aggressive and libidinal elements involved: one patient may conceive of it as his passively merging into the object, another as being engulfed by the object, another as forcefully getting into the object or being intruded into by the object, and so on. But in one way or another the ultimate result is seen as his being taken over totally by the object so that his anxiety is of total annihilation. This wish to merge and the consequent 'annihilation anxiety' invariably comes into the transference – for example, as a fear of being 'brainwashed' by the analyst, or as intensely claustrophobic feelings in the consulting-room.

Among the defensive reactions provoked by this 'annihilatory anxiety' is the obvious one of flight from the object, retreating emotionally to a 'safe distance' (that is, essentially, a narcissistic withdrawal). This is expressed in such attitudes as placing a premium on independence and self-sufficiency. In therapy, it may be encountered as a wish to terminate treatment, as a constant argumentativeness or negativism, as the development of an intellectual detachment, and so on.

However this 'flight to a safe distance' brings with it its own dangers and anxieties consequent on the implicit isolation. Such an isolated state may involve extremely painful affects and is, in my experience, one of the commonest reasons for the pervert seeking treatment. The relief from this state, or threat of it must ultimately be sought in renewing contact with the object. Both the nature of the anxiety and the intensity of the needs cause this contact to be conceived of in terms of an indissoluble closeness, security and gratification which could only be achieved by 'merging' with the object. And so the situation is back to the start of the vicious circle of the core-complex.

The emotional attitudes and fantasies I have described may well put one in mind of the 'symbiosis' and 'separation-individuation' stages of infant development (Mahler 1968) and since these stages are part of normal development it may be considered that I am not identifying anything specific to the pervert. I shall be taking up the discussion of the more specific factors later but at this juncture I would point out that the pervert differs from less severely disturbed individuals in that his core complex is fixated at these very early developmental stages. To envisage closeness and intimacy as annihilating, or separateness and independence as desolate isolation, indicates the persistence of a primitive level of functioning. What I have been referring to as the 'object' in my description of the core complex is thus ultimately the individual's mother (or the person who functioned in that capacity) during this very early period of development.

Most workers in the field in recent times identify this early period as critical to the development of perversions, also laying stress on the impulses towards merging or primary identification with, and separation and individuation from, the mother, as well as the influence of introjective-projective mechanisms, (see, among others, Bak 1956 and 1958; Chasseguet-Smirgel 1974; Freud A. 1968; Greenacre 1968; Khan 1962; Limentani 1977; McDougall 1970; Socarides 1973; and Stoller 1976). There is less agreement over what particular factor or factors determine the establishment of a perversion rather than other equally disturbed forms of psychopathology. I believe some light is thrown on this problem by the integral role aggression plays in the core complex; but before proceeding to discuss this I would like to clarify my understanding and usage of the term 'aggression'.

On the nature of aggression

In many psychoanalytic writings 'aggression' and 'sadism' have often been used interchangably and this has led to confusion, both theoretically and clinically. It must be acknowledged that there is still no agreed conceptualization of 'aggression'. Unlike 'libido', which is a defined, theoretical concept, 'aggression' is a term taken from everyday language and this carries with it the ambiguities of everyday usage. Too often it is not clear in theoretical or clinical presentations whether what is being referred to is a primary instinctual drive (as discussed, for example, by Hartmann, Kris, and Loewenstein, 1949); or a behavioural response to, say, frustration; or an affect, such as hostility; or an attitude, such as antagonism. Even when it *is* established that 'aggression' is being regarded as an instinctual drive, there is the well-known uncertainty whether to consider it as a basic drive in its own right or an outwardly-turned expression of a more fundamental 'death instinct'.

Since 'aggression' is central to my discussion, I consider it unavoidable to lay down at least a working definition and set out the boundaries of my usage of this term. In approaching such a task I take up the same viewpoint as Brenner (1971) when he states: 'An instinctual drive is a theoretical construct which serves the purpose of explaining the nature of basic motivation, of the prime impetus to mental activity', and later in the same paper: '...the evidence on which we base the concept of aggression as an instinctual drive is purely psychological.'

I would like to start by distinguishing 'aggression' from 'sadism'. The easiest and most reliable way of making this distinction is not by trying to identify the nature of the drive involved, or even the developmental level on which the individual might be functioning, but rather the *attitude to the object* at the time at which the act is carried out. In the aggressive act, the elimination, exclusion, destruction – in essence, *negation* – of the object is the cardinal factor (as I shall elaborate at some length below); the object's emotional reaction, the meaning of the behaviour to the object, in a sense the object's fate in any other context, is irrelevant. In the sadistic act, on the contrary, the emotional reaction of the object is crucial: the specific aim is to cause the object to suffer, physically or mentally, crudely or subtly. Domination and control are obviously critical features common to both aggression and sadism and it will become clear later how they differ in this respect. Needless to say, the expression of both aggressive and sadistic motives may be achieved in the most covert and disguised ways as can be shown by the amount of psychotherapeutic work needed to identify and assess them when they are factors in a clinical condition.

The distinction I am making between aggression and sadism may be illustrated by some simple examples. The bank-robber who takes hostages and then proceeds to derive pleasure in frightening them or humiliating them while negotiating his escape is being sadistic (quite apart, that is, from his initial act of robbery which may be aggressive or sadistic according to the nature of his motives); while the bank-robber who, in evading capture, shoots a guard dead, is being aggressive. An adolescent, who indulged in homosexual beating fantasies, spent a week having nothing to do with his parents, locking himself in his room and only opening it to receive trays of food and drink. He refused to talk to them, not even to explain why he was behaving in this way. His parents telephoned me to ask, in a troubled and exasperated way, what his behaviour was due to and what they should do about it. His behaviour was complexly motivated but it was clearly sadistic. In contrast we can consider his behaviour after a homosexual man had made advances to him. He performed compli-cated stone-throwing rituals which expressed, amongst other things, his wish to eliminate the homosexual. This motive should be identified as aggressive. These examples bear out the clinical observation that fear is always absent in sadism whereas it is consciously present, or denied, in aggression. This is the result of a primary function of the perversions as should become clear later when I elaborate how sadism is ultimately based on aggression.

Thus, crucial to the conception of aggression which I am proposing is that its aim is to remove or negate any element which stands between the individual and the meeting of his needs. This conception agrees rather closely with that put forward by Gillespie (1971) where he regards aggression from the viewpoint that 'all instincts (Triebe) are essentially homeostatic'. (See Cannon 1939). It is a fundamental task of the ego to guard the *psychic* homeostasis. The concept of psychic homeostasis is akin to, but not identical with, 'primary narcissism' which refers only to the disposition of libido. Taken from a physiological model, it implies a highly complex organization inter-relating all psychological systems and aimed at maintaining a *dynamic* balance, a steady state at optimum levels, rather than 'reducing [stimuli] to the lowest possible level; ... [maintaining itself] in an altogether unstimu-lated condition' (Freud 1915). I consider it is this way of thinking that led Freud to his formulation of the 'principle of constancy' and of the death instinct, concepts which my approach clearly rejects.

The concept of 'psychic homeostasis' which I am putting forward is rather similar to that of the 'ideal state' of Joffe and Sandler (1965) which they describe as 'a state of well-being, a state which is fundamentally affective and which normally accompanies the harmonious and integrated functioning of all the biological and mental structures .... It represents the feeling component which is attributed to the state of primary narcissism ....Much of the dynamics of ego functioning can be understood in terms of the ego's striving to maintain or attain a state of well-being, a state which even in the child who has been unhappy from birth exists as a biological goal.' But by 'psychic homeostasis' I mean something both broader and more complex than the 'ideal state', for not only is it not limited to the dimension of affectivity but it is also meant to refer to a multitude of systems with which the ego has to concern itself for psychic homeostasis to be achieved – such as self-esteem, biological needs, removal of castration threat, object relations fulfilment, to mention a few at random. In short, to maintain psychic homeostasis, the ego has to concern itself with demands and disturbances arising in the id, the super-ego, the external world, and within the ego itself. Maintaining a steady dynamic balance implies that over-gratification may be as disturbing as deprivation.

In considering aggression as an instinctual drive, we may follow the classical approach (Freud 1905, 1915) in regarding a drive as having *a source*, an *aim*, and an *object*. To this should be added that it also has a *stimulus*. In the context of psychic homeostasis, the stimulus of aggression would be any factor which threatens homeostasis; the aim of aggression is to eliminate the stimulus in one way or another; the object of aggression is the individual or thing responsible for the stimulus. I shall not attempt to identify the source of aggression but rather indicate its intrinsic nature by drawing attention to a quality of aggression which is not often appreciated, namely, how remorseless it is – how, if its initial ideational and affective expression does not bring about appropriate adaptive moves by the ego it will proceed to its ultimate aim of destroying the threatening factor, even if this is at the expense of murdering the object, developing a psychosis or committing suicide. This illustrates the relationship between psychic homeostasis and aggression – that, ordinarily, increasing intensity of need, or put more generally, increasing disturbance of psychic homeostasis, is accompanied by increasing aggressiveness. This applies as much to purely psychological considerations, such as self-esteem, as to matters of life-and-death. It will be recognized that any stimulus of aggression could also be regarded as a stimulus of anxiety (Freud 1926). This indicates how intimate a relationship there is between anxiety and aggression: anxiety may be the stimulus to aggression just as much as aggression may give rise to anxiety. This viewpoint differs from that of some schools of thought which consider aggression to be primary and basic anxieties a response to it (Klein 1948).

It is clear from the above that amongst the earliest capacities the ego has to aquire is a refinement in its perceptual functioning so that it is able to identify the stimulus to aggression with precision, that is, to be able to distinguish between the object's stressful aspect and the object as a whole. Perhaps the Kleinian school has drawn attention more than any other to the crucial implications of this in the early object relationships and this is complemented by the contributions of Anna Freud, Hartmann and others in stressing the importance of the ego, its autonomous functioning, maturation and, in short, its guiding and controlling role in the individual's development. To give a simple example of how important it is for the ego to refine its perceptual functioning: a man who is furious with his car because it will not start on a cold morning needs to be able to know that he does not want to destroy the whole car but rather its 'not-starting-ness'. It is precisely this capacity which severely regressed patients, such as perverts, lose to a greater or lesser degree, so that they feel that their rage against a feature or piece of behaviour of the object threatens its total destruction.

The view of aggression which I have been proposing is, in fact, rather close to that expressed by Freud in his 'Instincts and their vicissitudes' (1915) where, in considering *hate*, he states:

...the relation to *unpleasure* seems to be the sole decisive one. The ego hates, abhors and pursues with intent to destroy all objects which are the source of unpleasurable feelings for it, without taking into account whether they mean a frustration of sexual satisfaction or of the satisfaction of self-preservative needs. Indeed, it may be asserted that the true prototypes of the relation of hate are derived ... from the ego's struggle to preserve and maintain itself.

Perhaps it is necessary to emphasize that the aim of the aggressive instinct is not the infliction of pain. Too often this is implicitly or explicitly thought to be so. For example, in an otherwise admirable paper, Brenner writes (1971):

Aggressive aims vary with mental development and experience. They seem to be related to what hurts or frightens the child. Perhaps their close relationship to the aims of the libidinal component drives is due at least in part to the fact that the wishes connected with these sexual aims cause fear or pain, or both; the child hurts, or wants to hurt, someone else by doing to him what hurts or frightens the child himself.

I would say that Brenner is discussing sadism rather than aggression.

I have found the perspective given by regarding a threat to psychic homeostasis as the stimulus of aggression particularly useful clinically as the following example may illustrate.

At his initial interview a patient expressed great fear that his inability to control his temper would lead him to kill someone. He gave a number of illustrations of how he became 'fighting mad' and, making fists with both hands, said he would do anything I advised in order to overcome this threat to his future. The first illustration he gave was of how two men started teasing him in a public bar, commenting on the way he held his cigarette, the fact that he put his motorcar keys on the counter, the way he stood and so on. He replied in kind but kept quite calm. When he emerged a little later, he found the two of them waiting for him. They came at him and, feeling very frightened, he ran away. But after running about ten yards he had the thought 'Look what's happening to you!', whereupon he turned on his attackers in a wild rage and, in brief, assaulted them so fiercely that they both had to be taken to hospital. On another occasion, he was struck by the wing mirror of a careless driver. Before he knew what he was doing he was running after the car, calculating with a clear mind that he would reach it at the traffic lights. He did so and punched the driver in the face twice before the half-open window could be closed. He would have punched him through the window, heedless of any injury to himself, had he not calmed down. With great shame, he told me that on one recent occasion he had even punched his wife because of something she had said – something which he could not remember but which he thought implied humiliation. I shall not present any further clinical material except to mention that he was bullied by two older brothers in childhood and by older boys at school.

What stands out in this account is that it was of over-riding importance to the patient that something must immediately be put right by the aggressive 'eliminating' of it and that his behaviour had a quality of panic to it. This 'something' may be considered to be any of a number of 'dangers': the blow to his self-esteem; the assault on his masculinity; his denigration to the same lowly position as he experienced with his brothers; an impulse to respond with a passive, homosexual submission – no doubt further exploration in treatment would identify this; but the point relevant to the present discussion is that, whatever it might be, it constituted a serious threat to his psychic homeostasis and therefore provoked the extreme aggressive reaction he described. It is this which should initially guide the therapist in his management and approach to treatment, rather than a preoccupation with identifying the complex unconscious elements in the behaviour in question.

I would like to pursue this clarification further by distinguishing myself from those authors who consider aggression a special expression of a more fundamental instinctual drive of 'activity'; or, alternatively, those authors who consider 'activity' a derivation of the aggressive instinctual drive. They are no doubt influenced to such viewpoints by observing activities where aggression appears to be used constructively, for example in chopping down trees to build a log-cabin or hammering away fragments of rock to form a piece of sculpture. From my theoretical position, the aggressive behaviour remains a destructive one: in the act of sculpting, the shapelessness, the irrelevant parts of the rock, the parts of the rock which stand between the sculptor and his expression of his deepest feelings, are removed, negated; in the example of the log-cabin, it is the 'homelessness' of the environment that is attacked, much like the 'not-starting-ness' of the car.

Having elaborated how I consider aggression to be essentially part of the ego's response to a threat of psychic homeostasis, I would now like to turn to a discussion of the role of aggression in the core complex.

The part played by aggression in the core complex

Aggression is an integral feature of the core complex. Earlier I described how the intense need for the mother mounts to a wish to merge with her and how this carries the implicit concomitant of a loss of a separate existence as an individual – 'annihilation'. It will now be readily appreciated that this serious threat to psychic homeostasis will provoke an intense aggressive reaction on the part of the ego aimed at the preservation of the self and the destruction of the mother. Such a destruction, however, would bring about a condition of complete absence of the mother – abandonment; in this way aggression adds to the 'abandonment' anxiety consequent on withdrawal from the mother as described earlier.

With the limited resources the ego has at its disposal at this early stage of development, its efforts to deal with these conflicting considerations are inevitably crude and unsuccessful so that in the adult pervert one only discovers these features as components of a more developed clinical picture. Having only primitive mechanisms at its disposal, the ego may split its affective impulses towards the mother, attempting to deal with the aggressive component by denial. Often this aggressive component is then projected onto the mother so that she is experienced as engulfing or intrusive.

Another way in which the ego attempts to deal with the aggression is to split the internal representation of the object, so that it retains the loving relationship with one part of the object and is aggressive to the other part. Again it requires later development to sustain this position – for example, by displacing the aggressive feelings onto another person, such as the father (see below; also see McDougall 1970 and Chapter 8). In this early period the only direction in which the ego can displace the split-off aggression is onto the self and frequently this is done onto the individual's own body: what may be termed 'somatic displacement'. There it is felt to be safely contained. It is because of this primitive vicissitude of aggression that the pervert is able to treat his bodily contents not only as vehicles for the expression of affects but also as objects. An example of this is the transvestite patient discussed on pages 296/7. This basic mechanism of 'somatic displacement' is used in the establishment of psychosomatic conditions, so frequently found in the perversions.

The danger of 'abandonment' brought on by the need to destroy the engulfing, intrusive mother as much as by the wish to withdraw from her, will generally be dealt with by mechanisms which work towards enabling the re-establishment of contact with her; and the aggression will be focused on such factors as interfere with this aim. It is tempting to identify the energy utilized in the mechanisms which 'negate' such interfering factors, as neutralized aggressive energy, following Hartmann (1964) when he states: 'It is likely that defence against the drives [countercathexis] retains an element [fight] that allows of their description as being mostly fed by one mode of aggressive energy'. Some of the clinical features will be a result of these considerations. I have already discussed how the ego may seek to contain the aggressive intentions towards the mother by 'somatic displacement'. But it will also turn the aggression upon itself if other mechanisms seeking to re-establish contact with the mother are hampered by counter-considerations of the ego. For example, it may inhibit or negate its function of perceiving affects: the patient experiences a generalized 'numbness' so that there is no awareness of either missing the mother or wishing to destroy her. Such a 'numbness' is not the same as a later developmental capacity to repress affects, being much more gross and generalized and amounting almost to a body-state. Suicide may be seen as an ultimate expression of such processes. If the internalized aggression is sufficiently intense it may run amok, so to speak, and be directed in crude, gross ways at the ego's basic functions – perception, synthesis, and so on – much as an animal bites at its painfully wounded leg. I am, of course, alluding to the development of a psychotic, disintegrative breakdown (see page 283, see also Glover 1964).

It should be appreciated that the dynamics I have been discussing are solely in terms of a two-person relationship, the third person (ordinarily the father) is not involved. He is not utilized, as he may later be, as an object with whom to identify or onto whom aggressive and other feelings may be displaced. The vicissitudes of the core complex will naturally be influenced by the way the mother relates to her infant and I shall take this up more fully below. At this point I should simply like to put the reader in mind of the obvious ways in which the mother's attitudes and behaviour may disturb the psychic homeostasis of the infant and thus provoke further aggression, that is, by negligence or rejection on the one hand and by over-attentiveness and 'smothering' on the other (see Jacobson 1965).

The mental state of the infant in this core complex situation is far from placid and settled: it can be seen to be largely chaotic, fragmented, unintegrated and threatening a profound disruption of psychic homeostasis. This state is not, however, unique to the perversions; on the contrary, it is to be found in any condition involving the extreme degree of primitive, disrupted functioning that I have described. But what I am about to discuss *is* specific to the perversions and accounts, to some extent at least, for the 'choice' of psychopathology, that is, why it is that the individual developed a perversion rather than some other form of disturbance.

The establishment of the specific predisposition to perversions

In the perversions, then, the ego attempts to resolve the vicious circle of the core complex and the attendant conflicts and dangers which I have indicated by the widespread use of *sexualization*. Aggression is converted into sadism. The immediate consequence of this is the preservation of the mother, who is no longer threatened by total destruction, and the ensuring of the viability of the relationship to her. The intention to destroy is converted into a wish to hurt and control. Sexualization also acts as a binding, organizing force in the internal state of affairs, enabling defensive measures to be more effective and a certain stability to come about.

It is only when this process breaks down that sadism may revert to aggression. Sadism thus shades into sexual crimes, which in turn shade into crimes of violence, the appreciation of the object as a person decreasing in the process. When one works, as I do, psychotherapeutically with both delinquents and sexual deviants, one may observe how the patients may be graded on a continuum ranging from violence to true perversions. In some instances one may actually observe the process of sexualization taking place before one's eyes, so to speak, in the course of the treatment. It was a characteristic of a burglar I treated that at certain times he would impulsively run amok in a house he was in the process of burgling: he would pull out all the contents of cupboards and drawers, rip clothing to pieces, slash cushions, hurl pieces of furniture about the room, and run through the rooms throwing flour, sugar, eggs and other such things wherever he went. Finally he would leave the house without taking any of its valuables. The analysis of his housebreaking revealed that the main motives involved were those of the core complex. He would burgle at times when he felt particularly lonely. Entering the house represented entering his mother's body, and taking its valuables signified forcibly acquiring her precious love of which she had been so ungiving in his childhood. At the times he ran amok, some feature (such as an item of women's underwear) would have aroused his anger and his fear of being engulfed. His vandalizing behaviour was thus an expression of rage and panic in oral and anal terms, and his leaving the house reassured him he could escape being engulfed. At such times it was important not to take anything from the house since it would represent a claim of his mother on him. But what is of particular relevance to the present discussion is that, at the point in an extended treatment when he lost all desire to burgle, he started exposing himself indecently. This subsided with further therapeutic work when he established a satisfactory relationship with a woman whom he subsequently married.

With the contribution of other mental mechanisms, a more structured situation may be achieved, so that not only is there no evidence of aggression but even the sadism may not be immediately discernible. The favourite masturbation fantasy of a homosexual patient was to picture his lover sitting on a lavatory with himself astride his lap facing him and their both defaecating and urinating. Bearing in mind the aggressive meanings which can be attributed by the ego to excretion, as well as the ejective significance such activities may have, it can be seen from this brief clinical example how sexualization protects the object from the aggression of the core complex and preserves the relationship. In this instance, the sadism is not evident – it is safely deposited in the lavatory bowl and flushed away.

It is important to recognize that very often a crucial component in sadistic pleasure is the implication that the object is experiencing what the individual wants her to experience. This is reassuring in a number of ways. It removes the sense of uncertainty as to what the object may be feeling: this uncertainty is a significant element in the relationship with the mother, as I shall discuss below. It also conveys the sense of both participants being absorbed in the same affective situation: this approaches the longed-for merging with the object but contains the safeguard against loss of self in the process. It is for these reasons that it is so often a condition of the sadist that the object does not wish to suffer – often a masochist is of no interest to the sadist. The sadist's fantasy often requires that the object does not wish to participate in the sexual experience and is actually antipathetic to it, but because of the over-riding power or influence of the sadist, the object is carried away despite herself and ultimately participates passionately in the experience. The exhibitionist, for example, prefers to observe an initial expression of shock or disgust on the face of the woman to whom he exposes himself, and he may even be aware of a vicious quality to his affects at the time, but then, in his fantasy, she is overcome by the sight of his penis and comes to give herself to him enthusiastically. A further illustration of this is the homosexual patient who preferred to carry out acts of anal intercourse on young adolescent boys who had not experienced this before. It was important to him that they should feel his penetration as painful and struggle to free themselves but then find themselves beginning to enjoy the experience sexually and eventually delight in it and want to repeat it. When he met mature homosexuals who would happily offer themselves for anal intercourse he was quite uninterested. An important element in this 'seduction' of the object is that it implies that there is no doubt that he is intensely wanted by the object but at the same time he controls the object's want and his own passions (as he often demonstrates to himself by *coitus reservatus* and other such actions). Thus, through sexualization, all the disturbing components of the core complex are dealt with: the aggression no longer threatens destruction and loss and the dangers of both annihilation and abandonment are apparently averted. A further significance in the sadistic interplay with the object is that of revenge, basically on the mother. This is fully discussed by Stoller (1976). See page 110.

I would like to make it clear that I do not consider such sexualization of aggression results in the neutralization of the instinctual drives involved. I find myself unable to agree with those authors who seem to regard aggression and libido as 'equal but opposite', rather like acid and alkali, so that if they are mixed in suitable proportions they produce a 'neutral solution'. One can argue, for example, that the opposite of love is indifference rather than hate. This faulty approach is the result of allowing theoretical constructs to be applied too remotely from the clinical or behavioural phenomena they were set up to explain. It is also a clear implication of the viewpoint I have been elaborating that I do not regard sadism as part of the sexual drive, as Freud did and as many contemporary analysts still do – for example, Gero (1962). Undoubtedly the anal-sadistic stage is an integral part of normal psychological development, but to deem that a different quality of libido is involved is as misleading as maintaining that a different sort of libido is involved in homosexuality as opposed to transvestitism, as opposed to fetishism, as opposed to heterosexuality.

In the perversions, no psychic institution or function is free from being libidinized. The functions of the ego may undergo this fate. This may be observed most frequently in those ego-functions which are employed to make the earliest contact with the object. I must make it clear that I am not here referring to how the ego-function may subserve a perverse sexual aim, such as the importance of smell in fetishism or looking in voyeurism; it is the actual ego-function itself that becomes sexualized. For example, a patient developed eye symptoms which eventually came to be understood as being the result of the activity of looking being sexualized: it had the unconscious meanings of phallic intrusion into the object (as conveyed by such phrases as 'a penetrating gaze', 'a piercing look') and of visual incorporation ('taking things in through one's eyes'). Here the basic features of the core complex – being taken into the object, aggressive intrusion and so on – found expression in an ego-function through its sexualization.

I referred above to how internalization was one of the few courses the primitive ego could follow in attempting to deal with its aggression in the context of the early core complex. Perhaps this acts as a sort of facilitating pathway at a later stage of development when the super-ego is established, for the super-ego of perverts is characteristically sadistic. It is widely agreed (Freud 1930; Hartmann, Kris, and Loewenstein 1949) that aggression is internalized via the super-ego but in perverts this seems to be particularly so, the resultant sadism reflecting the nature of the object relations over the course of time that the super-ego is formed. I have discussed (Glasser 1978) how this relationship is a characteristic feature of exhibitionists where there is a general sub-missive masochistic attitude of the self to the super-ego, interrupted by spasmodic acts of defiance in the form of the exhibitionistic act; and I related this to the early relationship to the mother in which I identified the components of the core complex without explicitly referring to them as such. Such features are to be found in all perversions. This observation bears out how the sexualization of aggression permeates the whole of the pervert's personality structure.

I would now like briefly to indicate what part the mother plays in the vicissitudes of aggression in the context of the core complex. Frequently we have no objective information to corroborate the patients' depiction of their mothers, but one characteristic features so consistently in the accounts the true perverts give that one is safe to assume their veracity. This is that she has a markedly narcissistic character and relates to her child in narcissistic terms. To varying degrees with different patients, she is seen both to use her child as a means of gratification of her own needs and to fail to recognize his own emotional needs. She is both over-attentive and neglectful and thus disturbs his psychic homeostasis in both ways. Her narcissistic over-attentiveness, in treating him as part of herself, reinforces his annihilatory anxieties and intensifies his aggression towards her. Her neglect, emotional self-absorption and insensitivity to her child's needs will both frustrate him and arouse abandonment anxieties and again intensify his aggression towards her.

It may well be that the child's coming to deal with his aggression through sexualization is induced by his mother. There are many patients whose history contain accounts of manifest sexual stimulation of the child by his mother, this sometimes even extending into his adolescence: one patient will mention that his aunt told him how his mother used to play with his penis to stop him from crying; another will recall how, even at school-going age, he used to lie in bed with his mother fondling her bare breasts; another will mention in passing that his mother still baths him at the age of twenty-two. Even when the mother's sexual behaviour is less manifest, there is often the implication that the patient found his mother seductive. Many authors report such a finding. McDougall (1972) comments that 'complicity and seduction are attributed to the mother' and Bak (1968) describes the mother's seductiveness as being of a specific form: 'The boy is made to feel he is not only preferred, but closer to the mother through a bond of identity....In several instances the patients were close to the realization of incest'. Rosen (personal communication) stated his clinical findings were similar and expressed his view that the crucial factor was that while the mother was particularly seductive, she never fulfilled her promise.

However, Limentani (1976) draws our attention to the fact that such findings are not invariable when he states: 'In my own experience the mothers of bisexuals who have come to my attention were not seductive mothers, as we often meet in the case of homosexuals'. Indeed, the whole matter is put in doubt by patients' accounts which present their mothers as emotionally remote and they state that they are unable to remember ever being cuddled or embraced or in any way experiencing a physical communication of warmth from their mothers. But such mothers are not physically inattentive; on the contrary, one invariably finds evidence of a definite involvement with their son's bodies so that one is led to consider whether a special bodily cathexis, or an unconscious communication of sexuality, does not pave the way to the utilization of sexuality even in such cases. My account of the relationship between a transvestite and his mother (page 297) illustrates this.

However attentive the mother is, she is inconsistent and often even 'teasing'. This in itself promotes both the anxiety of uncertainty and aggression and can be seen as an important determinant of the subsequent sadistic need to control the object and determine exactly how she feels and responds. In fact in those patients with whom I have had the opportunity to study their early relationship to their mothers in detail, I have always found this to be predominantly sado-masochistic. Furthermore I have not encountered clinically a true pervert who has not had a close relationship with his mother (or an adequate substitute). The more distant the relationship the more likely is the sadism to be predominantly physically aggressive. Those patients who have had a motherless childhood, having been brought up in institutions or passed from one foster-mother to another without the opportunity to form any relationships in depth, invariably have a markedly disturbed sexuality which is either severely inhibited or involves viciously sadistic fantasies or behaviour showing little or no concern for the object. In my opinion such patients are not perverts but borderline or psychotic individuals manifesting a deviant sexuality. This may be recognized in their lacking the cohesion and integration of the pervert's make-up and in the impermanence of their form of sexual deviance, which now takes this form and now that.

Before concluding this section, I would like briefly to discuss the problem of masochism as a perversion. This may be discussed from many points of view (Freud 1924, Loewenstein 1956, Berliner 1958, Lihn 1971, de M'Uzan 1973); my comments are restricted to some aspects of the relation of masochism to the core complex. I think I can best convey my understanding of the role of masochism in this context by quoting a remark a female patient made when referring to the masochistic stories she read in her late teens, involving such events as a woman being raped by a group of conquering soldiers. 'Now I can only feel: Thank God she survived', she commented, 'but then I found it very exciting'. Sexualization preventing destruction again appears as the basic principle. The 'victim' in the above fantasy can be taken to be both the self and the object, with the different implications this carries; that is to say, it is not only 'seduction of the aggressor' (Loewenstein 1956) that is involved but also sexualization of the aggression directed towards the object in the context of the core complex.

It should be recognized that the masochist gives himself a sense of control of what transpires (as is most vividly illustrated in the paper by de M'Uzan). He is the master of operations, determining – often to the finest degree – in what he will suffer in the role of the victim. A masochistic patient gave me an account of his encounters with a prostitute whom he would visit once every eight weeks. For the whole of the day he would play the role of the prostitute's servant, cleaning out her flat from top to bottom, cooking her food, running her bath, addressing her deferentially and so on. At the end of the day, she would go on a walk of inspection of the flat and note any faults or oversights in his work – a trace of dust here, a fingermark there, an object not in place – and add these to the list of shortcomings he had displayed during the day. She would then make him stand submissively before her, reprimand him very sternly, and give him a cut on the hand with a cane for every fault found. Sometimes instead of this she would order him to stand in the corner with his trousers about his ankles and, after making him wait for some time, she would cane him on his bare bottom.

We can see that by and large he could determine what punishment he received. He could also be reassured that in this acted-out way his aggressive impulses were totally controlled, every fault being strictly noted and punished (thus, incidentally, giving externalized expression to his relationship to his super-ego, as discussed on page 292).

At the same time, he could feel he could control when he came and went, that is, the basic issue of moving towards or away from the object, in this way reassuring himself against both the annihilation and abandonment anxieties. It was relevant that while he was with the prostitute he would experience no sexual arousal whatsoever: only afterwards when he was at home would he masturbate with the memory of the day's events in mind – that is, when giving free expression to his passion did not carry the danger of his losing control of the situation in her presence. Studies of masochists bear out that they insist on laying down the conditions of their 'helpless suffering' most precisely. As Loewenstein states (1956): 'Masochists seek only certain specific and individually variable forms of suffering and humiliation. As soon as these reach greater intensity or take a different form, they are reacted to with the habitual fear and pain'.

Earlier (page 287) I discussed some of the consequences of aggression being turned inwards as a result of the flight from the object because of fear of annihilation; now we can consider how the individual seeks to retain the object via masochism. At one and the same time, he makes the aggression in both himself and the object innocuous. By means of masochism it seems indisputably established that he is not attacking the object, which is therefore secured against destruction. At the same time, masochism prevents the danger of abandonment: 'it attenuates her anger into domination precluding desertion (Loewenstein 1956). These features are well-illustrated in the account of the masochist patient just described.

From the preceding discussion it can be seen that there is always an element of deception in masochism, always an arrogant contempt and assertion of control hidden behind the humiliation and submission. Extrapolating from this, one is led to recognize that there is always an element of deception in any perversion since, for the reasons I have elaborated, sado-masochism is so ubiquitous a feature in the perversions. This is certainly substantiated by clinical experience and the therapist must be careful to watch out for it. One of the main areas in which such deception occurs is in relation to the super-ego and this is expressed in the transference. The fundamental motive for this deception is to ensure survival in terms of the core complex.

The contribution of aggression to the later developmental stages of perversions

True perversions are complex mental structures involving the whole of the personality. As such their ultimate form is shaped by the different stages of development that the individual must pass through, as well as by particular experiences. Consequently individuals cannot be diagnosed as suffering from a true perversion until they have passed through adolescence, only after which the structure of their psycho-pathology is firmly established. In each of the stages, development will be influenced by the particular way the conflicting needs of the core complex are resolved. I shall select aspects from different developmental periods to illustrate this.

The clinical material of a transvestite will be presented to indicate how, on the one hand, the anal phase contributed to the structure of the perversion and how, on the other hand, this phase was influenced by core-complex feelings. One of the important pleasures this patient felt when dressing in women's clothes was that it made him feel clean and fresh. This was related to a period in his childhood when he would retain the contents of his bowels to the point of incontinence, soiling his underpants and sometimes even defaecating in them. His mother was very annoyed about this as she had to wash his underpants. Analytic work established that one of his motives for faecal retention was his belief that in defaecating he would be giving expression to an explosive, obliterative rage towards his mother. He expressed this in a session when he said he felt like a hand-grenade that would explode and wipe us both out. This came about because he experienced me as not really caring for him and seeing him only as a therapeutic duty, just as his mother was depicted, in his accounts of his childhood, as emotionally remote yet conscientious in her physical care of him. But this symptom of retention and incontinence not only related to his rage; it also allowed him to derive sadistic pleasure by making his mother feel helpless and compelled to carry out the distasteful task of washing his soiled underpants. In this way he made her pay for her dutiful rather than loving attitude. This led to the severely traumatic experience of his being hospitalized. Many incidents occured there to provoke intense annihilation and castration anxieties, as well as feelings of abandonment, and the consequent terror and rage came close to overwhelming him. He reassured himself that all would be well because he would be discharged wearing girls' clothes, making use of his belief that women did not defaecate. Later, when he put on his mother's bloomers he felt delightfully cool and clean and relaxed. .

Much later in treatment we came to recognize a deeper, more primitive meaning to this anal behaviour. He made use of the sensation of a loaded rectum with its increasingly insistent 'statement' of something being inside his body, and then employed a split-identification characteristic of transvestites, that is, he identified his body with his mother's and at the same time identified with the stool in his bowel, thus giving concrete gratification to his wish to get inside his mother's body, to merge with her. By ultimately losing bowel control he could reassure himself that his faecal self could not be stopped from escaping from the containing mother, that is, that the rectal containment was not annihilatory.

All these various themes, then, are expressed in his adult perversion, dressing up symbolizing his getting inside his mother's body, and undressing the ability to escape whenever he so wishes.

It is true that the make-up of the child is fundamentally transformed by its passage through the 'prism' of the Oedipus complex but this prism is itself distorted in those children with a core complex of the sort I have been discussing. The emotional relationships have a predominantly sado-masochistic character. For example, the oedipal wish is not so much to destroy or castrate the father as to humiliate or denigrate him, that is, it is sadistic rather than aggressive, and castration-anxiety is frequently expressed in masochistic terms and may be dealt with, for example, by the development of beating fantasies.

In the oedipal relationships, the father invariably has a lesser status in the individual's emotional life than in the case of the normal child. The mother features more significantly in the patient's emotions so that the oedipal situation verges on a dual relationship rather than a triangular one. Thus mother is often the predominating, castrating figure; and this anxiety may often be traced to the core-complex anxieties. For example, anxieties of having his penis bitten off may be based on 'engulfing' anxieties. In the same way, I believe the so-called 'phallic mother' is a latter-day version of the powerful, executive mother of the core complex (for a different viewpoint, see Bak 1968).

It is interesting, in relation to these sorts of emotional issues, that the perverse patient may make use of a mechanism which resembles that seen in fetishism but which differs from it. Another transvestite patient of mine used to have a masturbation fantasy in which he would be seduced by a nun who would dress him in women's clothes, steal all his money and trick him in various unspecified ways. In the analysis he associated her black garb with a childhood memory of his mother, beautifully dressed in a long, black gown with elbow-length black gloves. From this material we can see that he regarded his internalized, childhood mother as being seductive, sadistic, and castrating. Implicit in the fantasy, however, is *his* tricking the nun by retaining his penis: while it appears that it is he who is being fooled in various ways and being castrated both by being turned into a woman and, in anal terms, having his money stolen, secretly he is triumphantly holding his sexually alive penis, and it is the nun who is deceived and tricked. This deception is a crucial element. It enables the patient to make use of splitting and give expression to the contradictory motives involved in the fantasy: 'I am being castrated' and 'I am being potent'; 'I am being ridiculed' and 'I am ridiculing'; ' I am helplessly surrendering myself' (merging) and 'I am retaining my independence and am in full control' (keeping separate). The oedipal father is not in evidence and his exclusion is emphasized through his mother featuring as a nun, thus denying the fact of parental intercourse and the father's sexual significance.

The father often seems to serve the function of a convenient figure for displacement of various drives, split-off from those directed towards the child's mother. This occurs particularly in adolescence (see page 300) but it may already be seen to be in operation in the oedipal phase. In defence against both oedipal and pre-oedipal desires and in an attempt to negate her seductiveness, the mother may be idealized and experienced as devoid of all sexuality, while the father is invested with all the dangerous attributes originally experienced in relation to the mother. In this way, the intensely aggressive feelings are deflected onto the father. This is a frequent post-oedipal course of emotional events in certain types of homosexuals (see also McDougall, Chapter 8). The clinical picture may consequently be superficially misleading in that the child may be understood to be reacting to his father as a frightening, castrating figure by adopting a placatory, passive posture and feminine identification. Unless the manifest state of affairs is considered in relation to the core-complex ingredients of the patient's life, treatment in such cases will remain ineffectual and this will be attributed to wrongly-conceived resistances.

It is now generally accepted that the latency period is not devoid of direct instinctual interest and expression. However, in perverts this period is often characterized by a much more evident instinctual activity. Aggressive behaviour, particularly in the form of minor delinquencies, is a very common feature. Their sexual history in this period often includes accounts of sexual seductions by older children or adults who are sometimes parents or close relatives, and masturbation often features as an activity consciously carried out. This is because the unsatisfactory resolution of the conflicts of the core complex and then, later, the Oedipus complex, does not let the instinctual life go to rest, so to speak. The interaction with, especially, the mother or her substitutes, continues to provoke intense aggressive reactions and sexuality must remain available to deal with this aggression along lines which were established in the original core-complex reactions.

There is some truth in Jones's statement (1923) that '...in adolescence the person lives over again, though on another plane, the development he passed through in the first five years of life', and that '...the precise way a given person will pass through the necessary stages of development in adolescence is to a very great extent determined by the form of his infantile development'. But the nature of the adolescent's make-up is altogether more complex and developed than that of the child and the impact of puberty occurs in such a different emotional context from that of infancy that the parallel cannot be too closely followed. We may well see the re-emergence of the Oedipus complex, the core complex and other regressive features but it would be wrong to regard these as simply unmodified recurrences. The ego may well be comparatively weak in the face of the intensified drives (Anna Freud 1936) but it is nevertheless an ego that has undergone a great deal of development in the years preceding puberty, and it has the super-ego both as an ally and as an extra factor with which to concern itself. Furthermore from the point of view of the object relationships, it can be said that the aim of the ego from birth to puberty is to establish and maintain a satisfactory relationship with both parents (and their imagos), a relationship which while involving a clear state of separateness is nevertheless a dependent one; from puberty inwards, in contrast, the aim of the ego is to bring about a harmoniously independent relationship with the parents. It is because of this that adolescence is sometimes described as the second, final period of individuation (Blos 1962).

Developments in adolescence are the inevitable consequences (unless interfered with by psychopathological factors) of the physical, psychological, and social forces which are brought to bear on the individual with the advent of puberty. Aggression, particularly in the context of the core complex, plays a crucial role in this.

The consequences of the maturational increase in instinctual drives in relation to the resuscitation of the oedipus complex at puberty have been extensively discussed in the literature (for example, Freud A, 1958). I shall limit my discussion to some of the implications of the remobilized core complex, not only because this aspect has not received sufficient attention but also because the true perversions become established as a result of the psychodynamic interplay around the forces of the core complex, while the perverse conditions which are more neurotic in nature develop out of a similar interplay around the Oedipus complex (Glasser 1977).

With the increase of sexual drives at puberty, the core complex desire to establish the absolute closeness to the mother, which I have referred to as 'merging', is greatly intensified. When this is allied to the increased capability of the ego to achieve its goals as well as, paradoxically, the weakened defensive strengths of the ego, the danger of absorption into the mother and consequent annihilation is a most intense and pressing one and the aggressive response appropriately extreme. In my opinion it is this dynamic more than any others which underlies the energetic rejection of parental influence that is characteristic of adolescence. The 'search for identity' of adolescence is as much a fight for self-preservation as it is for self-realization (ultimately these goals are synonymous).

Under suitable environmental and psychological conditions, the eventual outcome of this energetic reaction is the establishment of a comfortable, independent, appropriately affectionate relationship to the parents. This does not occur in the case of the pervert: even a comparatively superficial observation of his family relationships will reveal serious disturbance, the most common features being a mixture of excessive dependent involvement and violent pseudo-rejection. Because his sexualization of the core complex has bound him indissolubly to his mother, the pressures of early adolescence provoke particularly severe annihilation and abandonment anxieties, and the aggressive response is terrifyingly extreme. The danger of destroying the object is intense and imminent because of the intensification of drives and of anxiety, the sense of weakness of ego-control, the frequent provocativeness of the mother and the awareness that, as the result of maturational changes, the adolescent actually has the physical size and strength to bring about such destruction in reality. The fundamental guiding principles underlying the defensive reaction to this danger is to exploit the previously learnt measures of sexualizing the situation (making use of the newly-acquired sexual energies and capacities) and of seeking to establish a safe distance from the object.

The combination of sexualization and 'distancing' may take place in a number of different ways, employing various defence-mechanisms. For example, he may split his affectionate and destructive feelings for his mother, displacing one or other of these sets of feelings onto another object. As mentioned in discussing the oedipal stage, but taking place more regularly and characteristically in adolescence, it is here that the father may have an important role to play as a recipient of these split-off emotional attitudes. He may come to be regarded as a wickedly, libidinous individual intent solely on obtaining the satisfaction of his own needs, and he may seem to be particularly hostile to the adolescent as a result of the displacement onto him of the aggressive impulses originally projected onto the mother. The mother is then experienced as the virtuous, gentle victim of this brute, to be tenderly cared for by the patient. The aggressive feelings directed at and, as a result of projection, felt to be emanating from, the father may also be sexualized (and then further displaced) so that his sexual object-choice is a powerful, sadistic person. An illustration of this is a homosexual patient who had a lifelong caring relationship with his mother, with whom he lived, and whose sexual activities generally involved his being the masochistic recipient of violent homosexual activities. The success of the psychological manoeuvres is indicated by his being able to live in lifelong intimacy with his mother without consciously feeling any danger of being taken over by her in one way or another.

These dynamics may take a different course, as illustrated by some adolescent material from a patient who obtained sexual pleasure from being beaten by large, hairy men. In his early adolescence his father simply fell in with his mother's decision to send him to a boarding-school where he experienced intense loneliness. He decided to write an anonymous letter to one of his teachers recommending that he should cane the boys more frequently, anticipating that he would contrive to be one of the boys punished in this way. Since being beaten by his father as a child was the greatest form of emotional attention he obtained from his parents, being beaten by the teacher could be seen as a salve to his loneliness, being understood by him to be at least *some* expression of interest and attention.

The evolution of these feelings was as follows: initially he felt intense hatred and destructiveness towards his mother, who treated him with narcissistic exploitation and neglect, typified in his memory of her frequently suggesting they carry out some pleasurable activity together and then invariably letting him down. These destructive feelings were sexualized; and defensive and other considerations led to the now-sadistic feelings being displaced onto his father and inverted at the same time. The original sadistic feelings received expression in his seemingly gentle and genial personality through such subtle ways as his telephoning a girl-friend to cancel an evening out at the last moment.

On the other hand, the adolescent may not only intensify his antagonistic feelings towards his mother (maintaining her at a safe emotional distance in this way) he may also displace his tender feelings outside the family, the object being chosen on a narcissistic basis. For example, an 18-year-old paedophiliac, whose rejection of his mother became much more violent on the advent of adolescence, became at the same time more and more sexually absorbed in little girls ranging in age from three to twelve years. He regarded his sexual feelings for these girls as predominantly tender and aimed at making them feel contented.

The adolescent may use the perversion itself as a means of expressing his aggressive feelings towards his parents, particularly his mother. A fifteen-year-old homosexual insisted on making his homosexuality as widely public as possible to the mortification of his mother. He succeeded in getting himself expelled from school, because of grossly insubordinate behaviour, but then publicly protested, using the local mass media, that his expulsion was because of his homosexuality. He obtained the support of a homosexual liberation movement, and he became a leading member of the youth branch. He participated in making homosexual pornographic films. His mother was extremely ashamed and embarassed by this public display of his homosexuality and he took relish in telling her what new public action he had taken.

All this was indisputably sadistic and part of his perverse character structure but behind this one could observe a pathetic desperation, a panic-driven fight to push away a mother whom he continued to experience as constantly threatening engulfment. At the same time, one could observe at certain undefended moments his profound loneliness and his deep longing to feel loved 'safely'. This was the feeling to which he gave expression when he told me that the aspect of his homosexual activities he enjoyed most was being cuddled and held close. This patient serves to illustrate how important it is to distinguish between the sadistic and the aggressive motives in the pervert's relationships: sadism seeks to maintain the relationship, aggression to break it.

An obvious distinction between the child passing through the early phases of development and the youth moving through adolescence is the major bodily changes which follow on puberty and the consequent increased potential for real destructiveness. The pervert again deals with this danger by sexualization so that the narcissistic attitude to his body is intensified and henceforth plays an integral part in expressing the sado-masochistic feelings. This is obvious in the case of the exhibitionist who displays his penis sadistically to frighten, embarrass and humiliate. When the aggressive feelings are not adequately sexualized and threaten to find direct expression, the perversion may be used to contain them. The transvestite patient discussed on page 296 started dressing up in his early teens in direct relationship to his experiences at the hands of the severely punitive headmaster of the boarding-school he attended. Analytic work revealed that feelings about this headmaster repeated those he had had about his mother (the material already quoted illustrates this to some extent). When he put on the female garments he not only experienced sexual excitement, he also felt a profound sense of peace and security at having his intense destructiveness securely contained (it will be remembered that he likened himself to a hand-grenade). It should be noted how the development of a perversion may, in such emotional circumstances, be life-saving because the adolescent may commit suicide due to the fear of losing control of his body which he regards as a destructive instrument (Friedman, Glasser, Laufer, Laufer, and Wohl 1971).

Concluding remarks

I have made little mention of perversions in females because, although the early core-complex development is the same for both sexes, the later developmental paths diverge. The whole question of perverse sexuality in females is an unclear one and I did not feel confident that the points I made would necessarily apply to them. (See Chapter 8.)

It is the nature of mental functioning that no element can be discussed in isolation without distorting it: it acquires a different character with different implications according to the context in which it is being considered. I have placed my discussion of aggression in the inter-related dimensions of the core complex and psychic homeostasis and proceeded to examine how aggression in these contexts makes a fundamental contribution to the nature and structure of the perversions. Considered in this way, the perversions can be seen to serve the vital purpose of preventing the breakdown of the individual's object relations and the psychic disintegration that would come about as a result of the unremitting demand of aggression tó achieve its aim of negating the object which threatens psychic homeostasis.

References

Bak, R. C. (1956). Aggression and perversion. In *Perversions* (ed. S. Lorand and M. Balint). New York.

—— (1968). The phallic woman. *Psychoanal. Study Child* **23,** 15. London.

Berliner, B. (1958). The role of object relations in moral masochism. *Psychoanal. Quart.* **27**, 38.

Blos, P. (1962). *On adolescence*. New York.

Brenner, C. (1971). The psychoanalytic concept of aggression. *Int. J. Psycho-Anal.* **52**, 137.

Cannon, W. B. (1939). *The wisdom of the body*. London.

Chasseguet-Smirgel, J. (1974). Perversion, idealization and sublimation. *Int. J. Psycho-Anal.* **55**, 349.

de M'Uzan, M. (1973). A case of masochistic perversion and an outline of a theory. *Int. J. Psycho-Anal.* **54**, 455.

Freud, A. (1936). *The ego and the mechanisms of defence*. London.

—— (1958). Adolescence. *Psychoanal. Study Child* **13**, 255. London.

—— (1968). Studies in passivity. In *Indications for child analysis*. Aylesbury.

Freud, S. (1905). Three essays on the theory of sexuality. *Complete psychological works of Sigmund Freud*. Standard edition **7**, 125. London.

—— (1915). Instincts and their vicissitudes. *Complete psychological works of Sigmund Freud*. Standard edition **14**, 109. London.

—— (1924). The economic problem of masochism. *Complete psychological works of Sigmund Freud*. Standard edition **19**, 157. London.

—— (1926). Inhibitions, symptoms and anxiety. *Complete psychological works of Sigmund Freud*. Standard edition **20**, 77. London.

—— (1930). Civilization and its discontents. *Complete psychological works of Sigmund Freud*. Standard edition. **21**, 59. London.

Friedman, M., Glasser, M., Laufer, E., Laufer, M., and Wohl, M. (1972).

Attempted suicide and self-mutilation in adolescence. *Int. J. Psycho-Anal.* **53**, 179.

Gero, G. (1962). Sadism, masochism and aggression: their role in symptom-formation. *Psychoanal. Quart.* **31**, 31.

Gillespie, W. H. (1971). Aggression and instinct theory. *Int. J. Psycho-Anal.* **52**, 155.

Glasser, M. (1977). Homosexuality in adolescence. *Br. J. med. Psychol.* **50**, 217.
—— (1978). The role of the super-ego in exhibitionism. *Int. J. Psychoanal. Psychother.* In press.

Glover, E. (1964). Aggression and sado-masochism. In *The pathology and treatment of sexual deviation* (ed. I. Rosen). London.

Greenacre, P. (1968). Perversions: considerations regarding their genetic and dynamic background. In *Emotional growth*, (1971), New York.

Hartmann, H. (1964). *Essays on ego psychology.* London.
——., Kris, E., and Loewenstein, R. M. (1949). Notes on the theory of aggression. *Psychoanal. Study Child.* **3**, 4. London.

Jacobson, E. (1965). *The self and the object world.* London.

Joffe, W. and Sandler, J. (1965). Notes on pain, depression and individuation. *Psychoanal. Study Child* **20**, 394 London.

Jones, E. (1923). Some problems of adolescence. In *Papers on psycho-analysis.* London.

Khan, M. M. R. (1962). The role of polymorph-perverse body-experiences and object-relations in ego-integration. *Brit. J. med. Psychol.* **35**, 245.

Klein, M. (1948). A contribution to the theory of anxiety and guilt. *Int. J. Psycho-Anal.* **29**, 114.

Lihn, H. (1971). Sexual masochism: a case report. *Int. J. Psycho-Anal.* **52**, 469.

Limentani, A. (1976). Object choice and actual bisexuality. *Int. J. Psychoanal. Psychother.* **5**, 206.
—— (1977). The differential diagnosis of homosexuality. *Br. J. med. Psychol.* **50**, 209.

Loewenstein, R. M. (1956). A contribution to the psychoanalytic theory of masochism. *J. Amer. Psychoanal. Assoc.* **5**, 197.

Mahler, M. S. (1968). *On human symbiosis and the vicissitudes of individuation.* New York.

McDougall, J. (1970). Homosexuality in women. In *Female Sexuality* (ed. J. Chasseguet-Smirgel). Michigan.
—— (1972). Primal scene and sexual perversion. *Int. J. Psycho-Anal.* **53**, 371.

Socarides, C. W. (1973). Sexual perversion and the fear of engulfment. *Int. J. Psychoanal. Psychother.* **2**, 432.

Stoller, R. J. (1976). *Perversion: the erotic form of hatred.* Hassocks, Sussex.

11 Dynamic psychotherapy with sex-offenders†

Murray Cox

Introduction

This chapter has a readily discernible, though heterodox, structure and its content is based upon the clinical experience of working with a wide variety of sex-offenders in many settings. After defining 'dynamic psychotherapy' and 'sex-offender', there is an extended section on psychopathology. This is followed by a discussion of the setting and timing of the therapeutic alliance established between the sex-offender and the therapist. Setting and timing are inextricably involved with theoretical considerations which, in turn, underpin the indications for various therapeutic strategies. A rigorous structure is needed if a rambling, discursive approach is to be avoided in attempting to cover such a wide range of theoretical and practical considerations in the confines of one chapter. I hope the chapter will enable the reader to engage with its substance at the point of his need. For example, the following readers with widely differing needs may each justifiably hope to find relevant material in a chapter entitled 'Dynamic psychotherapy with sex-offenders'; the junior psychiatrist who is working for higher exams and yet has no personal forensic experience; the female probation officer counselling a rapist on parole; the psychoanalyst whose patient's sadistic fantasy is on the brink of erupting into reality, so that he fears his patient is about to become a 'sex-offender'; the experienced psychiatrist who, for the first time, is being called upon to undertake group therapy with sex-offenders either in a custodial or an out-patient setting; the general practitioner who finds that a patient, who ostensibly

---

†Based on lectures given in Helsinki, 1974, at the invitation of the Finnish Psychiatric Association.

The views expressed are those of the author and do not necessarily reflect those of the Department of Health and Social Security. Names, histories, settings, and other identifying features have been changed. Several incidents described are apocryphal, though they are based upon a corpus of experience. This camouflage does not diminish the human predicament of the disclosers and the clinical illustration they provide is not invalidated.

consulted him about organic illness, either discloses a fear of becoming a sex-offender or mentions that he has a record of such offences.

Any attempt to cover this field in one chapter necessitates the choice between a global, and inevitably superficial survey, and drastic selection with elaboration in depth of a few salient perspectives. I have chosen the second option, and hope that the discussion will act like a radiological tomogram, in which the subject is viewed from several angles, with varying degrees of penetration, so that contours and texture can be studied and a global appraisal attained.

Definition

Dynamic psychotherapy

I regard dynamic psychotherapy as a process involving a professional relationship, in which the patient is enabled to do for himself what he cannot do on his own. The therapist does not do it for him, but he cannot do it without the therapist. Such therapy may be conducted on an individual or a group basis. When the group-as-a-whole forms the therapeutic unit, the group is enabled to do for itself what the group-as-a-whole could not do on its own. There is a perennial debate amongst therapists as to whether the individuals who constitute the group, or the group-as-a-whole as an irreducible entity, form the therapist's prime object of concern. This debate, though of academic interest, seems far removed from the practical world of therapeutic strategy. No therapeutic group is created *ex-nihilo*, and each individual member of the group will have been referred to the psychotherapist by a general practitioner, a consultant psychiatrist, or other referral agency. Though the therapist may concentrate his attention upon resistance, mobility, patterns of interaction, and corporate defensive strategies (such as scape-goating) adopted by the group-as-a-whole, he is nevertheless responsible for the individual patient who was referred to him for psychotherapy. The professional colleague who has referred a sex-offender for psychotherapy is concerned to know whether his patient is showing evidence of dynamic change, or whether his endopsychic patterning is becoming more firmly entrenched, with hardening of his defensive position. The vicissitudes of the cognitive-affective life of the group-as-a-whole is solely of peripheral interest to the 'referrer'. I cannot envisage the possibility of running a mixed group of sex-offenders (say, four rapists and four female patients) and disclaiming any concern for the progress (or regression) shown by the individual patient. If, however, the therapist ever loses sight of the group-as-a-whole, he runs the risk of missing phenomena which can only occur in a group matrix. These phenomena may be 'therapeutic', but can become catastrophically destructive, if they are not perceived and handled in the right way, in the right place, at the right time.

Dynamic psychotherapy can be conducted as 'pure', small-group psychotherapy on an out-patient basis. It may therefore take place within the community and be part of an interdisciplinary collaborative effort, involving the probation officer, the psychiatrist, the family doctor, the social services, and so on. It may also be part of the therapeutic programme within the confines of a total institution such as a prison, or a secure hospital, such as Broadmoor.† Some institutions are run solely on group lines, so that every patient is a member of a small group, a larger group (such as the ward meeting), and, frequently, a global group in which all members of the unit or the institution participate. Individual psychotherapy, group psychotherapy, mileu therapy, and the therapeutic community are all therapeutic settings in which a therapeutic alliance may be established between the psychotherapist and the patient who is a sex-offender.

The theoretical approach which I adopt rests upon both psychoanalytic and existential premises. Though this may appear to be Janusian, I find that it provides me with a coherent frame of reference affording both the rigours of psychic determinism and the flexible openness to the exigencies of the present moment, which the sex-offender demands from the therapist. In my experience, this approach is self-authenticating and is equally appropriate for the inadequate exposer on probation and for the sadistic homosexual patient, found guilty of dismembering his sexual partner.

I wish to dissociate myself from the claim that any single psychodynamic conceptual scheme can possibly have an exhaustive monopoly of clinical truth. Such complex phenomena as sex-offences are always over-determined, and personality characteristics, organic factors, modified inhibition due to drugs or fatigue, the detailed circumstances of the offence (including the specificity of the victim), together with the

---

†The work described in this chapter would be impossible without the closest co-operation with staff colleagues at Broadmoor who refer patients, share in therapeutic work as co-therapists, assess patients' progress from many different perspectives, and, most important of all, spend long nursing hours in the life of the hospital when patients described in this chapter are *not* taking part in formal psychotherapy. Such work is possible only in a setting where the correct milieu is provided by a complex collaborative inter-disciplinary professional network. My gratitude to colleagues and patients is implicit on every page in this chapter, but it is made explicit here.

patient's previous life-experience, may all contribute to the patient's endo-psychic patterning at the particular moment when he assaulted his victim. One brief example of an important variable in the pattern of relationships of the sex-offender is furnished by Hitchens (1972), who describes denial as 'a major theme' in the marital relationships of such patients. For this reason, it must never be assumed that dynamic psychotherapy is the only *via therapeutica* appropriate for the sex-offender. Each patient must be assessed *ab initio,* and only after the fullest possible appraisal, from every conceivable angle, should a formal psychotherapeutic alliance be initiated. Physical treatments, medication, or behavioural modification (Bancroft 1976) may be appropriate, and frequently co-exist alongside dynamic psychotherapy as part of a total therapeutic policy. The integration of all therapeutic energies within the life of a total institution or, in the case of the out-patient, the wider community, must not be forgotten in the subsequent discussion, which concentrates upon one facet of offender-therapy. For example, the patient whose hypo-thyroid 'myxoedema madness' took the form of an escalating paranoid delusional system, in which a sexual assault was made upon a stranger, though construed by the patient as an act of self-defence against 'the attack in his eyes', would need appropriate medical treatment to render the patient euthyroid, as well as appropriate psychotherapy. The schizophrenic may need medication, but this does not absolve the therapist from trying to understand what the patient understands and is endeavouring to express or conceal.

Sex-offender

McGrath (1976) has indicated the difficulty of defining a 'sex-offender'. The problem becomes even more complex when inner world phenomena, such as the patient's fantasy of a sexual offence which may accompany a sexually 'neutral' action, are to be encompassed in the discussion. We are here concerned with what the offence means to the patient rather than the legal definition. There is the *'overt'* sex-offence such as rape, in which the patient knew he was committing rape, his victim would be painfully aware that she was being raped, and bystanders would be fully prepared to witness on oath to what they had seen and heard. There is also the *'displaced'* sex-offence, in which the offence is correctly legally classified as, say, 'larceny of milk bottles'. However, during the course of subsequent psychotherapy, the patient eventually discloses that his prevailing fantasies at the time of the incident were of grabbing breasts, humiliating and wounding women. Rubinstein (1965) has described sexual motivation in 'ordinary' offences. Thirdly, there is the sex-offence *'manqué'* which *appears* to be identical to that described above as 'overt'. The difference is that the 'offender' is out of touch with reality, so that he is not aware that he was involved in a violent assault 'against the person'. In these circumstances psychotic ideation may protect the patient. His prevailing delusional system might include the girl he was seen to 'rape', but his social construction of reality, at the material time, was that he was an estate agent showing a prospective buyer round a new house. Finding the door a little tight, he had to force his way in and was surprised at the screams of delight with which his client enjoyed looking at the new premises.

Thus the term 'sex-offender' covers a wide range of human activity and motivation, ranging from an almost harmless and trivial deviation from a socially acceptable norm, such as the *voyeur*, to the extremely disturbed and disturbing homosexual killing, such as that described by Marlowe in *Edward II*.

> I know what I must do. Get you away:
> Yet be not far off; I shall need your help.
> See that in the next room I have a fire,
> And get me a spit, and let it be red-hot...
> (Need you anything besides?)
> What else? a table and a feather-bed...
> So now must I about this gear: ne'er was there any
> So finely handled as this king shall be.
> Foh, here's a place indeed with all my heart!...
> If you mistrust me, I'll be gone, my lord.
> (No, no, for if thou mean'st to murther me,
> Thou wilt return again, and therefore stay.)
> So, lay the table down, and stamp on it,
> But not too hard, lest that you bruise his body.
>
> (*Edward II*, 2480)

This detailed description so accurately conveys the jarring incompatibilities of the sadistic enjoyment of using a red-hot spit, and the bizarre gentleness of the injuction that the table should be stamped upon... 'But not too hard, lest that you bruise his body'. It was a body already bruised by penetration with a red-hot spit, yet it should be protected from bruising. Othello describes another killing, completely different from the homosexual sadistic murder just described, but the sexual provocation leading up to the act and Othello's comment '...I will kill thee, and love thee after' (*Othello*, v, ii, 28.) mean that, in the widest sense, this cannot be removed from the realm of the sex-offence. After smothering Desdemona, Othello stabs himself and falling upon her, cries 'I kiss'd thee ere I killed thee ...' (v, ii, 358).

Psychopathology

There can be no unitary psychopathology underlying all sex-offences because of the over-determined, multicausal nature of the offence. There is no homogeneity of dynamic patterning behind the heterogenous offences 'against the person' known as sex-offences. The sex-offender is not confined to any single nosological classification. He (or she) may be appropriately diagnosed as neurotic, psychotic, psychopath†, or subnormal and all possible organic causes must be considered. Within three minutes of raising this topic with a group of colleagues at Broadmoor Hospital, the following organic factors were mentioned as being part of a precipitating constellation which had led to the release phenomenon of violence; a ruptured cerebral aneurysm, acute porphyria, a pineal tumour, post-epileptic automatism, and many cases of disinhibition due to alcohol or other drugs.

Learning theory and psychoanalytic theory, sadly frequently presumed to be uneasy bedfellows, may each contribute understanding to this complex over-determined constellation of predisposing and precipitating factors. For example, one rapist may be patently 'modelling' himself on his father who was an infamous rapist, whereas object-relations theory may account for other rapists' offences where 'modelling' played no part.

Freud's famous essay 'Criminals from a sense of guilt' (1916) is usually regarded as the *fons et origo* of psychoanalytic criminology. The offence may be regarded as the offender's adaption to social stresses in the environment (Halleck 1967), whereas Tuovinen (1973) considers *Crime as an attempt at intrapsychic adaptation*. This excellent monograph

---

†In this chapter, the term 'psychopath' is used to describe patients with a particular cluster of attributes, readily recognized by the clinician, though fashions in nomenclature change; for example, personality disorder, psychopath, sociopath, and sociopathic personality. However, narcissism and impoverished object-relations are core-elements in the psychopathology of such patients.

discusses the work of Kernberg (1970) and the 'criminal' outlet of narcissistic personalities, and that of Kohut (1971, see also Kohut 1977), with special reference to the development of the grandoise self and of the idealized-parent-image out of the original primary narciss-ism. Tuovinen links this to deviant activity. Tuovinen (1972) has written a key paper on *Schizophrenia and the basic crimes*. See pages 69–73.

Once it is accepted that patients with a wide range of organic factors, personality characteristics, socially influenced motivation, and prevailing endopsychic patterning may all commit sex-offences, then it clearly becomes impossible to do more than highlight certain features within the scope of one chapter. For example, the psycho-pathology of the psychopath who becomes a sex-offender is very different from that of the psychotic, who may commit an 'identical' offence. I am aware of the emotive quality of the word psychopath, but I use it as useful 'shorthand'; though, as I discuss further on, many 'psychopaths' subsequently prove to have borderline personality organization and may commit an offence during an ephemeral, micro-psychotic episode.

A useful concept is that of the *offence as a defence*. Bernheim (1976) has indicated that both acting-out and delusion may be a defence against anxiety for the psychopath who has relatively few inner conflicts. Primitive anti-social acting-out, involving assault, may be modified by psychotherapy into more acceptable styles of expression, and inner conflicts may be dealt with by increasingly differentiated and less anti-social defences.

The most ubiquitous and valuable concept in understanding the sex-offender is that of preservation of self. The *sense of self* of the sex-offender links so clearly with the work of Rosen (1968) on the self-esteem regulating quality of sexual deviation. In my experience, this profoundly influences the *genre* of appropriate psychotherapeutic management. Almost every mixed-group psychotherapy session in Broadmoor Hospital, where sex-offenders, say rapists, and female patients share in corporate group life, has moments of disclosure when a patient describes how his lost self-esteem was regained by committing the sex-offence or, for the first time, he experienced an enhanced sense of self – 'I really became somebody.' This remark might refer to sexual potency, or it might refer to the stigmatizing negative labelling by society so that girls in the neighbourhood were warned, 'watch him, you know what he's like!' Part of the essence of dynamic psychotherapy with sex-offenders is to find alternative avenues of self-esteem regulation, which can provide more than an ephemeral, aggressive genital climax as the basis for enhancing self-esteem.

The patient says that he feels there is a fault within him, a fault that must be put right. And it is felt to be a fault, not a complex, not a conflict, not a situation. Second, there is a feeling that the cause of this fault is that someone has either failed the patient or defaulted on him; and third, a great anxiety invariably surrounds this area, usually expressed as a desperate demand that this time the analyst should not – in fact must not – fail him.

(Balint 1968)

This quotation comes from *The basic fault*. There is a sense in which the sex-offender frequently suffers from an emotional deficiency disease, it is not so much a question of conflict as of primary deficiency. It is for this reason that third-level disclosures (see p.321) from sex-offenders are not always about psycho-sexual development, because sexual deviation itself may be a self-esteem regulator, and may cover a deeper pathology in which self-esteem is at risk, such as the threat of non-being. I have indicated (Cox 1973) the value of group psychotherapy as a *milieu*, in which fragile and negative self-definition can be 'redefined'. Such redefinition for the sex-offender lies in growing differentiation between who he is and what he does. 'I never thought anyone could love me. I couldn't believe I would get affection, so I took it'. 'I wanted to live so that I had my life and she [mother] had hers ... but it became her life. She pulled me back "with a rope" [an imperishable umbilical cord] ... and this stopped heterosexual adventures and the rope, like a dog lead, only allowed "friendships with children"'. In this instance the psychopathology of paedophilia was as simple as the umbilical rope which 'stopped me becoming me'. The patient's self-esteem had been so low that he did not think that he was worth anything to another person, except a child. Psychotherapy and the unfolding of life events, which can never be dissociated, freed the patient from the restrictions imposed by low self-esteem and a dominating mother. 'I feel safer with kids under five or people over sixty-five .... You really know that they want you'. 'Mum said she was going down the road for a loaf of bread and the bugger never came back ... I'm less value than a loaf of bread ... I hate women!' This disclosure speaks volumes and indicates key issues, such as low self-esteem and attitudes to women, which contributed to a violent assault.

A poignant aspect of precarious self-esteem is illustrated by the patient who said that no one had ever wanted a photograph of her and, in fact, she could never recall ever having her photograph taken. So that when her official photograph was taken for security purposes, she said to the photographer 'Can I have another copy please... to send to Dad?'. (See Chapter 3).

Balint's 'basic fault' is an important primary deficiency which is intensified by, and declares itself within, an inability to love and trust. People with such a basic fault frequently become patients because they misinterpret social cues, so that their sexual advances will be doomed to failure. It is easy to see how stigmatization can lead to the experience of rejection which soon finds the patient living within a paranoid 'pseudo-community' (Cameron, 1943).

In contra-distinction to Balint's 'basic fault', repressed infantile sexuality and the failure to negotiate maturational phases appropriately, on account of defective capacities for relinquishment and/or attachment, underlie the specific psychopathology of the majority of sex-offenders. Nevertheless, however much castration anxiety, the inability to negotiate the depressive position or libidinal fixation, may describe inner world phenomena of the sex-offender, these factors never operate *in vacuo*. There is always a social setting in which the offence actually takes place, although it may have taken place in the patient's fantasy on many occasions in other settings. Exactly why the offence was committed *in this place, at this time, with this victim* requires the most detailed analysis involving sociological factors, a thorough assessment of possible organic precipitating events, and, indeed, access to all possible sources of information about the patient's inner and outer world. A psychoanalytic dynamic formulation alone does not account for the complex interaction which constitutes a sex-offence. There may be other people with identical inner world phenomena who 'behave' differently in a particular setting. It is not as naive and simplistic as it may first appear, if I underline the fact that *the sex-offence always involves action between two people*. The therapist is therefore not solely concerned with fantasy. Many sober citizens have fantasies of committing sexual offences, yet relatively few put them into practice. The psychopathology of the sex-offender is different from that of the law-abiding citizen whose 'sex-offences' remain safely within his fantasy world.

Sometimes the psychopathology of the sex-offender patient is crystal clear, and represents a fugue with various subjects which are interwoven, recapitulated and lead to an almost predictable conclusion. On other occasions psychopathology has the characteristics of a primitive, undifferentiated, chaotic affective surge . . . . . . 'something came over me' . . . 'I had to do it' . . . 'I was powerless to resist'.

Victims may be 'killed again' if surrogates are sought and *it is therefore of cardinal importance that the therapist tries to reach the point of understanding what the offence means to the patient*. Only then is it possible for a realistic therapeutic policy to be formulated, because the goals of psychotherapy are inevitably influenced by the starting-point of the patient's predicament which must include his way of viewing the world. The victim must have been a focal point in the patient's perception of reality, although defence mechanisms may have blurred awareness and/or transposed location.

The sex-offender is frequently erroneously described as sadistic: this term should be restricted to the relatively small group of offenders in whom sexual arousal and orgasm only reach maximal proportions during the infliction of pain. Such a sadistic act may be homosexual or heterosexual and may be directed towards an adult or a child victim. True sadists should be distinguished from a different group of patients, frequently incorrectly called sadistic, whose expression of power and the assertion of dominance takes the form of humiliating and belittling another person. The first group only reach orgasm when inflicting pain (in fact or fantasy), whereas in the latter group the experience of sexual climax may not be associated with this personal statement of power, which may, however, lead to physical cruelty. The sex-offender may in fact occur in either category, though it should be noted that the sadistic sex-offender will have a different underlying psychopathology. In both categories the significance of emotional disclosure during the course of dynamic psychotherapy is central, though the content of the disclosure may vary. If the deviant behaviour is a self-esteem regulator, then it is likely that the deepest third-level disclosures (*vide infra*) will not be about the offence, but will refer to those other areas of experience where self-esteem was, at best, fragile and, at worst, shattered. This would clearly demonstrate that the offence had the function in the patient's psychic economy of recovering self-esteem.

The act designated as a sex-offence may be ego-syntonic or ego-dystonic for the offender. It may be prompted by conscious or unconscious factors. The latter may be exemplified by the patient who commits a sex-offence, ensures that he is detected, or actually gives himself up to the police. If such a patient subsequently enters psychotherapy, he may disclose the guilt which had previously been hidden. Such guilt is usually connected with forbidden acts, which led him to commit an offence which would be certain to attract a heavy sentence, and would thus give him the punishment which he felt he 'deserved', though never received. The exact nature of the early forbidden act will depend upon his early experience of socialization and is therefore culturally determined, although at root it usually stems from sexual taboos. The unconscious motivation behind the sex-offence explains the panic which some patients experience, if they are 'reprieved', or merely receive a token sentence, after an act which they unconsciously expect will merit severe punishment to match their hitherto undisclosed guilt. It is, therefore, not surprising that third-level disclosures (*vide infra*) from sex-offenders frequently contain such material. Nevertheless, it cannot be repeated too often that it must not be presumed that, because a patient is talking about a sex-offence he is, *ipso facto*, disclosing the deepest recesses of his inner world.

When the therapist makes an intervention of the right texture and at the right time, he 'catches' the patient as he talks of two different worlds of discourse simultaneously, though prior to the intervention he is only aware of one. For example, the patient describing his feelings leading up to an incident involving multiple stabbing, because of his 'fascination with the blade', is suddenly (after the intervention) aware that a knife, unlike his anatomical 'weapon', would never lose its erection, would always elicit fear, and would never fail to penetrate. Such clinical experience is unforgettable for the therapist and dynamic theory comes to life in a self-authenticating way.

Therapeutic alliance

Setting

Dynamic psychotherapy with the sex-offender may occur in several settings which inevitably have far-reaching consequences upon the patient's *modus vivendi* in general, and the nature of the psychotherapeutic alliance in particular. These vary from a custodial setting within a penal institution for a sentence of known duration (except for loss of remission or the granting of parole), to a time of unknown duration in the setting of a special hospital, such as Broadmoor. He may also be seen in an out-patient setting, which may involve psychotherapy in a hospital department or at a special unit, such as the Portman Clinic in London. Figure 11.1 illustrates at a glance the various settings in which patient and therapist may meet. The psychotherapy undertaken can

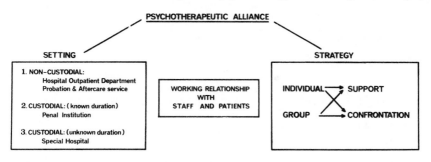

Fig.11.1   Reproduced by kind permission from *Brit. J. Crim.* (Cox 1974).

range from 'pure' individual psychoanalysis to, say, group therapy sessions within Broadmoor. It should not be forgotten that, in Broadmoor, the psychotherapeutic group is a very small part of the 'treatment' the patient receives; because such therapy takes place within the intense microcosm of life in the hospital, with its complex matrix of staff–patient, staff–staff, and patient–patient interactions which all form part of the on-going community life. Nevertheless, in whatever setting the patient and therapist meet, it is the patient's response as a whole person to the totality of therapeutic influences bearing upon him which guides prognosis. Psychotherapy may help him to understand and modify his inner world of fantasy and his idiosyncratic construction of reality, which led to an incident in his outer world of action and designated him as a sex-offender.

Timing

> Look to the lady:
> (*Lady Macbeth is carried out.*)
> And when we have our naked frailties hid,
> That suffer in exposure, let us meet,
> And question this most bloody piece of work,
> To know it further.
>
> (*Macbeth*, ii, iii, 126)

Figure 11.2 graphically portrays the chronological sequence of events from the pre-offence phase A to the post-trial phase C, where a patient may be, say, in Broadmoor 'without limit of time'. This brings a new set of variables into the discussion about dynamic psychotherapy with the sex-offender. For example, in phase A the patient is not, strictly speaking, an offender-patient because he has not yet committed an

TIME AND THE THERAPEUTIC ENCOUNTER

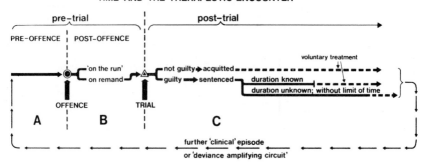

Fig.11.2   A deliberately simplified flow chart. Higher and Lower Courts, etc. are not distinguished.

offence. Nevertheless, he may present to his general practitioner or the social services department, saying that he feels he is going to stab someone 'if something is not done', or that he has read about 'baby batterers' and thinks that he may become one, if he is not rehoused. This front-line clinical situation, which the general practitioner or the social worker may have to face single-handed, demands almost impossible wisdom in differentiating the manipulative threat, from a genuine fear that 'if something is not done I will stab, rape, kill'. Some patients who ultimately commit sex-offences may give warnings of their intent, but there are vastly greater numbers whose thoughts of giving such warnings are not put into effect, and are subsequently dismissed by the comment 'I never really thought I'd do it'.

There is no easy rule of thumb to guide the general practitioner or the social worker in such situations, but an increased level of awareness grows from the assurance gained from inter-disciplinary staff support groups with experienced colleagues. These act as emotional resource points for the worker who battles with the need to 'worry along with each one'.

The timing of the first encounter between patient and therapist can have a critical effect on the subsequent course of the therapeutic alliance. It can be seen in Figure 11.2, phase B, that the patient 'on the run' may have very different disclosures to make from the patient who is on remand and being interviewed by a psychiatrist preparing a report for the court. The patient 'on the run' may have returned to his old, trusted family doctor and confessed 'I'm in dead trouble'.

Phase C, shows the circumscribed or extended duration of the therapeutic encounter upon which the therapist and patient may embark. Therapeutic space (see p.334) takes on entirely different qualities in the various post-trial patient-therapist alignments. The diagram speaks for itself, but it must be added that when a patient is resident without limit of time, both patient and therapist have long enough to share therapeutic space until it is no longer necessary. However, the bottom line in Fig. 11.2 indicates that one post-trial phase *may* usher in a future pre-trial phase. Recidivism is always an over-determined phenomenon. I have discussed group psychotherapy in a secure setting (Cox 1976), where this aspect of the work is amplified. There is a unique quality of relationship which can pervade therapeutic space and permeate the life of the group when therapist and patient are together 'without limit of time'.

The physical setting and timing of initiating the therapeutic alliance, shown in Figs. 11.1 and 11.2 respectively, are important in all psychotherapeutic work, though they have an added significance in psychotherapy undertaken with offender-patients including the sex-offender. For example, an entire chapter could be written on the dynamics underlying the optimal handling of the difficult therapeutic alliance in which a rapist on parole finds he is attracted towards his female probation officer. Both the setting and the timing of the encounter are of cardinal importance and, as with all supervision groups for, say, general practitioners or probation officers, the structuring of time, depth, and mutuality need to be rigorously scrutinized and constantly reappraised. The close interlocking of theory and clinical management makes an adequate conceptual scheme for structuring the therapeutic process mandatory (Cox 1978*a*).

General principles of dynamic psychotherapy

I regard the core datum of dynamic psychotherapy as the fact that movement always occurs in the direction of disclosure, as defences are gradually relinquished. Thus the classical Freudian concept of the Unconscious becoming Conscious may be extended, by saying that the Unconscious may become Conscious-but-withheld as a personal preserve of awareness. Further disclosure may therefore occur in a facilitating environment, when the patient is enabled to disclose, to others, material which he has hitherto kept as a 'secret'; though it may be a secret of which he is painfully conscious. The total process can therefore be stated as follows: Unconscious ⟶ Conscious-withheld ⟶ Conscious-disclosed. The final step is greatly facilitated in a group setting, where the safety mutual reciprocity with others, embarking upon the same risky business, can guarantee that the 'disclosure' is not 'solo'. This process is present in all group psychotherapy, wherever it is conducted, but when the patient is an offender-patient and, in particular, when he is a sex-offender, there is a snowball quality of escalation about disclosures. This means that a disclosure from one patient is frequently followed almost immediately by similar disclosures from other patients, 'I was waiting for you to start so that I could join in'...'Funny, I was just going to say that'. In actual fact, the patient who was *just* going to say that' was a reticent arsonist, terrified of making personal disclosures. But when, after eighteen months in a group, another patient admitted that he was an arsonist, the certainty of not being the odd man out allowed him to say something that he had 'just' been going to say! Examples of this disclosure-fostering quality of shared group life could be extended almost indefinitely: thus, a patient discloses that his impotence *preceded* his excessive drinking, a dramatic reversal of his earlier statement that he was impotent *because* he has been drinking. This has a facilitating effect upon other patients, who find it easier to disclose homosexual orientation as the 'reason' for using a knife, because of doubts about the penetrating ability of 'anatomical weapons'. When such disclosures occur in mixed groups, the therapeutic effect can be profound. 'I never thought I could say this to anyone...let alone a woman.' 'We used to need to read the blanks between the lines...but now you are writing them in for us!' This comment indicates a marked progression in reciprocal disclosure from an earlier phase of cautious non-commitment, such as 'If you're always talking, how the hell do we know when you want to say something?'

Dynamic psychotherapy with sex-offenders frequently confronts not only the patients, but also the co-therapists, with facts about the pervasive influence of unconscious mental processes which may have been previously dogmatically denied! For example, the cynical psychopathic rapist who may join a group because it will give the impression that he is co-operative, with the barely disguised determination to disclose nothing whatever about his personal world, is shattered when such events as a shared group-dream occur. He is immediately aware that 'something is going-on'. Another patient in the group describes, in considerable detail, a dream which she had during the previous night, and he, almost too shaken to hold a lighted match in one place long enough to ignite his cigarette, says 'Good God, that was my dream too!' In the same way, the junior therapist, who may be well trained academically but has comparatively little clinical experience, is startled when a patient who had certainly never read Freud says 'Hey, wait a minute, I know it sounds crazy, but could there be any connection between the feelings I had when I first broke into a house and when I first had sex with a girl? I know they are so different and yet in a funny way I had the same kind of feeling'. This is likely to be followed by disclosures from other patients in which 'forcible entry into forbidden territory', and the knowledge that the patient always chose to break into a locked house and had no interest whatsoever in entering an invitingly open door, plays a major part. Raping a prostitute might be equally uninviting. The trainee therapist is here confronted by clinical reality. Either this is a genuine third-level disclosure or the patient has 'read the right books and knows the right noises to make!'

Levels of disclosure

During the course of psychotherapy the words spoken by the patient, and the affective penumbra in which they are uttered, fluctuate across the boundaries between three levels of disclosure. The first is trivial, bus-stop 'chat': 'I thought I saw frost this morning'; the second is personal, but emotionally neutral: 'I am breeding budgies' (parakeets in the USA); the third is both personal and emotional: 'I never had a childhood'.

By definition, a third-level disclosure is difficult to make; it is either painful, shame-inducing and embarrassing, or 'precious' and not for public scrutiny. Thus, sadistic fantasies or the intimate information that 'I can never listen to Mahler without crying' could be third-level disclosures; though disclosures of sadistic fantasies are not *necessarily* third-level, a patient might enjoy recounting them.

The ability to distinguish between these levels depends upon the therapist's capacity to perceive what the disclosure means to the patient. It depends upon the clinical skill of experiencing 'vicarious introspection', which was Kohut's (1959) brilliant definition of empathy. For example, the disclosure 'I was born in Birmingham' is, for me, a second-level disclosure. I am neither particularly proud and want to publish the fact, nor anxious to conceal such information. Nevertheless, it is possible that the statement 'I was born in Birmingham' might be a third-level disclosure for someone other than myself, if, say, a strong Birmingham accent had blocked a life-long ambition to be a newsreader on television. The therapist learns to gauge what the disclosure means to the patient on the basis of the cognitive-affective qualities of the disclosure. It is the physiological concomitants of changing levels of anxiety, such as posture, gesture, rate of respiration, vocal rhythm and pitch, whether the direction and intensity of the gaze-pattern changes (either in the direction of becoming fixed or floating), which furnish evidence to confirm or contradict the overt affective 'statement' of feeling.

One of the axiomatic facets of psychotherapy training is to enable the trainee to be relatively 'uncluttered' by himself so that he has sufficient available energy, and the affective freedom, to recognize a patient's third-level disclosure and to distinguish it from what would be a third-level disclosure if he (the therapist) had said it.

The concept of disclosure levels is pertinent to all dynamic psychotherapy, but it is particularly relevant in offender-therapy. The fact that a sex-offender may be discussing rape does not, *ipso facto*, mean that he is making a third-level disclosure. A psychopath may discuss the incident with bland detachment or undisguised relish. The trainee therapist may be understandably impressed that the patient has been able to disclose such intimate phenomena, though, in fact, he needs to remember the caveat that such a disclosure may not be a genuine third-level disclosure for the patient. It is not infrequent for a third-level disclosure for such a patient to relate to various facets of an adolescent identity crisis; for example, he was teased at school because he had no pubic hair; he was the only boy in Borstal whose 'beard' did not register the fact that the daily distribution of razor blades had been withheld, because of a rumour that one had been stolen. Female sex-offenders often give overwhelming evidence that their third-level disclosures are concerned with the uncertainty of their sexual identity ('I didn't know if I was a man or a woman'), presenting as an adolescent identity crisis. For example, when a girl of twelve says 'I set fire to a convent', it is not unlikely that the most painful sense of emotional vulnerability and defencelessness might occur when she said 'The little girl in me still wanted to be cuddled but I felt torn apart because I hated the feeling that mum was superior and controlling... when I heard about *The* Mother Superior it was more than I could bear...' Another patient indicated that he could never share his life with another person, 'I could *never* share what I think of myself'.

Third-level disclosures of sex-offenders may be inextricably involved with self-esteem enhancement, and the offences often carry the secondary benefit of regaining peer group esteem or, if it has never been experienced previously, of establishing it for the first time.

It will be seen that levels of disclosure are intimately related to the psychoanalytic concept of the unconscious becoming conscious. Indeed, a third-level disclosure often occurs as the patient 'receives' into consciousness aspects of himself of which he was previously unaware. This has the effect of the disclosure having a novel 'startling' quality, not only for the other members of the therapeutic group, but for the discloser himself. 'Blimey, I never knew I felt like that before.' A third-level disclosure is rarely accessible to introspection, except in retrospect. (The hypothetical constructs of disclosure levels as elaborated in Cox (1977) and various visual display systems of disclosure phenomena are described in Cox (1978a, b)).

The phenomenon of the pseudo-disclosure merits a separate paragraph. In conventional psychotherapy it is important, though subsidiary, to the three levels already discussed; whereas in offender-therapy in general, and in sex-offender therapy in particular, it assumes major significance.

The psychopath and pseudo-disclosure. A third level disclosure is always a cognitive-affective phenomenon, and the non-verbal facets of communication, together with the physiological concomitants of change in the level of anxiety (either reduced or increased) are hall-marks of the affective components which accompany the cognitive 'statement'. Indeed, without such ancillary evidence, it is unlikely that third-level disclosure is occurring.

When the patient *seems* to be talking about disturbing, intimate, affect-laden material with simulated anxiety which does not 'ring true', then it is probable that the therapist is receiving a pseudo-disclosure. I regard the task of distinguishing pseudo-disclosure, beloved by the psychopath, as one of the most important skills in offender-therapy. Ultimately, the psychopath hopes to find that he cannot 'con' the therapist, though he may have an escalating life-long 'conning' pattern which enhances his defences, so that he may need fiercely incursive confrontation if his jealously guarded preserves of feeling are to be tapped. It must not be forgotten that 'confrontational therapy' is *confrontation with self,* facilitated by the therapist, not confrontation with the therapist.

The pseudo-disclosure of the psychopath is not a lie. Though this sounds a truism, it needs to be stressed, because it is so frequently presumed that because a particular patient is in the habit of lying, therefore whatever he may disclose about his inner world is, *ipso facto*, a lie. He may have lied about his involvement in a 'gang-bang' (a multiple rape), or about the number of robberies he has committed. Put bluntly, these are lies and not pseudo-disclosures. The essence of the pseudo-disclosure is that it is genuine in the sense that it describes certain facets of experience which are true, but which, nevertheless, are not related to the prevailing core psychopathology. The pseudo-disclosure is not a lie, but neither is it a third-level disclosure, although it may seem so to the therapist inexperienced in treating sex-offenders and, in particular, psychopaths who are sex-offenders. In my experience, it is possible to fail the patient precisely at the point where he is most vulnerable and indeed welcomes further confrontation with himself. For example, if the therapist diverts the attention of the group immediately a patient has described the incidents which led up to an incident of rape, there may be an implicit assumption that 'John has got it off his chest at last . . . he's been in the hot seat long enough . . . this is what we've been working towards for months'. He may have failed to discern that this was in fact a pseudo-disclosure. It may have been difficult for John to describe the incident of rape, and this pseudo-disclosure was most certainly not a lie, but an accurate account of what happened. Nevertheless, the crucial concept is that for John the genuine third-level disclosure, which lay behind the events which culminated in rape, would have related to impotence and homosexuality. 'I *know* I'm queer . . . I've known it for ages . . . it's a relief not to need to hide it any more' . . . this could easily be a rapist's third-level disclosure. The therapist can put the clock back almost indefinitely, if he misinterprets a pseudo-disclosure as a genuine third-level disclosure. What may be regarded as having 'struck oil' may in fact be nothing more than the removal of top soil.

The sex-offender frequently adopts the defensive manoeuvre of saying that he is now concerned to look ahead and 'face life' and it is not healthy to 'go back over the past and dig it all up'. The therapist's task is always that of facilitating disclosure, and I would never regard psychotherapy with a sex-offender as satisfactory if he discussed, with appropriate affect, everything *except* his offence. *Per contra*, it is equally unsatisfactory if he *only* discusses his offence. This always suggests that he is in fact making pseudo-disclosures because genuine third-level disclosures about a sex-offence always lead back to earlier relationships (in fact or fantasy) which were unsatisfactory. And, as in conventional psychotherapy, again and again the patient retraces his emotional footsteps to early life-experience. If he remains fixated at the point of discussing his offence it is either an indication of an unsuccessful attempt to 'con' the therapist, or it indicates that there are more painful earlier experiences which he is not yet able to tolerate so that he is therefore relatively more at ease 'living with' his offence.

'... where the crime's committed, the crime can be forgot'.

(*A woman young and old*: W. B. Yeats).

However, as far as psychotherapy with the sex-offender is concerned it is fallacious to assume that the crime can be, or should be, 'forgot'. In clinical practice the crime often needs to be renegotiated, almost to the point of tedium, until the patient not only understands what happened, but has been able to incorporate hitherto intolerable parts of himself which, prior to psychotherapy, may have been consciously denied and were often totally repressed.

Once the therapeutic alliance is firmly established, the patient no longer regards the therapist's incursive activity as an attack. It is gradually reconstrued as the necessary, though painful, co-operation of an 'ally'. When this stage is reached, the patient, himself, will be aware whether the 'crime can be forgot... [yet]'. '*I don't linger long* [in the traumatic past] *but the feeling comes back with me and lasts quite a long time.* It's very strong and tails off.' There is an entirely different ethos about the patient who is aware that he can safely turn to the future because 'the crime can be forgot' in the sense that, following in the wake of insight, endopsychic patterning has been changed. For example, when the rapist who had built up an infamous local reputation for being a 'lad with the girls' has become conscious of, and able to tolerate, his homosexuality, he can experience an emotional relief after years of emotional smoke-screens and pretending to be what he was not. Such a patient is in marked contrast to a fellow member of a therapeutic group, who still avoids the past at all costs, denies that he has any problems and is anxious to convince staff and fellow patients alike that 'all is well'. Such a patient may eventually begin to discover things about himself when, as a member of a mixed therapeutic group (four male and four female patients), he learns through the third-level disclosure of the most attractive girl in the group, that she has an exclusively lesbian orientation and is therefore impervious to his desire to impress her. An interesting question was raised in such a group: 'Is this really a mixed group if we are either male homosexuals or lesbians?'.

Nuclear disclosures. A nuclear disclosure is a third-level disclosure which so captures both core psychopathology and the process pattern of life predicaments that the therapist senses that what 'surfaced' during a transient, almost casual, disclosure, would furnish the 'skeleton' which extended interviewing or numerous therapeutic sessions would invest with detail. When a nuclear disclosure occurs, it makes such a vivid impact on the therapist that it is like reading a page of English literature, where five words 'stand out' because they are in another language. It is difficult to give examples of nuclear disclosures, because what would be a nuclear disclosure for one patient would not necessarily be so for another. Furthermore, sex-offenders are no more likely to make nuclear disclosures than any other patients in psychotherapy; though when they do, like all other nuclear disclosures, it is unforgettable. However, for three patients with different realms of experience, different psychopathology, and different clinical presentations, the following disclosures are examples of nuclear disclosures: 'we were her [mother's] life, so when we went there was nothing left'; '...the more things that are hurled at you, the less painful it becomes ...It's like scar tissue'; 'when I lost my temper, I seemed to *lose myself* in my temper'.

Disclosures such as these occur as individual patients and the group-as-a-whole free-associate. The way in which this process was described by a member of a group of sex-offenders to a new member, who had just joined a long-established group, exemplifies his awareness of psychic determinism and the existential exigency of the present moment. Though his description is in basic English, it is infinitely more articulate than any technical words used in this sentence. When he was asked what happened in the group, how did people know what to say, and so on, he replied '...in the group we do what happens'.

Probably the most frequent topic for discussion in the post-therapeutic session between co-therapists, revolves around the differential diagnosis of a genuine third-level disclosure and a psychopathic pseudo-disclosure, so eloquently described by a patient as 'a subscription to rent-a-mouth'! The problem is compounded by the psychotic whose disclosure may, paradoxically, appear to be 'too good to be true', that is a pseudo-disclosure, and yet, when perceived as part of a delusional system, may be a psychotic third-level disclosure.

The psychotic and the group-as-a-whole. Fascinating though the psychotherapy of the psychoses is as a topic in its own right, and particularly as many sex-offenders have psychotic phases, it can receive no more than a passing reference here. However, supportive psychotherapy with the psychotic sex-offender (alongside appropriate medication) must take the form of conveying to the patient by posture, gesture and word that he is taken seriously as a person. 'I'm blind because I see too much, so I study by a dark lamp' comes from a psychotic† arsonist with archetypal primitive disclosures and too little ego to defend. The therapist's role with such a patient is therefore that of acting as guardian for a man who cannot guard himself. I have frequently found that one such patient in a group confers a reciprocal benefit on both the psychotic and the non-psychotic. In an almost inexplicable way, the psychotic himself finds that the group is supportive, and this may be because of such 'trivial-significant' events as the sharing of sweets or cigarettes, and possibly because the psychotic's loose hold on reality protects him from the overt confrontation which may occur in such a group between, say, the sadistic paedophiliac and the psychopathic murderer. The non-psychotic patients gain, though painfully, by the blunt emotional broadside from the psychotic who has no customary defences of tact and caution which protect most of us in social situations, and therefore the question 'Why don't you talk about why you killed your mother?' takes on a strangely penetrating quality. The psychopath, who could bounce such a question back from a patient with similar psychopathology, does not know how to cope with a patient who is, in one sense, out of touch with reality, and, in another, able to penetrate defences with unerring accuracy.

When conducting small group psychotherapy with sex-offenders, there are advantages in making the group mixed, as far as the sex of the patients is concerned, and also in achieving the optimal, though heterodox, amalgam of having one psychotic in a group of psychopaths: though, for obvious reasons, the psychotic must be sufficiently stable and in touch with reality to be able to make the journey to the group room and to be aware of what is going on. The inherent buoyancy of a group constituted in this way offers both the psychotherapist and his colleague, the responsible medical officer, many advantages. First, it fosters more accurate diagnostic appraisal than is possible in the early stages of assessment. However appropriate the nosological classification 'psychopathic' may be, it frequently becomes clear that the patient exhibits borderline personality organization

---

†I know of no textbook which has so accurately captured the ethos of the psychotic's changing perception of the world as Hannah Green's novel, *I never promised you a rose garden* (1964).

(Wolberg 1973; Kernberg 1975) see also Hartocollis (1977). Such patients have capricious, mercurial, rapidly fluctuating defence organization, so that the sex-offence may have been committed during a transient psychotic micro-episode which, though catastrophic, was only a fragment of the patient's history which otherwise has the classical stamp of the psychopath. The presence of an overtly psychotic patient in the presence of a group of 'psychopaths' can evoke painful memories of the occasion when the 'cool, calculating' psychopath lost his 'cool' and was temporarily disorganized and chaotic.

Secondly, a group constituted in this way has an idiosyncratic orchestration so that the following vignettes are possible: 'I remember raping the girl next door', a pseudo-disclosure from a psychopath intent on impressing the group, and possibly succeeding, with all except the psychotic, whose reply follows: 'was she in a bungalow or a house?' The recipient of the disclosure is totally unimpressed, and this may push the discloser in the direction of genuine third-level disclosures. There is an infectious, escalating quality about genuine third-level disclosures, whether they come from the psychopath or the psychotic. Indeed, the following disclosure was from a psychotic patient, but it 'rang true' for almost every member of the group, though it was embedded in a jungle of disordered thoughts: 'the weakness I have in myself is what is in you . . . it's loneliness and desertion'.

No one in the group could deny that this, in part, had been their experience too, and a genuine sense of corporate solidarity was achieved in the group by the disclosure from the psychotic, which had acted as a Trojan Horse and taken the psychopaths from within.

Another example is furnished where a psychotic girl breaks into a psychopath's pseudo-disclosure and asks whether it matters if she has a spot on her dress. The ensuing free-association about blemishes; going through bad patches; having faults that people see; those that are hidden; having a 'stained soul' as being more disturbing than a stained dress; once again led the group to a disclosure level where the psychopaths were able to risk the vulnerability of disclosure. Such examples could be continued 'without limit of time', but I hope the few instances cited have indicated the vital fact that in conducting group psychotherapy with sex-offenders (as with all patients in group psychotherapy), the members of the group ultimately form their own best facilitators and become co-therapists for each other, though, for many technical reasons, there must always be professional co-therapists.

Ideally, there should be a therapist of each sex. Whenever possible members of the nursing staff should be fully integrated into a group therapy programme as co-therapists. The contribution of the nursing staff, who see the patient in formal 'small-group psychotherapy' as well as being intimately involved in the day-to-day events of his life within the total institution, is invaluable, and can never be exaggerated.

Brancale, Vuocolo, and Prendergast, (1971) describe a special treatment unit which is part of the New Jersey Program for sex offenders. The seven principles and guidelines they suggest are as follows:

1. Group therapy is more successful and longer lasting than individual therapy.

2. Sex offenders are generally too passive and inadequate for standard group therapy techniques and need more directive treatment, even to the point of reeducational methods.

3. Group therapy has to be supplemented by sex education sessions, since sex offenders are most often grossly misinformed or sexually naive or both.

4. Homogeneity of grouping by offense has been found to be useless and even potentially detrimental to successful treatment.

5. The sex offense itself must be understood by patient and therapist to be a symptom only and not the problem itself.

It then follows that:

6. The 'whole man' treatment philosophy should be employed.

7. Emotional release is an essential element in the treatment process.

Each one of these 'guidelines' is debatable, though they all raise issues which every therapist experienced in working with sex-offenders would acknowledge. Although I agree in general terms, my reservations are as follows (I use the same numbered paragraphs as Brancale).

1. A small minority of offender-patients, who have been exposed to the emotional pressures in a group and yet remain impervious, are referred to my colleagues who conduct individual psychotherapy. Occasionally individual psychotherapy 'strikes oil' where group therapy fails. Not surprisingly, there is also a reciprocal flow of patients in the opposite direction!

2 and 3. Not all sex-offenders are 'too passive and inadequate for standard group therapy techniques'. The great advantage of mixed group psychotherapy, with male sex-offenders and female patients, is that it not only demonstrates the way in which the offender relates (or

fails to relate) to the opposite sex, but it also provides 'education' in addition to the dynamic aspects of psychotherapy.

4. I entirely disagree with guideline 4 as a general statement. Group psychotherapy where the group is homogeneous as far as the offence of 'killing' (whether legally defined as murder or manslaughter) is concerned, can facilitate third-level disclosures at a rate rarely attained in heterogeneous groups. (There are, of course, other advantages in heterogeneous groups, but that is not being debated.)

5, 6, and 7. I agree with these guidelines, though methods of facilitation, participation and 'regulation' of 'emotional release' depend upon a complex network of 'domestic' relationships within the total institution.

Dynamic psychotherapy with sex-offenders brings into sharp focus two of the ubiquitous and perennial questions facing all psychotherapists. The first relates to the techniques of facilitating psychodynamic change so that movement in the direction of disclosure takes the following course: Unconscious $\longrightarrow$ Conscious-withheld $\longrightarrow$ Conscious-disclosed. The questions confronting the therapist are 'How can I facilitate disclosure in this individual or group setting?', and what are the risks for the patient and/or the community in which he lives, if the sex-offender is enabled to make such disclosures, which frequently relate to his offence, or, *per contra*, if he remains unable to do so?'. The second question is an inevitable consequence of the first. 'Having at last [in Broadmoor, we might substitute 'at long last'] enabled the patient to make third-level disclosures, what does the therapist do, that is, how does he respond to these disclosures from his patient?' This not a textbook on general psychotherapeutic theory or strategy, but once again the sex-offender patient presents, in an inescapable way, topics which arise with every patient in psychotherapy. How do I facilitate disclosure? How do I respond to the disclosures once they have occurred, and, even more important, how does the patient 'respond' to his own disclosures?

Special aspects of the therapeutic relationship with sex-offenders

I have discussed elsewhere (Cox 1974) the psychotherapist's anxiety with special reference to the offender-patient. Change in established defence patterns takes place in all dynamic psychotherapy, and that undertaken with the sex-offender is no exception. During individual psychotherapy, as transference is established and develops, the therapist is invested with feelings which the patient had previously invested in 'significant others'. The victim of his sex-offence may have been a specific 'target' whom the patient had been pursuing for many months; on the other hand, the victim might have been an unfortunate casualty who 'happened' to be present. During the course of dynamic psychotherapy, the therapist may have invested in him feelings transferred from this particularly significant 'significant other' in the life of the sex-offender—the victim. The therapist will be aware that, say, a victim has been killed, and there is no theoretical reason why this attack should not be repeated.

Arnold and Stiles (1972) write: 'Group methods have become one of the most widely used therapeutic techniques in our correctional institutions.' This, like conventional group psychotherapy, may have come about initially on economic grounds or because of the scarcity of trained personnel, though there is currently a striking shift in emphasis towards an appreciation of the intrinsic value of the group process itself. This applies both in terms of the facilities for enhanced dynamic understanding of the patient, and also as a therapeutic milieu. It may be that it was in a group setting that the patient originally established a deviant identity and, *ipso facto*, a group setting may also provide the re-defining process in which the patient's self-definition may be changed, in the direction of greater personal fulfilment in socially acceptable patterns. Group therapy therefore has an important re-defining function. Tuovinen (1973) writes: 'The only opportunity to study these problems is via individual psychotherapeutic work', which supports Ormrod (1975): 'Unless the study of offenders is undertaken on an individual basis, little progress will be made.' I disagree with these statements if they are taken to imply that it is *only* on an individual basis that the study of the individual can be furthered. In my experience, the greatest study of the individual is facilitated when he takes part in mixed group therapy and collateral individual appraisal is possible. It is in such settings that the rapist's relationship with women can be studied in great detail over a prolonged period of time. I am aware that this priveleged therapeutic opportunity is only likely to occur in hospitals such as Broadmoor, where mixed dynamic group therapy is an established part of the total therapeutic thrust of the hospital.

One special aspect of working with the sex-offender is the demand made upon the therapist to understand both the inner world of his patient, and the exact way in which his patient construed the context in which he committed the offence. To neglect either the inner world or the context betrays the patient. To concentrate solely upon the ambient circumstances of the offence and to rely upon objective, external sources of information about the offence fails the patient at his point of greatest need. It is one of the advantages of group psycho-therapy with sex-offenders that the patient is constantly finding his own inner world confronted by the external world of fellow-patients. They, better than any therapist, know the importance of the need to bring together their early blurred conception of 'how it was' with the undeniable facts, perhaps seen in legal depositions or even photographs, of how 'it really was'. The therapist needs both a macrocosmic and a microcosmic approach to the assessment of the significance of a sex-offence for a particular patient. The former is like a panoramic view, the latter like a zoom lens which closes-in. Thus for one patient a long-perspective macrocosmic view is necessary, if sense is to be made of his offence. His arson was no substitute sexual activity, but rather a way of getting his family, highly respectable and respected in the local Cornish village, into the headlines of the local paper, by ensuring that the reporters knew of his activity: 'Fancy one of them doing that. They were always such a good family!'. In such an event, the patient's com-ment that he set out to 'blacken the family name' by this form of indirect attack had succeeded. The microcosmic perspective may be needed for another patient, where the prevailing endopsychic pattern-ing of the sadistic homosexual killing, such as that described in such lurid detail by Marlowe (p.310), may be infinitely more important than the wider perspective of killing the king. The microcosmic perspective demands a close-up, detailed analysis of the context of the offence, and careful scrutiny of its relevance to the inner world of the patient; whereas the macrocosmic perspective involves standing back and seeing what the offence meant in its totality, such as 'blackening the family name'. Appropriate psychotherapy therefore depends upon the global appraisal of endopsychic patterning and its relation to *contextual analysis* which may need to be micro- or macro-cosmic.

In addition to such indubitably important topics as the relationship between transference phenomena developing during psychotherapy with the sex-offender and the possibility that the therapist may be perceived as a victim-surrogate, and the perennial debate between the value of individual and group methods of offender-therapy, there are other aspects of the therapeutic relationship with the sex-offender which must be discussed. I am referring to three phenomena which are of importance in all dynamic psychotherapy, but assume even greater significance when the patient is a sex-offender. These are the existential concept of Fragestellung, the concept of Therapeutic Space and the Weltanschauung of the Therapist. These will now be considered in turn.

Fragestellung†

There appears to be no English equivalent to this German term, which I am therefore retaining. It means literally 'the putting of the question', and refers to the totality of ideas which lead to the question being put in the first place. It implies that the answer to a question may be influenced by the way in which the question is asked, and can be demonstrated in the following example. The question, 'Why *did* you kill your mother?' may be asked forcefully in an early interrogation, or it may be asked with the greatest possible tact and diplomacy in a pre-trial psychiatric interview while the 'patient' is on remand. The question may be answered in several ways. The patient may be suffering from global or focal amnesia which may be organically or psychodynamically determined. He may be only too well aware of the event, but deny that he did it, or say that she was unduly provocative or that he was drunk and did not intend to do it. The same question, 'Why did *you* kill your mother?', asked by a fellow patient in the context of group psychotherapy at Broadmoor, where perhaps everyone else in the group was aware that it was a group of killers, might facilitate an entirely different answer. An identical question, but in a different setting, and with a totally different *fragestellung*. The first had the implication 'Come on, tell us ... we know you did it'; the latter was, in effect, asking the question 'Why did *you* kill your mother? ...I know why *I* killed mine!', and this obviously alters the ethos pervading therapeutic space. It is this facilitating process which allows third-level disclosures to occur. It must be remembered that the physiological concomitants of third-level disclosures usually enable the therapist to recognize them without difficulty, though the perennial trap for the therapist unaccustomed to working with offender-patients is to presume that, because a patient

---

†Part of this and the subsequent section are taken from *Structuring the therapeutic process: compromise with chaos* (Cox 1978a).

is talking about his offence, he is *ipso facto* making a third-level disclosure. For example, the patient who describes how he fatally stabbed a white-haired parish priest may be making a third-level disclosure, but on the other hand it may be a psychopathic pseudo-disclosure. Thus the patient might describe with disinterested, trivializing, detachment how he stabbed the priest, whereas he might find it almost overwhelmingly embarrassing, on a subsequent occasion, to disclose the fact that he was the only boy in his year at school whose voice had not broken. The trainee therapist might think that it was much easier to admit to a voice sounding feminine than to stabbing a priest, but he is not his patient. It is this ability to enter the inner world of the patient, and yet remain sufficiently detached to be objective, which is the hallmark of making progress in the growth of psychotherapeutic experience. Siirala has so admirably described psychotherapy training as a 'suffering-maturation process' (1974).

The concept of *fragestellung* is relevant to many aspects of psychotherapy with the sex-offender. It refers not only to the 'putting of the question' by the therapist to the patient but, to a much greater extent, to the putting of the question by one patient to another within the shared group. The therapist's task is to so modify disclosure depth that it is balanced between the invitational edge of the intolerable and the easily tolerable safety of inactivity. The poignant fact is that each patient in the group knows that, at some stage, he has to face the intolerable parts of himself. 'I have the burden of having no burden.' The *fragestellung* is a conceptual device which aids the therapist in monitoring disclosure potential, not only for the individual patient but for the group-as-a-whole.

Therapeutic space

This term is used in several ways by different authorities: Moreno uses it to describe the 'stage' upon which psychodrama in enacted; whereas others use it to describe intra-psychic space, that is that realm within the personality in which there is room for manoeuvre and growth.

There has recently been a growing interest in the concept of therapeutic space. Khan (1974) in a paper entitled 'The role of illusion in the analytic space and process' writes:

Clinically the unique achievement of Freud is that he invented and established a therapeutic space and distance for the patient and the analyst. In this space and distance the relating becomes feasible only through the capacity in each to sustain illusion and to work with it ... It is my contention here that Freud created a space, time and process which potentialize that area of *illusion* where symbolic disclosure can actualize.

The clinical experience of working with many patients whose lives have included incidents involving the 'basic' crimes, such as murder and incest, has convinced me that therapeutic space, though symbolic, is much 'firmer' and part of a joint reality than can be conveyed by the word 'illusion'. Khan writes 'the relational process through which the illusion operates is the transference'. The transference may be an illusion but it is not the whole content of dynamic psychotherapy, though its inherent dynamic pervades it.

Psychotherapeutic work with the offender-patient can provide a corrective emotional experience for the therapist! By this I mean that it reminds him that the ubiquitous and timeless fantasies of murder, and other destructive activity, may erupt into reality in a catastrophic manner. Much literature on psychotherapy often states explicitly, or conveys by an implicit *timbre*, that destructiveness is confined to intra-psychic fantasy or attenuated in the clinical presentation of verbal abuse or hostile silence. When the patient has actually killed someone, the conceptual boundaries between 'that area of *illusion* where symbolic discourse can actualize', and that area of *reality* where the 'hard' non-symbolic facts are disclosed, is of paramount importance. It is the merging of the *fact* that Donald killed his father with the *transference* '*illusion*' (when the therapist may transiently vicariously represent the un-killed father, or whoever Donald's father stood for in his social construction of reality) which sharpens the significance of reality testing. Such dynamic events are part of an established therapeutic alliance (whether on an individual or group basis) within therapeutic space. In my view, there is a danger of simplistic reductionism if the concept of therapeutic space is restricted to an illusion, on the one hand, or 'these four walls', on the other. In the same way that a patient who has actually killed his father reminds me that fantasy may become fact, so therapeutic space which may be an illusion can become 'factual' if enclosed within concrete boundaries.

The setting in which much offender-therapy takes place may be 'secure' so that therapeutic space takes on a literal 'concrete' quality, readily discernible in the form of bars at the windows and locks on the doors. These are constant reminders to both patient and therapist that therapeutic space has undeniable boundaries. Such therapy may be conducted in the 'group room' set aside for this purpose in a hospital, or prison, or a probation officer's office. In this sense, therapeutic space is the exact opposite of an illusion. My experience is that such custodial emblems as bars and keys intensify, rather than diminish, the affective flow of the therapeutic encounter. 'We are in this together' has a double meaning. There is the symbolic illusion of therapeutic space but this 'takes place' in a physical space (confined by a secure perimeter) which is also therapeutic. This existential blending, of the symbolic and the literal, intensifies transference phenomena and therefore facilitates individual and group dynamic psychotherapy when conducted within a secure setting.

In view of the many connotations of the term therapeutic space, it is essential that I clarify my own perspective. I regard it as a term which can be used metaphorically to describe an invisible boundary to the 'space' within which the therapist and patient meet, and where the phenomena of transference and counter-transference are 'housed'. It may therefore embrace both an individual therapeutic encounter or a total group matrix, involving eight patients and two co-therapists. In a more global sense it could include all the space within a hospital. Who would not regard the hospital football pitch, on which a patient might learn to improve physical co-ordination and at the same time learn the values of team-work and personal sacrifice, as therapeutic? However, the term usually refers to that space within and between those who share in a formal psychotherapeutic alliance. In other words, it includes the intra-psychic space of both patient and therapist and the inter-personal space between them. It is the shared air they breathe.

Even without bars and keys, I could not work if I felt that the therapeutic space which I shared with a patient was ever *solely* an illusion. I regard it as a 'concrete' existential fact that the patient and I are 'in this together'. Winnicott (1945) describing the feeding of the infant writes: 'I think of the process as if two lives came from opposite directions, liable to come near each other. If they overlap there is a moment of *illusion* – a bit of experience which the infant can take as *either* his hallucination *or* a thing belonging to external reality'.

Dynamic psychotherapy with sex-offenders frequently needs to get back to this early nurturing situation, and this implies that the therapist may become a transitional object. This links closely with Balint's (p.313) concept of the 'basic fault'. When the therapist is working at such a primitive level with his patients, he may be perceived as a transitional object, but this is only while his patients need to perceive him in this way. It is of the essence of psychotherapy training that the patient's prevailing needs determine the therapist's response. In this instance it would be disastrous if the therapist's personal 'need' to be seen as a transitional object, 'over-ruled' the fact that his patient had now reached a stage where he could safely relinquish such transitional maturation facilitation. It is logically impossible to be a permanent transitional object, and therapy has ceased to be dynamic if the patient's emotional needs and perceptions of the therapist do not change. Winnicott's comment about infant feeding is also exactly on target at the deepest level of dynamic psychotherapy with the sex-offender: the nourishing experience may be taken 'as *either* his hallucination *or* a thing belonging to external reality'.

Barker and Mason (1968) have taken Buber's theme *Between man and man* (1947) and look at the implications for treating patients 'confined by law, against their will, until they change' in *Buber behind bars*. The probation officer is literally in the same prison cell as his client, and the psychiatric nurse in a secure hospital shares therapeutic space in a more than symbolic sense. It is true that one member of the alliance has a key and the other does not, but both are locked in together, and it is in the intensity of this 'locked in-ness' that many of the dynamics I have already discussed take place. From my office at Broadmoor I have a panoramic view covering three counties, with the horizon eighteen miles away. From my desk I can only see the view, but when work is over I can, if I wish, enter and enjoy what I have previously only seen. My patient has the same view, he has no keys and the countryside can be nothing other than a view for him. In spite of the patient's knowledge that I alone have a key, he and I together share therapeutic space.

Hitherto the patient has been stigmatized as 'that bloody rapist', or 'that monster'. The judge, vicariously representing society, has pronounced him guilty of rape and he may, for example, have been admitted to Broadmoor under Section 60/65 of the Mental Health Act (1959) 'without limit of time'. He and I know the terms of reference within which we meet to share therapeutic space. It is no facile evasion or mere playing with words to state that, by his therapeutic presence, which may be conveyed by gesture, posture, and expression long before words have been necessary (and possibly also when they have ceased to be necessary), the therapist conveys to the patient with whom he shares therapeutic space the realization that '*one of us* has done this'. This is not to condone or in any sense approve of the offence, but there is a profound difference in therapeutic perspective when the patient senses that he is able to say 'I have done this', because the therapist is aware that 'one of us has done this'. This is in marked contrast to conditions previously obtaining when he was being confronted and challenged by 'you have done this', which may have made him retreat into the defensive position of rationalizing the particular episode of his history, deliberately denying it, or even being focally amnesic due to repression.

Within the context of a hospital such as Broadmoor, the fostering of the sense of therapeutic space occurs focally in the particularly intense cosmos of what would be formally known as 'small-group psychotherapy', and in wider life of the institution as a whole. This permeates the many-faceted staff-patient interactions, ranging from that with the football coach and the conductor of the choir, via that with staff undertaking more conventional nursing activities, to that with staff using specialized techniques such as dream interpretation or appropriately dealing with other 'pure' psychotherapeutic topics, such as group transference.

The concept of therapeutic space serves to counteract the previous stigmatizing experiences described by sociologists such as Goffman (1963), Chapman (1968), and Matza (1969). Merton (1949) warns us against the dangers of the 'self-fulfilling prophecy', and this is closely linked to the idea of 'controlling identity' elaborated by Matza. Attention is drawn to the risks inherent in limiting the patient's possible future by extrapolating from his past, though the clinician is always aware of the 'natural history' of disease processes. This applies, *a fortiori*, to the profound clinical and moral implications of decisions relating to the release of dangerous offenders such as the sex-offender, in whom there might be an 'outcropping' of violence after a five-year gap of impeccable social behaviour. The therapist is therefore warned against therapeutic nihilism implicit in the statement 'because the patient has behaved like this in the past, he will therefore continue to do so in the future', and the therapeutic naiveté implicit in the remark 'the patient now has insight into what he has done and therefore he will not do it again'! However, Matza's concept of the controlling identity, implicit in the stigmatization 'the patient is a thief, merits serious consideration. In fact this may only apply to one brief incident in the life of the patient, who may otherwise be a bank clerk, a psychotherapist, an out-of-work labourer or a retired general! Matza develops the argument that this indulgence in deviant activity incurs running the risk of intervention, apprehension, and signification. This leads to the enhancement of the identity in terms of the characteristics signified: that is to say, 'to be signified a thief is to lose the blissful identity of one who among other things happens to have committed a theft. It is a movement, however gradual, toward being a thief and representing theft'. It need scarcely be added that if the word 'arsonist', 'rapist', or 'murderer' replaces the word 'thief' in the preceding sentence, then an entirely different dimension of significance applies, not only to the individual concerned but to society as a whole.

Sociologists quite correctly point to the risks of labelling, though the clinician is aware that a firm diagnosis of schizophrenia has many more prognostic and therapeutic implications than the mere attachment of an appropriate 'label'. However, in day-to-day professional work a label such as 'psychopathic' is useful shorthand because it conveys 'infinite [diagnostic] riches in a little room'. By describing a patient as a psychopath, it is implied that there has been escalating anti-social behaviour, that he has low impulse control, and that he is not psychotic, but we must be careful that such a label does not lead to the implication that the patient will never improve, that he is always lying and therefore everything he tells you is untrue, and so on. In this way it is easy for a self-fulfilling prophecy to emerge which takes the following form: 'This patient is a psychopath. He will not respond to treatment. Therefore we will not offer him treatment'.

Many psychopaths do mature, and one of the functions of psycho-therapy with such patients is to hasten the maturational process, and to monitor and reappraise it as the patient encounters opposition and provocation, when he confronts 'himself' in other members of the group. Bolingbroke was describing the maturation of the psychopath with prophetic insight, though it was in the days before formal group psychotherapy could claim any share in the maturational process!

'As dissolute as desperate, yet thro' both I see some
Sparkles of a better hope, which elder days may happily bring forth.'
(*Richard II*, v, iii, 20)

In spite of Matza's strictures about the dangers of a controlling identity, it is perfectly true that if any staff member working in an institution concerned with treating the mentally abnormal offender-patient asks 'What did he do?' with reference to a particular patient, the answer is likely to be 'He shot his boss', 'He raped an usherette', or 'He set fire to a hotel'. This answer is of course only describing a fragment of the patient's history, but anyone who regards homicide, rape or arson as a fragment and unimportant for the patient or society, must be out of touch with reality.

Weltanschauung of the therapist

The psychotherapist sharing therapeutic space with the sex-offender comes closer to the inner life of the patient than the psychiatrist whose work is predominantly involved with over-all treatment strategies and administration. If an effective global therapeutic strategy is to be able to 'hold' a patient, the psychotherapist needs to work in a particularly close relationship with his colleague, the responsible medical officer. This has been discussed elsewhere (Macphail and Cox 1975). The responsible medical officer has to make many executive clinical decisions about his patient (Loucas and Udwin 1974), whereas the psychotherapist spends the majority of his time 'being with' the patient rather than 'doing to' the patient. When the patient is invited to 'say anything', then the therapist has, by implication, made the far-reaching claim that he can 'hear everything'. This may therefore stretch his personal emotional resources to the limit, and will inevitably call his *Weltanschauung* into play. The therapist never fully knows what content his patient's disclosures may carry. 'Looking back on it all now, do you see it very clearly or is part of it baffling and confusing?' Such an invitation to disclosure may yield material which is painful, though in a different way, to both therapist and patient. Yet he remains a human being, and there is no doubt whatever that his inner world may be invaded by that of his patients, and his own smouldering doubts and anxieties may be reignited by those with whom he shares therapeutic space. He is exposed to the awareness that his patients may be vicariously carrying his murderousness. He is not 'wholly other'. His patients therefore confront him with part of himself which is usually hidden. In the words of Prospero: 'This thing of darkness I acknowledge mine' (*Tempest*, v, i, 275). If he does not bring the sense of being a person and therefore partially vulnerable to the group, he will be construed as being 'remote and clinical'. If, on the other hand, he appears too soft and fragile, then the patients may feel either that he is unable to take their violence or aggression or, *per contra*, that if they 'go to pieces' the therapist will follow suit. This stretching of the therapist's personal *Weltanschauung* underlines the following paradox: he needs to be ruthlessly rigorous in diagnostic appraisal, alert for any disclosures, and aware of the risks of acting-out (particularly by patients who have known histories of violent offences against the person); yet, at the same, he needs to retain warmth and a sense of being at ease with himself. This is an ideal which no individual can ever achieve completely by either personal endowment or technical mastery. The longer I spend in therapeutic space with such patients, the more I feel that I am growing in two directions at once; namely by becoming more rigorous in my objective dynamic formulation of events and, *pari passu*, of accepting my patients as people who are in so many ways just like me. This links closely with the existential approach. It provides the therapist with an awareness of the dangers of foreclosing and pre-empting any fresh disclosures from a patient, if he has already made a cast-iron dynamic formulation based upon rigid psychic determinism. He may in fact run the risk of not hearing what does not fit into his presumed formulation of the patterning of the patient's endopsychic life. If the therapist is to be able to retain this Janusian quality of adopting both a deterministic and existential outlook, he will discover many surprising things. For example, he will learn that many psychopaths, far from being affectless people, have previously often been particularly vulnerable and formed strong emotional bonds on at least one occasion, but, having been betrayed, they have withdrawn from any further deep relationships. Third-level disclosures from psychopaths often take the form of personal reminiscence about tenderness, beauty, or the betrayal by a trusted ally, which frequently justifies the comment 'Never again, mister'. 'I can't get what I love, so I hate it.' I recall such a disclosure from a man with many violent offences 'against the person', who yet just withheld tears as he described scenes of fantasy from his childhood, which were not only Calibanesque but almost an exact paraphrase of '...the isle is full of noises,/Sounds and sweet airs, that give delight, and hurt not.../...that, when I waked,/I cried to dream again.' (*Tempest*, III, ii, 144). This patient, 'classified' correctly as an aggressive psychopath, showed a degree of tenderness which many would find it hard to believe, yet it was quite different from the incongruous tenderness of the sadistic homosexual killer, so vividly portrayed in the quotation from *Edward II*.

Bush (1975) in 'Sex offenders are people' describes her involvement as a volunteer therapist in a group of sex-offenders. There is a poverty of publications upon the role of the psychiatric nurse in forensic psychiatry, though in a hospital such as Broadmoor the weight of therapeutic initiative rests upon the relationship between the nursing staff and the patients. Consultants come and go. The nursing staff are involved 24 hours per day 'without limit of time'.

Caveat

No single theoretical approach holds a monopoly of truth in determining the predisposing and precipitating factors leading to a sex-offence. Therefore there cannot logically be a single therapeutic modality which is universally indicated.

It is for this reason that psychotherapy with the sex-offender is such an excellent *metier* for teaching both theory and clinical strategy. The trainee may indulge in elaborate psychodynamic hypotheses to account for his patient's behaviour, but he is brought down to earth by the personal confrontation with the question posed by the patient's legal representative, and society as a whole, 'Is John Smith "ready" to go yet?'. There is a paradigmatic quality about mixed-group psychotherapy when, say, rapists and female patients share therapeutic space. This makes the therapist tighten up his dynamic formulations with the utmost rigour, and yet, simultaneously, demands that he remains open towards the patients' unfolding disclosures. Dynamic psychotherapy with sex-offenders therefore makes particular emotional demands upon the therapist which, though present in every therapeutic alliance, here assume heightened significance. There is a need for constant re-appraisal of endopsychic patterning, and the monitoring of changes in defence organization which must occur within an emotional climate which facilitates disclosure and provides a therapeutic presence.

The 700 (approx.) patients in Broadmoor form a highly selected population and provide a unique opportunity for the psychotherapist. He is able to share therapeutic space with patients 'without limit of time', and at a depth of facilitated vulnerability impossible in any other setting. He is cautiously allowed to enter the outer world of his patients, and gradually, but only after repeated testing-out, is he accepted in their inner world. A therapeutic group slowly achieves an autonomous life of its own, and the paradoxical status of the therapist takes on its characteristically chameleon-like quality . . . 'He is one of us but he is not one of us . . . the group goes on without him, but not if he is not there . . . He is there at the beginning and the end, but seems to go away in the middle.' The long temporal perspective allows the 'trust-testing' see-saw to oscillate until it finally rests on trust, and the consequent disclosure of hitherto unconscious or 'conscious-withheld' material gives the therapist in Broadmoor unrivalled access to inner world phenomena of the sex-offender. It is from life within the intense arena of group psychotherapy, with male and female patients, when therapeutic space has been shared for literally thousands of hours, that the following dogmatically anti-dogmatic reflections come. Prolonged exposure to the inner and outer world of the rapist, the arsonist or the killer convinces me that any statement about 'The' psychopathology of such offences inevitably implies that the author must have limited personal experience and be basing such remarks upon the comparatively few such cases he has seen. There is a great danger in extrapolating from a few cases to assume that there is a universally applicable psychopathology of a particular offence. Nevertheless, there is clinical validation and an authenticating experience for the therapist, when disclosure at depth and of prolonged duration has occurred from hundreds of sex-offenders. A member of one such group, seeking reassurance, asked anxiously in a pre-therapy assessment interview 'It will be a group of killers, won't it?' and his question implied not only that there is 'safety in numbers', but also that group cohesion is fostered and disclosure facilitated if the murderer is exposed to the 'benevolent ordeal' (Haley 1963) of psychotherapy in a murderer's peer group.

Arson: a paradigm of over-determinism

'I shall love you horribly because you let me unlove you so soon...

I want horribly to burn a house, Alyosha, our house. You don't believe it, do you?...

Why not? There are even children about twelve years old who want very much to burn things, and they do.'   (*The Brothers Karamazov*. Dostoevsky)

'It is in the nature of extreme self-lovers, as they will set a house on fire, and it were but to roast their eggs.'   (*Of Age and Youth*.   Bacon)

'...thought-executing fires...'   (*King Lear*, III, ii, 4)

The arsonist may be diagnosed as subnormal, neurotic, psychotic, or psychopathic. The act may be of profound symbolic importance to the patient or almost incidental. It may be of overt sexual significance, and the patient will claim that he has his best ever orgasm as he watched the flames leaping up, or that his greatest moment of sexual excitement was when he was helping the fire service unsuccessfully to put out the fire which he had started. ('I started something which was so out of control that even I and the fire service could not deal with it.') In this instance the act is overtly and expressly sexual. On other occasions the act may be symbolically associated with love or hate ('My best flame, you set me on fire, burning anger' . . .) The arsonist may show psychotic concrete thinking so that self-immolation occurred when Charles Wesley's hymn, 'Kindle a flame of sacred love on the mean altar of my heart,' was taken literally. The act may be the quickest way of damaging the property of an enemy. It may be part of a deliberate sexual assault, either in fact or fantasy. One arsonist said that radio-therapy worked by the burning out of cancer, and therefore a really big blaze would destroy all the cancer cells in the vicinity and thus protect his children.

Thus the almost limitless range of clinical presentations means there is no neat unitary hypothesis which can underlie the behaviour of all patients convicted of arson, which may or may not be part of a sexual offence.

The endopsychic patterning and defence organization of patients committing arson recall us to the importance of studying the individual. However valuable statistical surveys may be, work at Broadmoor constantly reminds us that although we may have seen a hundred arsonists, we must remain open to what *this* patient is telling us about himself. Hurley and Monahan (1969) were unable to demon-strate any psychopathology specific to arsonists, which reinforces an editorial comment in the *British Journal of Delinquency* (1957) 'the dynamic approach to the individual aspects of crime is not yet ex-hausted', and more recently, Ormrod (1975), already quoted, 'unless the study of offenders is undertaken on an individual basis, little progress will be made'. The therapist working with such patients must welcome any possible exploratory avenue of research which might conceivably go some way towards answering the many unanswered questions.

Offender-victim alignments

Classical quotations can serve as a back-cloth to various sexual offences: the deliberately fostered morbid jealousy of Othello, or the 'textbook' homosexual sadistic murder of Edward II. The porter in Macbeth made comments about the effect of alcohol on sexual performance which have never been bettered:

'. . . much drink may be said to be an equivocator with lechery; it makes him, and it mars him; it sets him on, and it takes him off; it persuades him, and disheartens him; it makes him stand to, and not stand to ...' (*Macbeth*, ii, iii, 31.)

Many sex-offences are precipitated by alcohol or other drugs.

The following is a brief list of the range of clinical presentations: the psychotic killer who rapes and strangles a girl, he 'takes a life' because he needs a life; the woman who castrates her lover and then enucleates her own eye, because she sees what she has done and obeys the injunction 'If thine eye offend thee, pluck it out'; the anxious 'blameless' schoolmaster who confesses to the police that he has exposed himself to a 'sober-suited matron all in black' in the local park and admits that though he was not seen, let alone caught, he feels he ought to have been and has therefore given himself up; the ferocious homosexual dismemberment of a faithless partner; the man convicted of house-breaking who experiences the same excitement of forceful entry into forbidden territory as on his first illicit sexual adventure; the arsonist who burned her lesbian friend's flat, who now presents as psychotically deluded, claiming that her clitoris is protruding from her ear; the rapist whose victim had to be 'a stranger but look like Mum'; the unmarried man with a shoe fetish who can only masturbate when wearing stolen high-heeled shoes and who is charged with 'larceny of a pair of shoes'; the phobic housewife who stabbed a postman because the tubular parcel he handed in was 'too big to sqeeze through your letter-box'. Some are 'overt,' some are 'displaced', and some sexual offences 'manqué'. One of the least understood, but most pressing, problems is the relationship between the offender and his victim. This highlights the immense complexity of the subject and rules any simplistic interpretations out of court. Howells (1976), using a standard form of repertory grid, is studying the way in which mentally abnormally aggressive offenders perceive their victims subsequent to the actual offence. He uses a grid in which eighteen representative persons from the patient's life (including victim, mother, father, self, ideal self) are used to elicit fifteen constructs from the patient, so that it is possible to identify whom the victim resembles, and which constructs differentiate the victim from other people. Such information will be useful diagnostically and prognostically when used in conjunction with data from many other sources, not forgetting the primacy of the clinical presentation of the patient and the relationship he has with all members of the staff involved in his 'treatment'.

Whether or not the offence is victim 'specific', transference phenomena can induce the therapist, his colleagues, or other patients to be perceived as victim surrogates. Unremitting vigilance is therefore an inextricable facet of the therapist's use of self as he engages with a mentally abnormal sex-offender in therapeutic space. An additional complication is that of the masochistic victim who provokes assault.

'Disposal options'

These have been briefly indicated in figs. 11.1 and 11.2. In the interests of protecting society and the offender-patient himself, we are forced into making legal judgements and therefore deciding the appropriate 'disposal' of the offender-patient, while still very much in the dark as far as the individual patient's inner world is concerned. To describe him as being psychotic or psychopathic may have certain administrative and custodial implications, but it is often only after prolonged psychotherapy that we begin to understand what 'makes him tick'. Such executive decisions inevitably have to be made in the presence of incomplete knowledge. However, it is important to remember that such executive action must not be taken to imply that we know more about the patient than we do. Nosology may be administratively essential and yet be dynamically barren. We may have done what is right for society and for the patient at a particular time in his history, but this may mark the beginning of a psychotherapeutic encounter (Fig. 11.2) rather than the end of 'appropriate disposal'. Nevertheless, there is sometimes a marked contrast between the cautious, provisional statements of psychiatrists in executive positions of authority and the dogmatic certainty about inner world dynamics suggested by psychotherapists – which cannot be proved and is not put to the test! Scott (1964, 1969, 1970, 1974), Tennent (1971), Gunn (1976, 1977), together with editorials in professional journals, (such as, *Brit. med. J* (1975) Patients or Criminals) and the national press (for instance, *The Times* (2 October 1973) Therapy for Criminals) all draw attention to the dilemma with which the offender-patient confronts society. To punish or to treat? Scott (1977) underlines the crucial fact of 'involvement on a long-term basis' in 'Assessing dangerousness in criminals'.

It is undeniable that phenomenological identification and the gradual differentiation of syndromes, such as those recently demarcated by forensic psychiatrists, are of help in terms of assessing the outcome and the likely recrudescence of violence. I refer to the work of Mowat

(1966) and Brittain (1968 and 1970) who described morbid jealousy and sadistic murderers respectively.

The studies of Williams (1964) draw attention to a small group of sexual murderers who have similar psychopathology (though many do not). 'The idea of a focalized lesion breaking loose and taking over the whole personality in certain circumstances for a brief but crucial period would correspond to Wertham's catathymic crisis (1949).' Working with such patients can be one of the most testing experiences for those who share therapeutic space. The encapsulated enclave may be touched upon in a mixed group and, when the 'flash' occurs, the therapist tries to hold the group at a disclosure level where such primitive sequestrated energy can be discharged in safety. Other group members frequently act as 'hosts' for the temporary investment of the energy which streams out like volcanic lava. It is after such experiences that patients and therapists alike are aware that dynamic psychotherapy can be hard work!

'Listen to the patient, he is telling you the diagnosis' was William Osler's advice to clinical students, and it is equally applicable to those undertaking psychotherapy with the sex-offender patient. If we listen to the patient long enough, he may tell us not only the diagnosis but also disclose the dynamics of his inner world. Once the dynamics underlying a sex-offence are understood, an appropriate therapeutic policy can be initiated, though two caveats must be made. First, one of the paradoxes of psychotherapy is that disclosure proceeds as the therapeutic alliance matures; that is 'diagnosis' becomes more sharply delineated as 'treatment' progresses. Secondly, the mentally abnormal sex-offender may need psychotherapy for many reasons, such as coming to terms with his past, understanding himself, facing a prolonged period in a secure hospital, among others. Therapy may be 'effective' for such matters but this is *not* equivalent to stating that the patient is now 'safe' and will not rape again. *The reduction of re-offence potentiality is an extremely important parameter, but it is not the only reason why a sex-offender may need psychotherapy.* Dynamic psychotherapy with sex-offenders is likely to be a long and arduous process with many turbulent phases, though it is possible to reach a stage when therapeutic work is complete. Global generalizations about 'the' psychopathology of sex-offenders are doomed to failure; but the detailed 'close-up' of inner world phenomena disclosed in therapeutic space can furnish vital material which is impossible to glean in any other way. Tuovinen (1973) has drawn attention to *Crime as an attempt at intrapsychic adaptation* and psychotherapy may therefore be 'disturbing' to a balanced endopsychic system, with the result that the patient experiences new needs. In the long run, the patient may become 'safer' – but, during those unavoidable phases of the therapeutic process in which defence patterns are changing, he may become temporarily less stable and more dependent upon therapeutic proximity.

It is for this reason that the psychotherapist and the psychiatrist (responsible medical officer), who has over-all clinical and legal responsibility, work in a particularly close double-harness. Yet each operates within a preserve of autonomy, so that the patient's response to the responsible medical officer provides dynamic material for the psychotherapist and, *ipso facto*, the responsible medical officer can monitor the patient's adaptive response to a formal therapeutic 'session' and compare it with his response to other less structured encounters.

The implications of this chapter may only be fully understood when considered within the special milieu constituted by Broadmoor Hospital which, as a 'Special Hospital', provides the conditions for dynamic psychotherapy with serious sex-offenders.

References

Arnold, W. R. and Stiles, B. (1972). A summary of increasing use of group methods in correctional institutions. *Int. J. Group. Psychother.* **xxii**, 77.

Balint, M. (1968). *The basic fault: therapeutic aspects of regression.* London.

Bancroft, J. (1976). The behavioural approach to sexual disorders. In *Psycho-sexual problems* (ed. H. Milne and S. J. Hardy). London.

Barker, E. T. and Mason, M. H. (1968). Buber behind bars. *Canad. Psychiat. Ass. J.* **13**, 61.

Bernheim, J. (1976). Personal communications, Geneva.

Brancale, R., Vuocolo, A., and Prendergast, W. E. Jun. (1971). The New Jersey program for sex offenders. *Int. Psychiatry Clin.* **8**, 145.

Brit. J. Delinquency (1957), **8**, 82.

Brit. med. J. (1975), (**ii**), 70.

Brittain, R. D. (1968). In *Gradwohl's legal medicine.* 2nd Ed. (ed. F. E. Camps). Bristol.

—— (1970). Sadistic murderers. *Medicine, Science and the Law,* **10**, 198.

Buber, M. (1947). *Between man and man.* (Translated by R. Gregor Smith). London.

Bush, M. (1975). Sex offenders are people! *J. Psychiat. Nurse and Ment. Health Serv.* **13**, 38.

Cameron, N. (1943). The paranoid pseudo-community. *Amer. J. Sociol.* **46**, 32.

Chapman, D. (1968). *Sociology and the stereotype of the criminal.* London.

Cox, M. (1973). Group psychotherapy as a redefining process. *Int. J. Group Psychother.* **xxiii**, 465.

—— (1974). The psychotherapist's anxiety: liability or asset? With special reference to the offender-patient. *Brit. J. Crim.*, **14**, 1.

—— (1976). Group psychotherapy in a secure setting. *Proc. Royal Soc. Med.* **69**, 215.

—— (1978a). *Structuring the therapeutic process: compromise with chaos.* Oxford.

—— (1978b). *Coding the therapeutic process: emblems of encounter.* Oxford.

Freud, S. (1916). Some character types met with in psychoanalytic work. III Criminals from a sense of guilt. *Complete psychological works of Sigmund Freud.* Standard edition **14**.

Goffman, E. (1963). *Stigma: notes on the management of spoiled identity.* New Jersey.

Green, H. (1964). *I never promised you a rose garden.* New York.

Gunn, J. (1976). Sexual offenders. *Brit. J. Hosp. Med.* **15**, 57.

—— (1977). Criminal behaviour and mental disorder. *Brit. J. Psychiat.* **130**, 317.

Haley, J. (1963). *Strategies of psychotherapy.* New York.

Halleck, S. L. (1967). *Psychiatry and the dilemmas of crime.* New York.

Hartocollis, P. (1977). *Borderline personality disorders: the concept, the syndrome, the patient.* New York.

Hitchens, E. W. (1972). Denial: an identified theme in marital relationships of sex offenders. *Perspec. in Psychiat. Care* **x**, 152.

Howells, K. (1976). Personal communication, Broadmoor Hospital; PhD thesis, University of Birmingham.

Hurley, W. and Monahan, T. M. (1969). Arson: the criminal and the crime. *Brit. J. crim.* **9**, 4.

Kernberg, O. (1970). Factors in the psychoanalytic treatment of narcissistic personalities. *J. Amer. Psychoanal. Assoc.* **18**, 51.

—— (1975). *Borderline conditions and pathological narcissism.* New York.

Khan, M. M. R. (1974). The role of illusion in the analytic space and process. In *The Privacy of the Self.* London.

Kohut, H. (1959). Introspection, empathy and psychoanalysis. *J. Amer. Psychoanal. Assoc.* **7**, 459.

—— (1971). *The analysis of the self.* London.

—— (1977). *The restoration of the self.* New York.

Loucas, K. and Udwin, E. L. (1974). The management of the mentally abnormal offender. *Brit. J. hosp. Med.* **12**, 285.

McGrath, P. G. (1976). Sexual offenders. In *Psycho-sexual Problems* (ed. H. Milne and S. J. Hardy). London.

Macphail, D. S. and Cox, M. (1975). Dynamic psychotherapy with dangerous patients, Proc. 9th Int. Congress Psychother., Oslo 1973. *Psychother. Psychosom.* **25**, 13.

Matza, D. (1969). *Becoming deviant.* New Jersey.

Merton, R. K. (1949). *Social theory and social structure*, Chicago.

Mowat, R. R. (1966). *Morbid jealousy and murder.* London.

Ormrod, R. (1975). The debate between psychiatry and the law. *Brit. J. Psychiat.* **127**, 193.

Rosen, I. (1968). The basis of psychotherapeutic treatment of sexual deviation. *Proc. Royal Soc. med.* **61**, 793.

Rubinstein, L. H. (1965). Sexual motivations in 'ordinary' offenses. In *Sexual behaviour and the law* ed. R. Slovenko, Springfield, Illinois.

Scott, P. D. (1964). Definition, classification, prognosis and treatment. In *The pathology and treatment of sexual deviation* (ed. I. Rosen) London.

—— (1969). Crime and delinquency. *Brit. med. J.* (**i**), 424.

—— (1970). Punishment or treatment: prison or hospital? *Brit. med. J.* (**ii**), 167.

—— (1974). Solutions to the problem of the dangerous offender. *Brit. med. J.* (**iv**), 640.

—— (1977). Assessing dangerousness in criminals. *Brit. J. Psychiat.* **131**, 127.

Siirala, M. (1974). Personal communication, Helsinki.

Tennent, T. G. (1971). The dangerous offender. *Brit. J. hosp. Med.* **6**, 269.

The Times (1973) 2 October.

Tuovinen, M. (1972). Schizophrenia and the basic crimes. In *Psychotherapy of schizophrenia.* (ed. D. Rubenstein, and Y. O. Alanen). Amsterdam.

—— (1973). *Crime as an attempt at intrapsychic adaptation.* Oulu, Finland.

Wertham, F. (1949). *The show of violence.* New York.

Williams, A. H. (1964). The psychopathology and treatment of sexual murderers. In *The pathology and treatment of sexual deviation,* (ed. I. Rosen). London.

Winnicott, D. W. (1945). Primitive emotional development. *Int. J. Psycho-Anal.* **26**, 137.

Wolberg, A. R. (1973). *The borderline patient.* New York.

Since this chapter was written a report of a symposium on sex offenders has been published. Although not directly focused upon dynamic psychotherapy with sex offenders, it is an important source of collateral and complementary material: *Sex offenders: a Symposium* (ed. J. Gunn). Special Hospitals Research Report No. 14 (1978).

12 Behaviour therapy for sexual deviations

Michael Gelder

Introduction

The contribution of behaviour therapy to the treatment of sexual deviations has changed in important ways since the subject was reviewed by Coates in the last edition of this book. New methods have appeared, and more has been learnt about the value and limitations of the older techniques. The most important change, however, has been in the general approach to patients' problems. Only a few years ago the behaviour therapist was concerned mainly with the suppression of unwanted patterns of behaviour, often with aversion therapy; now more emphasis is placed on developing heterosexual behaviour and on attending to wider difficulties in social relationships using a combination of techniques. Unfortunately this change, while welcome, is so recent that there has not been time to accumulate research which answers all the questions the clinician must ask when he prepares to treat a patient. Nor, indeed are there, as yet, behavioural methods to deal with all the attendant problems in relationships which the behaviour therapist now recognizes as important. There will be times therefore when the clinician has to decide whether to combine techniques drawn from more than one approach. Hence, this review begins by considering the relationship between behavioural and psychodynamic forms of treatment, and it ends by suggesting the ways in which the clinician can make best use for his patients of the available, incomplete evidence from behaviour therapy research. We shall begin with the question of the relationship between the theories on which behaviour therapy and psychotherapy have been built.

The two systems of treatment share the assumption that sexual deviations arise as a result of some kind of disordered learning in early life. They differ in the view which each takes of the nature of this disordered learning. The behaviour therapist employs principles which have been established in the psychological laboratory. By contrast, the psychotherapist adopts one or other of the psychodynamic theories of development which originated in clinical observation rather than laboratory study. There are, of course, many points of overlap between these two theories, for to an extent they are based on observations of common phenomena. Nevertheless, over the years each has developed its own terminology and explanatory concepts which now are not always easy to reconcile. Moreover, the phenomena which have been studied, whilst similar, are far from identical. Dynamic psychology is founded on observations of patients and their problems, or people engaged in quite complicated activities of everyday life such as dreaming. Learning theories are based on observations of rather simple behaviour in the laboratory, and much stems from work with animals rather than man. It is not surprising, therefore, that the former provides a more extensive account of clinical phenomena, including those of the sexual deviations, than can yet be achieved by the learning theories. Nor is it surprising that it is sometimes difficult to extend learning theories to explain all the varied and complex phenomena which patients present. It is for just this reason that behaviour therapy has undergone important changes in the last few years. It is no longer so dependent on theories of learning, but draws its ideas from cognitive and social psychology as well. As a result there is more emphasis on changing thoughts and attitudes as well as outward behaviour, and a growing concern with social behaviour. At the same time, new developments are depending increasingly on observations of clinical phenomena rather than laboratory findings.

It is important from the start to recognize the strengths and limitations of these two approaches to the treatment of sexual deviations: the one is scientifically based but, despite the new developments, still somewhat remote from the complexities of psychopathology; the other is closer to clinical problems, but set out in a relatively unscientific way. The real task of behaviour therapists is not to defend their approach against criticism that is too narrow, but to push the explanatory principles to their limits, being prepared to revise them when they no longer accord with clinical observations. They must recognize that principles of learning and theories of social behaviour, although grounded in experiment, can as yet explain only a small fraction of the complexities of human behaviour and that it is not helpful to attempt to force clinical phenomena to fit them. Instead they must search for the point at which the principles cease to have explanatory power and then return to the laboratory to test them again and, if necessary, revise them. This is the approach that will be adopted in this chapter. It will enable us to avoid some of the fruitless arguments about the rival merits of psychotherapy and behaviour therapy which have marred so much of the literature. At the same time it will allow a constructive approach to the contribution to psychiatry of the behaviour therapies.

Having pointed to this common ground, it is important to make clear that there are three features which distinguish behaviour therapy from the usual psychotherapeutic approach. First, behaviour therapy is often said to be a 'symptomatic' treatment. In a sense it is, for it is usually concerned with the symptoms and maladaptive patterns of behaviour for which the patient seeks treatment, and not with their original causes. Undoubtedly, less attention is paid to underlying emotional disorders than is the case in psychotherapy, but they are certainly not ignored. Indeed, one form of behaviour therapy, desensitization, is directly concerned with modifying the anxiety which so often lies behind behaviour patterns such as frigidity, impotence, or homosexuality. Thus, although there is an important distinction here between the two forms of treatment, it is important to be clear about its real nature, and to realize that behaviour therapy is not restricted to the behaviour of which the patient complains when he first seeks treatment.

The second distinction concerns the assumption, sometimes made in behaviour therapy, that there is value in piecemeal treatment. It is implicit in many treatment plans that improvement in one part of a complex behaviour disorder will usually lead to improvement in other aspects of the patient's problems even though these are not treated directly. For example, the anxieties of a phobic patient are treated in the anticipation that attitudes and feelings will alter, and that relationships with family and friends will also improve, once fears subside. Equally, when frigidity is treated by desensitization it is assumed implicitly that changes will follow in attitudes, self-evaluation, and social relations. Of course, this is a difference in degree, not in kind, from the approach in brief psychotherapy where similar aims are limited and goals set in the expectation that further change will follow. The differences lie in the nature of the goals and in the amount of consequential change which is expected even in quite complex disorders. Moreover, it is another difference which may diminish as research in behaviour therapy progresses. Thus, although the original assumptions have been largely vindicated, certain failures of treatment have revealed specific instances in which the expected consequential changes do not take place. We shall return to these questions later.

Finally, the behaviour therapist, unlike the psychotherapist, is confident that he can identify the contingencies which control behaviour without first trying to find out how the condition developed. He goes about this by a minute enquiry into the circumstances of the patient's activities in his daily life, rather than by attending to past patterns of behaviour or by a detailed examination of transference phenomena, as in psychotherapy. Again these are differences of degree rather than a fundamental incompatibility of purpose.

Techniques of behaviour therapy for sexual deviations

For many years aversion therapy was the only behaviour therapy method that was used at all widely for sexual deviations. Now there is a choice of techniques that can be divided conveniently into those which suppress unwanted behaviour, and those which attempt to encourage alternative forms of behaviour. Many of the latter have been developed in the first place for the treatment of sexual inadequacy in men and women. Many are closely related to, and some are derived from, the methods described by Masters and Johnson (1970) whose starting-point was not, of course, that of behaviour therapy.

(a) *Methods for decreasing unwanted behaviour*

(i) *Aversion therapy*

Techniques. In aversion therapy, unwanted patterns of behaviour are linked repeatedly with unpleasant stimuli. Treatment was originally modelled on classical conditioning experiments in animals and emphasis was put on the need for careful timing of the aversive stimuli. However, it was subsequently suggested that a more appropriate model might be that of escape or avoidance learning, or alternatively a Skinnerian model. As a result there are several different procedures.

There used to be another division as well: some methods used chemical stimuli (usually emetic drugs), others relied on mild electric shock. With the exception of a report by Max (1935), most of the original aversion therapy used apomorphine or emetine to induce nausea, introducing the conditional stimulus just as vomiting was about to take place. It was a convenient model for treatment of alcoholism (and this was the principal use of aversion therapy until the 1950s) but it was much less appropriate for sexual deviations. There were other problems which were reviewed by Rachman and Teasdale (1969), and chemical methods should no longer be used to treat sexual deviations.

Mild electric shock has now replaced chemical methods of aversion. This method has the advantage that shocks can be timed accurately and repeated many times without danger. They need not be intense and the degree of unpleasantness can be chosen with the cooperation of the patient. Shock has the added advantage that it lends itself to patterns of reinforcement other than classical conditioning. Thus shock can be made to coincide with the *stimuli* for the behaviour pattern – for example the feel of women's clothes for the transvestite – or may be related to the *responses* to these stimuli – for example the development of sexual arousal or, in a transvestite, the act of crossdressing. And reinforcement can be given with every trial, or with only a proportion of trials. These variations have proved useful in allowing principles from operant conditioning experiments to be introduced into treatment, but they have led to a confusing variety of techniques with little uneqivocal evidence to indicate which is most effective.

The question of the part played by specific learning processes in aversion therapy is not simple. Bandura (1970) pointed out that too little attention has been paid to the role, in this context, of cognitive variables which are known to play an important part in human learning. Even the most successful aversive conditioning is known to have rather short-lived effects, and in humans its effects can be abolished quickly by giving the information that no further aversive stimuli will be received. If aversion treatment is simply applied aversive conditioning, it is difficult to understand why the effects of successful treatment for sexual deviations can last for years. Bandura suggested that the apparent paradox can be resolved by regarding aversion therapy as a technique for learning self-control which depends on cognitive, as well as on automatic reflexive, learning. This is not just an academic point, for if Bandura is right it suggests that aversion therapy could be replaced by other, less unpleasant, ways of learning self-control, and we shall see later that other methods are being tried. Bandura suggests that aversion treatment may be effective because it activates covert self-stimulation, that is the patient rehearses to himself the unpleasant experiences of the treatment sessions, and continues to do so long after they have finished. If this is so, then it is more important to ensure that treatment is arranged so that the patient can rehearse, easily and clearly, the events contained in it, than it is to attend to minute details of timing of stimuli or schedules of reinforcement.

A contrary view was held by Feldman and McCulloch (1965), who carried out a series of clinical experiments in which considerable attention was given to the precise pattern of learning. Their main innovation was to introduce the principles of anticipatory avoidance learning. In this technique, patients learn to avoid shocks by carrying out a predetermined response. The method is well tried in the laboratory and it was certainly appropriate to test it with patients. Unfortunately, however, Feldman and MacCulloch chose a somewhat unexpected avoidance response. Rachman and Teasdale (1969) remarked on this: 'When we look at the response trained, we find that is the depression of a button to remove a coloured slide of a naked male from a back projection screen. On the face of it, there is not the slightest reason to think that this response is in any way incompatible with the homosexual behaviour which is desired to eliminate'. It is difficult to argue with this assessment, despite the promising results originally described by Feldman and MacCulloch. Moreover, the second procedural innovation in their work is also open to challenge. They introduced partial reinforcement procedures (where shocks are omitted, unpredictably, from a proportion of trials), because there is good evidence that this makes the learning in laboratory studies more lasting. However, Bandura (1970) has pointed out that: 'Clients can easily recognise that the arbitary punishment contingency employed in the treatment is completely absent in the extra-therapeutic situation. Under conditions where schedules of reinforcement are highly distinguishable, the partial reinforcement effect would not be expected to carry over'. In the light of these comments, it is not surprising that Feldman and MacCulloch (1971) were unable to detect convincing differences, when they compared the therapeutic effects of their anticipatory avoidance method and another based on classical conditioning.

These variations of technique have been considered at some length, because they indicate that the links between practice and theory in aversion therapy are rather weak. Therefore the clinician must be guided by the results of clinical investigations and not by theory. We shall come to the results of such investigations in a later section.

Immediate effects. In a later section we shall consider the therapeutic results of aversion therapy; at this stage it is appropriate to examine the changes that take place during the treatment sessions. Such changes are of interest whether or not they persist as a useful therapeutic effect. Moreover an examination of the immediate changes brought about by different treatments can guide us when we come to decide how treatments should be related to the particular needs of individual patients, and how they should be combined.

Aversion therapy produces specific, and rather unexpected, effects. These can only be summarized here, but details are to be found in the article by Marks and Gelder (1968), and the book by Bancroft (1974). If patients are asked to imagine particular components of the deviant sexual behaviour, the time taken to produce a vivid mental image (the latency) changes very little however many times the task is repeated. If, however, shock is given each time a vivid image is reported, then the latency increases with each trial, until eventually about half of any group of patients report that they can no longer call up a mental image however hard they try, though they can still evoke unrelated mental images as quickly as before. Images which are related in meaning to that which was associated with shock, are delayed to an extent which seems in proportion to its similarity of meaning to the latter. Of course, these observations depend on self-report, but they are confirmed by measurements of erectile responses made at the same time, for these diminish in parallel. If the shocks are associated in time with the erectile responses (whether evoked by imagery or objects associated with the fetish) rather than the moment when a mental image is attained, then these erectile responses are also suppressed progressively. Moreover there is a similar degree of specificity – and a degree of generalization – to responses evoked by related stimulus objects. A further indication of the effects of aversion therapy is provided by the measurement of attitudes. Again, the changes are rather specific. Thus in one investigation (Marks and Gelder 1968) treatment was associated with one of the fetish objects of a patient who was aroused by more than one fetish. Attitudes towards the treated objects changed but those to unrelated matters did not.

These investigations, and others like them, show that aversion therapy has effects which are rather closely restricted to the aspect of behaviour which has been treated. They affect all 'levels' of that behaviour – physiological arousal, mental imagery, and associated attitudes – but they do not spread except to behaviour which has a closely similar meaning to the patient. This explains the observation, which has often been confirmed, that aversion therapy does not lead to general sexual inhibition – that is to impotence in heterosexual intercourse – when sexual deviations are treated. On the other hand the specificity might suggest that extensive treatment would be required to deal, in turn, with each separate aspect of the patient's deviant behaviour. Clinical trials indicate that this is not what has been observed in patients who respond to treatment, and this raises important questions about the way that improvement is brought about. But these are better deferred to a later section.

(ii) *Covert sensitization*

The technique. Bandura's suggestion that aversion therapy acts through cognitive processes, including rehearsal of the unpleasant events in treatment, leads naturally to the idea that the same cognitive changes might be brought about without electric shock. Cautela (1966) developed just such a method and applied it originally to compulsive behaviour. The essential points of the method can be stated quite briefly: Cautela (1965) reviewed the issues in detail for those who wish to employ the method. The patient is first taught to relax, with a method similar to that which is employed in systematic desensitization. This leads to a state in which it is easy to call up vivid mental imagery and to concentrate attention on this rather than on external events. He then imagines himself taking part in some part of the deviant behaviour. As in desensitization, it is important that he feels personally involved and does not merely imagine it as if he were a bystander. He is then instructed to imagine an unpleasant event coinciding with the sexual behaviour. Often this is a scene in which he feels nauseated, and then vomits just as the sexual behaviour becomes arousing. However, Harbert, Barlow, Hersen, and Austin (1974) used imagery which provoked feelings of shame: a priest was imagined to enter the room just as the deviant sexual behaviour was about to take place. Maletsky (1974) attempted to strengthen the effect by using the unpleasant smell of valeric acid to heighten the feelings of nausea brought about by the therapist's instructions to imagine events which are associated with these sensations. This is an interesting idea in view of the powerful effects which smell may have in patterns of sexual behaviour and it might repay further study.

Thus the procedure in covert sensitization is simple and, so far, used in much the same way in different reports.

Immediate effects. We are now ready to enquire what effects are brought about by covert sensitization and how far they depend on this specific treatment technique rather than the non-specific elements which inevitably accompany it when patients are treated. Barlow, Leitenberg, and Agras (1969) reported two individual case studies which demonstrated that, at least on measures derived from self-report, the procedure does not reduce deviant behaviour if the 'aversive imagery' is left out. In four further case studies, Barlow, Agras, Leitenberg, Callaghan, and Moore (1972) demonstrated that the results are not merely the result of the instructions given to the patient. Not only did 'therapeutic' instructions lead to no improvement if aversive imagery was absent, but aversive imagery led to improvement even when the patient was told that he was likely to experience an increase of sexual feeling in this part of treatment. In another series of single-case studies, Callahan and Leitenberg (1973) showed that the short-term effect of covert sensitization is comparable in magnitude to that of electric aversion therapy.

We do not yet have detailed information about the physiological and psychological changes after this technique which could be compared with that already discussed in relation to aversion therapy. However, there are some indications that they may also be rather specific. Thus, for example Harbert *et al.* (1974) report a single-case study in which changes in attitudes did not extend to non-deviant sexual behaviour.

Self-control techniques. Much attention has been given, in the treatment of subjects who over-eat or smoke too much, to methods of self-control. There is no standard technique but attention has been directed to the identification of the first stages of the unwanted behaviour, and to the use of self-reward and group pressures. We shall see later that there are reasons to think that such methods are also appropriate for sexual deviations, but they have been little used. At the time of writing only the study of Rooth and Marks (1974) need be mentioned. These authors treated a group of exhibitionists with a self-control procedure which emphasized control of the early parts of the behaviour which leads to exposure, and the results were, in most respects at least, equivalent to these of electric aversion therapy.

(b) *Methods of increasing alternative sexual behaviour*

Until a few years ago, these were limited to systematic desensitization and aversion relief. Now other methods are being tried, as it has become clear that lack of success in treatment is often due to failure to develop adequate alternative sexual behaviour. It is not possible to discuss these issues thoroughly in this chapter, but a useful review has been written by Barlow (1973). There is another recent issue which may become more important and which cannot be discussed fully here: whether the alternative behaviour need always be heterosexual. This question arises particularly in the treatment of paedophiliac homosexuals, and is exemplified by a report by Kohlenberg (1974) in which the treatment was intended to help such a patient change to satisfying homosexual behaviour with adults.

(i)   *Systematic desensitization*

This method of behaviour therapy is now well known and should require little description here. It is used to reduce pathological anxiety responses by presenting carefully graded stimuli in conditions which inhibit the anxiety which would normally follow – usually relaxation exercises are employed. Treatment is directed first to stimuli which normally evoke least anxiety. As these are presented repeatedly to the relaxed patient, anxiety responses diminish and eventually disappear. When this happens, the effect generalizes to those nearest in potency, and their power to evoke anxiety is reduced sufficiently to bring them within the range of the relaxation procedure. In this way, a hierarchy of stimuli can be ascended step by step. When sexual deviations are treated, attention is directed to anxiety responses to aspects of heterosexual behaviour which often accompany (and are, of course, thought by many to be casually related to) the sexual deviation.

It has usually been assumed that desensitization produces the predicted changes in anxiety about aspects of heterosexual behaviour. However, Bancroft (1974) has examined the matter in detail and found surprisingly similar changes in desensitization and aversion. Thus, although desensitization does lead to lessening of this anxiety, its effect is little more than that in aversion treatment. At the same time, recent work with phobic patients has cast doubt on the original ideas about the mode of action of desensitization. This is therefore one of a number of areas in which further work is required to clarify the psychological changes which are taking place in treatments used to encourage heterosexual behaviour.

(ii) *Aversion relief*

In aversion relief treatment, use is made of the laboratory finding that withdrawal from a noxious stimulus can act as a form of positive reinforcement. It is readily combined with aversion therapy: in treating homosexuals, for example, electric shock is associated with imagery about homosexual behaviour, withdrawal of shock with some aspect of heterosexual intercourse. The latter varies from single words (Gaupp, Stern, and Ratcliffe 1971) to pictures of women (Larson 1970). MacCulloch and Feldman (1967) also used aversion relief as part of their treatment of homosexuals, but it is not possible to separate clearly the effects of the two procedures in this study. Two investigations which have attempted to study the separate effect of aversion relief failed to obtain a clear positive finding (Solyom and Miller 1965; Abel, Levis, and Clancy 1970).

Doubts about the value of the treatment are increased by the finding of Marks and Gelder (1967) and Bancroft (1974) that heterosexual response may increase after aversion therapy without any use of aversion relief. Aversion relief has been used quite extensively – Barlow (1974) referred to 150 cases reported in the literature – but at the time of writing its value is doubtful at best. It is important to remember that treatment methods have to rest on the results of clinical investigations; a sound theoretical basis is not enough.

(iii) *Positive conditioning*

In this method, mental images of heterosexual behaviour are associated with a state of sexual arousal. This arousal can be set in train by fantasies of deviant sexual behaviour (Beech, Watts, and Poole 1971); but those who have used the method usually make use of the greater degree of arousal which follows masturbation (Davison 1968; Freeman and Meyer 1975). The procedure is based very loosely on the model of classical conditioning. Heterosexual fantasy is at first introduced at the moment of maximal arousal and then at progressively earlier stages.

In three single-case studies using 'backward conditioning' control periods, Herman, Barlow, and Agras (1974) found some evidence to confirm a specific role of classical conditioning in bringing about changes in heterosexual responsiveness in this procedure. However, they encountered difficulties over timing of stimuli and over voluntary inhibition of responses – both familiar problems in classical conditioning experiments in man – so that further work is needed before the mechanism of treatment is established with confidence.

A variant of this method borrows the ideas of 'shaping' and 'fading' from operant conditioning. The patient is encouraged to change gradually the nature of his masturbation fantasies, bringing them at each stage nearer to a fantasy of heterosexual intercourse.

For several reasons these methods are finding increasing interest. The increasing emphasis on masturbation in several forms of treatment for sexual inadequacy has reduced doubts about the appropriateness of this form of treatment. At the same time there has been a move in many forms of behaviour therapy towards treatments which are carried out by the patient at home, putting greater reliance on self-control and less emphasis on the need for the therapist to supervise personally every stage of treatment. Finally, there is the strong clinical impression, shared by many therapists, that deviant fantasies accompanying masturbation have a powerful effect in maintaining deviant behaviour, and in leading to relapse after treatment; thus treatment directed to this aspect of the behaviour disorder makes good clinical sense.

(c) *Other methods*

Two other methods must be mentioned briefly. All the procedures reviewed so far have attended to sexual behaviour in its narrow sense; they have ignored the wider social behaviour that is essential for satisfactory heterosexual relationships. We shall return to this important matter later; for the present it is sufficient to note the surprising lack of research in the training of the relevant social skills. This approach has of course been emphasized by Ellis (1956) but the reports by behaviour therapists are few and where it has been used it has been added to other behavioural procedures which were the main interest of the investigation.

Biofeedback is the second potential method. It was commended in a recent review (*The Lancet* 1973) but its use has not been explored systematically. This omission however is probably less important. Although biofeedback has been promoted with much enthusiasm, it is increasingly clear that the specific effect of feedback is quite small when care is taken to separate the influence of non-specific elements including the instructions given to the patient. Moreover, most subjects are reasonably well able to discriminate changes in penile response to sexual arousal without the addition of feedback information. The techniques may have something to add to procedures for conditioning heterosexual responses, but they seem unlikely to be a substantial addition to the other methods we have reviewed.

The results of behaviour therapy for sexual disorders

Some problems of evaluation

Before reviewing therapeutic results, we must consider some general issues about assessment. In the literature on behaviour therapy for sexual disorders, there is all too often a contrast between the careful attention which is given to technique, and the uncritical acceptance of evidence about the clinical outcome. It is often assumed, implicitly or explicitly, that the prognosis of sexual disorders is so uniformly bad, that evidence of improvement is proof that treatment has had a specific effect. Even Rachman and Teasdale (1969), after a searching review of the psychological problems posed by aversion therapy, adopt a less critical approach when they state (p.280): 'Any treatment procedure which produces even a modest success rate with sexual disorders is an improvement on existing treatment alternatives'. Yet the literature contains many claims for other treatments which are no less confident than those made for behaviour therapy, and it is certainly possible that the unwitting selection of patients with better-than-average prognosis may account for many of the results which have been reported.

How then can we be reasonably certain that a particular technique of behaviour therapy has a specific therapeutic effect for a sexual deviation? First, we must know the course of the disorder without treatment, and know any selection factors which pick out patients whose prognosis is better than average. Unfortunately, there is still much uncertainty about this. Luckianowicz (1959) in his comprehensive review of transvestism remarked: 'Only a few writers commit themselves on the question of outcome'. Likewise, Scott (1964), writing on homosexuality, commented: 'The whole subject is fraught with the most polar differences of opinion as regards prognosis'. There can be no doubt that patients, who share a common disorder, may differ widely in prognosis. It is essential, therefore, that the results of two treatments are compared only when reasonable steps have been taken to ensure that patients who receive each treatment would have a similar prognosis in the absense of treatment. Unfortunately few published reports meet this requirement. Comparisons between studies are even more dangerous. Thus the homosexuals whose psychoanalytic treatment was reported by Bieber *et al.* (1962) are quite unlikely to have been comparable with homosexuals treated by aversion treatment. However similar the two groups may appear on such easily measured variables as age and length of history, they are likely to have differed profoundly in their motivation, their expectations about treatment, and their social background – all factors which may affect prognosis.

The requirement for precise and objective indices of improvement is equally difficult to fulfil. With sexual disorders, subjective reports are particularly likely to be unreliable – it is difficult to be certain that the patient is not overstating improvement to please his doctor, or perhaps to avoid further treatment. With this in mind, investigators have tried to find more objective indices. There are fundamental difficulties in the way of establishing a system of assessment which is both reliable and valid. We can deal with them only briefly – for a more complete review the reader is referred to Bancroft (1974) and Zuckerman (1971).

There is certainly no single measure which is sufficient. Sexual behaviour has many components—physiological change, subjective feelings of sexual arousal, sexual activity fantasized and real, pleasure in and satisfaction with sexual behaviour, sexual preferences and, of course, the wider aspects of social behaviour which lead up to the sexual act. All may be affected in sexual deviations. One of the merits of behaviour therapy has been to draw attention to the complexity of this behaviour and the possibility of measuring these various components of the deviation. At the very least, a satisfactory assessment system should attempt to sample from more than one 'level' of behaviour.

Even at one level of complexity there are many problems. Thus physiological measures, although apparently objective, are far from satisfactory (Zuckerman 1971). Measures of penile erection (Bancroft, Jones, and Pullan 1966; Bancroft 1966) are the most direct reflection of sexual arousal, and the response to sexual stimuli has been shown to reflect the sexual preference of the subject quite closely (Freund 1967; McConaghy 1967). However, they can be modified by the voluntary effort of the subject, who may distract himself from the stimuli presented to him, and direct his attention to imagined sexual events. Thus they are not reliable with uncooperative patients. However, with suitable precautions, they have been used to study the immediate changes in treatment (Marks and Gelder 1967), and its longer course (McConaghy 1969).

Other investigations have measured autonomic changes such as pulse rate and pupil size (Hess, Seltzer, and Shlien 1965), which alter in sexual arousal but are less specific to it. The ease of measurement does not make up for the problems of interpretation.

Patients' attitudes to sexual and other topics can be measured, usually with a semantic differential technique (Marks and Sartorius 1968). These are convenient but require the complete cooperation of the patient, who can give a false impression on these tests almost as easily as he can in a clinical interview. Other investigators have used questionnaires about the frequency of sexual activities (Barlow *et al.* 1969); but the most important yardstick is careful clinical evaluation, with information from an independent source whenever this is possible.

Evidence about lasting therapeutic effects

The clinician needs more than evidence of short term changes if he is to decide to adopt a new treatment. He is interested in investigations which include an adequate period of follow-up – at least six months, preferably longer – and a well chosen control group. Few investigations can meet these requirements, and those which try to do so encounter difficult problems about the selection of control patients. Indeed, the objection is often raised, that people who share the same sexual deviation are so different in other ways that it is fruitless to compare two groups. While there is some force to this argument, it is true nevertheless, that if the clinician is to match treatment to patient then he must, intuitively if not explicitly, assess how far his patient shares the common characteristics of those who have responded to the same treatment in the past. Single-case studies can help to identify such factors, but a comparative study is needed to make certain that these features are specific to the treatment in question, and not merely prognostic factors common to all treatments, or factors that indicate improvement without treatment. It is necessary, therefore, to review the evidence from controlled studies. However, these cannot be the sole information which guides the clinician, and we shall need to draw this and other sources of evidence together in a later section.

Feldman and MacCulloch (1971) reported a controlled comparison of aversion therapy using anticipatory avoidance learning, aversion using classical conditioning, and psychotherapy. The patients were homosexuals. There were no differences between the two forms of aversion treatment, both of which were superior to the chosen form of psychotherapy. However, as Bancroft (1974) has pointed out, there were several factors militating against the effectiveness of psychotherapy in this study, so that the finding should not be generalized. With both behavioural treatments, patients who reported no previous pleasurable heterosexual experience did less well than the rest, and those who responded badly were also more likely to have evidence of personality disorder. McConaghy (1970) reported a related comparison, in 40 male homosexuals, of the aversion relief and 'chemical' forms of aversion therapy. Aversion relief was more effective at the end of treatment, though at two years the two groups did not differ. Again, however, it is difficult to generalize these findings, for it is not certain that the groups were well matched, and there were technical problems about measurement.

The most satisfactory controlled comparison to date is that of Bancroft (1974), who compared aversion therapy and desensitization given to 30 male homosexuals, assigned randomly to two groups. Both treatments led to significant changes in sexual behaviour, but their effects did not differ. This finding might be taken to indicate that both had only non-specific effects, but the investigation was notable for the detailed evaluation of the changes during treatment sessions, which indicated that the two treatments produced quite different immediate changes. Bancroft suggests that either can in turn provoke further cognitive changes which lead to clinical improvement.

A separate, though related, view of the value of aversion therapy, was put forward by Birk *et al.* (1971). Their trial compared a slightly modified form of Feldman and MacCulloch's technique, with a control procedure which differed only in having shocks omitted. The procedure with shocks led to more immediate change, but the long-term effects were no different. However, both sets of patients received group therapy in the follow-up period because the authors thought it important to 'use group therapy to maximise the chances of capitalising on a period of conditioning-induced response suppression'.

There are no comparative clinical trials of matched groups of patients other than homosexuals. It is clear, moreover, that the clinical trials with homosexual patients have provided no firm evidence on which to base clinical practice. The next section will consider how the therapist can best combine the evidence from clinical investigations with the experience of treating patients.

Behaviour therapy in clinical practice

Some ethical issues

Two questions about sexual deviations have been much debated recently. Is it in any sense the province of doctors – an illness? If so, should treatment be given? The use throughout this chapter of the word *patient* does not mean that homosexuality or any other sexual deviation is taken to be an illness. *Patient* is used in the sense of 'one who bears or suffers', and as a convenient single word for those sexual deviants who seek help from doctors, psychologists, and social workers. The sexual deviations are patterns of behaviour which can on occasion cause suffering to the individual, or occasionally to others (for example, paedophiliacs, exhibitionists, and sadists). This latter group provokes questions about compulsory treatment for those who cause suffering to others, and a misunderstanding leads to the further suggestion that behaviour therapy and particularly aversion treatment might be a suitable method. The misunderstanding is the commonly held idea that aversion treatment can act automatically – as a form of conditioning – in opposition to a patient's wishes. It cannot. It requires full cooperation and, as we have seen, its effect depends far more on cognitive processes than on conditioning. The view taken here is that it is appropriate to offer help to those who request relief for their suffering, and, if these patients request help in readjusting their sexual preferences, it is also appropriate to attempt this. This depends of course on the most careful assessment of a patient's motives for seeking help and this is the next topic we must consider.

Motives for seeking help

People who ask for treatment for sexual deviations may have mixed feelings and unrealistic aims. The transsexual who asks for his body to be changed to that of a woman presents an obvious example, but there are many situations in which the unrealistic nature of the patient's request to the therapist is less immediately obvious. A particular problem for the behaviour therapist is that patients are sometimes attracted to the treatment, because it appears to them to offer a way of bringing about a strictly limited change in sexual behaviour, without the need to undertake any wider readjustment in their lives. Needless to say this aim is as unrealistic, for the majority of patients, with behaviour therapy as it is with any other treatment; indeed, as we have seen, there is some evidence that behaviour therapy can lead to lasting effects only when it does provoke widespread changes in attitudes and social relationships.

At the other extreme, it is not uncommon to meet a patient whose wife is encouraging him to seek treatment, in the hope that he will not only cease his deviant sexual behaviour, but also undergo a major change in personality. She has, perhaps, focused all her dissatisfaction with her husband and with her marriage on the sexual disorder, and has led herself to believe that if specific treatment were to remove the sexual deviation everything else would be put right. Of course, if symptomatic treatment is effective, her discontent with her husband does not diminish, instead the true origin of her problems is revealed and divorce or separation may be brought nearer.

Such problems have, of course, long been known to psychotherapists, but they have been singularly ignored in the literature on behaviour therapy. Rycroft (1968), writing on the effects of psychoanalysis, summed up in these words: 'The patient loses his symptoms only if two conditions are filled: firstly, that he understands their origin, and secondly that his conscious wish to lose them is greater than his wish to maintain the status quo in his personal relationships. For instance, if a married man is impotent and perverted, his recovery depends on whether his wife really and truly welcomes his recovery.' Except that behaviour therapy stresses understanding of the present immediate causes of symptoms rather than their origins in early life, the quotation summarizes the problem equally well.

A last question about patients' motives for treatment is especially relevant to behaviour therapy. Some seek treatment because they feel guilty about their sexual practices or because they are depressed. Such patients may be led to aversion therapy because it represents to them a form of punishment which may help to allay guilt. This is another reason why a careful assessment of the patient's motives is required before any treatment, especially behaviour therapy, is offered.

Sometimes it is obvious that the patient has not come to the therapist on his own initiative, for example, he may have been placed on probation with a condition that he obtains treatment. On the other hand, it is not uncommon for a patient to appear to be coming on his own volition when he is not really doing so. Thus he may fail to reveal that he is seeking treatment because his wife has threatened to leave him if he does not; or he may be asking for treatment in order to prove that he cannot be changed, and to justify to himself or others that he should continue his pattern of deviant sexual behaviour. Patients who come for such reasons are as unlikely to respond to aversion therapy as to any other form of treatment. Moreover, threats by a spouse create a doubly unfavourable situation, for they usually indicate a strained marriage which may itself herald a poor response to treatment. It is important, therefore, to probe carefully into all these matters at the start of any treatment, not least with aversion therapy. Treatment – especially aversion therapy – should seldom be started until several sessions of history-taking have been completed and, whenever possible, an informant has been interviewed, even if this results in a few weeks' delay before the patient's motives and marital situation are understood clearly.

The prognostic importance of good motivation has been stressed by Bieber *et al.* (1962) in relation to psychoanalytic treatment and by Ellis (1956) in psychoanalytically-oriented psychotherapy. It has been demonstrated in aversion therapy by Feldman and McCulloch (1971) and by Marks, Gelder, and Bancroft (1970). It is easy to see how a poorly-motivated patient will fail to collaborate with treatment, and how easy it is for him to arrange his life afterwards in a way that encourages a return to his previous pattern of behaviour.

Analysis of the deviant behaviour

There is a need to combine the notions of behavioural analysis, common amongst behaviour therapists, with the psychiatrists' enquiry into the part which the sexual deviation plays in the patient's mental life. The behaviour therapist has much to offer in his detailed examination of the events which are associated with the deviant behaviour (and which in his terms reinforce it), but this detailed analysis is not enough.

What part is the disorder playing in the patient's mental life?

It is easy to assume that disordered sexual behaviour is always providing sexual gratification. Psychotherapists are well aware that this is not always true, and that disordered sexual behaviour sometimes acts as a regulator of self-esteem, or as a means of warding-off anxiety or depression. It is even more important to bear this possibility in mind when using behaviour therapy, which can sometimes produce quite rapid changes in sexual behaviour. This may provoke an equally sudden depressive reaction of the sexual behaviour was serving this original function. See Chapter 3.

Such interrelations between symptoms, sexual behaviour, and personality structure will usually be revealed if a careful account is built up of the circumstances in which aberrant sexual behaviour takes place (the behaviour analysis). The patient may be quite unaware of the interrelationships, and often does not reveal them clearly in the ordinary course of extended history taking, even when this is informed by psychodynamic concepts. If his day-to-day behaviour is examined over a number of weeks, a pattern can often be discerned. In such a case it would clearly be important to attempt to solve the problems which lead to loneliness, self-depreciation, or depression before administering treatment to suppress the sexual deviation.

Making the best use of behaviour therapy

When these criteria for assessment have been used, there remains the question of how to bring together behaviour therapy with other methods of treatment in a way which will be most helpful for the patient. To understand this, it is convenient to return briefly to the question of why the effects of aversion therapy outlast those which would be expected from laboratory data on conditioning.

Two pieces of evidence suggest an answer to this apparent paradox, and also help to explain why immediate treatment effects which are specific and limited can give rise to widespread changes in behaviour after treatment ends. Marks, Gelder, and Bancroft (1970) examined the relation between various changes observed during treatment and the final clinical outcome. No significant correlation was found between the amount of conditioned anxiety induced during treatment sessions and the final outcome. However, outcome was related to the extent to which attitudes to deviant sexual behaviour changed during the course of treatment. That these attitudes change at all must indicate that cognitive changes are provoked by the aversive conditioning, as Bandura (1970) suggested. Bancroft (1970) came to a similar conclusion in his investigation of homosexual patients, and a somewhat similar idea was put forward independently by Feldman and McCulloch (1971).

This leads readily to the idea that change in a sexual deviation requires not merely change in a single aspect of behaviour, but a chain of events. This chain begins with the immediate psychic and physiological response to sexual stimuli; continues through cognitive changes, and alterations in social behaviour; and, of course, depends as much on the development of heterosexual behaviour as on the suppression of deviant patterns. In some patients, attention to one point in the chain will be enough to provoke changes in all the others. In some patients, the relative strength of the unwanted and wanted sexual behaviour is such that it will be enough to encourage the latter; others will need help to suppress the unwanted behaviour. An analysis of this kind gives the best chance of matching the available methods of behaviour therapy to the needs of the individual patient and, more-over, the best chance of incorporating in a helpful way behavioural methods with approaches developed by psychotherapists and social workers.

If, after a suitable period of observation, it is clear that the patient requires assistance to suppress unwanted behaviour, while attempts are being made to develop heterosexual activities, then the choice lies between aversion therapy and covert sensitization. In the absence of clear evidence that aversion therapy is generally more effective than covert sensitization, and with evidence about the mode of action of each which was considered earlier, it is appropriate to begin with covert sensitization, only turning to aversion therapy for patients who do not respond. There is no definite evidence that one variant of aversion therapy is better than the others, and the technique described by Marks and Gelder (1967) is simple and acceptable to patients.

Of the methods of developing heterosexual behaviour, systematic desensitization is more acceptable than aversion relief, and there is no evidence that it is less effective. The commonsense presumption that it is most suited for patients who have specific anxieties about hetero-sexual intercourse is not supported by evidence, but is nevertheless an appropriate guideline. Patients will often also require counselling and training advocated by Masters and Johnson (1970). For those patients whose erotic imagery and sexual responses are almost exclusively tied to deviant behaviour, one of the methods of positive conditioning of heterosexual responses may be tried, with the proviso that its effective-ness has yet to be proved.

Attention must then be turned to wider aspects of sexual behaviour, and it is here that behaviour therapy has, so far, less to contribute. Some patients need to acquire social competence in their relationships with women. Behaviour therapy offers social-skills training methods, but none has been evaluated fully. Until they have, reliance must still be placed on procedures that are the result of clinical experience – counselling, social work, or psychotherapy, individually or in a group. It is sometimes argued that such an approach, which encourages the combination of behaviour therapy methods with clinical procedures derived more-or-less directly from psychodynamic ideas, is scientifically unsound. And it has been argued that the therapist or investigator must decide to which school he belongs – he can have psychotherapy or behaviour therapy but not both. Such an attitude not only ignores the limitation of learning principles in explaining and modifying complex behaviour, but it also ignores evidence about the psychological mechanisms by which conditioning procedures lead to clinical changes. It fails to deal with the whole question of how changes in simple psychological functions can be transformed into the complex modifications of social behaviour which we call clinical change. It is therefore wrong to think that no links should be made between different forms of treatment.

This chapter has deliberately refrained from attempting a comprehensive review of the literature about use of behavioural techniques in sexual deviations, for this would quickly become outdated. It is thought more important to establish a framework which can be tested against new observations, and to provide a guide to the way in which conditioning procedures can best be employed. If this model is accepted it becomes clear that the first step must be careful behavioural analysis and clinical assessment. At the end of this, it can be decided what changes may be expected if one of the behavioural methods is employed, and what other measures will be needed to ensure that the chain of subsequent changes takes place. Such a model may not stand the test of time, but for the present it is a practical aid both for the clinician and the research worker.

References

Abel, G., Levis, D., and Clancy, J. (1970). Aversion therapy applied to taped sequences of deviate behaviour in exhibitionism and other sexual deviations. *J. Behav. Ther. exp. Psychiat.* **1**, 59.

Bancroft, J. H. J. (1969). Aversion therapy for homosexuality: a pilot study. *Brit. J. Psychiat.* **115**, 1417.

—— (1971). A comparative study of aversion and desensitisation in the treatment of homosexuality. In *Behaviour Therapy in the 1970s* (ed. L. E. Burns and J. L. Worsley). Bristol.

—— (1974). *Deviant sexual behaviour: modification and assessment.* Oxford.

——., Jones, H. G., and Pullan, B. R. (1966). A simple transducer for measuring penile erection. *Behav. Res. Ther.* **4**, 239.

Bandura, A. (1970). *Principles of behaviour modification.* New York.

Barlow, D. H. (1973). Increasing heterosexual responsiveness in the treatment of sexual deviation: a review of the clinical and experimental evidence. *Behav. Ther.* **4**, 655.

——., Leitenberg, H., and Argas, W. S. (1969). The experimental control of deviation through manipulation of the noxious scene in covert sensitization. *J. abnorm. Psychol.* **74**, 596.

——., Agras, W. S., Leitenberg, H., Callahan, E. J., and Moore, R. C. (1972). The contribution of therapeutic instruction to covert sensitization. *Behav. Res. Ther.* **10**, 411.

Beech, H. R., Watts, F., and Poole, A. D. (1971). Classical conditioning of sexual deviation; a preliminary note. *Behav. Ther.* **2**, 400.

Bieber, I., Dain, J. H., Dince, P. R., Drellich, M. G., Grand, H. G., Gundlach, R. H., Kremer, M. W., Rifkin, A. H., Wilbur, C. B., and Bieber, T. B. (1962). *Homosexuality: a psychoanalytic study.* New York.

Birk, L., Huddleston, W., Miller, E., and Cohler, B. (1971). Avoidance conditioning for homosexuality. *Arch. Gen. Psychiat.* **25**, 314.

Callahan, E. J. and Leitenberg, H. (1973). Aversion therapy for sexual deviation: contingent shock and covert sensitization. *J. abnorm. Psychol.* **81**, 60.

Cautela, J. R. (1965). Covert sensitization. *Psychol. Rep.* **20**, 459.

—— (1966). Treatment of compulsive behaviour by covert sensitization. *Psychol. Rep.* **16**, 33.

Davison, G. C. (1968). Elimination of a sadistic fantasy by a client controlled counterconditioning technique. *J. Abnorm. Psychol.* **73**, 84.

Ellis, A. (1956). The effectiveness of psychotherapy with individuals who have severe homosexual problems. *J. cons. Psychol.* **20**, 191.

Feldman, M. P. and MacCulloch, M. J. (1965). The application of anticipatory avoidance learning to the treatment of homosexuality 1. *Behav. Res. Ther.* **2**, 165.

——, —— (1971). *Homosexual behaviour, therapy and assessment.* Oxford.

Freeman, W. and Meyer, R. G. (1973). A behavioural alteration of sexual preferences in the human male. *Behav. Ther.* **6**, 206.

Freund, K. (1967). Diagnosing homo- and heterosexuality and erotic age preference by means of a physiological test. *Behav. Res. Ther.* **5**, 209.

Gaupp, L. A., Stern, R. M., and Ratcliff, R. G. (1971). The use of aversion-relief procedures in the treatment of a case of voyeurism, *Behav. Ther.* **2**, 585.

Gold, S. and Neufield, I. L. (1965). A learning approach to the treatment of homosexuality. *Behav. Res. Ther.* **2**, 201.

Harbert, T. L., Barlow, D. H., Hersen, M., and Austin, J. B. (1974). Measurement and modification of incestuous behaviour: a case study. *Psychol.*

Rep. **34**, 79.

Herman, S. H., Barlow, D. H., and Agras, W. S. (1974). An experimental analysis of classical conditioning as a method of increasing heterosexual arousal in homosexuals. *Behav. Ther.* **5**, 33.

Hess, E. H., Seltzer, A. L., and Shlien, J. M. (1965). Pupil response in hetero and homosexual males to pictures of men and women. *J. abnorm. Psychol.* **70**, 165.

Kohlenberg, R. J. (1974). Treatment of a homosexual paedophiliac using *in vivo* sensitization; a case study. *J. abnorm. psychol.* **83**, 192–5.

Kolvin, I. (1967). Aversive imagery treatment in adolescents. *Behav. Res. Ther.* **5**, 245.

The Lancet (1973). Behaviour therapy for sex problems (leading article). *Lancet* **1**, 1295.

Larson, D. (1970). An adaption of the Feldman and MacCulloch approach to treatment of homosexuality by the application of anticipatory avoidance learning. *Behav. Res. Ther.* **8**, 209.

Luckianowicz, N. (1959). Survey of various aspects of transvestism in the light of present knowledge. *J. nerv. ment. dis.* **128**, 36.

Marks, I. M. and Gelder, M. G. (1967). Transvestism and fetishism: clinical and physiological changes during faradic aversion. *Brit. J. Psychiat.* **113**, 711.

Marks, I. M. and Gelder, M. G. (1968). Controlled trials of behaviour therapy, in *The role of learning in psychotherapy* (ed. R. Porter), London.

——, ——, and Bancroft, J. H. B. (1970). Sexual deviants 2 years after electric aversion. *Brit. J. Psychiat.* **117**, 173.

—— and Sartorius, N. H. (1968). A contribution to the measurement of sexual attitude. *J. Nerv. Ment. Dis.* **145**, 261.

Max, L. (1935). Breaking up a homosexual fixation by the conditioned reaction technique. *Psychol. Bull.* **32**, 734.

MacCulloch, M. J. and Feldman, M. P. (1967). Aversion therapy in the management of 43 homosexuals, *Brit. med. J.* **2**, 594.

—— (1970). Subjective and penile plethysmographic responses to aversion therapy for homosexuality: a follow-up study. *Brit. J. Psychiat.* **117**, 555.

Masters, W. H. and Johnson, V. E. (1970). *Human sexual inadequacy.* London.

Rachman, S. and Teasdale, J. (1969). *Aversion therapy and behaviour disorders.* London.

Rooth, G. and Marks, I. M. (1974). Persistent exhibitionism: short term response to aversion self regulation and relaxation treatments, *Arch. Sex. Behav.* **3**, 227.

Rycroft, C. (1966). *Causes and meaning in psychoanalysis observed.* London.

Scott, P. D. (1964). Definition, classification, prognosis and treatment. In *The pathology and treatment of sexual deviation,* (ed. I. Rosen). London.

Seligman, M. E. P. (1970). On the generality of the laws of learning, *Psychol. Rev.* **77**, 406.

Silverstone, T. (1970). The use of drugs in behaviour therapy, *Behav. Ther.* **1**, 485.

Solyom, L. and Miller, S. (1965). A differential conditioning procedure as an initial phase of behaviour modification of homosexuality, *Behav. Res. Ther.* **3**, 147.

Thorpe, J., Schmidt, E., and Castell, D. (1964). A comparison of positive and negative (aversive) conditioning in the treatment of homosexuality, *Behav. Res. Ther.* **1**, 357.

Zuckerman, M. (1971). Physiological measures of sexual arousal, *Psychol. Bull.* **75**, 297.

13 The law and sexual deviation

M.D.A.Freeman

Sexual mores vary from culture to culture, and there is an approximate correspondence between the law and the pattern of accepted behaviour. A survey of the world's legislation on sexual deviation and methods of treating it would thus present a variegated picture. The United States of America, according to Slovenko (1965), has more laws on the subject than all of the European countries combined. The world-wide trend is towards liberalization, 'decriminalization' as it is often called, and this is the tendency in the USA also. No purpose can be served by cataloguing the world's laws. This chapter, accordingly, concentrates on the law of England and Wales, though references are made where appropriate to other systems. Indeed, some of the discussion of the effects of legal intervention, whilst theoretically sound wherever the locale, are particularly apposite to the American situation.

The need for law

Every society must set up norms for the regulation of sexual conduct (Davis, K. 1971). In contemporary societies, the law is the principal vehicle of standard-setting. But such regulations must not be looked upon as altogether restrictive. In a broader sense, law is a programme for living together (Fuller 1969; Unger 1976): society is not a suicide club (Hart 1961), and much can be gained even from restrictions. Without limits upon sexual expression, there could be no civilization. As Balint (1957) has put it: sexual restrictions 'protect the structure of society against the onslaught of sexually highly excited individuals, that is, people "on heat". At the same time they protect the individual and allow him to enjoy a modicum of sexual pleasure in comparative peace and security'.

Sexual deviation, conflict, and interest groups

Generally speaking the law in this area is secondary. It follows; it does

376

not lead. It obtains its legitimacy, or seeks to do so, in a more primary reference point, the moral order. It is thus seen as re-institutionalizing custom (Bohannan 1967) and purports to act as a reinforcement agency. As such it will, in most societies, have the support of the majority and problems of law enforcement will focus on a deviant minority. There are exceptions to this; it is thought that the puritanical sex code in much of the USA (in some states all sexual behaviour, except for face-to-face intercourse with one's spouse, is proscribed) is completely out of touch with mainstream culture. The study by Kinsey, Pomeroy and Martin (1948) exposed the hypocrisy inherent in this by suggesting that nine Americans in ten were sex criminals.

But the American situation draws attention to what, in less acute form, is a very real problem. For, if the law follows conventional morality, *whose* standards is it following? Contemporary society is pluralistic, heterogeneous; there are numerous, often overlapping cultural standards and reference groups. Outside a practically universal core, one finds not consensus but conflict. It is clear that this problem has usually been glossed over. The morality of 'middle Britain' has been taken as a norm. As Troy Duster puts it (1970): 'so long as an activity is engaged in predominantly by those in the "center" social categories the likelihood of moral condemnation for the activity is miniscule.' He traced the history of narcotics legislation in the USA and showed how, until 1914, the taking of heroin was the prerogative of the upper and middle classes; legislation to outlaw its use followed the trend for medical journals to report that the 'overwhelming' majority of users came from 'unrespectable' parts of society. And his comment can be generalized. 'Middle America's moral hostility comes faster and easier when directed toward a young, lower-class, Negro male than toward a middle-aged, middle-class, white female.' And the middle classes are assumed to have a monopoly of moral indignation (Ranulf 1938).

This perspective has often been ignored in the past, because of the tendency to characterize the social problem in individualistic terms, to assume that it can be fully explained by reference to the supposed special characteristics or stigmata of the offender. Yet one cannot have violations without norms, and violations are relatively meaningless if they do not lead to action by social control agencies or members of society. Rule-makers, 'whistle-blowers' (Becker 1963), and rule-enforcers must, however, be upholding certain sets of values and collective interests, and this must redound to the detriment of other interest groups. Within the last decade, movements committed towards the 'politicization of deviance' (Horowitz and Liebowitz 1968) have grown up. Where once deviants accepted the prevailing definitions of their behaviour, and 'status degradation' (Garfinkel 1956) led to identity reconstruction (Schur 1971), now the tendency is to resist, to organize collectively, and to sound the trumpet of liberation (Humphreys 1972; Altman 1973; Millett 1973). Of course, 'if one accepts the view that dominant social and legal norms emerge out of conflicts or contests between competing interests and values, then it would seem to follow that the very meaning of the term "problem" is similarly problematic' (Schur and Bedau 1974). Lawyers working within the dominant positivistic paradigm are blind to the implications of this. Thus, legal treatises analyze sexual deviation as a 'given'. But a perspective which is sceptical of posited classifications will be used in this chapter.

The law and sexual morality

'When the mores are adequate, laws are unnecessary; when the mores are inadequate, the laws are ineffective' (Sutherland and Cressey 1970). This aphorism captures succinctly a contemporary dilemma. What ends should the law promote? Are there spheres of activity with which it would be wrong for the law to interfere? Are there areas where the law's intervention is self-defeating? What are the results of intervention and non-intervention? The debate has a long heritage, and has frequently found its inspiration in questions of legislation on matters of sexual morality. Mill argued that 'the only purpose for which power can be rightfully exercised over any member of a civilised community against his will, is to prevent harm to others' (1859). This essentially utilitarian approach was echoed in the Wolfenden report on Homosexual Offences and Prostitution (1957). The Committee stated: 'unless a deliberate attempt is to be made by society, acting through the agency of the law, to equate the sphere of crime with that of sin, there must remain a realm of private morality and immorality which is . . . not the law's business . . . .' (para. 61). 'It is not the duty of the law to concern itself with immorality as such . . . It should confine itself to those activities which offend against public order and decency, or expose the ordinary citizen to what is offensive or injurious' (para. 257).

This liberal position was challenged by the English judge, Lord Devlin (1965). His premise is that a society is not just a people but also a community of ideas. Shared attitudes about right and wrong and common standards of conduct are prerequisites of social life. So, he argues, a society is as morally justified in punishing immorality as it is in extirpating that most heinous of offences, treason, for failure to root out either will lead to the disintegration of that society. Devlin thus rejects pluralism (Wollheim 1959; Hart 1963). He would, however, tolerate a good deal of immorality before invoking the sanction of the criminal law. His criterion for intervention is widespread intolerance, indignation, and disgust of the particular activity. His model of rational judgment is the jury man. But Devlin had elsewhere (1956) described the jury as predominantly male, middle-aged, middle-class and middle-minded. The composition of the jury has changed since: eligibility for jury service no longer depends on a property qualification but on inclusion in the electoral register subject to exemptions and disqualifications.

Devlin's arguments have been attacked by Hart (1963; 1965; 1967), who takes a modified utilitarian position. He dismisses Devlin's disintegration thesis as lacking empirical foundation. His own assumption is that depriving individuals of their autonomy requires justification. Laws designed to enforce sexual morality interfere with sexual expression, and deprive individuals of sexual outlets. Such laws, and the coercive measures that may be used to enforce them, 'may create misery of a quite special degree' (Hart 1963). They, therefore, require justification of a weighty nature. He is not convinced by Devlin's arguments. Devlin appeals to the existence of laws that enforce morality. But this is merely to invoke 'the innocuous [sic] conservative principle that there is a presumption that common and long established institutions are likely to have merits not apparent to the rationalist philosopher' (Hart 1963). The present existence of such laws, and indeed their long history, says nothing about their normative value. Devlin asserts also that the function of the criminal law is only to enforce moral principles. He cites the conviction of a sadist who caned a masochist with her consent (*R* v. *Donovan* [1934] 2 K.B.498) as proof of this. But Hart argues that there may be another reason for invoking the criminal law in these circumstances, namely, paternalism. Hart supports legal paternalism on the ground that it is not always true that the individual is the best judge of his own interests. Laws 'excluding the victim's consent as a defence to charges of murder and assault may perfectly well be explained as a piece of paternalism, designed to protect individuals against themselves' (Hart 1963). But what is paternalism other than the enforcement of a moral principle? Can one support moral individualism and physical paternalism at the same time? As Devlin (1965) has written: 'What, alas, I did not foresee was that those who sailed under Mill's flag of liberty would mutiny and run the flag of paternalism up the mast'. To this, two comments may be offered. First, Mill himself recognized certain exceptions to his 'harm' principle: children, the feeble-minded, and backward peoples. In these cases he allows paternalism. These people may be restrained for their own good. Further, Mill qualifies his simple principle. He admits 'that the mischief which a person does to himself may seriously affect, both through their sympathies and their interests, those nearly connected with him, and, in a minor degree, society at large'. Such an injury would be contingent only, an 'inconvenience' which society must accept for the sake of the greater good of human freedom *unless* the individual violates a 'specific duty to the public' or a 'distinct and assignable obligation to any other person or persons'. But this admission would seem to cut the ground from under Mill's feet. Secondly, it has been argued (Ten 1969) in defence of Hart's stand on paternalism that it can be justified in terms of the individual's inability, because of his emotional or physical state, to make a rational decision. To argue this, however, is surely to invoke a moral principle.

The debate is inconclusive. The contestants do not define their terms clearly enough. Hart does not spell out the scope of paternalism — many socially useful activities and heroic acts of selfless abnegation are not self-interested. Mill seems to call for a 'weighing', but how can a balancing take place with such ill-defined concepts as 'harm', 'inconvenience', and the like? Each contains within itself certain unspecified moral and social assumptions (Nagel 1969; Golding 1975). Devlin seems to identify a society with its morality. The 'community of ideas' which he treasures is not to be found in contemporary, secular, heterogeneous society, and, though much separates the contestants ideologically, there are few substantive issues which divide them. Both Hart and Devlin favour privacy (another imprecise concept which limps badly out of the debate). Hart supports the use of the law to preserve a 'minimum content of natural law' (1961), 'universal values' (1963), and even particular institutions which are deeply embedded within a society – such as monogamy (1967). This is not to underestimate the importance of the debate, for the issues discussed here are never far below the surface when matters concerned with social policy in connection with sexual behaviour are disputed.

The law's concern with sexual deviation

Culture, in the sense of the public, standardised values of a community, mediates the experience of individuals. It provides in advance some basic categories, a positive pattern in which ideas and values are tidily ordered. And above all, it has authority, since each is induced to assent because of the assent of others. But its public character makes its categories more rigid ... They cannot ... easily be subject to revision. Yet they cannot ignore the challenge of aberrant forms. Any given system of classification must give rise to anomalies and any given culture must confront events which seem to defy its assumptions ... [Douglas, M. 1966].

The problem of anomaly may be solved in a number of ways; by settling for a different interpretation it may be reduced; it can be physically controlled; it can be avoided; and fourthly, anomalous events may be labelled dangerous. Sexual deviation may be construed as an anomaly and, as an event which disturbs reality, it constitutes a threat to the social order and occasions the intervention of social control.

A good example of this is our classification of sex identity. Sexual attributes are neatly categorized in contemporary society. One is either male or female and one's life is structured upon the classification. The hermaphrodite, the transsexual, the homosexual threaten this pattern and ordering; so, in similar ways, do the mentally ill and prostitutes (Lofland 1969).

This theme is pursued by Garfinkel in his study of the transsexual, Agnes (1967). He has constructed a list of 'properties of "natural, normally sexed persons" as cultural objects'. He argues that

the population of normal persons is a morally dichotomised population. The question of its existence is decided as a matter of motivated compliance with this population as a legitimate order. It is not decided as a matter of biological, medical, [or] sociological fact ... The adult member includes himself in this environment and counts himself as one or the other ... as a condition whereby the exercise of his rights to live without excessive risks and interference from others are routinely enforceable ... For normals, the presence in the environment of sexed objects has the feature of a 'natural matter of fact'. This naturalness carries along with it, as a constituent part of its meaning, the sense of its being right and correct; i.e. morally proper that it be that way.

This analysis of sexual typifications could be the inarticulate premise underlying Ormrod J's judgment in the April Ashley case (*Corbett* v. *Corbett* [1970] 2 All E.R.33). It could also explain attitudes towards prostitution—she does not behave as a 'normal' woman – .and homosexuality – he is a 'role-player, who attempts to refute the conception that the world is dichotomised into discrete sexes with their peculiar sets of characteristics. He poses the possibility of a midway position which is neither fully male nor fully female, and, by so doing, threatens the classification scheme with an anomalous case' (Rock 1973).

Some effects of legal intervention

Many reasons have been suggested why the law should interfere with sexual deviation. But what happens when it does? It is now generally accepted that legal intervention does not work. Thus, Packer (1968) describes the operation of the criminal process in this area as 'an extraordinarily difficult and costly method of social control'. Morris and Hawkins (1970) see it as an 'unwarranted extension' of the criminal law and as 'expensive, ineffective and criminogenic'. And Schur, describing much of this area as 'crimes without victims' (1965; 1969; 1973), has argued strongly for 'decriminalization'. A distinction has to be drawn between offences such as rape, indecent assault, and paedophilia on the one hand, where there are victims and where, on any test, the case for legal intervention is strong, and those such as homosexuality, prostitution, and some forms of incest. It is the latter category where the non-intervention school are on the strongest ground and, indeed, where on the whole they rest their case.

They argue that these are crimes without victims in the sense that the persons who are the objects of the crime do not see themselves as victims (see Quinney 1972; Schur and Bedau 1974). Schur (1965) defines a victimless crime as an offence arising in 'situations in which one person obtains from another, in a fairly direct exchange, a commodity or personal service which is socially disapproved and legally proscribed'. There are no complainants; so the police must ferret out those they intend to prosecute. How do the police decide which crimes, many of which such as obscenity and conspiracy to corrupt public morals are loosely defined, to discover and prosecute? It seems that customary morality (that is, middle-class morality) tends to define law enforcement. Thus, Lambert (1970) argues that 'the police force...tends to be an agency committed to establishing moral conformity; or in some instances achieving and maintaining social stability, by tolerating to a greater or lesser extent certain legal infractions – such as prostitution or some "social" violence – if such does not threaten the sense of well-being of the dominant moral community'. Offences such as these generate more work for the police (Reiss, 1971). 'Lacking direct complainants, law enforcers become dependent for evidence on a variety of unsavoury techniques—use of informers and decoys, clandestine surveillance, wiretapping and other types of "bugging", surprise ("no-knock") raids and the like' (Schur 1974). Skolnick (1966) found that half of the arrests of prostitutes resulted from decoy activity. Entrapment techniques are the norm to catch homosexuals (Gallo, Mason, Meisinger, Robin, Stabile, and Wynne 1966). Laws outlawing activities like prostitution and homosexuality cannot be enforced. The police recognize this. Arrests and prosecutions take place, but these are gestures 'to keep up the facade of public morality' (Millett 1973). Indeed, by using the informer system the police are giving indirect support to criminality. The laws can be harmful in another way. They 'can be used against those who violate inter-racial sex taboos, against political opponents and against welfare recipients and job applicants' (Sagarin 1974).

The economic effects of legislating in this area are equally great (Packer 1968; Rogers 1973). For 'regardless of what we think we are trying to do, when we make it illegal to traffic in commodities for which there is an inelastic demand, the effect is to secure a kind of monopoly profit to the entrepreneur who is willing to break the law' (Packer 1968). There is no doubt that the demand for illicit sex is inelastic. The result is the development of a black market and organized crime. A crime tariff is created and this has a number of unintended consequences.

The crimes under discussion are what is usually termed 'expressive' offences. That is to say that 'the act is committed because it is pleasurable in and of itself and not because, it is a route to some other good' (Chambliss 1967). There is evidence to suggest that punishment does not deter in this situation (Chambliss 1967). Looked at from the seller's point of view, for instance, the prostitute or purveyor of pornography, every increase in risk increases his potential gain. Packer therefore argues (1968) that the harder we strain to make sales risky 'the higher we drive the price that makes the risk worthwhile'. So 'the theory of deterrence, however useful it may be in the ordinary run of crimes, breaks down.' The inflation in the price and the absence of legitimate outlets, however, make it more difficult for the purchaser. He may be forced to commit other crimes. And there may begin a spiralling of deviant activities which sociologists of deviance have come to describe as 'secondary deviance' or amplified deviance (Lemert 1967; Wilkins 1964). A major consequence of legal intervention in this area is thus the creation of much additional crime that would not exist if the behaviour in question were not proscribed. A wide range of criminal occupations is given impetus: the opportunities for blackmail are increased; the customer, identified by the law as a criminal, takes on this imputation as his own self-identity. He becomes more and more antisocial. He is subject to constant discrediting processes, to exploitation, and discrimination. It should not, however, be thought that 'decriminalization' necessarily stems these deleterious effects. The legalization of consenting homosexual behaviour in England has not noticeably ameliorated the status of the homosexual (Plummer 1975). Social control continues unabated: there is still stigma, harrassment, and limited employment opportunities (see Humphreys 1970, 1972).

A final effect of the crime tariff, which cannot be ignored, is the impact it has on the credibility of the legal institutions. The opportunities for police corruption are wide. Police are known to take a 'cut', to accept protection money (Cox, Shirley, and Short 1977). The deviant pays rather as one pays an insurance premium. This breeds the inevitable cynicism and produces a backlash against the whole system. This is not helped when it is realized that the laws are unevenly enforced. There are socio-economic differentials as well as those grounded in race and sex. The rich not only get a better quality of illicit goods, but they also stand a greater chance of concealing their activity and not being subject to formal status degradation ceremonies. (See further Freeman (1974)).

Classification of deviant sexual behaviour

There are two types of classification that might be attempted. The legal approach is to characterize sexual deviation in terms of overt behaviour problems. The psychiatrist and psychoanalyst, on the other hand, are concerned to classify according to underlying clinical factors. It may be, therefore, that classification according to legally defined offences indicating the end behaviour will bear little relation to treatment requirements (Scott 1964). But, as James (1964) has remarked, 'the tracing of sexual perversions, which the law under various statutes or at common law proscribes, to infantile sexuality is too refined an approach to be incorporated on the statute books'. The Danish Penal

Code of 1930 (ss. 16 and 17) does make an attempt in this direction, but this is not the English approach. To the psychologist, the English lawyer's approach will appear crude and lacking in scientific foundation, rather as the psychologist would take exception to legal concepts concerned with mental health.

The official English Home Office publication *Criminal Statistics* is not particularly helpful. It lumps together one category—sexual offences. Many offences against the person and some offences against property can, however, be regarded as sexual offences in the widest sense of this term, since sexual motivation or an element of sexual perversion is the precipitatory factor (Schmideberg 1956). This complex dimension is omitted from the discussion which follows.

We do not, and cannot, know how many deviant sexual offences are committed. *Criminal Statistics* (1976, 1975) reveal that in 1975 23 731 sexual offences were recorded as known to the police, a decline of some 4 per cent from the figure of the previous year. The clear-up rate is high (78 per cent), exceeded only by offences involving violence to the person and fraud and forgery, which is an indication of the seriousness with which the police view such crimes. Criminal statistics are socially constructed and notoriously unreliable (Box 1971; Douglas, J. 1971). Estimates of sexual offences must be egregriously susceptible to error: perhaps only one-fifth of rape victims (or their families) notify the police, a large amount of incest goes undetected, and many other sexual offences do not come to the attention of control agencies.

The following classification is based on that of James (1964); and, as James stated, 'words such as "normal", "perverted", "homosexuality", etc. are here intended to indicate the overt behaviour problem, as seen by the court, and not the underlying clinical factors'. But, as James indicated, 'the law does seem to accept implicitly in its system of values that the genitally-oriented adult is the normal'.

Offences against the accepted standards of family life:
(a) bigamy
(b) incest
(c) adultery
(d) fornication

Offences which display the normal sex drive in a distorted or unacceptable manner:
(a) rape,

(b) indecent assault on a woman,
(c) unlawful sexual intercourse,
(d) sexual murder,
(e) paedophilia,
(f) prostitution by females to males.

Offences which display a perverted sexual drive:
(a) homosexuality (inc. indecent assault by males on males and importuning),
(b) lesbianism,
(c) transvestitism,
(d) fetishism,
(e) voyeurism,
(f) exhibitionism,
(g) bestiality,
(h) sodomy with a woman,
(i) necrophilia,
(j) sadism,
(k) making obscene telephone calls.

The historical background

In earlier times, the ecclesiastical courts exercised jurisdiction of a wide nature relating to the formalities of marriage, to problems arising from the status of marriage, and in connection with incontinence in general. Earlier still, the more primitive law punished the cruder sexual offences with great severity. Between 1558 and 1640 the Court of High Commission also dealt with sexual offences. It concerned itself with the immoral practices of the wealthy and the penalties imposed were accordingly more severe. Thus adultery, incest, excessive drinking, swearing and blasphemy came within its purview. Hale, in his *Ecclesiastical Precedents* (1736), reports cases relating to incest, bigamy, acting as a procuress, procuring abortion, and a case of assault with intent to ravish, amongst other offences.

The ecclesiastical jurisdiction gradually fell into decay. The ecclesiastical courts were abolished in 1640 and, though revived in 1661, were never a force again. The nineteenth century saw their final demise. Their jurisdiction in matrimonial causes was transferred to the secular courts in 1857, and by 1876 Lord Penzance was able to remark that 'a recurrence of the punishment of the laity for the good of their souls by ecclesiastical courts would not be in harmony with modern ideas, or the position which ecclesiastical authority now occupies' (*Phillimore* v. *Machon* 1 P.D.481).

However, even before Cromwell, incursions had been made into ecclesiastical jurisdiction. Thus in 1603 bigamy was made a crime by statute, and unnatural offences were proscribed under a statute of Henry VIII's day. The preamble to the latter statute states as justification for the new statutory offence that 'there is not yet sufficient and condign punishment appointed by the due course of the laws of this land'. There is a suggestion in earlier writers (Fleta, Britton both *circa* 1290–2) that burying alive or burning may have been the punishment, though this may be doubted (Stephen 1883). After 1640, the common law intervened to fill in the gaps left by statute. The judges assumed wider-ranging powers to protect society against what they deemed was immorality. Typical of the attitude was Lord Mansfield's judgement in *R.* v. *Delaval* in 1763 (3 Burr. 1435). The case concerned procuration. 'It is true', said the Lord Chief Justice. 'that cases of this incontinent kind fall properly under the jurisdiction of the ecclesiastical courts and are appropriate to it, but, if you accept those appropriated cases, this court is the *custos morum* of the people and has the superintendency of offences *contra bonos mores*'.

This reasoning is no longer acceptable. But it was used again in the notorious Ladies' Directory Case in 1961 (*Shaw* v. *D.P.P.* [1962] A.C.220), when the House of Lords convicted Shaw of conspiring with prostitutes to corrupt public morals by publishing a pamphlet which was a guide to their activities and contained vital information about them. Viscount Simonds asserted the existence in the court of

a residual power, where no statute has intervened to supersede the common law, to superintend those offences which are prejudicial to the public welfare ... No one can foresee every way in which the wickedness of man may disrupt the order of society ... Must we wait until Parliament finds time to deal with such conduct? ... If the common law is powerless in such an event, then we should no longer do her reverence. But I say that her hand is still powerful and that it is for Her Majesty's judges to play the part which Lord Mansfield pointed out to them.

Lord Reid powerfully dissented, but the other judges agreed. Lord Hodson, for example, saw no reason why a conspiracy to encourage fornication and adultery should be regarded as outside the ambit of a conspiracy to corrupt public morals. The existence of the offence was confirmed by the House of Lords in 1972, *Knuller* v. *D.P.P.* [1973] A.C.435, where advertisements in the *International Times* for homosexual contacts were held to come within its scope. Apparently, some 40 cases involving charges of conspiracy to corrupt public morals were brought in the decade between these two cases. One was the famous '*Oz*' case (*R* v. *Anderson* [1972] 1 Q.B.304). Two-thirds of the cases related to the showing of pornographic films in private, unlicensed premises to which members of the public were admitted on payment (Law Commission 1974).

Knuller's case is also important in that the majority of the House of Lords held that there was also a common law offence of conspiracy to outrage decency, and, perhaps, the generalized offence of outraging decency. It is not clear from *Knuller* precisely what meaning is to be attributed to 'outrage decency'. To Lord Morris, printed matter which 'could rationally be regarded as lewd, disgusting and offensive', and which would outrage 'the sense of decency of members of the public' would be caught by the offence. Lord Simon, on the other hand, argued that 'outrage' was a 'very strong word'. So "outraging public decency" goes considerably beyond offending the susceptibilities of, or even shocking, reasonable people'.

The Law Commission (1974) has recommended the abolition of both the conspiracy offences, as well as the general offences of corrupting public morals and outraging public decency. It recommends the filling in of various lacunae this would leave with new statutory offences. These recommendations have not been implemented. The Criminal Law Act 1977 (s.5(3)) has now expressly preserved both conspiracy offences referred to in this section (Smith 1977).

The history of the law in the area of sexual deviation thus presents a picture of an emergent statutory code swamping earlier ecclesiastical jurisdiction and powers cherished by the judges. But the common law lives on and ecclesiastical jurisdiction disappeared as recently as 1963, though it had long fallen into desuetude.

The offences

Bigamy

Bigamy was in earlier times exclusively an ecclesiastical offence. Only in 1603 did it become a felony. The 1603 statute recited that men had been committing bigamy 'to the great dishonour of God, and utter undoing of divers honest men's children'. The traditional rationale of the crime is well stated by Chief Justice Cockburn in *R* v. *Allen* ([1872] L.R. 1 C.C.R.367): 'it involves an outrage on public decency and morals, and creates a public scandal by the prostitution of a solemn ceremony, which the law allows to be applied only to a legitimate union, to a marriage at best but colourable and fictitious, and which may be made and too often is made, the means of the most cruel and wicked deception'.

The offence is committed by anyone who being married marries some other person during the life of the first spouse. It does not matter where the second marriage takes place. The maximum sentence for this is seven years' imprisonment. Glanville Williams (1945) has described bigamy as 'the only surviving offence ... based on word-fetishism'. He argues that 'the only anti-social consequences that are necessarily involved in the mere celebration of a bigamous marriage are (i) the falsification of the State records, and (ii) the waste of time of the Minister of Religion or Registrar'. He concludes that it 'does not make sense except on the supposition that the marriage ceremony is a magic form of words that has to be protected from profanation at almost any cost in human suffering'. The situation is the more striking in that no criminal offence is committed in deserting a spouse or committing adultery. But by making the position more regular the bigamist brings into potentiality the full opprobrium of the criminal law.

However, it is probable that few bigamists are detected. It is relatively easy in a country which shuns identity cards to disappear, and it is equally simple to effect a change of name. And there is a reluctance to prosecute, particularly where the second 'spouse' has not been deceived (Wilcox 1972). Of 155 offences known to the police in 1975, only 17, including 1 committed by a woman, were proceeded against. All were convicted, but only 7 were given an immediate custodial sentence, and nobody was sentenced to more than 2 years imprisonment.

The English law of bigamy has in recent years had to contend with the problem of immigrants whose own personal law permits polygamy. In the recent case of *R* v. *Sagoo* ([1975] 2 All E.R. 926) the Court of Appeal held that, where a potentially polygamous marriage has been converted (in this case both by legislation and a change of domicile) into a monogamous marriage, it prevents a man from contracting a valid union in this country and exposes him to a charge of bigamy. Many Muslims, however, remain domiciled in their own country of origin notwithstanding lengthy sojourns in England. A marriage contracted in England by such a person would be void, but it is probable that the second marriage would not be bigamous (Pearl 1976). It seems that the assumption of a Pakistan domicile of choice, together with a conversion to Islam by an Englishman would be sufficient to entitle him to marry in Pakistan a second 'wife' whilst still married to his first wife (*Cheni* v. *Cheni* [1965] P.85). Whether such a person commits bigamy is not settled: on principle, there seems no reason why he should.

Incest

Incest, also, was in earlier times exclusively (except for a short period from 1650 to 1660) an ecclesiastical offence. It was not made a criminal offence until the Punishment of Incest Act 1908. Stephen (1883) explains this in terms of the existence of ecclesiastical jurisdiction. But there is no evidence that the laity were being punished for such moral offences in the second half of the nineteenth century. So, as James (1964) has suggested, 'this leaves open an interesting legal and sociological consideration as to the incidents and legal control of incest between 1876 (the date of *Phillimore* v. *Machon*, referred to above), if not earlier and the statute of 1908'. However, it is thought such cases were frequently prosecuted as rape or unlawful sexual intercourse (West 1974).

In English law, a man commits incest if he has or attempts to have sexual intercourse with a female whom he knows to be his daughter, sister, half-sister, grand-daughter or mother (Sexual Offences Act 1956 s.10). It is also an offence for a man to incite to have sexual intercourse with him a girl under 16 whom he knows to come within these categories (Criminal Law Act 1977 s.54). A woman of 16 or over who permits a man, who stands in such a relationship to her, to have sexual intercourse with her also committs an offence (Sexual Offences Act 1956 s.11). In Scotland the law of incest is based upon Leviticus XVIII (Incest Act 1567) and was punishable by death until 1887 (Sellar 1978). Blom-Cooper and Drewry (1976) report a recent case where a man and his daughter-in-law were prosecuted under this Act, remanded in custody for a month and then 'admonished' for 'this wretched affair'. Incest by a man with a girl under 13 is punishable with life imprisonment: incest with an older person is punishable by up to seven years' imprisonment. Some legal systems, for example the French and the Dutch, do not punish incest as such, though the conduct concerned is covered by more generalized criminal law prohibitions.

We do not know how much incest there is. The incidents of incest which come to the attention of doctors or police or the courts tend to arise from situations of obvious family conflict. Where the behaviour involves adults and there is mutual consent and, hence, no victim, agencies of control are less likely to hear about it or take action. Even where cases are reported to the police, there is an almost constant ratio of nearly 2:1 between this number and the number subsequently convicted. There were 349 reported cases in 1975, and 188 convictions (9 of women). The laws of evidence require the victim's statements to be corroborated, and there is considerable discretion exercised by the police, and the Director of Public Prosecutions to whom all cases must be referred, in instituting proceedings (Manchester 1977). Some cases may also be dealt with informally by doctors, social workers, or the police. Flexibility is important for penal measures and, indeed, prosecution is sometimes inappropriate, as where, for example, brother and sister meet for the first time in adulthood and marry. In 1975, of 188 convictions for incest, only 33 offenders were under 21. So known cases are essentially adult. We do not know the ages of the victims, though we may surmise from the fact that over two-thirds of those convicted were men aged between 30 and 50 years that teenage daughters form a high proportion of the victims. This is borne out by Manchester's research (Manchester 1977). In Hall Williams' study (1974), the victim was the offender's own child in 53 per cent of the cases, and step-children were involved in 15 per cent of the cases: 60 per cent of the victims were in the 10–16 age group.

Sentences for incest are extremely variable and they can be most severe. In 1975, 80 men were sentenced to two years' imprisonment or more: 7 received sentences of over 5 years, and 1 over 10 years. Nobody received the statutory maximum sentence. It is thus possible that sentences are becoming less severe, for Thomas (1970) noted that in all cases involving parents and children sentences in the region of between 4 and 6 years imprisonment were commonly confirmed, even where there was no question of threat or force. For examples of more lenient treatment see *R*. v. *Huchison* ([1972] 56 Cr. App. R.307) and *R*. v. *Winch* ([1974] Crim. L.R.487). However, West (1974) believes that the Court of Appeal is more horrified by incest than the trial courts, for the sentences which it approves are much longer than those received by the majority of incest offenders.

There is strong revulsion felt against incest. Despite this, suggestions have been made that incest should not be a specially designated criminal offence when committed between mutually consenting persons over 14 (Sexual Law Reform Society Working Party Report 1975). Card (1975) argues that 'if incest is a crime because society finds it repulsive even among consenting adults this is an insufficient reason to invade their privacy' (see also Morris and Hawkins (1970); Packer (1968)). But other reasons are put forward in favour of the retention of incest as a crime. Anthropology suggests the origin of the taboo lies in the disruption and strife which incest generates in family groupings. There is evidence that this happens, though it is taken from prosecuted cases. The taboo is very widespread though not universal (Maisch 1973). The strongest argument for punishing adult, consensual incest is a dysgenic one: that inbreeding leads to a deterioration of the stock (see Lord Normand in *Philips' Trustees* v. *Beaton* (1938) S.C.733, 745–6). It is difficult to prove this. Allen (1969) has stated: 'studies of the offspring of incestuous unions among those of normal intelligence are probably impossible since they do not occur with any frequency'. (See also Aberle 1963) but there are findings which suggest a high risk of mental retardation (Carter 1967; Adams and Reed 1967; Seemanova 1971). The offspring of incestuous unions have a greater mortality and morbidity than the average. Further, Lukianowicz (1972) found a 4 per cent incidence of paternal incest amongst an unselected group of female psychiatric patients. Yet Weinberg (1963) suggests that most victims of father-daughter incest settle later to a normal heterosexual life.

The disruptive effect of a prosecuted incest on the family is not in doubt. Homes and marriages are broken up. The offender's chances of parole are adversely affected (Hall Williams 1974). His chances of being divorced are high. Even if the home is kept together the social service departments are under a statutory obligation to remove from the home of a convicted incest offender any child under 17 thought to be in moral danger. The repercussions of incest are thus manifold. Not surprisingly, therefore, the counselling programme in Santa Clara California has provoked much interest (Giaretto 1976).

Adultery

Adultery in English law connotes voluntary or consensual sexual intercourse between a married person and a person (whether married or unmarried) of the opposite sex not being the other's spouse (Cretney

1974). This definition has been criticized as 'legalistic' (Freeman 1971). Acts which do not constitute adultery in England have been held to do so in other systems. In New York sodomy constitutes adultery (Ploscowe, Foster, and Freed 1972). In New Zealand an attempt by a father to have sexual intercourse with his 9-year-old daughter was held to constitute adultery. He had failed to achieve penetration but had deposited sperm around her vaginal opening (*A* v. *A* [1943] N.Z.L.R.47). In England sexual familiarity or masturbation is not adultery. Insemination with the semen of a third party donor (A.I.D.) is probably not adultery according to English law. It is in Canada (*Orford* v. *Orford* (1921) 58 D.L.R.251), though it has been held not to be in Scotland (*MacLennan* v. *MacLennan* [1958] S.C.105).

It seems the public are equally bemused as to what constitutes adultery. In *Barnacle* v. *Barnacle* in 1948 ([1948] P.257), it transpired that one petitioner thought adultery involved illicit connection between two unmarried persons with the consequent production of a child. Others had thought that it was not adultery 'during the day-time', or it was 'drinking with men in public houses': yet another averred that it was not adultery if the woman was 'over 50' (Megarry 1955).

What is not in doubt is that adultery is quite common. Thus Kinsey found that 26 per cent of his sample of married women had had extramarital coitus by the age of 40. He estimated that 50 per cent of married men had committed adultery by that age (1948). De Wolf (1970) claims that 63 per cent of all husbands and 29 per cent of all wives have had an 'affair'. Johnson, on the other hand, reports that of those he interviewed only 24 per cent of the men and 13 per cent of the women had extramarital coitus (1970). To an extent adultery is acceptable. There is a double standard involved here. As Kinsey (1953) put it 'most societies recognise the necessity for accepting some extramarital coitus as an escape valve for the male, to relieve him from the pressures put on him by society's insistence on stable marital relationships. These same societies, however, less often permit it for the female'. Even then it may be 'covertly condoned if it is not too flagrant and if the husband is not particularly disturbed'. Gorer's studies of English life (1955; 1971) confirm this duality of standards. In his 1971 study he found that 22 per cent of his respondents disapproved of casual adultery in a man and 23 per cent disapproved of it in a woman. But men disapproved of women committing adultery more than they censured men (17 per cent and 27 per cent) and women also disapproved of female adultery more (18 per cent and 27 per cent). Confronted by serious adultery 29 per cent would 'talk it over with the spouse' and 24 per cent would 'analyze the situation'. Only 15 per cent advocated immediate separation and 7 per cent immediate divorce. Five per cent, on the other hand, believed in using physical violence on the spouse and another 2 per cent on the intervener.

Adultery is not a crime in England. It was at one time an ecclesiastical offence and was a capital crime in the period of the Commonwealth. Whether there were any convictions under the Commonwealth Act of 1650 seems doubtful (Megarry 1973). Ecclesiastical courts, however, certainly punished adulterers. There are records of a series of indictments and in at least one case a sentence is recorded, namely, that the male adulterer should be carted (Cleveland 1913). As recently as 1959, the Archbishop of Canterbury suggested that adultery could become 'such a public menace' as to necessitate it becoming a crime. Attempts were made in the late eighteenth and early nineteenth centuries to make it impossible for the *female* adulterer to marry her 'seducer'. Bills passed the Lords (but failed in the Commons) in 1771, 1779, and 1800.

In the USA, adultery is still a crime in a large number of states. Many, however, have abolished it in the last decade. But, where once the death penalty was imposed (see *Commonwealth* v. *Call*, 38 Mass. (21 Pick) 509 (1839)), to-day penalties vary from a ten dollar fine in Rhode Island to three years' imprisonment in Arizona. In most states adultery is rarely prosecuted. Thus, in New York between June 1959 and June 1960 there were 1700 divorce cases based on adultery (at that time the only ground), but no adultery prosecutions. But in some areas, such as Boston, prosecutions have been more frequent (Ploscowe 1962). Other countries have also regarded adultery as a crime; Sweden did until 1937 and Yugoslavia until 1945. In France, only a wife can commit the crime of adultery, though, if convicted, her sentence, which could be 2 years, is remitted if her husband agrees to take her back. (French Penal Code Arts 336–7). A husband who keeps a mistress at the matrimonial home also commits an offence but not one punishable by imprisonment (Art. 339).

This dual standard is common. It is found in countries influenced by Roman law. It is found also in Jewish law, under which a husband is obliged to divorce an adulterous wife, though such is not the case where he is the adulterer (Naamani 1963). It was also reflected in English law until 1923 (McGregor 1957): whilst a husband could divorce his wife on the ground of her adultery *simpliciter*, she had to prove aggravated adultery, for example, adultery accompanied by incest or bigamy. A double standard is still found in the law of Kentucky. There was an eloquent defence of the distinction by the English Lord Chancellor (Lord Thurlow) in 1779: adultery by a wife, he averred, 'not only subverts domestic tranquillity, but has a tendency, by contaminating the blood of illustrious families, to affect the welfare of the nation in its nearest interests'. Crozier (1935) argues that 'it is not immorality which is punished but theft. As the act of the wife, adultery is a revolt against the husband's property rights'. Neither argument is persuasive to-day.

English law then does not punish adultery as a crime. Indeed, since 1970 it has even been impossible to procure damages for adultery. It does, however, in common with most systems, permit the 'wronged' spouse to use the act of adultery as a vehicle for securing matrimonial relief. The standard of proof is high, though in most contested cases the court will have to infer adultery from circumstantial evidence. Once it was enough to prove adultery but, since the Divorce Reform Act 1969 came into operation in 1971, it has been necessary to prove additionally that one finds it intolerable to live with the respondent. However, the petitioner need not prove that cohabitation is intolerable as a result of the adultery, for the Court of Appeal, wrongly it is submitted (Freeman 1972), has held that the adultery and intolerability limbs must be construed disjunctively (*Cleary* v. *Cleary* [1974] 1 W.L.R. 73, *Carr* v. *Carr* [1974] 1 W.L.R.449). There is only one ground of divorce in England to-day: that the marriage has irretrievably broken down. Proof of adultery plus intolerability, however, raises a strong presumption of irretrievable breakdown. Some systems, such as California, do not specify individual grounds or facts such as adultery but require proof generally of irreparable breakdown. English law recognized adultery as the only ground until 1937. Now there are five facts which may be relied upon; these include separation periods, and adultery is no longer the most popular fact relied upon. More divorce petitions are now based on intolerable behaviour (the old cruelty). But husbands still rely on their wives' adultery to a much greater extent than any of the other facts. Thirty-six per cent of husbands' petitions are based on adultery, whereas only 22 per cent of wives' petitions are similarly based (Lord Chancellor's Office 1975). Whether this reflects less adultery by husbands, or their lower thresh-hold of tolerance cannot be determined.

Fornication

Fornication (or incontinence) was yet another offence that formerly fell within the jurisdiction of the ecclesiastical courts. In England today it is not in itself a criminal offence, though it may in certain circumstances amount to some specific crime such as indecent assault or procuration. Again, as with adultery and incest it was a crime under the Commonwealth. Blackstone (1765), referring to this, states that, 'when the ruling power found it for their interest to put on the semblance of a very extraordinary strictness and purity of morals', it made the commission of fornication upon a second conviction a felony without benefit of clergy.

It was also a crime under a statute of Elizabeth I to have a bastard child. Both the mother and reputed father were punishable. A statute of James I provided for her committal to a House of Correction. The rationale of the offence was economic rather than moralistic: the offence was only punishable if the child became chargeable to the parish.

Fornication is still a crime in many of the states of the USA. As with adultery the penalties vary from nominal to severe. But the offence is rarely prosecuted.

Although fornication is not a crime in England to-day it is 'regulated' in a number of ways. An incontinent girl under 17 years of age may be held to be 'in moral danger' and taken into the care of the local authority (Children and Young Persons Act 1969 s.1(2)). She cannot be 'in moral danger' if she is married, even if she is under the minimum age for marriage. Thus, a 13 year old Nigerian girl was held not to be 'in moral danger' in cohabiting with her Nigerian husband in Southwark. They were domiciled in Nigeria (*Mohamed* v. *Knott* [1969] 1 Q.B.1). A boy who is similarly promiscuous is less likely to be regarded as 'in moral danger' by the relevant control agencies (Schur 1973).

Fornication need not lead to the birth of a child and, with improved contraceptive techniques and abortion facilities, it rarely does (Illsey and Gill 1968). Should it do so, and it seems the lower down the socio-economic scale one goes, the more likely is such an occurrence (Bones 1973; Wynn 1974), the mother is permitted to take the man, she alleges is the father, to court for an affiliation order. Blood tests may be used to elicit the truth (Family Law Reform Act 1969) (see also Hayes 1971; Krause 1970). If the mother cannot show that a particular man out of several with whom she has had intercourse is the father, the court cannot make an order. In South Australia, on the other hand, contribution orders may be made against men admitting intercourse in circumstances in which, in the court's opinion, that man might possibly be the father of the mother's child (Finlay and Bissett-Johnson 1970). In addition to the mother, the Supplementary Benefits Commission, in some cases a local authority caring for the child, and a custodian can seek an affiliation order. Few affiliation orders are sought. The whole process is rather demeaning and most orders are not worth the paper they are written on (Marsden 1973; McGregor *et al.* 1970).

Rape

Of all behaviour which exhibits sexual deviation, rape is the one which currently excites most interest. The interest is world-wide (Fargier 1976; Solat 1977) and the literature voluminous. Of the many collections of materials on the subject, perhaps the best, and certainly the most representative, is that by Chappell, Geis, and Geis (1977). Rape has become a rallying subject for the Women's Liberation movement and much of the literature is accordingly feminist in orientation (see Griffin 1971; Medea and Thomson 1974); Brownmiller 1975; Reynolds 1974; Schwendinger 1974; Weis and Borges 1973; Toner 1977)). This is certainly one of the main reasons for the dramatic shift in emphasis in recent materials. Where once they were 'largely concerned with the difficulties of protecting a man accused of rape from a spurious or vindictive charge', now they 'emphasize the problems involved in protecting raped females from what is seen as particularly odious behaviour on the part of components of the criminal justice system' (Chappell, Geis, and Fogarty 1974). In England, attention was focused on rape by the decision in *D.P.P.* v. *Morgan* ([1975] 61 Cr. App. R. 136). This held that a man could not be convicted of rape if he in fact believed the woman consented, even if he had no reasonable grounds for so believing. This decision engendered widespread concern, though it is perfectly consistent with existing English criminal law principles (Smith 1975; Glanville Williams 1975). *Morgan* led to a Home Office enquiry (Heilbron Report 1975) and ultimately to legislation but, on the issue of the substantive elements of the offence, this merely confirmed what the House of Lords had said (see Sexual Offences (Amendment) Act 1976).

Rape 'consists in intentionally having sexual intercourse with a woman who does not consent, knowing that she does not consent or being reckless whether she consents or not' (Smith 1976). 'Rape, by definition, cannot exist within marriage, although the behaviour itself—forced intercourse—may be functionally equivalent to a comparable behaviour committed outside the bounds of marriage and given the official label of rape' (Philipson 1974). A husband may, however, be convicted of raping his wife if magistrates have made a non-cohabitation order in favour of the wife (*R* v. *Clarke* [1949] 2 All E.R.448), if a decree *nisi* of divorce has been pronounced (*R* v. *O'Brien* [1974] 3 All R.E.663), if the husband has given an undertaking to a court not to molest his wife (*R* v. *Steele* (1977) Crim. L.R.290). and possibly if they have agreed to separate, particularly if there is a separation agreement containing a nonmolestation clause (*R.* v. *Miller* [1954] 2 Q.B.282). In *R* v. *Reid* ([1972] 2 All E.R.1350), Cairns L. J. opened that 'the notion that a husband can, without incurring punishment, treat his wife ... with any kind of hostile force is obsolete'. He held that the crime of kidnapping could thus be committed by a husband against his wife. Kidnapping and rape are not *in pari materia*, but Cairns L. J's dictum is wide enough to cast doubts on the propriety of exempting husbands from prosecution for rapes upon their wives. Despite the existence of the immunity, it is clear that a husband, though at liberty to have sexual intercourse with his wife, may not use force or violence to exercise that liberty. If he does he may be charged with assault or some other offence. The law rests on a fiction and is clearly inconsistent with civil law principles: a wife, for example, is not bound to submit to inordinate or unreasonable remands by her husband (*Holborn* v. *Holborn* [1947] 1 All E.R.32) and she may refuse intercourse if he is suffering from a venereal disease (*Foster* v. *Foster* [1921] P.438). It has also been repudiated in the criminal codes of Sweden and Denmark (Livneh 1967), as well as in Delaware and in the USSR and a number of other countries in the communist bloc. An attempt to abolish the exemption failed in England in 1976. The logic of Soames in *The Forsyte Saga* is thus preserved: 'women made a fuss about it in books, but in the cool judgement of right thinking men ... he had but done his best to sustain the sanctity of marriage, to prevent her from abandoning her duty' (Galsworthy 1906; Freeman 1978; Maidment 1978).

Rape as an offence is also limited in that it can only be committed by a male upon a female. 'In reality', as McCaghy (1976) notes, 'despite the daydreams of many men, females rarely force sexual intercourse on males'. The rape of males by males is, however, not so unusual. Both Genet (1951) and T. E. Lawrence (1935) describe personal incidents, and prison rapes are known to be common (Brownmiller 1975). Davis's study (1970) of Philadelphia prisons found that 'virtually every slightly built young man committed by the courts is sexually approached within a day or two after his admission to prison. Many of these young men are repeatedly raped by gangs of inmates'. If we search for reasons why such acts should not be regarded by the law as rape we find three.

There is, first, the historical argument and the supposed novelty of homosexual rape. Secondly, there is, what one may call, a structural argument. Rape involves penetration by a penis of a vagina. According to Brownmiller (1975) 'one inch is the usual standard'. Oral and rectal insertions, whether the victim be male or female, are not, therefore, rape. And thirdly, the legal approach to rape categorizes its motivation as sexual. But much rape is not sexual at all. Eldridge Cleaver in *Soul on Ice* (1968) describes his rapes of white women as 'insurrectionary'. 'It delighted me that I was defying and trampling upon the white man's law, upon his system of values, and that I was defiling his women'. The Schwendingers (1974) argue: 'it should be kept in mind that the rapist's motives involve feelings of domination, regardless of whether the "victim" is a man or woman. Rape is a power trip – an act of aggression and an act of contempt – and in most cases is only secondarily sexual'. Much homosexual rape, then, is not overtly sexual. Davis (1970) did not find homosexual rape in prison to be primarily motivated by the need for sexual release: autoerotic masturbation to orgasm being 'much easier and more normal'. The greatest proportion of assaults in his study involved blacks attacking whites. 'A primary goal of the sexual aggressor . . . is the conquest and degradation of his victim . . . Sexual assaults . . . are expressions of anger and aggression prompted by the same basic frustrations . . . summarised as an inability to achieve masculine identification and pride through avenues other than sex.' Feminist writers generalize this assertion. To them the act of rape is a cameo of male–female relationships, forcible penetration being at one end of a spectrum of male sexual dominance (Greenwood and Young 1975). 'It is the final expression in a series of indignities and prejudices heaped on women' (Melani and Fodaski 1974), 'a form of mass terrorism' (Griffin 1971). In other words, they see rape as representing conflict, the supreme act of domination.

The other critical element of the offence of rape is the absence of the woman's consent. The test is not 'was it against the woman's will?' but 'was it without her consent?' So the prosecution does not have to prove positive dissent: it is enough that she did not assent (Smith and Hogan 1973). It is not rape if she consents even if her will is weakened, unless fraud or threats are used to that end (*R*. v. *Lang* [1976] Crim. L.R.65). Seduction is not rape: 'the seducer may resort to various devices in order to obtain the consent of his victim – soft lights, sweet music, flattery, and drink' (Smith 1976). An apparent consent arising from a fundamental error, induced by fraud is no consent: so it is rape where a man induces a woman to have sexual intercourse with him by impersonating her husband, or where he deceives her as to the nature of the transaction. Thus, the choir master master of a Presbyterian church, who had intercourse with a 16-year-old pupil under the pretence that it was a surgical operation which would improve her voice was convicted of rape (*R*. v. *Williams* [1923] 1 K.B.340). 'She was persuaded to consent to what he did because she thought it was not sexual intercourse and because she thought it was a surgical operation' (*per* Lord Hewart C. J.).

The question of consent will often turn on conflicting testimony and the question then becomes one of whom to believe. Thus, a jury's concept of 'consent' is likely to be based on its interpretation of the events leading up to the incident and on its opinion of the woman's moral character. Kalven and Zeisel (1966) note in their monumental study of *The American Jury* that 'the jury . . . does not limit itself [to the law]: it goes on to weigh the woman's conduct in the prior history of the affair. It . . . scrutinizes the female complainant and is moved to be lenient with the defendant whenever there are suggestions of contributory behaviour on her part'. Leaving aside cases where there was extrinsic violence, or where the victim and defendant were total strangers, as well as group rapes, they found that, whereas judges would have convicted in 22 out of 42 cases, the jury convicted in only 3. But, as Brownmiller (1975) argues, 'while most rational people might be able to agree on what constitutes rash, reckless, or precipitant behaviour leading to a homicide, in rape the parameters are indistinct and movable'. The USA National Commission on the Causes and Prevention of Violence (1969) found less victim precipitation in rape than other crimes of violence (4·4 per cent, as against 22 per cent in homicide and 10·7 per cent in armed robbery). Brownmiller quotes the case of a girl on a 'date' confronted with 'if you don't let me, I'll put it in your mouth'. She gave in and then his two friends took their turn. 'I wasn't screaming or fighting anymore. I just wanted to get it over with and not have anything worse happen to me', she said. Was she raped? It is certainly arguable that, according to legal definitions, she consented to sexual intercourse taking place. A study of 80 rape victims found their primary reaction to be fear (Burgess and Holmstrom 1973). They later documented what they called a 'rape trauma syndrome' (Burgess and Holmstrom 1974). 'A *quid pro quo*—rape in exchange for life, or rape in exchange for a good-faith guarantee against hurtful or disfiguring physical damage – dominates the female mentality in rape' (Brownmiller 1975). Nor do potential victims behave rationally under stress: 'all I could think of was my new dress' . . . 'I kept saying over and over "Don't rip my nylon stockings"' (quoted in Brownmiller 1975). In this light consent is an artificial concept. The law is crude and glosses over dimensions of the female psyche.

Some of these difficulties are reflected in the statistics. Thus, of 1040 offences reported as known to the police in England and Wales in 1975 (a 24 per cent increase over 1971's figures), only 409 suspects came before the courts: 328 were convicted. Although the maximum sentence is life imprisonment, only 280 were even sentenced to imprisonment or borstal training. Five got life, 8 over 7-years, and another 34 over 5-years' imprisonment, but the commonest sentences were between 2-and 5-years' imprisonment. The occasional sentence provokes critical comment. Thus, when a man who raped a student hitch-hiker got a suspended sentence from Mr. Justice Melford Stevenson (known as one of the severest of contemporary judges), the Press was very critical. But the judge had opined, for what it is worth, that it was, 'as rape goes, a pretty anaemic affair. The man had made a fool of himself but the girl was almost equally stupid'. An MP commented that perhaps he would like to have handed down a sentence for the grievous crime of hitch-hiking! (Philip Whitehead MP, H.C. vol. 905 col. 822). Another recent case, which provoked angry press and backbench comment, was that of the self-confessed, double rapist who assaulted women at knife point and whom Judge Christmas Humphreys saw no reason to send to prison. Fifty-four per cent of the victims in the cases tried, on the other hand, had to go through the ordeal of seeing their names and other details printed in the Press (Southill and Jack 1975). This latter practice has now been proscribed by the Sexual Offences (Amendment) Act 1976: anonymity will now be preserved in nearly all cases. The injustice of denying anonymity to rape defendants (Mairs 1975) was recognized by the same Act, though defendants to other charges are not protected.

The women, it is often said, are made to feel that it is they who are on trial. Brownmiller (1975) quotes one victim as saying: 'I don't understand it. It was like I was the defendant and he was the plaintiff. I wasn't on trial. I don't see where I did anything wrong. I screamed. I struggled. How could they have decided that he was innocent, that I didn't resist'. The tendency in trials is to scrutinize the victim's past sexual history. The theory is that this is suggestive of whether she is likely to have consented. It is said to reflect on her credibility, even her predisposition to tell the truth. Women are made to feel their own moral characters are on trial (Berger 1977). In English law it has been long recognized that evidence may be adduced as to the victim's 'notorious bad character' (*R. v. Clarke* (1817) 2 Stark. 241), and she may be cross-examined as to such character (*R. v. Barker* (1829) 3C and p.589). She can also be asked questions as to her previous relationship with the accused, as her answers may throw light on the issue of consent (*R. v. Cockcroft* (1870) 11 Cox 410). As far as cross-examination as to the victim's relationship with other men is concerned, the law has been that she might be asked questions about her previous sexual activities, but if she denied their existence evidence could not be called to rebut what she said (*R. v. Holmes* (1871) LR 1 CCR 334). But, as Heilbron (1975) conceded, 'the difficulty in practice [was] that her denials may not be believed by the jury, and they may react adversely to her demeanour which may possibly be caused by the shock and dismay of this line of questioning'. Heilbron recommended 'that [such] questions ought not to be asked, not evidence admitted, except with the leave of the trial judge on application made to him in the absence of the jury'. A total ban was, therefore, not advocated as situations were foreseen (for example, where the victim was a prostitute) where such evidence would be relevant. This recommendation has now been implemented by the Sexual Offences (Amendment) Act 1976.

The trial, however, is only the culmination of a process that begins with the decision to report the rape. Women claim that their complaints are met by insensitive, often hostile policemen. Police manuals warn that rape is one of the most falsely reported crimes (Payton 1966). It probably is, but the consequences of such a warning are alarming. 'The tragedy for the rape victim is that the police officer is the person who validates her victimization' (Brownmiller 1975). But if the police believe that complaints are 'prostitutes who didn't get their money' (quoted in Brownmiller 1975), women can hardly expect a sympathetic response. A study in the University of Pennsylvania Law Review (1968) showed that the police declared one-fifth of complaints to be unfounded. Rapes reported promptly, and cases involving strangers, weapons, and violence stood the highest chance of being validated. Rapes in cars were considered dubious and where the man was a 'date' every instance in a car was held to be false. The police were more ready to believe a complainant who screamed than one who silently struggled. The veracity of black women, and women who had been drinking was frequently doubted.

In addition to police interrogation, there will be further questioning by a police surgeon, and an intimate gynaecological examination. Apparently, the facilities for such examinations are sometimes inadequate and unsuitable (Heilbron 1975). Against this background it is not surprising that only one-fifth of rape incidents are reported to the police. In spite of Hale's 'old saw' (Le Grand 1973), women do not find it 'an accusation easily to be made'. But this myth persists. As do others: that women need to be raped (Gebhard 1965), or deserve to be raped (Kanin 1967; Amir 1971), or even want to be raped (Russell 1973). Yet the statistics suggest the number of rapes is rising, that half of the victims are raped by acquaintances, and that a larger pro- portion of reported rapes involve more than one offender (Geis and Chappell 1971). The 'gang-bang' rape may well be the pattern for the future.

Indecent assault on a woman

Under the Sexual Offences Act 1956, it is an offence punishable with two-years imprisonment to commit an indecent assault on a woman (s.14). Generally, consent is a defence, but neither persons under 16 years of age nor defectives can give any consent. Consent is not a defence where it is exacted by force, or fraud as to the nature of the transaction, nor is it where the probable consequence of the assault is the infliction of bodily harm. (*R.* v. *Donovan* [1934] 2 K.B.498). Boys under 14 cannot be convicted of rape (*R.* v. *Groombridge* (1836) 7 C & P 582), but they can be convicted of indecent assault on evidence that they did in fact have intercourse (*R.* v. *Waite* [1892] 2 Q.B.600).

Indecent assault is an aggravated assault and, accordingly, requires an attempt to apply force of some kind to another person. There will usually by physical contact but this is not necessary (*R.* v. *Rolfe* [1952]

36 Cr. App R.4). There must be an act done to the person of the defendant, as distinct from an accepted invitation to do something to the person of the accused. So in *Fairclough* v. *Whipp* ([1951] 2 All E.R.834), the accused was acquitted where he invited a girl of 9-years-of-age to touch his exposed penis. However, a new offence has been created by the Indecency with Children Act 1960: committing an act of gross indecency with or towards a child *under the age of 14 years*, or inciting a child under that age to such an act with him or another (for example, another child) is punishable by two-years imprisonment. A man who allowed a girl of 8 to touch his penis for 5 minutes was recently convicted, the court holding that inactivity could amount to an invitation to the child to do the act (*R* v. *Speck* (1977) Crim. L.R.689). The law as stated in *Fairclough* v. *Whipp* is still applicable so far as persons over 14 are concerned.

The meaning of 'indecent' has also caused problems. It has been held that an act decent in itself but committed for the purpose of sexual gratification, does not in itself amount to an indecent assault. For example, George (*R.* v. *George* [1956] Crim. L. Rev. 52) had attempted to remove girls' shoes from their feet because it gave him sexual gratification. So, an indecent motive cannot convert an objectively decent act into an indecent assault. A decent motive, however, may justify what would otherwise be an indecent act. Medical examinations are, therefore, not indecent assaults, irrespective of consent. In the Supreme Court of Canada, there was held to be no assault where a doctor obtained a patient's consent to his friend's presence at her vaginal examination by falsely pretending he was a medical student. The court said the fraud did not go to the nature and quality of what was done (*R.* v. *Bolduc* and *Bird* (1967) 63 DLR (2d) 82). English principles suggest he would have been convicted in this country.

The number of cases reported to the police is declining. In 1975 there were 11 809. Less than one-third were proceeded against and of these 232 men and 1 woman were sent to prison. Some, notably the Sexual Law Reform Society (1975), would like to see the offence abolished as a separate offence. It advocates charges relating to sexual assaults being dealt with as common assaults or assaults occasioning actual bodily harm, as appropriate. The maximum sentence for assaults occasioning actual bodily harm is five years. But most indecent assaults will only be common assaults, on this criterion, and attract a maximum of one-year's imprisonment.

Unlawful sexual intercourse

This offence is known as 'statutory rape' in the USA. There, ages of consent vary from the ludicrously low (it was 7 in Delaware until 1973), to ages well above that provided by English law (for example, it is 21 in Tennessee). According to English law, a man may not have intercourse with a girl under 16 years of age (s.6 of Sexual Offences Act 1956). If she is under 13 years of age, the offence is punishable with life imprisonment (s.5). The girl cannot, by law, consent. Belief that the girl is over 13-years-old, no matter how reasonable it may be, is no defence to a charge (s.5): belief that the girl is over 16-years-old is a defence to a charge (s.6) only if it is reasonable, and held by a man under 24 who has not previously been charged with a like offence (s.6(3)). The offence dates from 1885. It was tied then, as it is now, to the minimum age of marriage. Intercourse with a girl under 16 will not be unlawful where she is validly married under her personal law (*Mohamed* v. *Knott* [1969] 1 Q.B.1), nor where the man reasonably believes that the girl, who is under age, is his wife (s.6(2) of S.O.A. 1956).

Under s.6, 4533 offences were recorded as known to the police in 1975 (a decline of 10 per cent from 1971): 327 offences under s.5 were also recorded (a 47 per cent increase from 1971). Eighty-four men went to prison for unlawful sexual intercourse with girls under 16 years of age (65 for a year or less), and another 48 where the girl was under 13 years of age (the sentences here were stiffer—7 years' imprisonment being the longest). This crime is one which is never long out of press comment. There is a regular crop of notorious prosecutions, usually involving a man little older than the girl, and judgements tend to be humane. One case that recently attracted attention concerned a man of 22 years of age who had intercourse with a 15-year-old girl. The judge, Judge McKinnon Q.C., said of the girl: 'she has no complaints at all; it was a thoroughly satisfactory experience so far as she is concerned'. The judge was strongly critical of the law. Indeed, he went on television to say so. 'How on earth any society can delude itself into thinking that this sort of law can have any sort of success baffles me', he commented. The defendant was conditionally discharged for 12 months (*The Times*, 23 June 1976). The case sparked off a debate about whether the age of consent should be lowered. Whatever age the law selects must necessarily be arbitrary for physical and mental maturation vary so much. Any change would be resisted by powerful lobbies. What is therefore to be preferred is retention of the existing age with a flexible approach to invocation of the law. The police should be encouraged to caution rather than prosecute, and sentencers should exercise their powers flexibly, taking account of the circumstances of the individual case. This has been recognized by the Court of Appeal in the case of *R*. v. *Taylor* ([1977] 3 All E.R.527). Lawton L. J. said that the offence covered a wide spectrum of guilt and accordingly the penalties appropriate to the offence will vary in different cases. The court confirmed short prison sentences on adult men who had used the village whore of fourteen. The law, said Lawton L. J., 'exists for the protection of girls', and was particularly necessary in the case of 'wanton girls'.

Many cases of 'unlawful sexual intercourse' are paradigm examples of 'crimes without victims'. In this light, the comment of Skolnick and Woodworth (1968), though generally applicable, is particularly apposite. 'It does not matter very much if criminal law forbids various erotic activities, so long as it is impossible to see through walls. When such vision becomes possible, however, the totalitarian potential is enormous because ... the surveillance potential of those performing police functions will be extraordinary.' They found that in one town on the west coast of the USA, the greatest single source of information in statutory rape cases was the family support division of the prosecutor's office: the adolescent girl applying for maternity assistance was sent as a matter of routine to the police, who urged her in the strongest terms to present a complaint. The impact of the cybernetic revolution on an area of law like statutory rape is thus profound. Further, it means that crimes like statutory rape are punished mainly among the poorer sections of the community: their actions surface to visibility on applications for welfare benefits.

Sexual murder

English law, in common with every other system of law, proscribes murder and it does not distinguish between different motivational causes. Nor, so far as is known, does any other system. But any crime can have sexual gratification as an underlying motivation. One must distinguish between cases where killing is done for sexual pleasure, and cases where killing takes place in the course of some other crime or otherwise lawful action which has sexual motivation. The former type of case may result in prosecutions, or convictions for manslaughter, rather than murder, on the basis that the killer is suffering from diminished responsibility. This entails the existence of 'abnormality of mind' which 'substantially impairs . . . mental responsibility for acts or omissions' (Homicide Act 1957 s.2). In effect, the law recognizes that sexual drives may irresistibly impel one to murder. Thus in *R*. v. *Byrne* ([1960]) 2 Q.B.396), the accused strangled a girl in a YWCA hostel and then committed horrifying mutilations on her body. There was evidence that Byrne had, from an early age, been subject to perverted sexual desires, and that the urge of those desires was stronger than normal sex-impulses, so that he found it difficult, if not impossible, to resist putting the desire into practice. It was suggested that this girl was killed under such an impulse. Lord Parker C. J. held that it was wrong to say that these facts did not constitute evidence which would bring Byrne within the purview of diminished responsibility. 'Abnormality of mind' included 'the ability to exercise will-power to control physical acts in accordance with . . . rational judgment'.

Examples of the latter category are murders committed in the course of rape or assault. An example is the case of *Bedder* v. *D.P.P.* ([1954] 2 All E.R.801). Bedder was 18-years-old, and sexually impotent. He attempted unsuccessfully to have sexual intercourse with a prostitute. She jeered at him and attempted to get away. When he tried to hold her, she kicked him in his genitals. He stabbed her with a knife and killed her. The House of Lords held this was murder. When considering provocation as a defence (which would reduce the crime to manslaughter), it was the effect that the prostitute's acts would have had on an ordinary person, not one invested with the physical peculiarities of Bedder, that was relevant. A rather different illustration is the case of *R*. v. *Sharmpal Singh* ([1962] A.C.188). He killed his wife in the course of sexual intercourse with her. She had consented to intercourse but he used excessive force and death resulted. He pressed on his wife's neck much too hard and went 'beyonds the limits of the normal accompaniments of intercourse'. The Privy Council held his actions to constitute manslaughter.

Paedophilia

Paedophilia connotes sexual attraction to children or young persons. It can take a number of varieties: it can involve rape or unlawful sexual intercourse with young girls. Both these offences have been separately considered; it can also cover indecent assault of children and indecency with them, again, both of these offences in relation to young girls have already been consisdered. Paedophilia, however, is usually understood to mean homosexual fixation on young boys. As the Sexual Offences Act 1967 excuses homosexual behaviour in private between consenting adults (the age of consent is 21 years), the main interest of the law in relation to homosexual practices lies in paedophilia.

According to West (1974), paedophiliacs account for about 30 per cent of all homosexuals. Two types exist (i) those fixated upon sexually immature children, and (ii) those who choose physically responsive pubertal children. Power (1976) states that 'the paedophiliac is usually shy and timid and may show a wide range of psychopathological behaviour.... Fear has prevented the development of adult heterosexuality and they tend to seek comfort and sexual gratification with children'. Curran and Parr (1957) found paedophiliacs to be older than the other homosexuals they studied and a higher proportion were married: many are middle-aged and have experienced heterosexual intercourse over long periods. They tended to isolate themselves from other homosexuals.

The traumatic effect on the child-victim has often been noted (Ferenczi 1949). Power (1976) suggests they suffer 'permanent psychological harm and sexual maladjustment' and he lists some of the complications: but this need not happen. Children do not automatically recognize the experience as adults classify it. The child may experience a sexual assault in a totally 'non-sexual' way 'because [he] has not yet been fully socialized into the motives and feelings that adults routinely come to associate with sexuality: thus a child is merely 'playing', 'being attacked' or 'playing with an adult'. Whatever meanings people come to associate with sexuality, they are always learnt and constructed meanings' (Plummer 1975).

A number of crimes are associated with paedophilic tendencies. These offences are better treated under the classification of homo-sexuality (discussed below). It may be noted here that the offences of indecent assault and indecency with children do apply equally to male victims as female.

Prostitution by females to males

In English law prostitution is not of itself an offence against the law. It is, however, in the opinion of the Wolfenden Report (1957) 'a social fact deplorable in the eyes of moralists, sociologists and . . . the great majority of ordinary people'. At least as far as sociologists are concerned, the accuracy of this statement may be doubted (Davies 1937; Lemert 1967; Gagnon and Simon 1974). Davis (1971), for ·example, argues that prostitution is not only inevitable but necessary. Feminists challenge views like these: they contend that prostitution is merely another example of the general exploitation of women in sexist-society. Thus, they argue, elimination of sexist biases will do away with prostitution (Klein 1973; Millett 1973; Feminist Group 1973). What such a thesis ignores is the phenomenon of male prostitution. Davis's arguments seem, therefore, to have greater force.

The literature on prostitution is strangely biased. It deals almost exclusively with the prostitutes. Their clients 'are fleeting shadows not only to prostitutes, but to researchers as well' (McCaghy 1976). The Kinsey studies (1948) are an exception. He documented the male clients' motivations and found that, incredibly, 69 per cent of the white male population had had some experience with prostitutes.

In some countries, including the USA, prostitution is proscribed. In England, on the other hand, it is legal but positively discouraged. Thus, it is criminal to cause or encourage a woman to become a prostitute; it is an offence to keep a brothel; it is a crime to live on the earnings of prostitutes; it is, above all, a criminal offence to loiter or solicit for the purposes of prostitution. No statute, however, defines prostitution. Winick and Kinsie (1971) say it is 'the granting of non-marital, sexual access, established by mutual agreement of the woman, her client and/or her employer, for remuneration which provides part or all of her livelihood'. The definition commonly used in English law is more value-laden, and wider: it is the offering by a woman of 'her body for purposes amounting to common lewdness for payment in return' (*per* Darling J. in *R*. v. *de Munck* [1918] 1 KB 635). This definition was approved in *R*. v. *Webb* ([1964] 1 Q.B.357): there a girl was employed as a masseuse and was expected, as part of her employment, to masturbate clients who so desired. In her defence, it was argued that the role of the prostitute must be passive, and active indecency of this type could not amount to prostitution. This argument was rejected: 'it cannot matter whether she whips the man or the man whips her, it cannot matter whether he masturbates himself on her or she masturbates him'. In Utah a woman has been held to be a prostitute even if she takes no reward (*Salt Lake City* v. *Allred* 430 P 2d

371 (1967). Some of the offences connected with prostitution will now be surveyed.

It is an offence to procure a woman to become a common prostitute (s.22. of Sexual Offences Act 1956). Procure is widely defined by the courts (See *R* v. *Broadfoot* (1976) 3 All E.R.753 where it was held that a woman employed for massage in a massage parlour is procured by her employer for prostitution if she is masturbating clients. The offence is not complete until the woman becomes a common prostitute. According to Wolfenden (1957) very few cases of procuration come to the notice of the police, presumably because most women who become prostitutes do so because they want to and need no persuading (Davis 1971). Sections 33 to 36 of the 1956 Act deal with the use of premises for prostitution. Thus, it is an offence to keep or manage a brothel ('a place resorted to by persons of both sexes for the purpose of prostitution' *per* Wills J in *Singleton* v. *Ellison* ([1895] 1 Q.B.607); 'a nest of prostitutes' in *Donovan* v. *Gavin* ([1965] 2 Q.B.648): there must be at least two prostitutes in the place). It is also an offence to let premises knowing they are to be used as a brothel, or to sub-let with that knowledge.

The prostitute's employer (the pimp) commits a crime in knowingly living, wholly or in part, on her earnings (Sexual Offences Act 1956 s.30). If he lives with her or is habitually in her company or exercises control, direction, or influence over her movements, he is presumed to be knowingly so living. These methods of proof are not exhaustive and the prosecution can adduce other evidence to show that a man is living on the earnings of a prostitute (see *R* v. *Clarke* (1976) 2 All E.R.696). This offence can only be committed by a man. The offence has caused interpretational problems (Smith and Hogan 1973). For example, does the landlord who lets premises for prostitution commit an offence? It seems that he does if he charges an exorbitant rent but not otherwise. Wolfenden (1957) considered whether this ought to be an offence. It thought not for 'as long as society tolerates the prostitute, it must permit her to carry on her business somewhere'. However, a landlord who lets premises for prostitution cannot recover the rent however reasonable, nor can he recover possession of the premises until the lease is terminated (*Alexander* v. *Rayson* [1936] 1 K.B.169).

The one relevant offence that is directed against the prostitute herself is found in the Street Offences Act 1959 s.1: 'it shall be an offence for a common prostitute to loiter or solicit in a street or public place for the purpose of prostitution'. It has been recommended (Home Office 1976*b*) that two other offences be repealed as being obsolete (*viz.* s.3 of Vagrancy Act 1824 – a common prostitute behaving in a riotous or indecent manner; and s.3 of the Universities Act 1825 – a common prostitute found wandering in Oxford University and not giving a satisfactory account of herself deemed to be an idle and disorderly person!). The retention of neither of these provisions can be justified and it is expected that both will soon be repealed. The Home Office Working Party Report recommends that the existing offence in s.1 should be retained. But the law on loitering and soliciting is neither without its problems nor its criticisms.

The expression 'common prostitute' is said to be at best derogatory and at worst prejudiced. It is, however, only applied to someone who has been twice formally cautioned by the police for loitering or soliciting and who has to some extent invited the label. But she has not been convicted of any offence: as such the procedure offends against the principle of equality before the law. The cautioning system is extra-statutory, and its impact is somewhat attenuated by the ease with which new aliases can be adopted and new environments sought. In a Working Paper, the Home Office (1974) suggested a power of arrest for cautioning, a power to fingerprint, and a national cautions register. It now concedes that such innovations would be far too draconian.

The word 'solicit' has not caused many problems. It is clear that the prostitute must be physically present. The offence is, therefore, not committed where she displays a card on a notice board, inviting men to visit her for the purpose of prostitution (*Weisz* v. *Monahan* [1962] 1 All E.R.664). The owner of the notice board may be convicted of conspiring to corrupt public morals (*Shaw* v. D.P.P. above) publishing an obscene article (*idem*), and, if a man, living on the earnings of a prostitute. Further, solicitation may be by acts done and it is unnecessary to prove that the prostitute used any words. In *Horton* v. *Mead* ([1913] 1 K.B.154), a case on importuning, it was enough that he 'smiled in the faces of gentlemen, pursed his lips and wriggled his body'. And in *Behrendt* v. *Burridge* ([1976] 3 All E.R.285), a prostitute, who sat still on a stool in a bay window in a low-cut top and mini-skirt with a red light in the window, 'might as well have had a notice saying she was available'. It was held that she was soliciting in the sense that she was tempting and alluring prospective customers.

She made no gesture or other form of communication with men in the street.

The question as to whether solicitation has taken place *in* a street or public place has also caused problems. In *Smith* v. *Hughes* ([1960] 2 All E.R.859) a prostitute attracted the attention of men in the street by tapping on her window pane. She was convicted of soliciting.

Other criticisms levelled at the soliciting offence are: (i) that it is differently drafted from comparable legislation controlling male importuners and there is no offence of a man importuning a woman, so that it is in effect discriminatory; and (ii) that the necessity to prove annoyance or nuisance (which existed until 1959) showed a concern for the liberty of the individual which is now missing. As far as (i) is concerned offensive propositioning of women by men for sexual intercourse could, until 1966, be prosecuted as soliciting or importuning in a public place for immoral purposes (s.32 of Sexual Offences Act 1956). But in *Crook* v. *Edmondson* ([1966] 2 Q.B.81) the Divisional Court ruled that heterosexual intercourse was not an immoral purpose. Since then the police have used s.5 of the Public Order Act 1936 (which deals with threatening, abusive, or insulting words or behaviour in a public place and was passed to deal with Mosley's 'Blackshirts'), as well as road traffic legislation on obstruction, and binding over to keep the peace. None of these expedients has been totally successful. The Home Office Report (1976) recommends the introduction of a new offence of kerb crawling to deal with this problem. The same Report regards any re-introduction of the 'annoyance' element in soliciting as retrograde: it would lead to the return of prostitutes to the streets, the very mischief which the Street Offences Act tried to remove.

English legislation is directed mainly against the old-fashioned street-walker and those who sponge on her. In reality, of course, the true professional has found newer, safer, and more profitable pastures. The growth of massage parlours and escort agencies, call girls, and clip-joints has assumed major importance. The law tackles none of these directly though it intervenes when, as often happens, crimes are committed as incidents of these institutions. Thus, owners of escort agencies have recently been convicted of living off immoral earnings.

There are some who argue for the total repeal of all laws against prostitution. The feminist movement is to the fore in the agitation for decriminalization. It finds itself in a difficult position: on the one hand, its philosophy dictates that a woman should be able to do whatever she likes with her body; on the other hand, it sees prostitution as dehumanizing and sexist. Prostitutes themselves also support decriminalization and, in the USA and France, have formed pressure groups geared towards that end. *Coyote* (Call Off Your Old Tired Ethics) is one such American organization (Anderson 1975). In England, the Sexual Law Reform Society (1975) is also pledged to decriminalization. The law, it argues, should be based on 'annoyance, injury or nuisance to specific citizens and no person should be convicted of such annoyance without the evidence of the person aggrieved'.

There is also a rather different movement committed to regularization of prostitution. It envisages government licensing of prostitutes, statutory medical examinations, and other controls. In this country such a movement is very much in its infancy, though it recalls similar movements in the nineteenth century. There is no evidence that regulation is successful at controlling prostitution (Sion 1977). France abolished controls in 1946, Italy in 1958 (Honoré 1978).

Homosexuality

Homosexuality, according to Plummer (1975), 'refers to sexual experience, actual or imagined, between members of the same sex, which may be accompanied by emotional involvements'. As a clinical entity it does not exist, for its forms are as varied as heterosexuality (Hooker 1957; Sagarin 1974). Discussion of homosexuality is usually found within the rhetoric of either sin or mental health – the American Psychiatric Association dropped it from its list of mental disorders as late as 1974 (see chapters 7 and 9). Gagnon and Simon (1974) who are critical of these approaches, attack the existing literature for being 'ruled by a simplistic and homogeneous view of the psychological and social contents of the category of "homosexual"' and at the same time for concentrating on the 'least rewarding of all questions, that of etiology'. There is too much emphasis on 'homosexuality' as a condition and too little understanding of it as process (Plummer 1975). It may well be that our very sense of boundary derives from the existence of legal sanctions (Gagnon and Simon 1974).

Kinsey's studies (1948) demonstrate that homosexuality and heterosexuality are not polar concepts. He showed that the behaviour of many was not an either – or proposition. He found that only 4 per cent of the male white population were exclusively homosexual throughout their lives, yet 37 per cent had had at least one homosexual experience to the point of orgasm: 50 per cent had had some homosexual experience during their adult life. The figures for females were lower, respectively 2, 13, and 28 per cent in 1953. 'Legal literature commonly thinks of homosexual activity as being performed for orgastic pleasure whereas this may be insignificant . . . The mutual dependency, which is often intense, may be far more important than sexual activity' (Slovenko 1965).

The lot (pun unintended) of the homosexual has been graphically described by Plummer (1975).

Around the subject of homosexuality has emerged a vast superstructure of beliefs and imagery which help to conceal an underlying relationship by which dominant heterosexual groups tacitly but persistently oppress and attack homosexual groups. Whether this domination takes the form of being burnt at the stake as a heretic or murdered on a common by 'queer-bashers'; whether it takes the form of penitentials in medieval cloisters or exclusion from employment and country; whether it takes the form of being pilloried in the market square or mimicked and mocked on television and radio; whether it takes the form of trial and imprisonment or psychiatric examination and therapy; whether it is devalued as sin, sickness, crime or simply a sorrowful state – in each and every case the structure of the relationship is politically similar: a dominant group, probably unwittingly, coerces and controls a subordinate one.

To this may be added exposure to blackmail (Gagnon and Simon (1974) suggest as many of 15 per cent of all homosexuals have been blackmailed at some time: the Dirk Bogarde film *Victim* did much to bring this evil to public attention), police harassment (Gallo, *et al.* 1966), entrapment (Szasz (1970) suggests the episode in Sodom is the earliest account of entrapment of homosexuals, the law enforcement agents being 'God's plain-clothesmen'), and ostracism. Homosexuals appear to be victimized with considerable frequency (Sagarin and Macnamara 1975).

Other societies have been more tolerant of homosexuality. Ford and Beach (1952) found that in 64 per cent of the 72 simpler societies they studied, homosexuality was considered acceptable for some groups. Gebhard's survey of 193 world cultures showed that only 14 per cent rejected homosexuality (1969). Yet in England and the USA the reaction has been extremely hostile. Simmons (1965) asked American respondents: 'What is deviance?' More identified homosexuals than any other stereotypical category. Gorer's English study (1971) found that over half his male respondents, and just under half his female respondents, viewed homosexuality in strong, negative terms of disapproval. Another one-third saw them as sick. Schofield (1973) found the young to be more tolerant.

The law in England no longer punishes homosexual behaviour in private between consenting adults (Sexual Offences Act 1967). Nor does it in Illinois, New York, Connecticut, or six other states in the USA. It has not been a crime in France, Belgium, or the Scandinavian countries for some considerable time. In England, homosexuality came within the province of the ecclesiastical courts until 1533. They handed over convicted homosexuals to the civil authorities for burning. Apparently, this rarely happened (Pollock and Maitland 1898). The 1533 Act, part of Henry VIII's campaign to assert royal supremacy against the authority of the church (Hyde 1970), imposed the death penalty for buggery. The death penalty was removed in 1861 (the maximum sentence then became penal servitude for life). The scope of the law was extended from buggery (that is anal connection) to all homosexual practices by the Criminal Law Amendment Act 1885. The change was the result of a peripheral amendment to a bill which aimed to protect women and girls and suppress brothels. Though a major alteration in the law it was not debated. 'It is extremely doubtful if either parliament or the government of the day were aware of the substantial change they had directed in the law against homosexuality' (Robinson 1964; see also Hyde 1948). Then in 1898, the Vagrancy Act made it an offence for a male to solicit persistently in a public place for an immoral purpose. The Act was intended to prevent men from trying to obtain clients for prostitutes but it came to be widely used to stop solicitation for homosexual purposes. The equivalent Scottish Act (the Immoral Trade (Scotland) Act 1902) has not been so used (Wolfenden 1957).

The law began to be questioned in the early 1950s, and the Wolfenden committee was appointed in 1954. Its report, issued in 1957, concluded: 'we do not think it proper for the law to concern itself with what a man does in private unless it can be shown to be so contrary to the public good that the law ought to intervene in its function as the guardian of the public good'. It was another 10 years before legislation was passed to implement the proposal that the taint of criminality should be removed from homosexual acts by consenting adults committed in private (Richards 1970). 'The one determined lobby against the Bill came from the National Maritime Board and the National Union of Seamen and this was designed to exclude the Merchant Navy from its provisions' (Richards 1970). The sponsors of the Bill yielded, otherwise the whole Act could well have been lost.

Current English law is particularly complicated. One must distinguish buggery involving anal penetration and gross indecency. Buggery with a boy under 16 years of age (or with a woman or animal) carries a penalty of life imprisonment. Buggery with an unwilling male over 16 carries a maximum penalty of 10-years' imprisonment. Buggery with a consenting partner carries only a two-year penalty, provided that the participants are both over 21 years, or both under that age (subject to the exception listed below). Where one of the partners is over and the other is under 21 years of age, the older man becomes liable to 5-years imprisonment.

An act of gross indecency (which is not further defined) between two consenting males is punishable by two-years' imprisonment (five years if the defendant is over 21 and his partner under 21 years of age). If a male procures or attempts to procure a male under 21-years-old to commit an act of gross indecency with a third party he may also be sentenced to five-years' imprisonment. If the partner is a boy under 16 the maximum sentence is 10-years' imprisonment.

The Sexual Offences Act 1967 introduced one important exception to all this. It provided that in England and Wales, but not in Scotland or Northern Ireland, buggery and gross indecency by male couples are not offences, provided both participants are consenting civilians over 21 years of age, and provided their conduct occurs in private with no third party present. Members of the Forces are still subject to court-martial for homosexual conduct. The crews of UK merchant ships are also still exposed to the criminal sanctions listed above.

Males are also subject to criminal penalties for persistently soliciting or importuning for immoral purposes (s.32 of Sexual Offences Act 1956 and see *R* v. *Ford* (1977) Crim. L.R.688). The maximum penalty is two-years' imprisonment. The Home Office Report on Vagrancy and Street Offences (1976) recommends the offence be retained with lower maximum penalties. In practice it means that men who loiter in the vicinity of public lavatories or 'gay' bars are liable to prosecution. It is not necessary to prove evidence of annoyance. There is no doubt that the police use decoys to secure arrests.

The law, though an improvement on the pre-1967 situation, is unsatisfactory on several counts. The law still discriminates against homosexuals (Sexual Law Reform Society Report (1975)).

(i)   The age of consent is 21 years: a girl can consent to heterosexual intercourse at 16; heterosexuals can marry at 16; and, of course, the age of majority is 18.

(ii)   Males can solicit women with impunity (*Crook* v. *Edmondson* above) but not other men. Indeed, women can solicit men, but not if they do so in the streets for the purpose of prostitution.

(iii) The definition of what constitutes a homosexual act 'in private' is far more narrowly drawn than in the case of heterosexual acts. Privacy requires that only two persons shall be present. Since the 1967 Act was passed the recorded incidence of the offence of indecency between males has doubled, and the number of persons prosecuted for the offence has trebled (Walmsley 1978).

(iv)   The Armed Forces and Merchant Seamen are still penalized by the old provisions, even where off-duty or on leave.

(v)   The penalties are still severer than those for equivalent heterosexual offences.

(vi)   It is still an offence for a third party to procure a homosexual act, even one legalized by the 1967 Act.

(vii) Advertisements in a magazine inviting homosexual acts may amount to a conspiracy to corrupt public morals (*Knuller* v. *D.P.P.* [1973] AC 435).

(viii) Scotland and Northern Ireland are still excluded from the liberalization of the 1967 Act.

The effects of all this are that blackmail, for example, is still possible. Thus, a mature 18-year-old man who chooses to participate in homosexual conduct with a man of 21 can blackmail the older man, knowing that his victim will not complain for fear of a trial and potentially heavy prison sentence. However, it is thought that blackmail is still prevalent even where the behaviour no longer constitutes a criminal offence: the threat is no longer to expose to the police but, for example his employers. In a society where stigma still attaches to homosexuality, such threats are very potent.

Another effect is that social workers, psychiatrists, marriage guidance counsellors, and others cannot easily provide the guidance that they might wish to give for fear of being accused of encouraging what the law still regards as a crime (Sherwin 1965). It is true that the Director of Public Prosecutions must be consulted before proceedings are taken involving a homosexual offence and a person under 21. But prosecutions nevertheless take place, even where both participants are under that age. The *Criminal Statistics* do not distinguish between the different offences clearly enough to draw any conclusions but we do know that, in 1975, 125 men were sent to prison for buggery, another 152 men (and 1 woman) for attempting to commit buggery, and 27 more for indecency between males. Sentences for deterrent purposes can be severe. (See *R* v. *Gillespie* (1977) Crim. L.R.429; *R* v. *Meadows* (1977) Crim. L.R.429). It is to be assumed that the victims of few if any of these men were consenting adults under 21: the statistics do not classify the age, sex, or willingness of the victim (nor, for that matter, do they tell us how many and what animals were involved!).

The situation in much of the USA, however, is worse. The Supreme Court has recently ruled that it is constitutional for states to forbid unnatural acts by consenting adults in private. The court, without comment, ruled by 6 to 3 that a Virginia Appeals court was correct in sustaining the constitutionality of a law of that state prohibiting sodomy. The Virginia court had quoted Leviticus, and then stated that the prohibited conduct was likely to end in a contribution to moral delinquency (*Doe* v. *Commonwealth's Attorney for City of Richmond* 44 U.S.L.Week3545 (1976) Even though enforcement of these laws is rare (McGaghy 1976), the police apparently rely on statutes of lesser severity to deal with homosexuality. Thus '"vagrancy" laws are a convenient catchall used ... to harass homosexuals' (Weinberg and Williams 1974). The sentence may not be severe but its consequences are still grave.

Lesbianism

Lesbianism is, of course, homosexuality. It is separated here from male homosexuality not to romanticize or minimize it (Socarides 1965), but because the attitude of the law towards female homosexuality is so very different from that towards the male counterpart. Lesbianism may be seen as less of a problem than male homosexuality. Female homosexual-paedophilia is rare. Society is probably offended less by lesbianism than male homosexuality. Less is known about it and the literature is scanty (Gagnon and Simon 1974). Today it is often a 'political act' (Hite 1977). Lesbianism has never been a crime in England, nor anywhere else, so far as is known. Socarides (1965) says he has known of no instances in which female homosexuals were trapped by the police using female detectives and unmarked police prowl cars, and one suspects that this almost never happens.

The expression of lesbianism may amount to a common assault, an indecent assault, or an offence under the Indecency with Children Act 1960. If lesbian activities are carried out in the street, or any public place to the annoyance of residents or others, they would probably be classed as one of the offences created by the many by-laws which regulate conduct offensive to the public sense of decency. Lesbians are penalized by the law in other ways. Thus, it has recently been alleged (Stephens 1976) that courts are reluctant to give custody of a child to a lesbian mother. Further, it is clear that lesbian activities would be regarded as 'unreasonable behaviour' for the purposes of divorce (Rayden 1974). An allegation that a woman is a lesbian is actionable as slander without proof of special damage (Slander of Women Act 1891, as interpreted in *Kerr* v. *Kennedy* [1942] 1 K.B.409).

Transvestism

Transvestites are usually males, heterosexual, and married. But marriage relationships may not be very important for them. Transvestism tends to assert itself where there is a 'perceived difficulty in establishing successful masculine and heterosexual identity, combined with a blockage of the possibility of achieving a homosexual identity' (Taylor Buckner 1970).

There are two types of transvestite: exhibitionistic and non-exhibitionistic (Enelow 1965). In the exhibitionistic form the individual, male or female, has the need to be viewed by others in the clothes of the opposite sex, and is probably less inclined to masturbatory gratification than the non-exhibitionist. The exhibitionist transvestite may be homosexual. The non-exhibitionist is usually not and is less likely to be psychotic. Masturbatory fantasies are a feature of this type of transvestism. See Chapter 5.

Karpman (1954) says 'transvestism as such is not likely to be involved with the law but there is a definite law against it, and there are transvestites who dress up and parade the streets and are apprehended by the police'. But, as Enelow indicates (1965), 'this group of transvestites who come into conflict with the law, that is, the exhibitionist group, are apparently in the minority. The majority of people with this disorder are usually not discovered, or if they are discovered are not brought to the courts'. Men are more likely to run foul of the law than women. This is the result of greater cultural acceptance of women dressing as men that vice versa.

In England, transvestites may be charged with a number of offences ranging from behaviour likely to cause a breach of the peace, or loitering with intent to commit a felony (Vagrancy Act 1824 s.4), to importuning (s.32 of Sexual Offences Act (1956). It is also possible that dressing in the clothes of the opposite sex may amount to fraud or deception for the purpose of various offences of dishonesty.

Fetishism

Fetishism is a sexual affective state held by an individual towards an object or part of a person of such intensity that the object or part of the person serves as a primary source of arousal and consummation (Storr 1964; Epstein 1965). Fetishes tend to be feminine symbols: the high-heeled shoe is probably the commonest fetish of all. Nearly all fetishists are men: minor degrees of fetishism can be detected in all men. Fetishism becomes a sexual deviation when the fetish is totally substituted for the person, and becomes the end in itself rather than a means. Fetishism is neither rare nor exotic (Becker 1963). Fetishism often involves 'theft', the 'borrowing', for example, of women's panties. If they belong to a friend, relative, or lover nothing may be said: 'it is only when [the fetishist] goes outside into the community and "steals" that the fetishist and his work becomes visible' (Plummer 1975). In the same way if a wife willingly dresses in rubber wear for her husband, the problematic nature of her husband's deviation decreases (North 1970). See also Chapter 4.

In itself fetishism is not a crime. Most fetishists do not run foul of the law. But fetishistic behaviour may lead to a whole gamut of crimes. A fetishist may feel an overpowering desire to grasp the object to which he is sexually attracted. Stealing women's underwear from washing lines is common. The case of *R*. v. *George* has been considered. In his pursuit of sexual gratification via girls' shoes, he was found guilty of assault. He had also been charged with attempted larceny (now theft). Potentially the cause of any crime can be attributed to fetishistic motivation. (Haines and Zeidler 1961). There is a well-documented case of a variety of murders committed by an individual who exhibited fetishistic behaviour (Kennedy, Hoffman, and Haines 1947).

Voyeurism

Voyeurism or scopophilia is very widespread. As with fetishism, it can properly be described as a deviation only where it substitutes for normal sexual activity. According to Storr (1964), in one study 65 per cent of males admitted to have engaged in voyeuristic activity, whilst 83 per cent would have liked to do so. Striptease shows will always be popular amongst men. Rosen (1965) distinguishes three types of 'looking': compulsive looking, looking and touching which may involve frotteurism, and voyeurism.

The pathology of compulsive looking and 'fully developed voyeur-istic perversion' (Rosen 1965) may be distinguishable, but the law does not distinguish them. Neither is in itself a crime but both may involve a number of offences. The behaviour of 'peeping toms' is apt to occasion a breach of the peace, and voyeurs may be bound over to be of good behaviour. They may be charged with being a public nuisance, but this charge will only be sustained where a large number of people has had to complain, and this will be rare. Burglary and attempted burglary are other possible charges (Theft Act 1968 s.9). Neither are particularly likely as the voyeur would have to enter a building as a trespasser with intent to commit a specified offence, such as, theft, rape, grievous bodily harm, or criminal damage. But voyeurs who are also fetishists (for example, on a pantie raid) or pyromaniacs (Rubenstein 1965; Lewis 1965), which is also often connected with voyeurism, could find themselves accused of burglary or its attempt.

Looking and touching may involve other offences. It may result in the man exposing himself and then inviting the female to touch or masturbate him. This would constitute the crimes of indecent exposure (an offence at common law and under s.4 of the Vagrancy Act 1824) and, if the female is under 14 years of age, indecency with children (Indecency with Children Act 1960). It may lead to mutual stimulation or frottage with the man stimulating himself to the point of orgasm: in so doing, the offences of common assault and indecent assault would be committed.

Exhibitionism

Exhibitionism is probably the commonest sex offence. In addition to that which comes to attention, a vast amount is unreported (Coleman 1964). Perhaps 20–35 per cent of all sex offenders are exhibitionists. Radzinowicz (1957) found that 80 per cent of exhibitionists were first offenders. The other 20 per cent had been convicted of previous sexual offences but 78 per cent of these offences were also for indecent exposure. Thus, there is a high rate of recidivism for exhibitionists. Most exhibitionists are non-violent. Fifty per cent of their victims are under 16 years of age: but in most of those cases where sexual assault also takes place, the offence is of a minor nature and no physical injury is done to the child (Allen 1969). See Chapter 6.

At common law it is a misdemeanour to commit an outraging of public decency in public and in such a way that more than one person sees, or is at least able to see, the act (*R.* v. *Sedley* (1663)). Sir Charles Sedley was indicted for exposing himself naked on a balcony 'in Covent Garden and urinating on the crowd beneath. The offence is in the nature of a public nuisance. The essential element is publicity. It may or may not involve a sexual motive and it is not necessary that there be any intent to insult or offend any other person. A wide view is taken of 'in public' and private premises may be so regarded, provided more than one person must at least have been able to see the act (*R.* v. *Mayling* [1963] 2 Q.B.717).

It is an offence under s.4 of the Vagrancy Act 1824 'wilfully, openly, lewdly and obscenely' to expose ones 'person with intent to insult any female'. 'Person' means penis (*Evans* v. *Ewels* [1972] 2 All E.R.22), 'The exposure of the backside' is not within the section (Radzinowicz 1957). The offence may be committed in public or in private (Criminal Justice Act 1925 s.42), and the exposure is committed 'openly' even if it occurs in the exposer's own bedroom (*Ford* v. *Falcone* [1971] 2 All E.R.1138). A specific intent to insult must be proved.

It is also an offence under the Town Police Clauses Act 1847 s.28 and under numerous local acts and by–laws, some of which are set out in Radzinowicz (1957). Thus, the Hyde Park Regulations 1932 provide: 'no person shall sit, lie, rest or sleep on any seat or any part of the Park in any indecent posture or behave in any manner reasonably likely to offend against public decency.'

The latest criminal statistics show that, in 1975, 2495 persons (all male) were found guilty of indecent exposure. Fifty-seven were sent to prison, 1348 fined, 21 bound over, and hospital orders under s.60 of the Mental Health Act 1959 were made in the case of 15 offenders. We do not know how many were first remanded for medical and psychiatric reports. In many cases fines and short terms of imprisonment may do little harm. But where there are 'well-developed perversions' neither fines nor imprisonment 'diminish the repetition compulsion especially in the impulsive type of exhibitionist' (Rosen 1965).

Both the Law Commission (1974) and the Home Office (1976*b*) have made recommendations to reform this area of law. They are broadly in agreement that the existing law should be repealed and replaced by an offence, the ingredients of which would be that a man has exposed his genital organs knowing that it is likely that other people will see him, in circumstances where those who are likely to see him are likely to be offended. The Home Office also suggests that female nudity in public in circumstances likely to cause offence should be made a criminal offence.

Bestiality

Bestiality can be committed by both men and women. It consists in having any kind of sexual intercourse with an animal. Most cases occur in the country, where farm labourers have been known to have intercourse with a wide variety of domestic animals. There are also reported instances of women having sexual relations with dogs and other animals. In *R.* v. *Bourne* ((1952) 36 Cr. App.R.125), a man compelled his wife to submit on two occasions to the insertion of the male organ of an Alsatian, which he had excited, into her vagina. He was convicted of aiding and abetting her to commit buggery. She was not charged with any offence but the Court of Criminal Appeal assumed she was entitled to be acquitted.

Under the Sexual Offences Act 1956 s.12, bestiality carries a maximum of life imprisonment. It has been argued (Brazier 1975) that the crime as such should be abolished. Its retention is justified on two grounds: (i) that it is repulsive and (ii) that it is cruel to animals. The first justification is not sound and the second could be taken care of by prosecuting the offender under cruelty to animals legislation. There is also a school of thought which claims that animals have 'rights', one of which might be their sexual freedom (Clark 1977). It must be assumed that few cases are detected: the 'victims' do not usually report the offences to the police. However, if the offence were to be abolished, which is unlikely, it is difficult to see with what Bourne could have been charged.

Sodomy with a woman

This consists in sexual intercourse *per anum* by a man with a woman. It can be committed by a husband with his wife. Penetration must be proved: emission is not necessary. Consent is no defence: indeed, the consenting party is also guilty of the offence, as a principal offender. The law is thus in the highly anomalous situation that two consenting males may do with impunity what a husband and wife risk a sentence of life imprisonment for doing. Though not uncommon – for reasons suggested by Storr (1964) – it is still regarded by many with horror. Apparently, sodomy and heresy were frequently associated in medieval times. It has even been suggested that an act of sodomy is described in *Lady Chatterley's Lover* and that, if the jury had realized this, they might have found Lawrence's novel to be obscene. Many psychiatrists and social workers must break the law regularly by knowing about, or even encouraging for therapeutic purposes, acts of sodomy between husband and wife. It is impossible to defend the retention of this crime where adults consent to it, particularly in the light of the 1967 reform in relation to homosexual practices.

Necrophilia

Necrophilia is assumed to be rare. It is not specifically proscribed by English law. There may be an offence of 'outraging decency' (*Knuller* v. *D.P.P.* [1973] A.C.435), and necrophilia might come within its contours. If carried out in public or with intent to insult a female in private, it could fall within one of the exhibitionism offences outlined above.

Sadism

Hartwich (1962) defines sadism as 'the experiencing of sexual desire up to the pitch of orgasm, when accompanied by humiliations, chastisement and all manner of cruelties inflicted upon a human being or an animal', and also as 'the impulse to evoke such feelings of desire by means of the appropriate treatment'. Sadism and masochism are bipolar manifestations of the same drive (Rothman 1968, Klein 1972; The history of flagellation is now well documented (Gibson 1978) see also Chapters 2 and 10). As was indicated in the discussion of rape, not all violent sexual crimes are sadistic in motivation. Sado-masochistic practices are found in conjugal relations and in homosexual practices, and are common activities for the prostitute and her client. Flagellations do not usually cause undue physical pain for 'the environment is one of controlled violence' (Leigh 1976). There is, of course, the possibility that 'the lines of communication between the partners will become blurred, resulting in the inflicting of greater violence than was in the customer's contemplation' (Leigh 1976). It is these cases that are more likely to come to the attention of the police.

Many crimes, and not just sexual offences, may be expressions of sadism. 'Sadism *per se* is not a mental disorder within the meaning of the Mental Health Act 1959 and does not legally excuse or mitigate murder or other serious crimes against the person. It may be an expression of psychopathic disorder, psychosis, subnormality or organic brain disease' (Power 1976). But sadism more commonly expresses itself in actions which amount to common or indecent assault, or assaults occasioning actual (or more rarely) grievous bodily harm. In English law, 'the infliction of some harm is not criminal provided that the victim consents to the harm' (Leigh 1976). What the law is saying in effect is that consent is a defence to an otherwise criminal assault (*R* v. *Donovan* [1934] 2 K.B. 498). If, on the other hand, the blows are likely or intended to cause bodily harm, the act is criminal whether the victim consents or not. the court said 'there were many gradations between a slight tap and a severe blow'. This leaves the law in a very uncertain state. The Canadian solution is preferable: Canada defines assault as the non-consensual application of force (Criminal Code (1970) sec.244).

Making obscene telephone calls

This may be described as the 'symbolic equivalent' of voyeurism (Power 1976). Offenders are almost exclusively male; many are young and timid, the majority are probably harmless. Offenders are difficult to trace but, if located, may be charged with insulting behaviour, or behaviour likely to cause a breach of the peace. Making obscene telephone calls is also an offence under the Post Office Act 1969 s.78 (and see *R* v. *Norbury* (1978) Crim. L.R.435). The sending of any message by telephone that is 'grossly offensive, or of an indecent, obscene or menacing character' is punishable by a £50 fine, 1-month imprisonment or both.

A note on transsexualism

The transsexual is someone who adopts totally the identity of the other sex. The majority of transsexuals are born into the male sex but have taken on a feminine gender role. Many also undergo surgical treatment to remove, what for them, are redundant appendages. There have been a number of well-publicized cases: April Ashley and Jan Morris are two of the better known, the latter has written up her experiences in *Conundrum* (1974). (See also Chapter 5.)

As far as the law is concerned, the transsexual raises two major problems. The first concerns legality of the surgical operation. The second relates to the question of the transsexual's status. How is the law to classify him/her? Is it to characterize him/her in the same way for all purposes?

It may be doubted whether surgical operations, involving converting someone from one sex to a state where they present a convincing picture of the other, are lawful in England. In principle there is no reason why they should not be: one is entitled to consent to surgery at 16 years of age. But surgery to remove sexual organs has for public policy reasons been excluded from the general principle. As a result most transsexual surgery tends to take place outside England, commonly in Casablanca. However, there are now hospitals in England where the necessary operative work is undertaken in spite of the seeming unlawfulness of such action.

There is no doubt as to the transsexual's status in English law. Sex is fixed at birth and cannot be changed thereafter. Thus, in the only case to reach an English court, *Corbett* v. *Corbett* ([1970] 2 All E.R.33) Ormrod J. held that April Ashley, 'a convincing feminine pastiche' was still of the male sex in spite of 'her' undoubted adoption of a feminine gender role. The judge held that sex was tested by chromosomal, gonadal, and genital factors and possibly by hormonal (secondary sexual) characteristics. Psychological considerations were irrelevant. He recognized the phenomenon of inter-sex, the classic case of the hermaphrodite, where there was an absence of congruence between the first three factors. In such a case, Ormrod J. opined, he would place greatest emphasis on genital considerations. But April Ashley was 'male' because there was no doubt as to the congruence of the primary factors at 'her' birth, and that was the latest time (mistakes apart) when sexual classification could be made. Ormrod J. did, however, limit himself to pronouncing on April Ashley's sex for the purpose of marriage. He was, he said, not concerned with her status 'at large'. Her marriage was declared to be no marriage (her husband was a transvestite male). Statute now declares that a marriage is void if the marriage partners are not respectively male and female (Matrimonial

Causes Act 1973 s.11 (c)). Thus, the marriage of a transsexual like April Ashley or Jan Morris to a woman would be upheld as valid by an English court. It would, however, be voidable at the option of the 'wife', certainly for incapacity and more doubtfully for wilful refusal to consummate the marriage (M.C.A. 1973 s.12 (a) (b)).

Ormrod J.'s judgment, however, leaves open the status of a transsexual for purposes other than marriage. It is thought that for most other purposes, there will be recognition of gender. Thus, she would get a woman's national insurance card, go to a women's prison, etc. She could be charged with soliciting and could be the victim of rape.

The law is most unsatisfactory. It may, with justification, be asked what interest the state has got in preserving a citizen's sexual identity. One can change one's name easily and one's nationality without too much trouble, but not one's sex. Other countries, Switzerland, for example, take account of psychological considerations and the English law should follow their example. The gravest error in Ormrod J.'s reasoning was to tie the essential role of woman in marriage to the task of procreating children. The fallacies of this line of reasoning are numerous and obvious (Kennedy 1973, Smith 1971).

Treatment of sex offenders

The word 'treatment' is used to conform with contemporary terminology. Medical imagery has replaced the legal-punitive in discussions about the disposition of offenders. The therapeutic model is now all-powerful: but it should not be forgotten that looked at from the viewpoint of the offender treatment may be brutal punishment. Locking up a person's mind with drugs is at least as harsh as confining his body within prison walls. Advancing technology may eventually enable us to do away with the fabric of prisons: human warehouses may be replaced by sophisticated monitoring devices (Cohen 1974). However effective this may be, we cannot pretend that it is humane.

Treatment assumes that there is something wrong with the offender: that his behaviour is inherent to his condition. 'The very fact that a person is seen to need rehabilitation implies that he was once habilitated and now needs the process to be repeated' (Bean 1976). Further, no one is quite sure what constitutes rehabilitation. Decisions are, of course, based on 'a reliance of professional judgement' (Matza

1964). It is difficult for the 'patient' to refuse treatment (Plotkin 1977). The prisoner or patient is said to be rehabilitated 'when a specifically defined goal has been reached' (Rapaport 1971). Implicit in this is a sense of values and moral ordering, and a consensus. Psychiatric diagnoses are moral evaluations (Goffman 1961). But therapists act as· if there were no conflict between them and their patients. For these reasons it is wrong to suppose a qualitative difference between the penal and the therapeutic, whatever the supposed difference of approach (Pearson 1975).

The legal systems of the world, together with medical and psychiatric professions of each society, have developed numerous ways of tackling sexual deviance (Bancroft 1974). One must, of course, distinguish between those who offend against the law and those who do not, or rather, given the vast amount of hidden sexual deviation, between those labelled deviants by agents of control or who identify themselves as such and those who do not surface to the attention of 'significant others'. The latter, who constitute the greatest number of sexual deviants, are not 'official deviants' (Box 1971) and do not attract treatment, though informal social control is insidious enough to affect all of us from cradle to grave. One must also distinguish different types of sexual deviation. For a start they provoke different reactions. Rape may call forth a need for vengeance and a sense of horror. Living off immoral earnings may evoke anger and disgust. The public, aided by the press (Cohen 1972), conjures forth stereotypes of each. On any criterion such disparate offences merit different treatment.

The Cambridge Report on Sexual Offences (Radzinowicz 1957) found that 4 in 10 of all sexual offenders who were tried were fined; one-quarter were sent to prison; and 16 per cent were put on probation. The period since this report has been one of innovation in the penal system: it has seen the development of suspended sentences and the community service order as well as an increased emphasis on the social enquiry report, on psychiatric treatment and on the rehabilitative ideal. We have, however, no more recent study of the disposition of sexual offenders. Disparities in sentencing are common and frequently commented upon (Hood 1962; Bottomley 1973). This is not the place to account for these though it must be noted that severe sentences are sometimes engineered by moral panics when a particular offence is prevalent in a certain place at a particular time. Offenders may be given medical or psychiatric treatment once in prison. There is, however, little provision made for sentences with specifically medical aims. One exception is the probation order with a condition for mental treatment. Hospital and guardianship orders may be made by courts under the Mental Health Act 1959, but they rarely do this and decisions to transfer a prisoner to a mental institution tend to be left to the prison administration. Such a transfer needs the approval of the Secretary of State.

In much of the USA, there is specific legislation to deal with sexual psychopaths (Bowman and Engle 1965; Swanson 1960; Slovenko and Phillips 1962). Sexual psychopaths are defined as persons who lack the power to control their sexual impulses or who have criminal propensities towards the commission of sex offences. Most of the states require a person to have been convicted of some offence, but some simply demand that cause be shown that he is probably a sexual psychopath. The legislation is coming under increasing attack. As Slovenko (1965) puts it:

the vagueness of the definition of a sexual psychopath has resulted in the commitment for long periods of time – at state expense – of many nuisance-type, non-dangerous sex offenders, such as the homosexual, the exhibitionist, and the peeping tom. The legislation has resulted in a round-up of the nuisance-type offender and left untouched the dangerous, aggressive offender. The purpose of the legislation has been lost in its application.

Sentences are indeterminate, and presuppose the existence of adequate psychiatric assistance, which is not always available. Perhaps, the most serious criticism of this type of legislation is that it lacks 'scientific foundation', thus 'if one uses the medical framework, sexual deviation simply refers to a symptom, but, if one however uses a psychosocial framework, it refers to a type of behaviour' (Slovenko 1965). It has been held constitutional to detain a sexual psychopath for treatment for a longer time than that for which he might have been sentenced if he were so classified. (*Trueblood* v. *Tinsley* 366 P 2d 655 (1961)). Reforms have recently been suggested. Sidley and Stolarz (1973) have argued that what is required is a 'dangerous sex-offender' law. Commitment of such an offender would depend on (i) the commission of the sexual offence in which his victim was injured (but what constitutes injury? is the willing partner in a statutory rape injured?); and (ii) a convincing demonstration by the person making predictions about the offender's future behaviour, that the offender will, within a period of one year, unless he is incarcerated or treated, commit a sexual offence that will result in physical injury to his victim.

But how does a psychiatrist determine this? We are told that a heterosexual aggressor 'who has no insight' satisfies the second limb. What is 'insight'? The moral overtones of evaluations like this are undeniable. The truth of the matter is that legislation of this nature is apt to be dangerously vague: indefinite commitments on such criteria offend the rule of law and should be repealed. Hospital orders in this country are subject to similar criticisms. (Gostin 1977, Honore 1978). The Butler report (1975) has recommended amending the Mental Health Act so that a psychopathic disorder consisting of a sexual deviation alone should not be a ground for a hospital order. Report of the Committee on Mentally Abnormal Offenders, Cmnd 6244, London.

Sexual deviation is treated in a number of other ways. Bieber *et al.* (1962) say that analytical psychotherapy is an appropriate treatment for sex criminals in general, but, as judged by the reduction in the reconviction rate, its practical value may be doubted (Field and Williams 1971). Aversion therapy is used mainly to 'treat' homosexuality, transvestism, and fetishism (Gibbens 1967). Storr (1964) thinks 'it is too early yet to say whether it is a permanently effective treatment, or what disadvantages may accompany it'. Many will think it totally repellent (see Chapter 12). Hormonal 'treatment' is a similarly repulsive approach (see Chapter 1). Field and Williams (1970), for example, advocate subcutaneous implants of oestradiol. This induces testicular atrophy. Field and Williams's study shows that 16 out of 25 of their implant group were not reconvicted of a sex offence over a 2-year period: 8 were, however, convicted of non-sexual offences. It is, however, difficult to define a non-sexual offence. These individuals may now be expressing their general frustration through other criminal outlets. Twenty out of 37 of a control group, who were given a placebo, were similarly not reconvicted of a sexual offence; 8 were reconvicted of a non-sexual offence; and 9 reconvicted of sex offences. Defenders of these inhuman experiments argue that 'these individuals appreciate treatment', whilst conceding 'dosage should be adjusted to allow some sexual activity' (Power 1976). What makes this form of experimentation all the more unacceptable is the belief that 'objective conclusions' may be reached and that 'this procedure could help decide when a sexual offender who has killed may be safely released. The view may be taken that such men should be detained until physiological waning of the sex drive occurs in old age' (Power 1976). Power is a Senior Medical officer in H.M. Prison Service. Other drugs used include Benperidol and

Cyproterone Acetate, which Power (1976) tells us 'is *alleged* not to cause any *significant undesirable* effects' (my italics). It is used apparently in the 'treatment' of sexual exhibitionism, excessive masturbation, paedophilia, and 'to relieve depression secondary to abnormal sexual practices'. See Chapter 1 page 21.

In Scandinavia, castration of sexual recidivists is performed fairly extensively. It is usually carried out with consent (*sic*), often influenced by promises of earlier release from prison or security hospital. Not surprisingly, 'some castrated individuals remain embittered and resentful' (Power 1976). The value of castration may be doubted for of 900 men castrated in Denmark between 1929 and 1959, 10 committed sex crimes after the operation. The average relapse rate is 20 per cent. Castrated adult males may still remain capable of erection and orgasm (Bremer 1959). Sturup (1968) reports that, of 284 men castrated at Herstedvester between 1935 and 1967, 5 committed suicide within 5-years of their operations. He also indicates that few regretted being castrated. That this is punishment and not treatment is quite clearly expressed in statements which abound in the literature like this one from Power: 'three male patients had hypothalamotomy *for* repeated homosexual offences with pubertal boys' (1976) (italics mine). They were doctored because they had committed criminal offences.

The public probably approves of this inhumanity which masquerades as treatment. It also approves of hanging and flogging – incidentally still used in the Isle of Man for sex offences (Kneale 1973). Legislators have taken a lead and abolished corporal and capital punishment. The time will come when hormonal and surgical 'treatment', if not other forms described above, will also be removed from the battery of the prison medical officer.

Addendum

As this book was going to press the Home Secretary's Advisory Council on the Penal System published a controversial report in which it was recommended that statutory maximum sentences be reduced. The proposed new maximum for rape is 7 years, sexual intercourse with a girl under thirteen 5 years, buggery with a boy under sixteen, a woman, or an animal 7 years, and bigamy 4 years. A judge would have discretion to impose a higher sentence in exceptional cases. In defence of the report it may be said that judges anyway rarely exceed the suggested new sentences (Home Office 1978).

References

Aberle, D. W. (1963). The incest taboo and the mating pattern of animals. *Amer. Anthropol*. **65**, 253.

Adams, M. S. and Reed, J. V. (1967). Children of incest. *Paediatrics,* **40**, 55.

Allen, C. (1969). *A textbook of psychosexual disorders.* 2nd edition. London.

Altman, D. (1973). *Homosexual: oppression and liberation.* New York.

Amir, M. (1971). *Patterns in forcible rape.* Chicago.

Anderson, M. (1975). Hookers, arise!. *Hum. Behav.* 40.

Balint, M. (1957). *Problems of human pleasure and behaviour.* London.

Bancroft, J. (1974). *Deviant sexual behaviour: modification and assessment.* Oxford.

Bean, P. (1976). *Rehabilitation and deviance.* London.

Becker, H. (1963). *Outsiders.* London.

Berger, V. (1977). Man's trial, women's tribulation: rape cases in the court-room. *Columbia L. R.* **77**, 1.

Bieber, I., Dain, H. J., Dince, P. R., Drellich, M. G., Grand, H. G., Gundlach, R. H., Kremer, M. W., Rifkin, A. H., Wilbur, C. B., and Bieber, T. B. (1962). *Homosexuality: a psychoanalytical study of male homosexuals.* New York.

Blackstone, Sir W. (1765). *Commentaries on the Laws of England.* London.

Blom-Cooper, L. and Drewry, G. (1976). *Law and morality.* London.

Bohannan, P. (1967). The differing realms of law. *Amer. Anthropol.* **67**, 33.

Bones, M. (1973). *Family planning services in England and Wales.* HMSO, London.

Bottomley, K. (1973). *Decisions in the penal process.* London.

Bowman, K. and Engle, B. (1965). Sexual psychopath laws. In *Sexual behaviour and the law.* (ed. R. Slovenko).

Box, S. (1971). *Deviance, reality and society,* London.

Brazier, R. (1975). Reform of sexual offences. *Criminal Law Review* 421.

Bremer, J. (1959). *Asexualization: a follow-up of 244 cases.* London.

Britton, J. (1865). Laws of England (Original French 1290–2). (ed. F. M. Nichols). Oxford.

Brownmiller, S. (1975). *Against our will—men, women and rape.* London.

Burgess, A. W. and Holmstrom, L. L. (1973). The rape victim in the emergency ward. *Amer. J. Nursing* **1740**, 73.
—— and —— (1974). Rape trauma syndrome. *Amer. J. Psychiat.* **131**, 981.

Card, R. (1975). Sexual relations with minors. *Criminal Law Review* 370.

Carter, C. D. (1967). Risk to offspring of incest. *Lancet* (**i**), 436.

Chambliss, W. (1967). Types of deviance and the effectiveness of legal sanctions. *Wisconsin L. Rev.* 703.

Chappell, D., Geis, G., and Fogarty, F. (1974). Forcible rape: a bibliography. *J. Crim. Law*. **65**, 248.

——, Geis, R., and Geis, G. (1977). *Forcible rape*. New York.

Clark, S. L. R. (1977). *The moral status of animals*. Oxford.

Cleaver, E. (1968). *Soul on ice*. New York.

Cleveland, A. (1913). Indictments for adultery and incest before 1650, *Law Q. Rev.* **29**, 57.

Cohen, S. (1972). *Folk devils and moral panics*. London.

—— (1974). Prison as human warehouses *New Society*. (14 November).

Coleman, J. C. (1964). *Abnormal psychology and modern life* (3rd ed.). London.

Cox, B., Shirley, J., and Short, M. (1977). *The fall of Scotland Yard*. Harmondsworth.

Cretney, S. (1974). *Principles of family law*. London.

Crozier, B. (1935). Marital support. *Boston University Law Review*. **15**, 28.

Curran, D. and Parr, D. (1957). Homosexuality: analysis of 100 male cases seen in private practice. *Br. med. J.* (**i**), 797.

Davis, A. J. (1970). Sexual assaults in the Philadelphia prison system. In *The sexual scene* (eds, J. H. Gagnon and W. Simon). Chicago.

Davis, K. (1937). The sociology of prostitution. *Amer. Soc. Rev.* **45**, 215.

—— (1971). Sexual behaviour. In *Contemporary social problems* (eds, R. K. Merton and R. Nisbet). New York.

Devlin, P. (1956). *Trial by jury*. London.

—— (1965). *The enforcement of morals*. London.

Douglas, J. (1971). *American social order*. New York.

Douglas, M. (1966). *Purity and danger*. London.

Duster, T. (1970). *The legislation of morality*. New York.

Enelow, M. (1965). Public nuisance offences. In *Sexual behaviour and the law* (ed. R. Slovenko). Springfield, Illinois.

Epstein, A. W. (1965). Fetishism. In *Sexual behaviour and the law* (ed. R. Slovenko). Springfield, Illinois.

Fargier, M. O. (1976). *Le viol*. Paris.

Feminist Group (1973). Prostitution: A non-victim crime. *Issues in criminology* **8**, 137.

Ferenczi, S. (1949). Confusion of tongues between the adult and the child. *Int. J. Psychiat.* **30**, 225.

Field, L. and Williams, M. (1970). The hormonal treatment of sexual offenders. *Med. Sci. Law* **10**, 27.

—— (1971). Note on scientific assessment and treatment of sexual offenders. *Med. Sci. Law* **11**, 180.

Finlay, H. and Bissett-Johnson, A. (1972). *Family law in Australia*. Melbourne.

Fleta. (1290–2). (In Latin. Ed. H. Richardson and G. O. Sayler) 1953, 1972. London.

Ford, C. S. and Beach, F. (1952). *Patterns of sexual behaviour*. London.

Freeman, M. D. A. (1971). The search for a rational divorce law. *Current Legal Problems* **24**, 178.
—— (1972). Adultery and intolerability. *Modern Law Review* **35**, 98.
—— (1974). *The legal structure*. London.
—— (1977). Le vice anglais—Some responses of English and American law to wife abuse. *Family Law Quarterly* **11**, 199.

Fuller, L. L. (1969). Human interaction and the law. *Amer. J. Jurispr.* **14**, 1.

Gagnon, J. H. and Simon, W. (1974). *Sexual conduct*. London.

Gallo, J. J., Mason, S. M., Meisinger, L. M., Robin, K. D., Stabile, G. D., and Wynne, R. J. (1966). The consenting homosexual and the law: an empirical study of enforcement and administration in Los Angeles County. *UCLA Law Rev.* **13**, 647.

Galsworthy, J. (1906). *The man of property*. London.

Garfinkle, H. (1956). Conditions of successful degradation ceremonies. *Am. J. Sociol.* **61**, 420.
—— (1967). *Studies in ethnomethodology*. New Jersey.

Gebhard, P. (1965). *Sex offenders: an analysis of types*. London.
——. In *The same sex: an appraisal of homosexuality* (ed. R. W. Weltge). Boston

Geis, G. and Chappell, D. (1971). Forcible rapes by multiple offenders. *Abstracts on Criminology and Penology* **11**, 431.

Genet, J. (1951). *The miracle of the rose*. London.

Giaretto, H. (1976). Humanistic treatment of father-daughter incest. In *Child abuse and neglect* (eds R. Heffer and C. H. Kempe).

Gibbens, T. C. N. (1967). Is aversion therapy wrong? *New Society* **10**, 42.

Gibson, I. (1978). *The English vice*. London.

Goffman, E. (1961). *Asylums*. Harmondsworth.

Golding, M. P. (1975). *Philosophy of law*. New Jersey.

Gorer, G. (1955). *Exploring English character*. London.
—— (1971). *Sex and marriage in England today*. London.

Gostin, L. (1977). *The law relating to mentally abnormal offenders*. London.

Greenwood, V. and Young, J. (1975). *Notes on the theory of rape and its policy implications*. Paper to London Group on Deviancy.

Griffin, S. (1971). Rape: the all American crime. *Ramparts* (September issue), 28.

Haines, W. H. and Zeidler, J. C. (1961). Sexual fetishism as related to criminal acts. *J. Soc. Ther. Corrective Psychiat.* **7**, 187.

Hale, Sir M. (1736). *Ecclesiastical precedents*. London.

Hart, H. L. A. (1961). *The concept of law*. London.

—— (1963). *Law, liberty, and morality*. London.

—— (1965). *The morality of the criminal law*. Jerusalem.

—— (1967). Social solidarity and the enforcement of morality. *University of Chicago Law Rev.* **35**, 1.

Hartwich, A. (1965). *Aberrations of sexual life*. London.

Hayes, M. (1971). The use of blood tests in the pursuit of truth. *Quart Law Rev.* **87**, 86.

Heilbron Report (1975). *Advisory group on law of rape*, (Cmnd 6352) London, HMSO.

Hite, S. (1977). *The Hite Report*. London.

Home Office (1974). Working Paper.

—— (1975). *Civil judical statistics*. HMSO, London.

—— (1976a). *Criminal statistics*. (Annually). HMSO, London.

—— (1976b). *Report of the working party on vagrancy and street offences*. HMSO. London.

—— (1978). *Sentences of imprisonment—a review of maximum penalties*. HMSO, London.

Honoré, T. (1978). *Sex law*. London.

Hood, R. (1962). *Sentencing in magistrates' courts*. London.

Hooker, E. (1957). The adjustment of the male overt homosexual. *J. Projective Techniques* **21**, 18.

Horowitz, I. L. and Liebowitz, M. (1968). Social deviance and political marginality: towards a redefinition of the relation between sociology and politics. *Soc. Problems* **15**, 282.

Humphreys, L. (1970). *Tea room trade: impersonal sex in public places*. Chicago.

—— (1972). *Out of the closets: the sociology of homosexual liberation*. New Jersey.

Hyde, H. M. (1948). *The trials of Oscar Wilde*. London.

—— (1970). *The other love*. London.

Illsey, R. and Gill, D. (1968). New fashions in illegitimacy. *New society*, 709.

James, T. E. (1964). Law and the sexual offender. In (ed. I. Rosen). *The pathology and treatment of sexual deviation* London.

Johnson, E. (1970). Extramarital sexual intercourse: a methodological note. *J. Marr. Fam.* **32**, 279.

Kalven, H. and Zeisel, H. (1966). *The American jury*. Boston.

Kanin, E. J. (1967). Reference groups and sex conduct norm violation *Sociological Quarterly* **8**, 495.

Karpman, B. (1954). *The sexual offender and his offences*. New York.

Kenedy, F., Hoffman, H. R., and Haines, W. H. (1947). A study of William Heirens *Amer. J. Psychiat.* **104**, 113.

Kennedy, I. M. (1973). Transsexualism and the single sex marriage. *Anglo-Amer. Law Rev.* **2**, 112.

Kinsey, A., Pomeroy, W. B., and Martin, C. E. (1948). *Sexual behaviour in the human male*. Philadelphia.

——, ——, ——, and Gebhard, P. H. (1953). *Sexual behaviour in the human female.* Philadelphia.

Klein, D. (1973). The Etiology of Female Crime. *Issues in Criminology* **8**, 19.

Klein, H. (1972). Masochism. *Medical Aspects of Human Sexuality* **6**, 32.

Kneale, A. (1973). *Against birching.* London.

Krause, H. (1971). *Illegitimacy—law and social policy.* Indianapolis.

Lambert, J. (1970). *Crime, police, and race relations in Birmingham.* London.

Law Commission (1974). *Working Paper 57—Conspiracies relating to morals and decency,* §50–56. HMSO, London.

Lawrence, T. E. (1935). *Seven pillars of wisdom.* London.

Le Grand, C. E. (1973). Rape and rape laws: sexism in society and the law. *California L. Rev.* **61**, 932.

Leigh, L. (1976). Sado-masochism, consent and the reform of the criminal law. *Mod. Law Rev.* **39**, 130.

Lemert, E. (1967). *Human deviance, social problems and social control.* New Jersey.

Lewis, N. (1965). Pathological firesetting and sexual motivation. *Sexual behaviour and the law* (ed. R. Slovenko). Springfield, Illinois.

Livneh, E. (1967). On rape and the sanctity of matrimony. *Israel L. Rev.* **2**, 415.

Lofland, J. (1969). *Deviance and identity.* New Jersey.

Lord Chancellor's Office (1975). *Civil Judicial Statistics,* London.

Lukianowicz, N. (1972). Incest. *Br. J. Psychiatry* **120**, 301.

McCaghy, C. H. (1976). *Deviant behaviour.* London.

McGregor, O. (1957). *Divorce in England.* London.
——, Blom-Cooper, L., and Gibson, C. (1970). *Separated spouses.* London.

Maidment, S. (1978). Rape between spouses, *Family Law* **8**, 87.

Mairs, W. (1975). Letter to *The Times,* 15 July.

Maisch, H. (1973). *Incest.* London.

Manchester, A. H. (1977). *Incest and the law.* Paper presented to 2nd World Conference of International Society on Family Law, Montreal.

Marsden, D. (1973). Mothers alone. Harmondsworth.

Matza, D. (1964). *Delinquency and drift.* Chichester.

Medea, A. and Thomson, K. (1974). *Against rape.* London.

Megarry, R. (1955). *Miscellany-at-law.* London.
—— (1973). *A second miscellany-at-law.* London.

Melani, J. and Fodaski, S. (1974). Rape: the first source book for women. In (eds N. Connell and C. Wilson).

Mill, J. S. (1859). *On Liberty.* London.

Millett, K. (1973). *The prostitution papers.* New York.

Morris, J. (1974). *Conundrum.* New York.

Morris, N. and Hawkins, G. (1970). *The honest politician's guide to crime control*. Chicago.

Nagel, E. (1969). The enforcement of morals. In *Moral problems in contemporary society* (ed. P. Kurk).

North, M. (1970). *The outer fringe of sex: a study in sexual fetishism*. London.

Naamani, I. T. (1963). Marriage and divorce in Jewish law. *J. Fam. Law* **3**, 177.

Packer, H. (1968). *The limits of the criminal sanction*. Stanford University Press. London.

Payton, G. T. (1966). *Patrol procedure*, Los Angeles.

Pearson, G. (1975). *The deviant imagination*. London.

Pearl, D. (1976). Polygamy and Bigamy. *Cambridge Law Journal* **35**, 48.

Philipson, M. (1974). *Understanding crime and delinquency*. Chicago.

Plummer, K. (1975). *Sexual stigma*. London.

Pollock, F. and Maitland, F. (1898). *A history of English law*. London.

Power, D. J. (1976). Sexual deviation and crime. *Med. Sci. Law* **16**, 111.

Ploscowe, M. (1962). *Sex and the law*. New York.

——, Foster, H., and Freed, D. (1972). *Family law*. (2nd ed.). Boston.

Plotkin, R. (1977). Limiting the therapeutic orgy: mental patients' rights to refuse treatment. *Northwestern Univ. L. Rev.* **72**, 461.

Quinney, R. (1972). Who is the victim? *Criminology* **10**, 315.

Radzinowicz, L. (1957). *Sexual offences*. London.

Ranulf, S. (1938). *Moral indignation and middle class psychology*. Munksgaard, Copenhagen.

Rapaport, L. (1971). Crisis intervention as a mode of treatment. In *Theories of Social Casework*. (Eds Roberts, R. W. and Nee, R. H.). Chicago.

Rayden, N. A. (1974). *On divorce*. London.

Reiss, A. (1971). *The police and the public*. New Haven.

Reynolds, J. (1974). Rape as social control. *Catalyst* **8**, 62.

Richards, P. G. (1970). *Parliament and conscience*. London.

Robinson, K. (1964). Parliament and public attitudes. In *The pathology and treatment of sexual deviation* (ed. I. Rosen). London.

Rock, P. (1973). *Deviant behaviour*. London.

Rogers, A. J. (1973). *The economics of crime*. Hinsdale, Illinois.

Rosen, I. (1965). Exhibitionism and voyeurism. In *Sexual Behaviour and the law* (ed. R. Slovenko). Springfield, Illinois.

Rothman, G. (1968). *The riddle of cruelty*. New York.

Rubinstein, L. H. (1965). Sexual motivations in ordinary offences. In *Sexual Behaviour and the Law* (ed. R. Slovenko). Springfield, Illinois.

Russell, D. (1973). *Rape and the masculine mystique*. Paper presented at American Sociological Association Meeting.

Sagarin, E. C. (1974). Sexual criminality. In *Current prospectives on criminal behaviour* (ed. A. Blumberg). Knopf, New York.

Sagarin, E. C. and Macnamara, D. (1975). The homosexual as a crime victim. *Int. J. Criminol. Penol.* **3**, 13.

Schmideburg, M. (1956). Delinquent acts as perversions and fetishes. *Brit. J. Delinq.* **7**, 1 and 44.

Schofield, M. (1973). *Sexual behaviour of young adults*. London.

Schur, E. (1965). *Crimes without victims*. New Jersey.
—— (1969). *Our criminal society*. New Jersey.
—— (1971). *Labelling deviant behaviour*. New Jersey.
—— (1973). *Radical non-intervention*. New Jersey.
—— and Bedau, H. (1974). *Victimless crimes: two sides of a controversy*. New Jersey.

Schwendinger, J. and H. (1974). Rape Myths. *Crime and Social Justice* **1**, 18.

Scott, P. A. (1964). Definition, classification, prognosis, and treatment. *The pathology and treatment of sexual deviation*. (1st edn) (ed. I. Rosen). London.

Seemanova, E. (1971). A study of children of incestuous matings. *Hum. Her.* **21**, 108.

Sellar, D. (1969). Leviticus XVIII, the forbidden degrees and the law of incest in Scotland. *Jewish Law Annual* **1**, 229.

Sexual Law Reform Society (1975). Working Party Report. *Criminal Law Review* 323.

Sherwin, R. V. (1965). Sodomy. In *Sexual behaviour and the law* (ed. R. Slovenko). Springfield, Illinois.

Sidley, N. and Stolarz, F. (1973). A proposed 'dangerous sex offender' law. *Am. J. Psychiat.* **130**, 765.

Simmons, J. (1965). *Deviants*. Los Angeles.

Sion, A. (1977). *Prostitution and the law*. London.

Skolnick, J. (1966). *Justice without trial*. Chichester.
—— and Woodworth, R. (1968). Morality enforcement and totalitarian potential. In *Orthopsychiatry and the law* (eds I. Levitt and M. Rubinstein). Detroit.

Slovenko, R. (1965). *Sexual behaviour and the law*. Springfield Illinois.
—— and Philips (1962). Psychosexuality and the criminal law. *V. and L. Rev* **15**, 797.

Smith, D. K. (1971). Transsexualism, sex reassignment, surgery and the law. *Cornell Law Rev.* **56**, 963.

Smith, J. C. (1975). Note on D. P. P. v. Morgan. *Criminal Law Review*, 717.
—— (1976). The Heilbron Report. *Criminal Law Review*, 97.
—— (1977). Conspiracy under the Criminal Law Act 1977. *Crim. L. R.* 598.
—— and Hogan, B. (1973). *Criminal law* (3rd ed.). London.

Socarides, C. (1965). Female homosexuality. In *Sexual behaviour and the law* (ed. R. Slovenko). Springfield, Illinois.

Solat, M. (1977). Les feministes et le viol. *Le Monde*, 18–20, October, Paris.

Soothill, K. and Jack, A. (1975). How rape is reported. New Society **32**, 663; 702.

Stephen, J. (1883). *A history of the criminal law of England*. London.

Stephens, E. (1976). Out of the closet into the courts. *Spare Rib* September 1976, 6.

Storr, A. (1964). *Sexual deviation*. Harmondsworth.

Sturup, G. K. (1968). Treatment of sexual offenders in Herstedvester, Denmark, *Acta Psychiat. Scand.*, Supp. **44**, 1.

Sutherland, E. and Cressey, D. (1970). *Principles of Criminology.* (8th ed.) Philadelphia.

Swanson, A. H. (1960). Sexual psychopath statutes—summary and analysis. *J. Crim. L, Crimin, and Police Sci.* **51**, 215.

Szasz, T. (1970). *The manufacture of madness*. New York.

Taylor Buckner, H. (1970). The transvestite career path. *Psychiatry* **30**, 381 (also in *Deviance, Reality and Change* (1971), New York).

Ten, C. L. (1969). Crime and immorality. *Mod. Law Rev.* **32**, 648.

Thomas, D. A. (1970). *Principles of sentencing*. London.

Toner, B. (1977). *The facts of rape*. London.

Unger, R. M. (1976). *Law in modern society*. London.

University of Pennsylvania L. Review (1968). Police discretion and the judgment that a crime has been committed. **117**, 277.

U.S.A. National Commission on the causes and prevention of violence (1969).

Walmsley, R. (1978). Indecency between males and the Sexual Offences Act 1967. *Criminal Law Review* 400.

Weinberg, M. and Williams, C., (1974). *Male homosexuals: their problems and adaptation*. London.

Weinberg, S. K. (1963). *Incest behaviour*. New York.

Weis, K. and Borges, S. (1973). Victimology and rape: the case of the legitimate victims. *Issues in Criminology* **8**, 101.

West, D. (1974). Thoughts on sex law reform. In *Crime, criminology and public policy* (ed. Hood). London.

Wilcox, A. (1972). *The decision to prosecute*. London.

Wilkins, L. (1964). *Social deviance*. London.

Williams, G. (1945). Language and the law. *Law Quarterly Review* **61**, 71.

—— (1975). Letter to *The Times*, 3 October.

Williams, J. Hall (1974). The neglect of incest. *Med, Sci. Law* **14**, 64.

Winick, C. and Kinsie, P. (1971). *The lively commerce—prostitution in the United States*. Chicago.

de Wolf R. (1970). *The bonds of acrimony*. Philadelphia.

Wolfenden, J. (1957). *Report on homosexual offences and prostitution*. HMSO, London.

Wollheim, R. (1959). Crime, sin and Mr Justice Devlin. *Encounter* 1 November, 38.

Wynn, A. and M. (1974). *Can family planning do more to reduce child poverty*. London.

14 Biological factors in the organization and expression of sexual behaviour

Richard P.Michael and Doris Zumpe

Introduction

No single physical, chemical, or biological factor is responsible for the expression of sex. On the contrary, the more complex the organism, the more numerous the factors that influence the phenomenon. In some very simple forms of motile, water-dwelling plants, the addition of a chemical to the medium causes the population to fall into two groups: those which attract and those which repel each other. This type of chemistry no longer holds in higher forms; and in the human, subtle cultural and educational influences may be quite as important in determining sexual role and orientation as the genetic and endocrine factors.

One of our tasks in this chapter is to trace this increasing complexity in phylogenetic and ontogenetic terms, and as it would be impossible to do this here in any systematic fashion, we shall simply take illustrative examples of the factors to be dealt with, progressing from simple to more complex levels of organization, ascending gradually the evolutionary scale, in the hope that certain general statements may emerge. The aim, then, is to place human sexual activity, together with its distortions, in its proper setting against a more general biological background.

Phylogenetic aspects

Reproduction in primitive forms of life – viruses, bacteria, and protozoa – is carried on by binary fission, the whole organism simply dividing into two. There is no sexual differentiation into morphological males and females, although with newer data from electron microscopy even this statement is no longer quite true. In metazoa, this asexual division is supplemented by a stage in which two cells first fuse in order later to multiply. This represents the beginning of sexual differentiation, neither cell being capable of reproduction without the stimulus

441

of prior fusion. This characteristic union between gametes is found in all but the most primitive forms of life. It opens the possibility of inherited variation and permits evolutionary development in place of the endless replication of progeny that are identical with parents (clones). The physical basis of such inheritence are the genes and sexual characteristics, like all others, have a genetic basis. The sexual characteristics are, therefore, subjected in the same way as any other characteristic to selection pressures that mould the process of evolution.

Tinbergen has recently given a beautiful example from the work of Crossly of an artifical selection pressure resulting in the development of sexual isolation within the laboratory. Using the technique of micro-evolution with ebony (winged) and vestigal (non-winged) mutants of *Drosophila melanogaster* (a fruit fly) and anti-hybrid selection to 40 generations, it was found that this artifical selection pressure resulted in decreased hybrid matings and increased homogamic matings. An analysis of the mating behaviour of the selected lines indicated that this depended upon the development of a mating preference, resulting in a greater sensitivity of the females to strange males, which were repelled more readily, and a greater sensitivity of males to the repelling movements of the females. Thus, development of reproductive isolation appeared to be due to the selecting of specific sexual behavioural characteristics – clearly an important factor in the isolation of species.

Similar sorts of situations are found in nature. Four species of poeciliid fishes (the guppy and some relatives) are sympatric in the waters of British Guiana and, although closely related, show complete sexual isolation without hybridization. Working in the laboratory, it has been shown by Liley that the lack of interbreeding between these species, which have a true copulation and are viviparous, is due to a selective mating preference shown mainly by the females. As Tinbergen has been careful to point out, experiments of the type conducted with *Drosophila* indicate only a possible mechanism by which such a situation could have come about. At the present time we have no reliable information on whether or not behavioural characteristics and preferences have played any part in isolating the races of man.

Genetic considerations

Because of its special suitability, much of the early experimental work on inheritance was carried out with *Drosophila*, and the view developed that the action of genes in sex determination was expressed through inter-chromosomal balances, including factors in the cytoplasm as well as in the chromatin material. Though changes in chromosome numbers were found to be associated with abrupt differentiation of new sexual types, the concept that chromosome differences are all-important has been replaced by that of balance within the haploid set. In this, sex determination does not differ from what is known of the determination of any other organ or characteristic. McClung (1902) first suggested that a single chromosome was associated with the differentiation of fertile eggs into those with specifically male or female features. In addition to a set of homomorphic pairs of autosomal or 'A' chromosomes, the number being specific for the species, a common arrangement in the male is a single 'X' paired with a 'Y' sex chromosome, the latter being variable in size or even absent. In the common female arrangement two X sex chromosomes are present: the females being homogametic for sex whereas the males are digamic or heterozygous.

In amphibia and certain species of fishes and birds the situation is reversed, the female being XY and the male 2X, usually designated ZW and 2Z to avoid confusion. The basic theory that sex determination is the result of the quantitative interaction of two sets of genes present in separate chromosomes is due to the work of Morgan, Bridges, and Sturtevant (1925) working with *Drosophila* and of Goldschmidt (1931) working with *Lymantria dispar*, a moth. They succeeded in producing every grade of sex reversal and of intersexuality by subspecies crosses resulting in the proper combination of genes. The bi-potentiality was proved to result from two types of genetic sex determining agents, the balance between them determining the balance between maleness and femaleness. It is now recognized that certain aspects of this genetic control rest in the autosomes and more especially in the ratio between autosomal and X chromosomal characteristics. Although the major sex genes are carried in the sex chromosomes, gene mutations influence every aspect of sexual morphology and physiology and genes with this type of influence, whether recessive or dominant, have been found in all of the autosomes of *Drosophila*, and a similar situation occurs in other forms. In amphibia and fish the addition of hormones to the medium in which they live during the developmental period results in marked morphological changes and sex reversal. The phenotypic modifications are not accompanied by corresponding changes in the chromosomal constitution of the cells, the animals retaining their original genotypes. Among mammals, intersex states are encountered not infrequently. The classic example, the calf freemartin, is not primarily genetically determined and will be referred to later. Goat hermaphrodites range in phenotype from almost normal males to almost normal females with frequent persistence of both male and female internal structures in a single individual. These types are due to a recessive autosomal gene acting only upon the female zygote (Kondo 1955) so that homozygous embryos simultaneously develop male and female characteristics; a condition with particular interest for intersex states in the human.

In 1956 Tjio and Levan, using colchicine-induced metaphase arrest and newer methods of fixation with hypotonic saline, observed that the number of chromosomes in somatic cells in human tissue-culture was 46; 22 paired autosomes plus X and Y sex chromosomes. Although there are probably some minor racial variations, prior to this discovery it had been widely accepted that 48 was the normal karyotype in man. Sexual dimorphism has now been detected within the nuclei of human somatic cells (Moore and Barr 1954) and in those of many other mammals (Barr and Bertram 1949; Barr 1956, 1957) including monkey, cat, dog, ferret, and, less reliably, in rabbit and rodents. In up to 80 per cent of the somatic nuclei of females a granule of nuclear chromatin can be identified adjacent to the surface of the nuclear membrane. This material is present in only 10 per cent of the cell nuclei of males. The test has high reliability in assigning presumed genetic sex and can be carried out easily upon buccal smears or skin biopsy material. In difficult cases sex chromatin determination is supplemented by investigation of the full chromosome complements. Genetically determined abnormalities of sexual differentiation in the human leading to abnormal phenotypes, are especially similar to those occurring in other species and some of these will now be considered.

The testicular feminization syndrome (Morris 1953; Jacobs *et al.* 1959) consists of female external genitalia together with testes which are to be found either in the labia majora or abdomen. There is a typically feminine body habitus at puberty except that pubic and axillary hair is sparse and there is primary amenorrhoea, the vagina is underdeveloped, and the uterus and Fallopian tubes are rudimentary or absent. Epididymi and vasa deferentia are frequently present. The somatic cells are chromatin negative and the chromosome complement is $XY + 44A$. However, the phenotype, apart from the suppressed testes, is almost entirely feminine. The syndrome is familial and maternally transmitted. The evidence indicates a simple autosomal dominant acting in the male zygote. The testes secrete testosterone in the low, normal, male range but there is a failure of male target tissues to respond: testosterone injections are also without effect. It is thought that the female breast development is due to oestrogen secreted normally by testes and adrenals, and castration before puberty, to prevent malignancy in the ectopic testes, prevents mammary gland development.

In Klinefelter's syndrome (Klinefelter, Reifenstein, and Albright 1942) there are small, hard, but functionless scrotal testes and male differentiation of the genital tract. The habitus is eunuchoid with gynaecomastia, sparse facial hair, and a high-pitched voice. The nuclear chromatin is positive in 60 per cent of cases; XXY sex chromosomes and a total complement of 47 have been described. Sixty-three cases were investigated by Ferguson-Smith *et al.* (1960) and at least two distinct types of the condition described.

Another genetically determined intersex state in the human is Turner's syndrome or ovarian agenesis which substantiates further the feminizing effect of the X chromosome, usually designated XO; the absent chromosome could have been either X or Y. The gonads consist merely of connective tissue but the reproductive tract is female. There are no female puberty changes and the secondary sexual features of the adult are missing. There is a wide gradation of defects from the near normal. In full development the syndrome is associated with multiple congenital defects – abnormal skeletal development, heart disease, webbing of the neck, and mental defect (Bishop, Lessof, and Polani 1960). The condition may be familial, nuclear chromatin is negative in 80 per cent of cases. There is a lone X chromosome and a total of 45 (Polani, Lessof, and Bishop 1956). True human herm-aphroditic phenotypes are very rare but some 108 are on record (Polani 1970); they are probably mostly non-genetic. Ovotestes were found on the right in 50 per cent of cases in association with either a left testis or ovary in about equal numbers. In only a few cases have separate ovaries and testes been found.

Sexual behaviour possesses an hereditary basis and can be modified by selective breeding; the operation of a genetic factor being clearly evident in the development of strain differences (see Goy and Jakway 1962). Grunt and Young (1952) have shown that the behavioural differences between high- and low-drive strains of male guinea-pigs is independent of the amount of androgen administered after castration.

Differences in the sexual behaviour of female guinea-pigs of different inbred strains were found to persist after ovariectomy and the administration of oestradiol benzoate and progesterone (Goy and Young 1957). These findings indicate that the sensitivity of the soma rather than the level of hormone present is the determining factor. Rasmussen (1952) used selective breeding to separate strains of rats with high and low sex drives as measured by the frequency of crossing an electrified grid in order to reach a sexual partner. The inherited basis of the low sexual activity of certain strains of rats was established by Craig, Casida, and Chapman (1954) and similar observations have been made in many different breeds of farm animals.

Embryological development

The hormonal control of sexual differentiation during embryogenesis was opened as a field for experimentation by the studies of Keller and Tandler (1916) and of Lillie (1917) upon the freemartin condition in the calf. Although the effects of castration have been known since antiquity, the concept of a blood-borne agent produced by the gonads capable of controlling the development of sexual characteristics was not given experimental validity until the transplantation studies of Berthold (1849). The work of Bouin and Ancel (1903) and of Lillie extended this concept to the problem of sexual differentiation in the embryo. The freemartin is an intersex condition occurring in one of a pair of dizygotic twin calves, the other twin always being a normal male. The external genitalia and mammary glands of the freemartin are female but there may be an enlarged penis-like clitoris. Elements of both male and female genital tracts persist internally, male duct structures usually being well preserved while female duct structures are often rudimentary. The gonads are usually sterile testes but may be poorly developed ovotestes. The freemartin is genetically female and chromatin positive. The essential prerequisite for this condition is some degree of anastomotic communication between the placental circulations of the twins, the extent of the vascular interconnection determining the extent of the abnormality. These studies raised the possibility that a substance produced by the normal male embryo was exerting a masculinizing effect upon the zygotically female twin via the common circulation and led to the theory that embryonic hormones or similar morphogenetic substances control sexual differentiation during the embryonic period.

In 1925 Burns, working with amphibia, was able to graft together two embryos so that they developed a common circulation and came to be in parabiotic union; an experimental imitation, in fact, of the freemartin situation. The grafting procedure and the cross-circulation of hormones can be arranged so that there is either a large or small intercommunication. The grafting of gonads themselves can be carried out in the embryonic or early larval stage and results depend upon the extent to which the grafts become re-vascularized. An improved technique was developed for transplanting gonad primordia removed from one embryo to identical sites in hosts from which the corresponding parts had been previously removed (Humphrey 1928). Embryos bearing these orthotopic transplants can be reared to maturity along with the donor embryos enabling their sex to be established with certainty. When pure hormone preparations became available in the mid 1930s, their administration to some extent replaced grafting methods. The addition of hormone to the water in which larval forms of amphibia are developing or their injection directly into the incubating eggs of birds has resulted in almost complete morphological transformations. In placental mammals, also, the administration of hormones to the pregnant mother has produced marked changes in the developing young and this will be referred to below. The pouched young of certain marsupials are in an unusually under-developed state at birth, they are readily accessible to hormone treatment and morphological sexual differentiation is largely post-natal. Almost complete sex reversals have been produced in the North American opossum (*Didelphis virginiana*) by hormonal means. The results of early embryonic castration in both birds and mammals also support the hormone theory, for animals so treated fail to show normal sexual development. Some of these experimental findings will now be considered in more detail.

Sex reversals within the gonads

The hilar or medullary part of the amphibian undifferentiated gonad is derived from the mesonephric blastema as medullary cords which grow into the embryonic genital ridge. This hilar portion has the developmental potential of a testis. Surrounding it is a cortical zone with the developmental potential of an ovary. Sexual differentiation under genic influences results in the ascendancy of either the medullary component, with incorporation of germ cells centrally (future testes) or ascendancy of the cortical component, the germ cells remaining more peripherally (future ovary). The presence, in the undifferentiated state, of cortex and medulla and the gradual development of ascendancy of one component over the other led to the theory of corticomedullary antagonism (Witschi 1932, 1939). The testis appears to be the dominant gonad in amphibia for, in parabiotic animals and in transplantation studies with embryonic gonads, the testes induce reversal in ovaries, in some cases causing complete ovarian suppression, but are not themselves reversed. To effect predominance of the ovary, it is necessary to employ heteroplastic ovarian grafts from species with large ovaries and greater rates of growth; under these conditions transformations of host testes result (Humphrey 1942). The administration of oestradiol or testosterone to higher Anurans brings about complete reversal and the transformed gonad may become functional. The administration of sex hormones is not without paradoxical effects and results depend upon the duration and level of dosage as well as the species and stage of differentiation.

Among birds, the chick (Willier 1933) and duckling (Wolff and Haffen 1952) have been most investigated. The situation is somewhat complicated by the lateral asymmetry of the genital tract; this is particularly marked in the female in which the left ovary is large with marked cortical development while the right ovary is rudimentary. In *Aves* generally it appears that the ovary dominates the testes. Removal of the left ovary in the chick causes the rudimentary right one to develop into an ovotestis. Indifferent avian gonads when transplanted at the genital ridge stage into another embryo, or when cultured *in vitro*, differentiate according to genotype, and sex reversal in birds was not achieved until potent hormone preparations became available (Dantchakoff 1935; Willier, Gallagher, and Koch 1935). The injection of oestrogens into incubating eggs has little effect upon developing ovaries but testes are transformed. This is particularly marked in the left testis, which is normally more developed in the adult, and becomes an ovary; the right testis, which is normally undeveloped, is more difficult to transform (Wolff 1948). Male hormones are less effective upon the embryonic ovary than are female hormones upon the embryonic testis; the left ovary can be transformed into an ovotestis but the effect upon the rudimentary right ovary is less marked. These successes with hormone treatment led to renewed interest in grafting. It was found that transformations could be obtained in the gonads of 50-hour-old hosts when the gonadal grafts were from embryo aged 10 days (Wolff 1946). Similar results have been obtained *in vitro* when gonad primordia are cultured in close contact so that they fuse during growth. Here again the ovary has proved dominant. Although gonad primordia in tissue culture develop and differentiate autonomously according to genotype, the process is susceptible to moulding by heterologous hormones.

In general, the administration of steroidal sex hormones has failed to produce similar transformations in the gonad primordia of placental mammals. Pregnant females have been treated with hormones during the period of gestation when sexual differentiation in the embryo takes place. In the rat (Greene 1942), guinea-pig (Dantchakoff 1936), mouse (Turner 1940), rabbit (Jost 1947, 1955), and monkey (Wells and van Wagenen 1954) treatment has failed to bring about transformations within the gonads themselves, although marked changes may be produced in the accessory structures and this will be referred to again. Although the bisexual stage is brief and the recessive sexual component weaker, the mammalian embryonic gonad shows histological evidence of a bisexual structure similar to that found in lower vertebrates. In the embryonic testes the germinal epithelium soon disappears and with it the cortical potential, while in embryonic ovaries the medullary cords soon become vestigial. Testes primordia in the rat are extremely stable and develop as such under many conditions of transplantation and of hormone administration. In contrast, ovarian primordia are extremely labile, the cortex frequently fails to develop and then the medullary component over-balances it. As a result many intermediate types are produced but they appear to be quite unrelated to the sex of the host (Moore and Price 1942; Holyoke 1949).

Because of its ready accessibility, much experimental work has been done with a marsupial, the opossum. At the stage of separation of the primary sex cords from the germinal epithelium, embryonic testes are readily transformed into ovotestes and ovaries by oestradiol adminis-tration from birth to 30 days of age (Burns 1955, 1956). The develop-ment of the germinal epithelium is enhanced by this treatment, with the production of secondary sex cords and a cortical zone; testicular differentiation is suppressed. Involution of the germinal epithelium normally occurs during the 24 hours after birth and if the administra-tion of oestradiol is delayed beyond this time it has no effect. Low dosages of the order 0.2 µg oestradiol per day must be given or sterility results. Apart from these remarkable findings in the opossum, the only other instance of transformation of the gonad in a mammal is that of the freemartin and here the predominant type is male whereas in the opossum it appears to be the female. In the experiments referred to, hormones of adult type were employed and it may well be that hormones derived from embryonic gonads would have more profound effects.

Differentiation in the accessory sexual structures

The embryonic sex ducts are derived from the primitive nephric system while the lower part of the genital tract and associated out-growths are derived from the urogenital sinus, itself originating from the primitive gut. Full development of the secondary sexual characteristics only occurs after puberty. In male embryos, the duct of the primitive kidney or mesonephros becomes the Wolffian duct and eventually the male genital tract. The female or Müllerian duct develops as a furrow in the thickened lateral portion of the urogenital ridge and eventually becomes the female genital tract. The development of these accessory structures is in two stages; the early stage appears to be independent of genetic sex and it is then that the primordia of both sexual systems are laid down (bisexual potential). The second stage, that of sexual differentiation, follows the period of differentiation in the gonads themselves and it is then that the tissues of both sex ducts become reactive to hormones.

Certain over-simplified generalizations may be made concerning the development of male and female genital tracts. In bird embryos, the destruction of gonads of both sexes leads to the anhormonal development of a mainly male accessory sexual system, penis and syrinx being developed, but the Müllerian ducts are retained and persist independently of the genetic sex. The presence of a testis, a testis graft, or androgen administration inhibits development of the Müllerian duct (an ovarian graft or oestrogen administration has little effect). However, when the gonads compete, the ovary is dominant. In mammalian embryos, and most work has been done in the rabbit (Jost 1947, 1953), destruction of the gonads of either sex results in the anhormonal development of a mainly female accessory sexual system, the Müllerian duct persists and differentiates, the Wolffian duct disappears, and the external genitalia are female. Again, the testis inhibits Müllerian duct development and stimulates differentiation of the Wolffian system but, in contrast to birds, the mammalian testis in direct competition dominates the ovary. However, in the mammals so far studied, there is an interesting discrepancy between the effect of a foetal testis and that of the administration of androgen. The latter treatment, though stimulating the Wolffian system, fails to produce any more than a patchy and partial suppression of the Müllerian system. *In vitro* experiments confirm that effects cannot be attributed to the influence of hormones derived from the maternal circulation (Jost and Bozic, 1951; Wolff, 1953), and organ cultures of rat mesonephric bodies and ducts of both sexes have revealed that the Müllerian duct survives and develops while the Wolffian duct degenerates.

The external genitalia and the structures derived from the urogenital sinus are sensitive to the administration of hormone in many mammals, providing this is done at the appropriate stage of development. Androgens administered to female embryos result in the suppression of vaginal development, prostatic hypertrophy, and an external masculinization. The administration of oestrogens to male embryos produces some degree of vaginal development and stratified metaplasia, complete prostatic suppression, and an external feminization. The effects of castration upon the developing urogenital sinus and its derivatives in mammals resemble the effects upon the sex ducts. The female is not greatly affected whereas male structures fail to develop and the female type predominates. The female pattern is independent of hormone and genetic sex, but it appears that the embryonic testes are essential for male differentiation of these structures. The genital tubercle, the simple primordium present in both sexes from which the copulatory organ develops, is itself highly susceptible to modification by sex hormones and complete transformations can occur in reptiles, birds, and mammals.

Although the male phenotype appears to be basic in birds, the female type is basic in mammals. The avian ovary is the dominant gonad but in mammals the testes dominate the ovaries. It happens that, in each case, the basic type is the homogametic sex. Except in the marsupial, experimental reversal of the mammalian gonad is very incomplete, but reversal in the accessory sex structures is readily obtained and many of these remarkable transformations, once produced at the appropriate moment in development, cannot be reversed. The crucial importance of timing is very evident throughout the process of embryological maturation. The disappearance of the bisexual potential of the gonad would be a good example of this and there are others. Embryological development proceeds according to genetic determinants, but it is clear that at certain stages the organism passes through phases of special vulnerability or sensitivity to morphological, and perhaps psychological, modification by hormonal substances.

Sensitive periods during development

Most of what has been said already concerning the effects of administering hormone to the developing organism has referred to the induction of structural modifications in the sexual apparatus. These will obviously affect the behavioural capacities of animals so treated, but it is now becoming increasingly clear that equally profound modifications may be produced in the behavioural mechanisms which are themselves responsible for the expression of sexual activity. Here, too, the concept of sensitive or critical periods has emerged and, of great interest in the field of sexual behaviour, effects may not become fully apparent until maturity is reached. W.C.Young and his colleagues have pioneered experimentation in this area. Pregnant guinea-pigs have been treated with intramuscular injections of testosterone propionate between the 30th and 65th day of gestation and this has induced masculinization of female young. Although males in the litters appear unaffected, the external genitalia of the genetic females are, in some cases, completely masculinized, vaginae are absent, and the Wolffian duct structures are hypertrophied. When such females reach maturity they fail to show normal ovarian function and, of great interest, their capacity to display the normal feminine sexual behaviour appropriate to the species is grossly disturbed. Androgen administration to these mothers results, then, in female offspring whose subsequent pattern of sexual behaviour is permanently impaired. The female components of the pattern are suppressed as revealed by a decrease in the number of tests positive for oestrus, a decrease in the duration of oestrus, and, also, in the duration for which the maximum lordosis response can be elicited. The masculine elements of the females' oestrous behaviour (see below), present normally in 85 per cent of guinea-pigs, are much enhanced which is shown by an increase in male-like mounting activity (Phoenix *et al.* 1959; Goy, Bridson, and Young 1961). This striking masculinization of the behavioural repertoire cannot be attributed solely to disordered pituitary and ovarian function, since administration of the appropriate regimen of oestrogen and progesterone to ovariectomized animals fails to restore the behaviour to normal.

It is inferred from evidence of this kind that the changes in sexual behaviour induced by exposure to androgen during intrauterine development are due to an effect upon mechanisms within the brain itself which are responsible for the expression of normal sexual activity. It is noteworthy that these androgen-treated animals also show in adult-hood an increased responsiveness to androgens which is comparable to that shown by normal males. Permanent effects are obtained only if treatment is given before birth in the guinea-pig, the critical period probably being the middle trimester, and no permanent effects upon adult sexuality result if treatment is delayed until the 50–65th day of gestation.

The notion that embryonic hormones can influence sexual differentiation of the brain, especially of the hypothalamus, stems from the observations of Everett, Sawyer, and Markee (1949) and Harris (1955). These workers were mainly concerned with the differentiation of cyclic patterns of gonadotrophin release from the pars distalis that characterize the female mammal compared with the continuous pattern of release that is characteristic of the male. Although Pfeiffer (1936), in a beautiful series of grafting experiments in rats, had demonstrated that males, castrated at birth and transplanted with an ovary when adult, would ovulate and develop corpora lutea from granulosa cells, that is, they became capable of a luteinizing hormone surge (as in females), he attributed this consequence of neonatal castration to changes in the hypophysis rather than to changes in the hypothalamus. We know now from pituitary grafting experiments (Harris and Jacobsohn 1952) that the pituitary does not undergo sexual differentiation, but takes its secretory patterns from the sex of the hypothalamus to which it is juxtaposed.

The role of embryonic hormones on sexual differentiation within the brain has been developed further by the work of Segal and Johnson (1959), Barraclough (1961), and Barraclough and Gorski (1961). Gestation is shorter in the rat than in the guinea-pig, young are born in a less mature condition, and effects can be obtained with post-natal hormone administration: a single injection of testosterone propionate (0.1–1.25 mg) to female rats between birth and 4 days of age produces permanent infertility. After puberty, not only do these testosterone-treated females develop polycystic ovaries and fail to ovulate, but they show few signs of oestrous behaviour when caged with active males for prolonged periods. Comparable findings have been reported in oestrogen-treated males by Harris and Levine (1962) who found that in 50 per cent of cases all signs of male sexual behaviour were abolished. Although the critical period in the rat extends post-natally, the overall picture is closely similar to that found in the guinea-pig, and when treatment is delayed to 20 days after birth no irreversible behavioural changes result.

Clinical observations upon the children of mothers receiving 17-ethinyl-testosterone for threatened abortion during the middle trimester of pregnancy have indicated that pseudohermaphroditism may be similarly produced in the human infant. Eighteen such cases have been reported by Wilkins *et al.* (1958). The congenital adreno-genital syndrome in genetic females is a naturally occurring condition that results in hormonal masculinization and pseudohermaphroditism (see below). Attention has been drawn to the similarity between the critical period for hormone action in the morphogenesis of the genital tissues and the critical period for hormone action in the neural tissues mediating the eventual expression of adult sexual behaviour. These actions of hormones during the developmental period are quite different from those seen in mature individuals. Harris has referred to *inductive* effects on the undifferentiated brain and to *excitatory* effects on behaviour in adult life. Young has also put this aptly by contrasting their *organizational* and *activational* roles. He has speculated upon the pos-sibility of there being two neural substrates, corresponding to the two primitive sex ducts, susceptible to the organizational influences of the foetal gonads; in fact, a sexual dimorphism in the neural tissues. The hypothesis of a basic bisexuality in the brain is certainly an attractive one, and some evidence to support it is beginning to emerge. Raisman and Field (1971) have demonstrated by quantitative electron micro-scopy that a sexual dimorphism exists in the dendrites of the pre-optic area and ventromedial hypothalamic nucleus of rats.

The concept of periods of special sensitivity during development has come to be of importance in the fields of behaviour and of psycho-analysis. It seems possible that while hormonal and chemical changes in the internal environment have great importance before birth, the effects of changes in the external environment and the effects of early experiences may have equally profound organizational effects in the neonatal period. This is clearly seen in the critical period for the phenomenon of imprinting, first systematically studied by Lorenz (1937). This term describes the process by which first experiences very rapidly result in the formation of fixed behavioural responses and need not be described again in any detail. It is not intended to enter the controversy concerning its nature but it is clearly a specialized type of learning occurring in early life and of the highest importance in species recognition, in the formation of the bond between mother and young, and in the organization of later social behaviour including the pair-bond. A critical period for primary socialization appears to be quite general and has been identified in birds and also in mammals (howling monkey: Carpenter (1934); dog: Scott (1945), Scott, Frederickson, and Fuller (1951); mouse: Williams and Scott (1953)).

The recent studies of Harlow and the Wisconsin group (Harlow 1962*a*, *b*), because they are concerned with the maturation of behaviour in a primate, must be of special theoretical importance to clinicians. Harlow's investigations have been concerned with the so-called 'affectional system' in the monkey, with a particular emphasis upon the nature of the infant's relationship to its mother. Although this topic has engaged the interest of psychiatrists and psychoanalysts for many years (Freud and Burlingham 1942; Klein 1948; Spitz 1950; Robertson, Bowlby, and Rosenbluth 1952; Winnicott 1958), it is by studies in a sub-human primate, paralleling those in the child, that this whole area has become susceptible to effective experimentation. Studying the development of play behaviour in heterosexual groups of infant rhesus monkeys, the following phases in sexual development have been recognized: an infantile heterosexual stage, a pre-adolescent stage, and both adolescent and mature sexual stages. The infantile stage in the rhesus monkey appears to last throughout the first year and is characterized by inadequate sexual play and inappropriate sexual posturing. An outstanding finding is that male and female infant monkeys show differences in sex behaviour from as early as the second month of life onwards. The infant males show earlier and more aggress-ive sexual behaviour and very rarely assume the female sex posture; females, on the other hand, display both male and female patterns.

Although these early expressions of sexual behaviour are fragmentary and short-lived, they appear to be of the highest importance in the eventual development of a capacity for adult sexuality. This is revealed by Harlow's observations upon infant primates reared in states of semi-isolation. Infants were separated from their mothers shortly after birth and spent the first year of life in cages so arranged that, although the sight and sound of other infants was possible, physical contact with other monkeys was not (Mason and Harlow 1958; Harlow and Zimmermann 1959). When mature, animals so reared were found to exhibit a wide range of grossly disturbed behaviour including such autistic patterns as self-sucking, stereotyped movements, persistent masturbation, uncontrolled episodes of frenzy and self-mutilation, and other distortions of behaviour which have seemed to many observers to be analogous to austistic and psychotic behaviour in the human child. Of interest in the present context is the failure of these deprived animals to socialize and relate to others in the group. They also show an almost total loss of all sexual activity other than masturbation. Sexual behaviour involves relating to another member of the species and this they are incapable of doing. The females may show normal menstrual cycles and appear to ovulate normally but the normal pattern of female receptive behaviour is lost. Instead, the overtures of the male are met by an aggressive reaction which is quite foreign to the normal female macaque. Laboratory-raised infants, either permitted contact with their mothers or permitted opportunity for play with peers, develop normal male and female sexual behaviour when adult. The importance of experiential factors and learning processes during the period of maturation in the primate could not be more convincingly demonstrated. These expressions of sexuality during infancy and prior to puberty in lower primates are in line with many observations made on children.

The role of such factors during the developmental period upon the subsequent sexual function of the adult human has been recognized by psychiatrists and, in this context, the clinical observations of the Hampsons (Hampson 1955; Hampson, Money, and Hampson 1956; Hampson and Hampson 1961) have a special interest. These workers have studied many types of ambisexual incongruity and different forms of pseudohermaphroditism (congenital hyperadrenocortical females, pseudohermaphrodites with masculinized external genitals, cryptorchid hermaphrodites of different types, and simulant females with feminizing inguinal testes, etc.). In the congenital adrenogenital syndrome (AGS), which is a familial, autosomal, recessive hereditary disease, there is defective cortisol synthesis because of a 21- or 11 ß-hydroxylase deficiency (Eberlein and Bongiovanni 1955). This leads to increased ACTH release and excessive production of testosterone, androstenedione, and 17-hydroxyprogesterone with virilization of the genetically female foetus. In these cases of doubtful sexual status, the chromosomal sex, gonadal sex, hormonal sex, the condition of the internal and external accessory organs, and the assigned sex and type of upbringing have all been taken into account.

The striking fact emerges that the psychological sex and sexual orientation or, as we would now say, the gender role, coincides in the majority of instances with the assigned sex and type of rearing. It would seem from these studies that the human infant's orientation as a male or female does not depend solely on the chromosomal and hormonal factors outlined above, but also on the psychological experience of being reared as, and regarded as, a boy or a girl. In cases where mistakes are made in assigning sex at birth, reassignment may be undertaken without difficulty during the first year of life. However, when reassignment is delayed very much beyond this period, severe psychological damage appears to result. This is an observation of great importance and surely links with the idea of a critical period which is seen to be so widespread in lower mammals. Nevertheless, pathological androgenization (AGS) of girls was found to be associated subsequently with increased tomboyism and high energy expenditure in rough outdoor play (Erhardt and Baker 1974), and the effects of foetal hormones could be clearly discerned. See Chapter 5, page 131.

Finally, some mention should be made of critical period effects in genetic males. If male rats are deprived of androgen in the perinatal period, their behaviour patterns tend to be both demasculinized and feminized, and this can be brought about experimentally by severely stressing the pregnant mother from day 14–21 of gestation (Ward 1972). Since female litter-mates were hardly affected, this raises the question of the special vulnerability of the male's behavioural patterns to stress *in utero*.

Sexual behaviour in laboratory mammals

In 1923 Allen and Doisy described the extraction of a hormone from the ovaries which was responsible for the manifestation of mating instincts in ovariectomized rats and mice. This discovery was the beginning of the biochemistry of sexual behaviour. There followed a large number of publications in which were described the behavioural changes induced by the administration of both androgens and oestrogens, over a wide dose-range, to intact and gonadectomized animals of both sexes and varying degrees of maturity. The early work of Calvin Stone formed a prototype for experimentation in this area and his distinguished successors, William C.Young (1941) and Frank A.Beach (1948), have reviewed the field. Marshall, in 1922, was writing 'little or nothing is known concerning the chain of causation leading to that disturbed state of the nervous mechanism, the existence of which during oestrus is so plainly manifest in the display of sex feeling'.

Although Stone drew attention to the two important factors underlying sexual behaviour, the central nervous system and the endocrines,
it is doubtful whether a great deal more is known about the 'chain of
causation' today. It has been shown that states of sexual receptivity
result from the administration of oestrogens in many mammalian forms
(spayed mouse: Marrian and Parkes (1930); Wiesner and Mirskaia
(1930); spayed rats: Allen *et al.* (1924); Hemmingsen (1933); dogs:
Kunde *et al.* (1930); ewe: Cole, Hart, and Miller (1945); cow:
Asdell, de Alba, and Roberts (1945)). It has also been shown in the
case of the female guinea-pig (Dempsey, Hertz, and Young 1936) that
while 31 per cent of spayed females become receptive when given
oestrogen alone, mating invariably occurs if the oestrogen administration is followed, some 36 hours later, by a small dose of progesterone.
With this treatment the latent period to mating is reduced from 35
hours to 4.8 hours. The oestrogen-progesterone combination results
in a more complete and normal pattern of sexual behaviour as well as
in a higher percentage of animals showing the response. Although a
synergism between these hormones has been demonstrated in the
mouse, rat, and guinea-pig, the reverse is true in the ferret (Marshall
and Hammond 1945). In this species, the administration of progesterone inhibits oestrogen-induced receptivity. In the ewe, progesterone
and oestrogen again act together but in this case progesterone
administration must precede oestrogen administration (Hammond,
Hammond, and Parkes 1942; Moore and Robinson 1957); thus, the
time relationship is the reverse of that in the rat.

These examples have been given in order to demonstrate the high
degree of species specificity in the hormonal control of mating
behaviour and the difficulty of making generalizations. This is also true
for the effects of androgens in the male. It is particularly unwise to
extrapolate information from lower to higher mammals. Just as the
hormonal basis of sexual receptivity in female mammals differs in different species, so the exact pattern of behaviour exhibited varies in a highly
specific manner. It is impossible to enter into details in the present
context, but several relevant points can be exemplified by considering
the sexual cycle of the female cat. This is a polyoestrous form in which
cycles of about 14 days' duration recur regularly throughout most of
the year, unless interrupted by a fertile mating. In London, cats
housed under laboratory conditions are seasonally anoestrous in
October and November. The 14-day cycle is divided into four phases –
dioestrous, pro-estrus, oestrus, and metoestrus. Each phase is associated

with a particular state of ovarian activity and a particular condition of the uterus and vagina which can easily be demonstrated by assessing the cornification response of vaginal smears (Scott and Lloyd-Jacob 1955).

The period of oestrus (heat) usually lasts 2–3 days and it is during this time that the female is receptive and, if mating occurs, fertilization of ova is possible. While many forms, such as the mouse, rat and guinea-pig, ovulate rhythmically like the human female, in cat, rabbit, and ferret ovulation is reflex and the stimulus of coitus is necessary to bring it about. If coitus does not take place, the ripe follicle simply regresses. The female cat in heat adopts a highly characteristic lordosis posture, the basic characteristics of which are shared by many laboratory and farm quadrupeds. In the case of the feline, mating can only take place if this posture is adopted and it has been shown to be specifically dependent upon the presence of oestrogens (Michael 1958, 1961a). The change in behaviour from the aggressive refusal reaction, typical of anoestrus, to acceptance of the male's coital efforts, typical of oestrus, is under the chemical control of the oestrogens. Mating never occurs after bilateral ovariectomy and the whole sequence of mating behaviour in the cat is known to be hormone-dependent. The central nervous system clearly mediates these behavioural changes and consideration will now be given to some of the neurological structures involved.

Neurological factors

Evidence has accumulated indicating that certain parts of the brain are of special importance in organizing the total pattern of sexual behaviour.

It has been shown that the presence of the genital tract itself is not necessary for the manifestation of sexual excitement. Rats with congenital absence of uterus and ovaries show oestrous responses after hormone administration (Beach 1945). Similarly, surgical removal of the uterus and vagina in rats does not prevent the expression of oestrous behaviour (Ball 1934) and total deafferentation of the pelvic erogenous zones, by combined sacral cord section and abdominal sympathectomy, does not inhibit sexual behaviour in either male or female cats (Bard 1935; Root and Bard 1937). Further, heat behaviour can occur in the absence of the olfactory bulbs and neocortex, and after destruction of the labyrinths, the cochlea and after removal of the eyes (Brooks 1937; Bard 1939). Thus, it seems that neither the distance receptors nor any one modality of sensation is essential for the expression of sexual excitement in lower mammals although all, obviously, may contribute to it. Money (1961) has collected data from patients following penectomy, vulvectomy, and from both paraplegics and quadriplegics. In general, the data are in line with the animal observations and indicate that sensory input from the genitalia is not essential for sexual activity, sexual fantasy, and even sexual climax.

Bard (1940) has reviewed the evidence relating certain parts of the brain to the expression of mating behaviour. It has been shown that spinal and low mid-brain animals do not show integrated oestrous behaviour (guinea-pig: Dempsey and Rioch (1939); cat: Bromiley and Bard (1940)) and that after complete removal of the neocortex, part of the rhinencephalon, striatum and rostrolateral thalamus, the female continues to exhibit oestrous behaviour (cat: Bard and Rioch (1937); rabbit: Brooks (1938); rat: Davis (1939)). Male animals appear to be somewhat more dependent upon neocortical mechanisms than female animals, and following large neocortical ablations the mating efficiency of males is markedly diminished. This is probably due to loss of motor and mechanical efficiency rather than a direct reduction of sexual drive. Attention has been directed to subcortical regions of the brain and, with the advent of modern stereotaxic methods, particularly to the diencephalon. Large localized lesions within the hypothalamus were found, in some cases, to block the behavioural effects normally associated with the administration of gonadal hormones. However, the hypothalamus is, relatively, a very small area of the brain and it is known to be importantly concerned with many behavioural, autonomic, and endocrine regulatory mechanisms (feeding, drinking, temperature regulation, fluid balance, pituitary control, etc.). The profound general disturbances that sometimes follow the placement of hypothalamic lesions make for difficulties in interpreting the significance of the loss of a behavioural pattern.

A more fruitful approach to the problem of determining the regions of the brain responsible for the manifestation of mating behaviour has been the implantation of minute fragments of solid hormone directly into the brain substance (Harris, Michael, and Scott 1958; Harris and Michael 1958; Michael 1961*b*). A study has been made of the activation of oestrous behaviour in ovariectomized cats by implants of stilboestrol ester in various intracerebral sites. The use of solid implants was preferred to the injection of solutions of oestrogens since they provide a higher degree of localization and a more prolonged period of action. The female cat was chosen because it possesses a highly stereotyped pattern of sexual behaviour which is remarkably constant in individual animals, and because the oestrous pattern of behaviour can be evoked only by the administration of oestrogens. Stainless steel brain needles are prepared, the tips of which can be coated with a small amount of hormone (50–150 μg). After weighing, the implant of hormone on the needle tip can be examined microscopically to measure its shape and dimensions. Needles can be inserted into the brain at any desired site by means of the Horsley-Clark stereotaxic apparatus and secured permanently in position by means of stainless steel screws and cold-curing acrylic cement. Animals prepared in this fashion make a quick recovery from operation and can be tested with the male cat daily for many weeks in order to assess any behavioural changes that the implant brings about. It has been found that hormone implants in the hypothalamus result in the production of sustained states of sexual receptivity. Identical implants placed elsewhere in the brain, in the majority of instances, fail to produce any changes in sexual behaviour. It is of interest that a high proportion of animals brought into continuous heat by the hypothalamic implants fail to show any signs of an oestrogen effect upon the genital tract – the uteri remain atrophic and the vaginal smears show no cornification response. Since low-level doses of oestrogens given systemically always result in full vaginal cornification prior to the occurrence of mating, there are good grounds for believing that the sexual behaviour consequent upon hypothalamic implantation is due to the local action of the stilboestrol ester upon a nervous mechanism.

Since these original studies in cats, the implantation of hormone in the brain has been used to evoke sexual behaviour in birds (Barfield 1965), and in both female (Lisk 1962) and male (Davidson 1966) rodents. The problem of localizing hormone action in the brain has been followed up by using [^{14}C]-diethylstilboestrol di. *n*. butyrate and an autoradiographic technique (Michael 1962*a*). It has been found that only a thin shell of brain, immediately adjacent to the implant, is exposed to a high concentration of hormone and, of much interest, there is evidence that cells in the vicinity of the implant selectively accumulate the labelled material. Since only a small proportion of neural elements seem to possess this capacity it becomes necessary to postulate that certain cells possess a selective biochemical affinity for the oestrogen.

One of the most difficult and perplexing problems confronting investigators in this field is the identification and localization of the particular neural elements upon whose altered activity must depend the altered behaviour patterns which, in many female mammals, we recognize as the state of oestrus. An approach to this problem became possible by making use of [³H]-hexoestrol of very high specific activity (Michael and Glascock 1961; Glascock and Michael 1962). This material undergoes rather rapid radiolysis and is purified by chromatography prior to administration. Injections were made subcutaneously in ethyl oleate in the dose range 1–20 µg per kg of body weight. Animals were killed from 1 to 72 hours after the oestrogen administration and the uptake of radioactivity in a wide range of tissues was investigated by both isotopic gas analysis of tissue samples and by autoradiography. The autoradiographic data reveal a bilaterally symmetrical system involving the septal area, pre-optic region, and hypothalamus of the cat (Michael 1962*b*). These results have now been confirmed and amplified in both rodents and rhesus monkeys using more refined methods. There is considerable agreement between the results obtained by the implant method and those obtained by the use of radioisotopes. It seems that the concept of a highly localized sexual 'centre' should perhaps now be replaced by that of a rather more diffuse sexual system. The use of tritium permits of very high resolution in the autoradiograph since these low energy ß-particles travel only a few micrometres in soft tissue. This has made possible the successful autoradiography of single cells, and neurones have been identified in the areas referred to which have selectively accumulated the hormone reaching them via the systemic circulation. Although it has not yet been possible to prove that some of these neurones are directly connected with sexual behaviour, this seems quite probable and, if so, the 'chain of causation' between the endocrine system and the brain seems nearer to being understood.

Studies in higher primates

One of the most significant developments in studies on sexual behaviour during the past decade has been the increasing number of high-quality field and laboratory studies on primates. There is quite a widely held view that as one ascends the phylogenetic scale, the role of hormones in behaviour is correspondingly decreased. While this generalization has considerable validity, recent field and laboratory studies nevertheless indicate that the endocrines may play a very significant role in the behavioural interactions between male and female higher primates. Old World (catarrhine) monkeys and apes alone among mammals (except for the human) have true menstrual cycles of about 30 days' duration. There is much evidence that many anthropoid monkeys show heightened sexual activity near midcycle, that is, around the time of ovulation. Such periods may be fairly well-circumscribed, particularly in some mangabeys, macaques, baboons, and apes in which females show marked perineal swelling. In some quite closely related species, however, sexual activity may continue throughout most of the menstrual cycle.

Under free-ranging conditions, rhesus monkeys live in troops of up to 100 animals. Males are generally dominant over females, and adults of each sex exhibit hierarchical rank orders with the male hierarchy being rather more linear and well-defined than that of the female. During the autumn mating season, females begin to approach males, and a given female will then form temporary consort- (pair)-bonds with a male and mate exclusively with him for several days. Thereafter, the female may mate with other males in the troop before becoming sexually inactive until she again starts approaching males in her next menstrual cycle. Copulation consists of a very variable number of mounts made by the male on the female, each mount being associated with intromission and pelvic thrusting, the series of mounts being terminated by one in which ejaculation occurs. The male's mount may be initiated either by the male or by the female. The female may refuse the male's mounting attempt or herself initiate a mount by making sexual invitational gestures to the male. We have used adult, oppositely-sexed pairs of animals as the basic unit for study. This eliminates several important variables, such as the effects of other conspecifics, but simplifies the situation although inevitably impoverishing it. During standard, 60-minute behaviour tests, all social, sexual, and agonistic behaviours were recorded in sequence and timed to the nearest 30 seconds. As a rule, males were tested on consecutive days with each of two female partners in order to control for individual differences and partner preferences. At all other times animals were housed together in the same cage room in individual cages to exclude the possibility of unobserved behavioural interactions influencing the test results. Despite the artificial testing situation, the behaviour observed was remarkably similar to that seen under free-ranging conditions, with the exception that its frequency was usually higher in the laboratory than in the field.

Behaviour during the menstrual cycles

When males are paired with intact females whose oviducts have been ligated to prevent pregnancy, rhythmic changes in several behavioural indices occur in relation to the menstrual cycle of the female of the pair (Michael, Herbert, and Welegalla 1966, 1967; Michael and Welegalla 1968): these include changes in grooming activity, in mounting activity, in female sexual invitations, in the number of ejaculations, and in the time taken for ejaculation to occur. Considering now just the changes in the number of ejaculations by the male per test, it has been found that they reach a maximum about 17 days prior to the start of the next menstruation. These data are shown in Fig. 14.1, which also makes a comparison with the frequency of sexual intercourse in a human population (Udry and Morris 1968). The similarity between the timing of the behavioural changes in the two species may point to the existence of a neuroendocrine mechanism that is common to both. As in women, plasma oestradiol levels in the female rhesus monkey rise sharply to a maximum 24–48 hours before ovulation but then decline to low levels in the luteal phase. Plasma progesterone levels are low during the follicular phase, start to increase just before the oestradiol peak, and reach high levels in the luteal phase of the cycle. Plasma testosterone levels in the female are fairly low throughout but reached a maximum on the same day as the oestradiol peak.

The precise relation between the changes in plasma hormone levels in the female and changes in her interactions with the male has now been examined in 5 female rhesus monkeys during 33 menstrual cycles by using an operant conditioning situation. To obtain a measure of the female's readiness to approach the partner, she was required to press a lever 250 times in order to obtain access to his cage. Blood samples were collected from females throughout their cycles and analysed by radio-immunoassay techniques for progesterone, oestradiol, testosterone, and dihydrotestosterone. When the hormone and behaviour data were aligned on the days of the oestradiol peaks, it was found that the highest ejaculatory frequency and the fastest access times by females for males both occurred one day after the oestradiol peak, namely, on the expected day of ovulation (Fig. 14.2) (Michael and Bonsall 1977). Thus, the neuroendocrine mechanisms responsible for synchronizing the behaviour of the sexes with the timing of ovulation optimize the chances for successful fertilization.

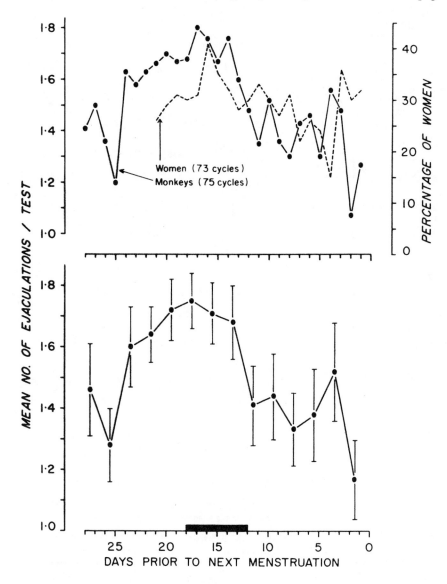

Fig. 14.1   *Upper*: comparison of the copulatory activity of the rhesus monkey and man in relation to the menstrual cycle. ●—●, Mean number of ejaculations per test (32 pairs of rhesus monkeys); --- percentage of women reporting sexual intercourse (40 women, Udry and Morris (1968). *Lower*: rhesus monkey data smoothed by plotting means of two consecutive days. Horizontal bar gives expected time of ovulation (Hartman 1932); vertical bars give standard errors of means. (From Michael and Zumpe (1970*a*), with permission.)

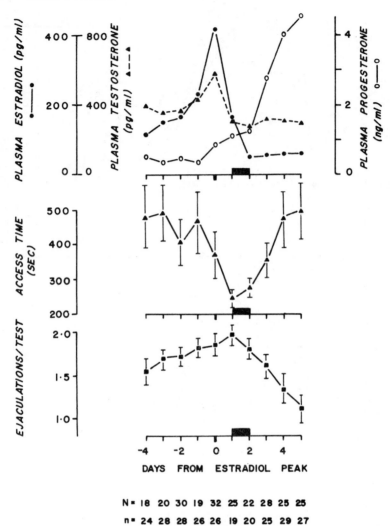

Fig.14.2   Peri-ovulatory synchronization of the behaviour of male and female rhesus monkeys. When the behavioural and hormone data were aligned on the day of the oestradiol peak (day 0), it was found that female access times were shortest, and numbers of ejaculations by males greatest, on the expected day of ovulation (solid horizontal bars) (33 menstrual cycles). Vertical bars give standard errors of means. N = number of plasma samples; n = number of behaviour tests (9 pairs, 252 tests). (From Michael and Bonsall (1977), with permission.)

Ovarian hormones and sexual behaviour

Bilateral ovariectomy usually results in the eventual cessation of sexual activity of the pair; however, the time taken for this to happen is very variable. The administration of small subcutaneous doses of oestradiol benzoate to the female (5–10 µg per day) invariably results in a rapid reappearance of mating behaviour. As in rats and cats, this effect is in part due to a localized action of oestrogen on the brain, since behavioural effects were more marked when small amounts of oestrogen were implanted into the upper tegmental region than when they were implanted into the frontal sub-cortex (Michael 1971). Subcutaneous administration of progesterone to ovariectomized, oestrogen-treated females seems to antagonize the behavioural effects of oestrogen and there is a marked decline in mating activity (Michael, Saayman, and Zumpe 1968).

Since oestrogen and progestins are constituents of oral contraceptive preparations, the observation that these substances affected sexual behaviour raised the possibility that oral contraceptives might have similar effects. This, was, indeed, found to be the case, and treatment of female rhesus monkeys with various oral contraceptive agents (mestranol, ethynodiol diacetate, chlormadinone diacetate) depressed the sexual activity of male partners with which she was paired (Michael and Plant 1969). These observations in a higher primate may have some implications for the long-term use of oral contraceptives by women.

Communication between the sexes

In the preceding section, it was shown that treating the female with different hormone preparations could produce major changes in the behaviour of her male partner and this immediately raises the question of how the information is transmitted from the female to the male and vice versa. At least two forms of distance receptors are involved, namely, the eye and the nose. It has been established that the female signals her readiness to copulate by means of a number of different gestures and postures (sexual invitations), and these are observed by the male which responds accordingly. Similarly, it is now known that the female produces substances that are volatilized from the genital region which are received by the male and stimulate his sexual interest. Auditory communication probably plays a role but less is known about it at present.

The female of many species of anthropoid primates use the quadrupedal presentation posture, in which the hindquarters are directed toward the male, as a means of stimulating the male to mount. Rhesus monkeys also initiate mounting by three other gestures, the 'hand-reach' (a slap on the ground with one hand), the 'head-duck' (a quick lowering of the head relative to the shoulders), and the 'head-bob' (a rapid upward jerk of the head) (Michael and Zumpe 1970*b*). On the other hand, the unreceptive female may refuse the male's mounting attempts by pulling away or fleeing. By using these sexual invitations and refusals as measures of female sexual motivation, it was found that ovariectomy decreased it, oestrogen treatment enhanced it, and additional progesterone again had a depressing effect. These findings were confirmed in a lever-pressing situation in which a female was required to work in order to obtain access to a male (Michael, Zumpe, Keverne, and Bonsall 1972), and the results in ovariectomized animals given hormones were very much in line with those in intact females with normal menstrual cycles.

Olfactory communication between individuals of the same species is well-known to be important in the control of reproductive processes in lower mammals, particularly mice, and this subject has been adequately reviewed (Bronson 1974). In higher primates, the possible role of chemical signals in the communication of information about the sexual condition of the partner has received experimental attention only recently. Our attention was drawn to olfactory mechanisms by observations of the following types. Males frequently sniff at the perineal region of their female partners and under certain experimental conditions, females appeared to be very interesting to males yet quite unreceptive to their mounting attempts. Under other circumstances, female sexual motivation appeared to be quite high, and yet the level of the males' sexual interest in them remained quite low. From this, we developed the notion of female attractiveness as a separate entity from that of female receptivity. Now, female attractiveness no doubt depends on a combination of several different factors, but important among them are olfactory cues emanating from the vagina (Michael and Saayman 1968). This matter was investigated by again using the operant conditioning situation, only this time males were required to press a lever 250 times for access to female partners. Generally, males will not press with any consistency for ovariectomized females, but do so rapidly and reliably when the females are treated with oestrogen. If males are made anosmic by the bilateral insertion of nasal plugs, they fail to detect that their female partners have been oestrogenized (Michael and Keverne 1968). On the other hand, when males are pressing for access to oestrogen-treated females, the additional administration of progesterone rapidly causes the males to cease lever-pressing, and this effect can be blocked by making males anosmic (Michael, Bonsall, and Zumpe 1976). These and other experiments have clearly demonstrated the involvement of the male's olfactory pathways in the communication of information about the female's endocrine status. Gas chromatography and mass spectrometry have now characterized the principal behaviourally active substances as a series of volatile aliphatic acids that are present in oestrogen-stimulated vaginal secretions (Curtis, Ballantine, Keverne, Bonsall, and Michael 1971). Synthetic mixtures of these acids (copulins), when applied to the hindquarters of ovariectomized female rhesus monkeys, are effective in stimulating the sexual activity of their male partners. However, not all males respond to these olfactory stimulants and the overall effect seems to depend upon many variables including the relationship between the partners (Michael, Zumpe, Richter, and Bonsall 1977).

Copulins are found in the vaginal secretions of several other primate species, including the human. Secretions were collected on alternate days from 47 women during a total of 86 menstrual cycles, and it was found that the volatile aliphatic acid content of these secretions increased significantly during the late follicular phase and then declined progressively during the luteal phase of the cycle. Women with normal menstrual cycles showed a well-marked mid-cycle maximum whereas those taking oral contraceptives, in whom ovulation was blocked, failed to show any signs of such rhythmicity (Fig. 14.3) (Michael, Bonsall and Warner, 1974). While we have no direct evidence that these substances have communicatory significance in the human, we know that the human olfactory detection threshold is well below the concentrations found at midcycle. Furthermore, human testers can discriminate the sex of the owners of garments by their odour, and even identify those of their sexual partners (Hold and Schleidt 1977).

Social organization: the roles of sex and aggression

Social organization and behaviour may be regarded as the resultants of a number of species characteristics (e.g. size, mobility, nutritional needs, reproductive physiology) that interact with certain environmental factors (e.g. distribution of food, density of cover, presence of predators) so as to produce life-support strategies that are optimal for the survival of the individual and of the species. A given species in its

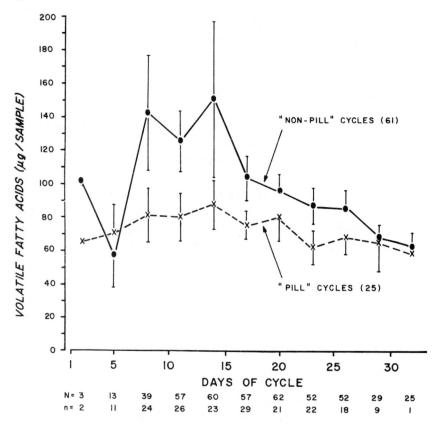

Fig. 14.3   Changes in volatile aliphatic acid content of the vaginal secretions of 47 women (86 cycles) during 3-day periods of the menstrual cycle. The rise before mid-cycle found in normal women was absent in those taking oral contraceptives ('pill' cycles). Vertical bars give standard error of means. N = number of 'non-pill' samples; n = number of 'pill' samples. (From Michael, Bonsall, and Warner (1974), with permission.)

habitat will be subjected to different selection pressures that may operate in opposition to each other. For example, in a physically small species with restricted mobility, the distribution of food in the environment might promote territoriality that serves to space individuals over the available resources. To reproduce, however, a male and female come together (often seasonally) for mating and their usual agonistic (aggressive and flight) responses must not prevent this. Studies on a number of vertebrates, particularly fishes and birds, have shown that there is a close relationship between reproductive activity and agonistic behaviour, and there is evidence that many courtship displays have originated in evolutionary terms from the conflict between agonistic tendencies towards, and sexual attraction for, the partner (Tinbergen 1959). Thus, the behavioural ambivalence with which our own species has daily to contend is a characteristic that is shared by many much simpler vertebrates. The onset of the breeding season is often associated with increased aggressivity, especially by males, and, rather remarkably, when females first approach males in their territories, they are often repeatedly attacked; this initial aggression towards the female is widely observed in fishes, birds, and many mammalian species. However, as the courtship proceeds, this aggression begins to be redirected from the female onto some other aspect of the environment. In some cases, this may involve other conspecifics not involved in the courtship of the pair. All species of primates studied exhibit intraspecific aggression, and its frequency and intensity appear to vary widely between species and between different groups of the same species. Within the group itself, the frequency of agonistic interactions increases with social change (Bernstein, Gordon, and Rose 1974), and changes with the level of sexual activity, increasing at the start of the mating season and varying in relation to the female's reproductive cycle. Thus, in a great many vertebrates, and certainly in primates, intraspecific aggression is the rule and mechanisms exist that modify its level of intensity. It seems highly probable that the human is no exception and that in man, too, there are mechanisms for modifying agonistic tendencies to ensure the formation and maintenance of social and sexual bonds. Important as it is, the study of these mechanisms is difficult in the human, but some understanding may be gained from experimentation in infrahuman primates.

Under our laboratory testing conditions, about half the males and females exhibit aggressive gestures and movements that are characterized by being directed *away from*, rather than towards, the partner (Zumpe and Michael 1970). An animal (the male or the female) will suddenly stare fixedly at some spot either inside or outside the cage and will start making threats in that direction (threatening-away). Between threats, it will briefly glance over its shoulder at the partner that is sitting beside or behind it. Eventually, the partner may join in and start making threats also, so that both animals are threatening together in the same general direction. This behaviour usually begins just before the start of a mounting series, continues between and even during mounts, and invariably stops after ejaculation has occurred.

Threatening-away by the male is closely associated with his sexual interest in the female; increasing when mounting attempts increase and decreasing when they decline. However, the female threatens-away only when receptive: her threatening-away behaviour increases with oestrogen treatment and declines with progesterone-induced un-receptivity.

Joint threatening-away by sexual partners is obviously a useful mechanism for directing onto the environment the aggression existing between the pair. In a social species under free-ranging conditions, such threats will almost invariably be directed towards other conspecifics in the vicinity; this helps to isolate the sexually interacting pair from interference from other group members and will consolidate consort-(sexual pair)-bonds. Threatening-away from the partner is high when direct aggression between the pair is low, and this lends further support to the view that it may be regarded as redirected aggression. Further, there is evidence that individual components of redirected aggression in the rhesus monkey have become ritualized into specifi-cally female invitational gestures, namely, the hand-reach, head-duck, and head-bob. Thus, mechanisms that exist in a large number of lower vertebrates are also clearly operative in a highly evolved primate with a complex social organization. Of course, in human societies and within the human family, instances of the utilization of analogous mechanisms abound, for instance, the 'scape-goat', the 'straw man', 'identification with the aggressor', the use of 'an external threat' by national leaders, etc.

Field observations and laboratory data suggest that the periodic making and breaking of consort-bonds are in large part the result of changes in sexual attraction and agonistic tendencies which are both under hormonal control. This proposition was investigated experiment-ally in intact females undergoing normal menstrual cycles by permitting them to express their readiness to gain access to each of two male partners by pressing a lever. All females consistently pressed faster for the male that (1) groomed them more (grooming being an index of social bonding in this species), (2) made fewer aggressive gestures, and (3) elicited fewer submissive gestures (Michael, Bonsall, and Zumpe 1978). In addition to reflecting a female's readiness to copulate, access times also seem to reflect the strength of social bonds which increase during the follicular phase of the cycle, reach a peak on the expected day of ovulation, and weaken markedly during the luteal phase when declining sexual attraction leads to a resumption of agonistic exchanges.

What, one may now ask, is the function subserved by fluctuations in these aggressive and sexual interactions? We have been led to the view that these variations are important for the maintenance of adequate levels of arousal and sexual potency in primates. Rhesus monkeys were subjected to regular testing with constantly receptive partners over a period of 3 years. Fig. 14.4 shows that after the first year, the numbers of ejaculations by males progressively declined, particularly in the third year of testing (1975 A). However, replacing the familiar females with a similarly treated group of unfamiliar females (with which the males had not been tested previously) resulted in an abrupt return of male potency to the high, initial levels (1975 B). Suddenly confronting the males in this way with unfamiliar partners resulted in a great deal of excitement, direct, and redirected aggression, particularly during early tests, and along with this went the increase in sexual activity. One month later, re-introduction of the original females was associated with an immediate deterioration in male potency (1975 C) (Michael and Zumpe 1978). Similar results were obtained with a group of castrated, testosterone-treated males, so that the behavioural effects could not have been mediated by the gonads. Thus, it seems that although excessive aggression between partners may totally disrupt the sexual interactions, some agonistic tension is necessary to maintain optimal levels of sexual excitement in this species.

In modern man, shielding from environmental changes and the virtual lack of breeding seasonality are now associated with diminished menstrual cyclicity and birth periodicity because of the wide-spread use of contraceptive techniques; these factors make for an almost continuous sexual life in our own species. Under such conditions, one might expect that social and cultural devices would be employed to provide the needed variability. This is seen (1) in the imposition of periodicity on sexual activity (menstrual and pregnancy taboos, Lent, safe period, etc.), (2) in the use of cultural means for periodically altering one's stimulus properties (clothing, adornment, coiffure, odour), and (3) in a tendency to break and remake consort bonds (new partners and easier divorce).

Bisexuality

In 1905 Freud proposed the theory of bisexuality, itself partially derived from the writings of Krafft-Ebing (1895) and others, to account for

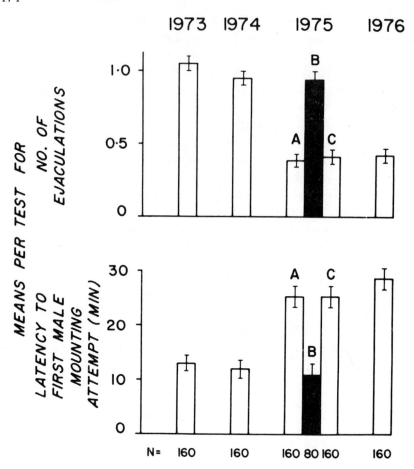

Fig.14.4　The potency of male rhesus monkeys gradually declines during successive years of testing with the same, constantly receptive, female partners (1973, 1974, 1975 A). Replacing these females with similarly treated new females with which the males were unfamiliar, immediately restored male sexual activity (1975 B). When the original females were reintroduced (1975 C), there was an abrupt deterioration in potency. Vertical bars give standard errors of means; N = number of tests. (From Michael and Zumpe 1978, with permission.)

some of the vagaries of human sexuality. This hypothesis has now received some confirmation from the field of general biology, and it was mentioned earlier that the bisexual potential of the embryonic gonad is now well established in many experimental forms. More recent work, already referred to, has indicated that a similar bisexual potential may exist in the diencephalic structures controlling both the pattern of sexual behaviour and the pattern of gonadotrophin secretion. Comparative studies in the field of sexual behaviour further illumine this area. Examples can be found throughout the vertebrates of some of the sexual behavioural characteristics of the opposite sex being exhibited in an animals' *normal* repertoire of sexual behaviour. It is not proposed here to deal further with effects produced experimentally by the administration of heterologous hormones during the perinatal period. In general, it is more common to find elements of the male pattern in the female than vice versa. Thus, mounting activity towards males and other females is *normally* shown by the oestrous guinea-pig and is used as a criterion when sexual behaviour is measured quantitatively in this species. Similar behaviour is sometimes shown by the rat (Beach and Rasquin 1942), and the mounting activity of cows in heat, towards other members of the herd, is a common observation. The sudden assumption of the male pattern (neck grip, mounting, and pelvic thrusts) by one of a pair of oestrous cats has been described by Beach (1948) and Michael (1961a); closely similar behaviour has been reported in the African lioness (Cooper 1942). Under natural or semi-natural conditions, many female primates (tree shrews, squirrel monkeys, talapoins, macaques, baboons, chimpanzees) have been observed to mount and execute pelvic thrusts on other females or males, and such mounting activity seems to occur most frequently at a time when females are also sexually receptive to males. This behaviour, by those who object to it, is sometimes attributed to abnormal caging conditions (zoos, circuses, etc.), and is thought of as an aberration of captivity; but this is untrue, as the many field observations can document. In our laboratory, where observations are made on heterosexual pairs of feral-born and -reared rhesus monkeys, about 37 per cent of females have been observed to make mounts or attempted mounts on their male partners (Michael, Wilson, and Zumpe 1974). Whether or not a female's mounting attempts result in a mount depends on the persistence of her efforts and the tolerance of the male. In some cases, the male responds aggressively and the female never attempts to mount that male again. However, in 5 out of 40 females, mounting behaviour occurred with sufficient frequency and regularity to warrant numerical treatment. Several mounting postures are adopted, but females frequently assume a typically male pattern in which they clasp the backs of the male's legs with their feet and his hips with their hands while making male-like pelvic thrusts. In intact females, changes in the frequency of mounting are closely related to the menstrual cycle, increasing during the follicular phase to reach a peak on day 17, and declining again thereafter. Ovariectomy results in a decrease in female mounting, whereas oestrogen replacement restores it. Castration and testosterone replacement treatment of males also affect the mounting behaviour of their ovariectomized, oestrogen-treated female partners. When ejaculatory activity reached very low levels some 10 weeks after castration, there was a marked increase in the number of mounts by female partners, and this effect was reversed when testosterone replacement treatment restored the males' ejaculatory activity. This, together with the observation that female mounts often appear to stimulate the male to mount, and that a series of female mounts may, albeit rarely, culminate in rigidity and muscular spasms similar to those seen during orgasm in the male, suggests that mounting by females may serve both sexual initiating and masturbatory functions.

Acknowledgements

The original work reported here was supported by grants from the Medical Research Council, U.K., the Bethlem–Maudsley Research Fund, the Foundations Fund for Research in Psychiatry, the Population Council and Grant MH19506, National Institute of Mental Health, U.S. Public Health Service – all these are very gratefully acknowledged.

References

Allen, E. and Doisey, E. A. (1923). *J. Amer. med. Assn.* **81**, 819–21.
——, Doisy, E. A., Francis, B. F., Robertson, L. L., Colgate, C. E., Johnston, C. G., Kountz, W. S., and Gibson, H. V. (1924). *Amer. J. Anat.* **34**, 133–81.
Asdell, S. A., de Alba, J., and Roberts, J. B. (1945). *J. Anim. Sci.* **4**, 277–84.
Ball, J. (1934). *J. comp. Psychol.* **18**, 419–22.
Bard, P. (1935). *Amer. J. Physiol.* **113**, 5–6P.
—— (1939). *Res. Publ. Ass. nerv. ment. Dis.* **19**, 190–218.
—— (1940). *Res. Publ. Ass. nerv. ment. Dis.* **20**, 551–79.
—— and Rioch, D. M. (1937). *Johns Hopk. Hosp. Bull.* **60**, 73–147.
Barfield, R. J. (1965). *Amer. Zool.* **5**, 203.
Barr, M. L. (1956). *In modern trends in obstetrics and gynaecology*, p.117. London.
—— (1957). *Prog. Gynec.* **3**, 131.
—— and Bertram, E. G. (1949). *Nature (Lond.)* **163**, 676–7.
Barraclough, C. A. (1961). *Endocrinology* **68**, 62–7.
—— and Gorski, R. A. (1961). *Endocrinology* **68**, 68–79.
Beach, F. A. (1945). *Anat. Rec.* **92**, 289–92.

—— (1948). *Hormones and behavior*. New York.

—— and Rasquin, P. (1942). *Endocrinology* **31**, 393–409.

Bernstein, I. S., Gordon, T. P., and Rose, R. M. (1974). *Folia primat.* **21**, 81–107.

Berthold, A. A. (1849). *Arch. Anat. Physiol. Lpz.* **16**, 42–6.

Bishop, P. M. F., Lessof, M. H., and Polani, P. E. (1960). *Mem. Soc. Endocrin.* No. 7, 162–72.

Bouin, P. and Ancel, P. (1903). *C. R. Soc. Biol. (Paris)* **55**, 1682–4.

Bromiley, R. B. and Bard, P. (1940). Quoted by Bard (1940).
Bronson, F. H. (1974). *Frontiers in Biology* **36**, 344–65.

Brooks, C. McC. (1937). *Amer. J. Physiol* **120**, 544–53.

—— (1938). *Amer. J. Physiol.* **121**, 157–77.

Burns, R. K. (1925). *J. exp. Zool.* **42**, 31–89.

—— (1955). *Proc. Nat. Acad. Sci.* **41**, 669–76.

—— (1956). *Amer. J. Anat.* **98**, 35–67.

Carpenter, C. R. (1934). *Comp. Psychol. Monogr.* **10**, 1–168.

Cole, H. H., Hart, G. H., and Miller, R. F. (1945). *Endocrinology* **36**, 370–80.

Cooper, J. B. (1942). *Comp. Psychol. Monogr.* **17**, 1–48.

Craig, J. V., Casida, L. E., and Chapman, A. B. (1945). *Amer. Naturalist* **88**, 365–72.

Curtis, R. F., Ballantine, J. A., Keverne, E. B., Bonsall, R. W., and Michael, R. P. (1971). *Nature (Lond.)* **232**, 396–8.

Dantchakoff, V. (1935). *C. R. Acad. Sci. (Paris)* **201**, 161–3.

—— (1936). *Bull. Biol. France Belg.* **70**, 241–307.

Davidson, J. M. (1966). *Endocrinology* **79**, 783–94.

Davis, C. D. (1939). *Amer. J. Physiol.* **127**, 374–80.

Dempsey, E. W., Hertz, R., and Young, W. C. (1936). *Amer. J. Physiol.* **116**, 201–9.

—— and Rioch, D. M. (1939). *J. Neurophysiol.* **2**, 9–18.

Eberlein, W. R. and Bongiovanni, A. M. (1955). *J. Clin. Endocrinol. Metab.* **15**, 1531–4.

Erhardt, A. E. and Baker, S. W. (1974). *Sex differences in behaviour*, pp.33–51. New York.

Everett, J. W., Sawyer, C. H., and Markee, J. E. (1949). *Endocrinology* **44**, 234–50.

Ferguson-Smith, M. A., Lennox, B., Stewart, J. S., and Mack, W. S. (1960). *Mem. Soc. Endocrin.* No. 7, 173–81.

Freud, A. and Burlingham, D. (1942). *Young children in wartime*. London.

Freud, S. (1905). *Three essays on the theory of sexuality*, Standard Edition, Vol. 7. London.

Glascock, R. F. and Michael, R. P. (1962). *J. Physiol.* **163**, 38–9P.

Goldschmidt, R. B. (1931). *Quart Rev. Biol.* **6**, 125.

Goy, R. W., Bridson, W. E., and Young, W. C. (1961). *Anat. Rec.* **139**, 232.
—— and Jakway, J. S. (1962). *Roots of behavior*, pp.96–110. New York.
—— and Young W. C. (1957). *Behaviour* **10**, 340–54.

Greene, R. R. (1942). *Biol. Symp.* **9**, 105–23.

Grunt, J. and Young, W. C. (1952). *Endocrinology* **51**, 237–48.

Hammond, J., Jr., Hammond, J., and Parkes, A. S. (1942). *J. Agric. Sci.* **32**, 308–23.

Hampson, J. G. (1955). *Johns. Hopkins Hosp. Bull.* **96**, 265–73.
——, Money, J., and Hampson, J. L. (1956). *J. Clin. Endocr.* **16**, 547–56.

Hampson, J. L. and Hampson, J. G. (1961). *In Sex and Internal Secretions,* pp.1401–30. Baltimore.

Harlow, H. F. (1962*a*). *Amer. Psychol.* **17**, 1–9.
—— (1962*b*). *Sci. Amer.* **207**, 137–46.
—— and Zimmermann, R. R. (1959). *Science (N.Y.)* **130**, 421–32.

Harris, G. W. (1955). *Neural control of the pituitary gland.* London.
—— and Jacobsohn, D. (1952). *Proc. Roy. Soc. (Biol.)* **139**, 263–76.
—— and Levine, S. (1962). *J. Physiol.* **142**, 26P.
——, Michael, R. P., and Scott, P. P. (1958). *Ciba Foundation Symposium: The neurological basis of behaviour.* pp.236–51.

Hartman, C. G. (1932). *Contrib. Embryol.* **23**, 1–161.

Hemmingsen, A. M. (1933). *Skand. Arch. Physiol.* **65**, 97–250.

Hold, B. and Schleidt, M. (1977). *Z. Tierpsychol.* **43**, 225–38.

Holyoke, E. A. (1949). *Anat. Rec.* **103**, 675–99.

Humphrey, R. R. (1928). *Biol. Bull.* **55**, 317–39.
—— (1942). *Biol. Symp.* **9**, 81–104.

Jacobs, P. A., Baikie, A. G., Court Brown, W. M., Forrest, H., Roy, J. R., Stewart, J. S. S., and Lennox, B. (1959). *Lancet* **ii**, 591–2.

Jost, A. (1947). *Arch. Anat. micr. Morph. exp.* **36**, 242–70.
—— (1953). *Recent Progr. Hormone Res.* **8**, 379–418.
—— (1955). *Mem. Soc. Endocrin.* No. 4, 237–48.
—— and Bozic, B. (1951). *C. R. Soc. Biol. (Paris)* **145**, 647.

Keller, K. and Tandler, J. (1916). *Wien. Tierarztl. Wschr.* **3**, 513.

Klein, M. (1948). *Contributions to psycho-analysis,* 1921–45. London.

Klinefelter, H. F., Reifenstein, E. C., and Albright, F. (1942). *J. Clin. Endocrin.* **2**, 615.

Kondo, K. (1955). *Jap. J. Genet.* **30**, 139–46.

Krafft-Ebing, R. von (1895). *Jb. Psychiat. Neurol.* **13**, 1.

Kunde, M., D'amour, F., Carlson, A., and Gustafson, R. (1930). *Amer. J. Physiol.* **95**, 630–40.

Lillie, F. R. (1917). *J. exp. Zool.* **23**, 371–452.

Lisk, R. D. (1962). *Am. J. Physiol.* **203**, 493–6.

Lorenz, K. (1937)..*Auk* **54**, 245–73.

Marrian, G. F. and Parkes, A. S. (1930). *J. Physiol.* **69**, 372–6.

Marshall, F. H. A. (1922). *The physiology of reproduction,* London.
—— and Hammond, J. (1945). *J. Endocr.* **4**, 159–68.

Mason, W. A. and Harlow, H. F. (1958). *Psychol. Rep.* **4**, 79–82.

McClung, C. E. (1902). *Biol. Bull.* **3**, 43–84.

Michael, R. P. (1958). *Nature (Lond.)* **181**, 567–8.
—— (1961*a*). *Behaviour* **18**, 1–24.
—— (1961*b*). *Regional Neurochemistry,* pp.465–80. Oxford.
—— (1962*a*). *Science (N.Y.)* **136**, 322–3.
—— (1962*b*). *Exerpta med. (Amst.), Int. Congr. Ser.,* No. 47, 650–2.
—— (1971). *Frontiers in Neuroendocrinology,* pp.359–98. London.
—— and Bonsall, R. W. (1977). *Nature (Lond.)* **265**, 463–5.
—— and Glascock, R. F. (1961). *Proceedings of the Fifth International Congress on Biochemistry,* 10 (Abstract).
—— and Keverne, E. B. (1968). *Nature (Lond.),* **218**, 746–9.
—— and Plant, T. M. (1969). *Nature (Lond.)* **222**, 579–81.
—— and Saayman, G. S. (1968). *J. Endocr.* **41**, 231–46.
—— and Welegalla, J. (1968). *J. Endocr.* **41**, 407–20.
—— and Zumpe, D. (1970*a*). *J. Reprod. Fert.* **21**, 199–201.
—— —— (1970*b*). *Behaviour* **36**, 168–86.
—— —— (1978). *Science* (N.Y.) **200**, 451–3.
——, Bonsall, R. W., and Warner, P. (1974). *Science (N.Y.)* **186**, 1217–19.
——, ——, and Zumpe, D. (1976). *Vitam. Hormones* **34**, 137–86.
——, ——, —— (1978). *J. comp. physiol. Psychol.* In press.
——, Herbert, J., and Welegalla, J. (1966). *J. Endocr.* **36**, 263–79.
——, ——, —— (1967). *J. Endocr.* **39**, 81–98.
——, Saayman, G. S., and Zumpe, D. (1968). *J. Endocr.* **41**, 421–31.
——, Wilson, M. I., and Zumpe, D. (1974). *Sex differences in behaviour,* pp.399–412. New York.
——, Zumpe, D., Keverne, E. B., and Bonsall, R. W. (1972). *Recent Progr. Hormone Res.* **28**, 665–706.
——, Zumpe, D., Richter, M., and Bonsall, R. W. (1977). *Horm. Behav.* **9**, 296–308.

Money, J. (1961). In *Sex and internal secretions,* pp.1383–9. Baltimore.

Moore, C. R. and Price, D. (1942). *J. exp. Zool.* **90**, 229–65.

Moore, K. L. and Barr, M. L. (1954). *Acta anat. (Basel)* **21**, 197.

Moore, N. W. and Robinson, T. J. (1957). *J. Endocr.* **14**, 297–303.

Morgan, T. H., Bridges, C. B., and Sturtevant, A. H. (1925). *Bibl. Genet.* **2**, 1–262.

Morris, J. McL. (1953). *Amer. J. Obstet. Gynecol.* **65**, 1192–211.

Pfeiffer, C. A. (1936). *Amer. J. Anat.* **58**, 195–221.

Phoenix, C. H., Goy, R. W., Gerall, A. A., and Young, W. C. (1959). *Endocrinology* **65**, 369–82.

Polani, P. E. (1970). *Phil. Trans. roy. Soc. London B***259**, 187–204.

——, Lessof, M. H., and Bishop, P. M. F. (1956). *Lancet* **ii**, 118–20.

Raisman, G. and Field, P. M. (1971). *Science (N.Y.)* **173**, 731–3.

Rasmussen, E. W. (1952). *Proceedings of the Second International Congress on the Physiology and Pathology of Animal Reproduction* **1**, 188–91.

Robertson, J., Bowlby, J., and Rosenbluth, D. (1952). *Psycho-analytic Study Child*, **7**, 82.

Root, W. S. and Bard, P. (1937). *Amer. J. Physiol.* **119**, 392–3.

Scott, J. P. (1945). *Comp. Psychol. Monogr.* **18**, 1–29.

——, Frederickson, E., and Fuller, L. J. (1951). *Personality*, **1**, 162–83.

Scott, P. P., and Lloyd-Jacob, M. A. (1955). *Stud. Fertil.* **7**, 123–8.

Segal, S. J., and Johnson, D. C. (1959). *Arch. Anat. micr. Morph. exp.* **48**, 261.

Spitz, R. A. (1950). *Psycho-analytic Study Child*. **5**, 66.

Tinbergen, N. (1959). *Behaviour* **15**, 1–70.

Tjio, J. H., and Levan, A. (1956). *Hereditas* **42**, 1–6.

Turner, C. D. (1940). *J. exp. Zool.* **83**, 1–31.

Udry, J. R., and Morris, N. M. (1968). *Nature (Lond.)* **220**, 593–6.

Ward, I. L. (1972). *Science (N.Y.)* **175**, 82–4.

Wells, L. J., and van Wagenen, G. (1954). *Contr. Embryol. Carneg. Inst.* **35**, 93–106.

Wiesner, B. P. and Mirskaia, L. (1930). *Quart. J. exp. Physiol.* **20**, 274–9.

Williams, E. and Scott, J. P. (1953). *Behaviour* **6**, 35–64.

Willier, B. H. (1933). *Wilhelm Roux' Arch. Entwickl-Mech.* **130**, 616–49.

——, Gallagher, T. F., and Koch, F. C. (1935). *Proc. nat. Acad. Sci.* **21**, 625–31.

Wilkins, L., Jones, H. W., Holman, G. H., and Stempfel, R. S. (1958). *J. clin. Endocr.* **18**, 559–85.

Winnicott, D. W. (1958). *Collected Papers*. London.

Witschi, E. (1932). In *Sex and internal secretions*, Chapter 5. Baltimore.

—— (1939). In *Sex and internal secretions*, Chapter 4. Baltimore.

Wolff, E. (1946). *Arch. Anat. micr. Morph. exp.* **36**, 69–91.

—— (1948). *C. R. Acad. Sci. (Paris)* **226**, 1140–1.

—— (1953). *Experientia* **9**, 121–33.

—— and Haffen, K. (1952). *J. exp. Zool.* **119**, 381–404.

Young, W. C. (1941). *Quart. Rev. Biol.* **16**, 135–56, 311–35.

Zumpe, D. and Michael, R. P. (1970). *Anim. Behav.* **18**, 11–19.

Bibliography

Each chapter contains a selected list of references. The following additional bibliography is of the last five years. Because publications often cover many specific areas, particular writings as well as the fullest references may be obtained by widely consulting this bibliography in conjunction with the relevant chapter reference lists.

Psychoanalytic theory of perversion

BLÉDER, J. (1973) [The polymorphous sexual deviant: a reading of Freud and the Bible.] *Ann. Med. Psychol. (Paris)* **2**, 274–81 (Fre.)

DEMOULIN, C. *et al.* (1973) [Perverse structure and sexual perversion. I. A clinical approach.] *Acta Psychiatr. Belg.* **73**, 725–46 (Eng. Abstr.) (Fre.)

DENKO, J. D. (1976) Amplification of the erotic enema deviance. *Am. J. Psychother.* **30**, 236–55.

LEVINE, E. M. *et al.* (1977) Sexual dysfunctions and psychoanalysis. *Am. J. Psychiatry* **134**, 646–51.

McDOUGALL, J. (1972) Primal scene and sexual perversion. *Int. J. Psychoanal.* **53**, 371–84.

MARCHAIS, P. (1975) [Process of perversion. Methodological and clinical study.] *Ann. Med. Psychol. (Paris)* **2**, 241–66 (Eng. Abstr.) (Fre.)

PETO, A. (1975) The etiological significance of the primal scene in perversions. *Psychoanal. Q.* **44**, 177–90.

STOLOROW, R. D. *et al.* (1973) A partial analysis of a perversion involving bugs. *Int. J. Psychoanal.* **54**, 349–50.

STOLOROW, R. D. (1975) Addendum to a partial analysis of a perversion involving bugs: an illustration of the narcissistic funtion of perverse activity. *Int. J. Psychoanal.* **56**, 361–4.

Fetishism

BADER, A. (1976) [Modern images of womanhood and their relationship to fetishism.] *Schweiz. Arch. Neurol. Neurochir. Psychiatr.* **119**, 49–72 (Eng. Abstr.) (Ger.)

BAK, R. C. (1974) Distortions of the concept of fetishism. *Psychoanal. Study Child* **29**, 191–214.

BETHELL, M. F. (1974) A rare manifestation of fetishism. *Arch. sex. Behav.* **3**, 301–2.

EPSTEIN, A. W. (1975) The fetish object: phylogenetic considerations. *Arch. sex. Behav.* **4**, 303–8.

FURLAN, P. M. *et al.* (1975) [A case of autoerotic fetishism: psychodynamic evaluation (author's transl.).] *Riv. Patol. Nerv. Ment.* **96**, 287–300 (Eng. Abstr.) (Ita.)

HAMILTON, J. W. (1977) The evolution of a shoe fetish. *Int. J. Psychoanal. Psychother.* **6**, 323–37.

McSWEENY, A. J. (1972) Fingernail fetishism: report of a case treated with hypnosis. *Am. J. clin. Hypn.* **15**, 139–43.

MARKS, I. M. (1972) Phylogenesis and learning in the acquisition of fetishism. *Dan. med. Bull.* **19**, 307–10.

MARSHALL, W. L. (1974) A combined treatment approach to the reduction of multiple fetish-related behaviours. *J. consult. clin. Psychol.* **42**, 613–16.

PETO, A. (1973) The olfactory forerunner of the superego: its role in normalcy, neurosis and fetishism. *Int. J. Psychoanal.* **54**, 323–30.

PONIKLEWSKA, W. *et al.* (1973) [Fetishism in the course of simple schizophrenia.] *Psychiat. Pol.* **7**, 645–7. (Eng. Abstr.) (Pol.)

ROLPHE, H. *et al.* (1975) Some observations on transitional object and infantile fetish. *Psychoanal. Q.* **44**, 206–31.

TAYLOR, B. *et al.* (1976) Amputee fetishism: an exclusive journal interview with Dr. John Money of Johns Hopkins. *Md State med. J.* **25**, 35–9.

WAKEFIELD, P. L. *et al.* (1977) The hobbyist. A euphemism for self-mutilation and fetishism. *Bull. Menninger Clin.* **41**, 539–52.

ZAVITZIANOS, G. (1972) [Fetishism and exhibitionism in women and their relations with psychopathy and kleptomania.] *Rev. Fr. Psychoanal.* **36**, 475–89 (Fre.)

—— (1977) The object in fetishism, homovestism and transvestism. *Int. J. Psychoanal.* **58**, 487–95.

Gender disorders

ADKINS, E. K. (1976) Embryonic exposure to an antiestrogen masculinizes behaviour of femail quail. *Physiol. Behav.* **17**, 357–9.

ARRIGONI, G. *et al.* (1977) [Stenosis of the urethral neo-meatus in surgery for transsexualism. Observation of 2 man–woman cases.] *J. Urol. Nephrol (Paris)* **83**, 240–3 (Fre.)

ATTARDI, B. *et al.* (1976) Androgen and estrogen receptors in the developing mouse brain. *Endocrinology* **99**, 1279–90.

Australian Medical Journal (1973) Editorial: Transsexualism. *Med. J. Aust.* **2**, 251–2.

BAKER, H. J. (1975) Male transsexualism. Confirmation of a hypothesis? *Arch. gen. Psychiat.* **32**, 1587–8.

BARAMKI, T. A. (1974) Embryology of the urogenital system in man and genetic factors in intersex problems and transsexualism. *Clin. plast. Surg.* **1**, 201–13.

BARLOW, D. H. *et al.* (1973) Gender identity change in a transsexual. *Arch. gen. Psychiat.* **28**, 569–76.

—— *et al.* (1977) Gender identity change in a transsexual: an exorcism. *Arch. sex. Behav.* **6**, 387–95.

BARR, R. *et al.* (1976) Autonomic responses of transsexual and homosexual males to erotic film sequences. *Arch. sex. Behav.* **5**, 211–22.

BATES, J. E. *et al.* (1973). Measurement of deviant gender development in boys. *Child Dev.* **44**, 591–8.

—— (1974) Gender role abnormalities in boys: an analysis of clinical ratings.

J. abnorm. Child Psychol. **2**, 1–16.

—— *et al.* (1975) Intervention with families of gender-disturbed boys. *Am. J. Orthopsychiat.* **45**, 150–7.

BAUDER, E. S. *et al.* (1976) Report of a male transsexual. *Pa. Med.* **79**, 48–9.

BELL, J. I. *et al.* (1977) Haemoperitoneum in a transsexual [letter]. *Lancet* **2**, 817.

BELLI, M. M. (1978) Transsexual surgery. A new tort? *J. Am. med. Ass.* **239**, 2143–8.

BELLINGER, C. G. *et al.* (1973) Secondary surgery in transsexuals. *Plast. reconstr. Surg.* **51**, 628–31.

BENJAMIN, H. *et al.* (1973) Transsexualism. *Am J. Nurs.* **73**, 457–61.

BENTLER, P. M. (1976) A typology of transsexualism: gender identity theory and data. *Arch. sex. Behav.* **5**, 567–84.

BOILLY-MARER, Y. (1976) [Stability of determination and differentiation of the somatic sexual characters in *Nereis pelagica* L. (Annelida, polychaeta).] *J. Embryol. exp. Morphol.* **36**, 183–96 (Eng. Abstr.) (Fre.)

BOMBA, J. (1972) [Therapeutic problems in transsexualism.] *Psychiat. Pol.* **6**, 569–75. (Eng. Abstr.) (Pol.)

BRAÜEROVA, E. *et al.* (1976) [Problems of transvestism manifestations in childhood.] *Cesk. Pediat.* **31**, 207 (Eng. Abstr.) (Cze.)

British Medical Journal (1974) Editorial: Transvestism and transsexualism. *Br. med. J.* **2**, 289–90.

—— (1974) The management of transsexualism. *Br. Med. J.* **2**, 289–90.

BRODY, J. E. (1973) Transsexual surgery: 10 000 helps mind match body. *Can. Hosp.* **50**, 32–3.

BUHRICH, N. and McCONAGHY, N. (1978) Two clinically distinct syndromes of transsexualism. *Br. F. Psychiat.* **113**, 73.

—— *et al.* (1976) Transvestite fiction. *J. nerv. ment. Dis.* **163**, 420–7.

—— (1977) A case of familial heterosexual transvestism. *Acta Psychiat. scand.* **55**, 199–201.

—— (1977) Brief communication. Transvestism in history. *J. nerv. ment. Dis.* **165**, 64–6.

—— *et al.* (1977) Can fetishism occur in transsexuals? *Arch. sex. Behav.* **6**, 223–35.

—— *et al.* (1977) Clinical comparison of transvestism and transsexualism: an overview. *Aust. N. Z. F. Psychiat.* **11**, 83–6.

—— *et al.* (1977) The clinical syndromes of femmiphilic transvestism. *Arch. sex. Behav.* **6**, 397–412.

—— *et al.* (1977) The discrete syndromes of transvestism and transsexualism. *Arch. sex. Behav.* **6**, 483–95.

BUHRICH, N. (1976) A heterosexual transvestite club: psychiatric aspects. *Aust. N.Z. J. Psychiat.* **10**, 331–5.

BULLOUGH, V. L. (1974) Transvestites in the middle ages. *Am. J. Sociol.* **79**, 1381–94 (Eng. Abstr.) (Jap.)

—— (1975) Transsexualism in history. *Arch. sex. Behav.* **4**, 561–71.

CALNEN, T. (1975) Gender identity crises in young schizophrenic women. *Perspect. psychaiat. Care* **13**, 83–9.

CHILDS, A. (1977) Acute symbiotic psychosis in a postoperative transsexual. *Arch. sex. Behav.* **6**, 37–44.

CLINGMAN, J. *et al.* (1976) Gender roles and human sexuality. *J. Pers. Assess.* **40**, 276–84.

CROVITZ, E. (1976) Treatment of the transsexual and medicolegal issues. *Forensic Sci.* **7**, 1–8.

DAVENPORT, C. W. *et al.* (1977) Gender identity change in a female adolescent transsexual. *Arch. sex. Behav.* **6**, 327–40.

DE WOLF, M. (1976) [The transsexual enigma. Apropos of the work of Jan Morris 'Enigma'.) *Acta. Psychiat. Belg.* **76**, 860–81 (Eng. Abstr.) (Fre.)

DEROGATIS, L. R. *et al.* (1978) A psychological profile of the transsexual. I. The male. *J. nerv. ment. Dis.* **166**, 234–54.

DIAMOND, M. (1974) Letter: Transsexualism. *Med. J. Aust.* **1**, 51.

DÖRNER, G. *et al.* (1967) On the evocability of a positive oestrogen feedback action on LH secretion in transsexual men and women. *Endokrinologie* **67**, 20–5.

DOSIK, H. *et al.* Y-chromosomal genes in a phenotypic male with a 46XX karyotype. *J. Am. med. Ass.* **236**, 2505–8.

EBERLE, A. (1974) Male transsexualism. *West. J. Med.* **120**, 376–86, (Transsexualism in the tension field of medicine and law. Errors and confusion.) *Med. Klin.* **69**, 304–8.

EDGERTON, M. T. (1973) Transsexualism—a surgical problem? *Plast. reconstr. Surg.* **52**, 74–6.

—— (1974) The surgical treatment of male transsexuals. *Clin. plast. Surg.* **1**, 285–323.

EISSLER, K. R. (1977) Comments on penis envy and orgasm in women. *Psychoanal. Study Child.* **32**, 29–83.

FABER, H. (1973) Specifics of physical care after transsexual surgery. *Am. J. Nurs.* **73**, 463.

FALICKI, Z. *et al.* (1975) [Female transsexualism in psychiatric diagnosis.] *Psychiat. Pol.* **9**, 647–51. (Pol.)

FEINBLOOM, D. H. *et al.* (1976) Lesbian/feminist orientation among male-to-female transsexuals. *J. Homosex.* **2**, 59–71.

FELDMAN, W. S. (1977) The transsexual imbroglio. *J. Leg. Med.* **5**, 16E–16G, 16K, 16O–16P.

FINNEY, J. C. *et al.* (1975) A study of transsexuals seeking gender reassignment. *Am. J. Psychiat.* **132**, 962–4.

FLORES, J. R. *et al.* (1971) (The transsexual syndrome.) *Rev. Neuropsiquiat.* **34**, 37–57 (Eng. Abstr.) (Spa.)

FLUMARA, N. J. *et al.* (1973) Gonorrhoea and condyloma acuminata in a male transsexual. *Br. J. vener. Dis.* **49**, 478–9.

FØGH, M. *et al.* (1978) Serum-testosterone during oral administration of testosterone in hypogonadal men and transsexual women. *Acta Endocrinol.* (KGh) **87**, 643.

FRANZINI, L. R. *et al.* (1977). Detectability and perceptions of a transsexual: implications for therapy. *J. Homosex.* **2**, 269–79.

FREUND, K. *et al.* (1974) The transsexual syndrome in homosexual males. *J. nerv. ment. Dis.* **158**, 145–53.

——— *et al.* (1974) Parent–child relations in transsexual and non-transsexual homosexual males. *Br. J. Psychiat.* **124**, 22–3.

FRIEDMAN, R. C. *et al.* (1976) Reassessment of homosexuality and transsexualism. *Ann. Rev. Med.* **27**, 57–62.

GEORGE, G. C. *et al.* (1972) Transsexualism in a fourteen-year-old male. *S. Afr. med. J.* **46**, 1947–8.

GILBERG, A. L. (1977) Gender-specific therapy problems in male youths. *Am. J. Psychoanal.* **37**, 253–5.

GODLEWSKI, J. (1976) [Some comments on the particular features of incest and transsexualism.] *Psychiat. Pol.* **10**, 559–63 (Pol.)

——— (1977) [Postoperative functioning of transsexualists] *Wiad. Lek.* **30**, 1891 (Pol.)

GRANATO, R. C. (1974) Surgical approach to male transsexualism. *Urology* **3**, 792–6.

GREEN, R. (1970) Little boys who behave as girls. *Calif. Med.* **113**, 12–16.

——— (1974) *Sexual identity conflict in children and adults.* New York.

HABERMAN, M. *et al.* (1975) Gender identity confusion, schizophrenia and a 47 XYY karyotype: a case report. *Psychoneuroendocrinology* **1**, 207–9.

HASTINGS, D. W. (1974) Postsurgical adjustment of male transsexual patients. *Clin. plast. Surg.* **1**, 335–44.

HEIMAN, E. M. *et al.* (1975) Transsexualism in Vietnam. *Arch. sex. Behav.* **4**, 89–95.

HENRIK, H. *et al.* (1973) [Surgical construction of a vagina in primary agenesis and transsexualism.] *Tidsskr. Nor. Laegeforen.* **93**, 1042–3 (Eng. Abstr.) (Nor.)

HERSCHKOWITZ, S., *et al.* (1978) Suicide attempts in a female-to-male transsexual. *Am. J. Psychiat.* **135**, 368.

HEREMANS, G. F. *et al.* (1976) Female phenotype in a male child due to 17-alpha-hydroxylase deficiency. *Arch. Dis. Child.* **51**, 721–3.

HIGHAM, E. (1976) Case management of the gender incongruity syndrome in childhood and adolescence. *J. Homosex.* **2**, 49–57.

HOENIG, J. *et al.* (1973) Epidemiological aspects of transsexualism. *Psychiat. Clin. (Basel)* **6**, 65–80.

——— *et al.* (1974) Sexual and other abnormalities in the family of a transsexual. *Psychiat. Clin. (Basel)* **7**, 334–46.

——— *et al.* (1974) The nosological position of transsexualism. *Arch. sex. Behav.* **3**, 273–87.

——— *et al.* (1974) The prevalence of transsexualism in England and Wales. *Br. J. Psychiat.* **124**, 181–90.

——— (1977) The legal position of the transsexual: mostly unsatisfactory outside Sweden. *Can. med. Ass. J.* **116**, 319–23.

HOFFMAN, B. F. (1977) Two new cases of XYZ chromosome complement: and a review of the literature. *Can. Psychiat. Ass. J.* **22**, 447–55.

HOLLOWAY, J. P. (1974) Transsexuals: legal considerations. *Arch. sex. Behav.* **3**, 33–50.

HOOPES, J. E. (1974) Surgical construct of the male external genitalia. *Clin. plast. Surg.* **1**, 325–34.

HORE, B. D. *et al.* (1973) Male transsexualism, two cases in a single family. *Arch. sex. Behav.* **2**, 317–21.

—— *et al.* (1975) Male transsexualism in England: sixteen cases with surgical intervention. *Arch. sex. Behav.* **4**, 81–8.

HYDE, V. *et al.* (1977) A male MZ twin pair, concordant for transsexualism, discordant for schizophrenia. *Acta psychiat. Scand.* **56**, 265–75.

HYNIE, J. *et al.* (1975) [The transsexual female (author's transl.).] *Cesk. Psychiat.* **71**, 48–52 (Eng. Abstr.) (Cze.)

IMBER, H. (1976) The management of transsexualism. *Med. J. Aust.* **2**, 676–8.

IMIELINSKI, K. *et al.* (1976) [Transsexualism and partnership. A clinical case.] *Psychiat. Pol.* **10**, 565–9 (Pol.)

—— *et al.* (1976) [The sex disapproval syndrome.] *Pol. Tyg. Lek.* **31**, 1803–5 (Eng. Abstr.) (Pol.)

JONAS, S. P. (1976) Transsexualism and social attitudes. A case report. *Psychiat. Clin. (Basel)* **9**, 14–20.

JONES, J. R. *et al.* (1973) Plasma testosterone levels and female transsexualism. *Arch. sex. Behav.* **2**, 251–66.

JÖRGENSEN, G. *et al.* (1976) [Transsexuality—medical and legal aspects (author's transl.).] *Munch. Med. Wochenschr.* **118**, 639–44 (Eng. Abstr.) (Ger.)

JUCOVY, M. E. (1976) Initiation fantasies and transvestitism. *J. Am. psychoanal. Ass.* **24**, 525–46.

KANDO, T. (1973) *Sex change: the achievement of gender identity by feminized transsexuals.* Springfield, Illinois.

KÖBBERLING, J. *et al.* (1972) [Transsexualism in testicular feminization.] *Klin. Wochenschr.* **50**, 696–701 (Eng. Abstr.) (Ger.)

KOCKOTT, G. *et al.* (1976) [Cerebral dysfunction in transsexualism.] *Nervenarzt* **47**, 310–8 (Ger.)

KONERT, H. *et al.* (1977) [Acute form of idiopathic transsexualism.] *Psychiat. Pol.* **11**, 241–3 (Pol.)

KONIG, P. (1973) [A case of transsexualism in a female schizophrenic patient.] *Wien. Z. Nervenheilkd.* **31**, 167–75 (Eng. Abstr.) (Ger.)

KRUEGER, D. W. (1978) Symptom passing in a transvestite father and three sons. *Am. J. Psychiat.* **135**, 739–42.

KUBIE, L. S. (1974) The drive to become both sexes. *Psychoanal. Q.* **43**, 349–426.

KUHR, M. D. (1977) Neural-tube defects and mid-cycle abstinence: a test of the 'over-ripeness' hypothesis in man. *Dev. Med. Child Neurol.* **19**, 589–92.

LAHL, R. *et al.* (1977) [Multiple sex drive abnormalities in a patient with Klinefelter's syndrome.] *Psychiat. Neurol. med. Psychol. (Leipz.)* **29**, 152–63 (Eng. Abstr.) (Ger.)

Lakartidningen (1977) [Transsexualism.] **74**, 3857–60 (Swe.)

LANGEVIN, R. *et al.* (1977) The clinical profile of male transsexuals living as female vs. those living as males. *Arch. sex. Behav.* **6**, 143–54.

LA TORRE, R. A. *et al.* (1976) Cognitive style, hemispheric specialization, and tested abilities of transsexuals and nontranssexuals. *Percept. Mot. Skills* **43**,

719–22.

LAUB, D. R. *et al.* (1974) A rehabilitation program for gender dysphoria syndrome by surgical sex change. *Plast. reconstr. Surg.* **53**, 388–403.

LESTER, W. (1973) Transvestitism and transsexualism. *Practitioner* **210**, 677–8.

LEVINE, E. M. *et al.* (1976) Behavioural differences and emotional conflict among male-to-female transsexuals. *Arch. sex. Behav.* **5**, 81–6.

—— (1976) Male transsexuals in the homosexual subculture. *Am. J. Psychiat.* **133**, 1318–31.

LINDGREN, T. W. *et al.* (1975) A body image scale for evaluating transsexuals. *Arch. sex. Behav.* **4**, 639–56.

LOTHSTEIN, L. M. (1977) Psychotherapy with patients with gender dysphoria syndromes. *Bull. Menninger Clin.* **41**, 563–82.

—— (1978) The psychological management and treatment of hospitalized transsexuals. *J. nerv. ment. Dis.* **166**, 255–62.

LUNBERG, P. O. *et al.* (1975) Sella turcica in male-to-female transsexuals. *Arch. sex. Behav.* **4**, 657–62.

McKEE, E. A. (1976) Transsexualism: A selective review. *South. med. J.* **69**, 185–7.

—— *et al.* (1976) Transsexualism in two male triplets. *Am. J. Psychiat.* **133**, 334–40.

McKELLAR, A. (1978) Request for sex change. *South. med. J.* **7**, 265, 270.

MALLOY, T. R. *et al.* (1976) Experience with the 1-stage surgical approach for constructing female genitalia in male transsexuals. *J. Urol.* **116**, 335–7.

MARKLAND, C. *et al.* (1974) Vaginal reconstruction using cecal and sigmoid bowel segments in transsexual patients. *J. Urol.* **111**, 217–19.

—— (1975) Transsexual surgery. *Obstet. Gynecol. Ann.* **4**, 309–30.

MARSHALL, W. A. (1974) Growth and secondary sexual development and related abnormalities. *Clin. Obstet. Gynaecol.* **1**, 593–617.

MARTEL, P. G. (1974) [Case study of a transsexual male.] *Can. psychiat. Ass. J.* **19**, 13–16 (Eng. Abstr.) (Fre.)

MEDVECKY, J. *et al.* (1973) [A case of transsexualism.] *Cesk. Psychiat.* **69**, 236–9 (Eng. Abstr.) (Slo.)

MEYER, J. K. (1974) Psychiatric considerations in the sexual reassignment of non-intersex individuals. *Clin. plast. Surg.* **1**, 275–83.

—— (1974) Sex assignment and reassignment: intersex and gender identity disorders. Foreword. *Clin. plast. Surg.* **1**, 199–200.

—— *et al.* (1974) The gender dysphoria syndromes. A position statement on so-called 'transsexualism'. *Plast. reconstr. Surg.* **54**, 444–51.

MILLER, H. J. (1973) A case of transsexualism exhibiting intersexuality having a possible XXY-sex determining mechanism. *J. Am. Soc. psychosom. dent. Med.* **20**, 58–60.

MONEY, J. *et al.* (1970) [Transsexuals after the change of sex. Experiences and findings in Johns Hopkins Hospital.] *Beitr. Sexualforsch.* **49**, 70–87 (Ger.)

—— (1971) Sex reassignment therapy in gender identity disorders. *Int. Psychiat. Clin.* **8**, 197–210.

—— *et al.* (1975) 47, XXY and 46, XY males with antisocial and/or sex-offending behaviour: antiandrogen therapy plus counseling. *Psychoneuroendocrinology* **1**, 165–76.

—— *et al.* (1976) Iatrogenic homosexuality: gender identity in seven 46 XX chromosomal females with hyperadrenocortical hermaphroditism born with a penis, three reared as boys, four reared as girls. *J. Homosex.* **1**, 357–71.

MONTAGUE, D. K. (1973) Transsexualism. *Urology* **2**, 1–12.

MUNROE, R. L. *et al.* (1977) Male transvestism and subsistence economy. *J. soc. Psychol.* **103**, 307–8.

NELSON, C. *et al.* (1976) Medicolegal aspects of transsexualism. *Can. psychiat. Ass. J.* **21**, 557–64.

NEUMANN, F. (1970) [Animal experimental studies on transsexualism.] *Beitr. Sexualforsch.* **49**, 54–69. (Ger.)

NEWMAN, L. E. *et al.* (1974) Nontranssexual men who seek sex reassignment. *Am. J. Psychiat.* **131**, 437–41.

NOE, J. M. *et al.* (1974) The surgical construction of male genitalia for the female-to-male transsexual. *Plast. reconstr. Surg.* **53**, 511–16.

NUSSELT, L. *et al.* (1976) [Electroencephalographic changes in transsexualism (author's transl.).] *EEG. EMG.* **7**, 42–8 (Eng. Abstr.) (Ger.)

OLES, M. N. (1977) The transsexual client: a discussion of transsexualism and issues in psychotherapy. *Am. J. Orthopsychiat.* **47**, 66–74.

OVESEY, L. *et al.* (1976) Transvestism: a disorder of the sense of self. *Int. J. Psychoanal. Psychother.* **5**, 219–36.

PANDYA, N. J. *et al.* (1973) A one-stage technique for constructing female external genitalia in male transsexuals. *Br. J. plast. Surg.* **26**, 277–82.

PANIKIEWSKA, W. *et al.* (1975) [Homosexuality with transvestism in a mentally retarded person.] *Psychiat. Pol.* **9**, 465–6, (Pol.)

PARKS, J. S. (1977) Endocrine disorders of childhood. *Hosp. Pract.* **12**, 93–102, 107–8.

PAULY, I. B. (1974) Female transsexualism: part I. *Arch. sex. Behav.* **3**, 487–507.

—— (1974) Female transsexualism: part II. *Arch. sex. Behav.* **3**, 509–26.

PERSON, E. *et al.* (1974) The transsexual syndrome in males. II. Secondary transsexualism. *Am. J. Psychother.* **28**, 174–93.

—— *et al.* (1974) The psychodynamics of male transsexualism. In *Sex differences in behaviour* (Friedman, R. C. *et al.* eds) New York.

—— *et al.* (1974) The transsexual syndrome in males. I. Primary transsexualism. *Am. J. Psychother.* **28**, 4–20.

—— (1976) Initiation fantasies and transvestitism. Discussion. *J. Am. psychoanal. Ass.* **24**, 547–51.

PLOEGER, A. *et al.* (1976) [Synopsis of transvestism and transsexualism (author's transl.).] *Fortschr. Neurol. Psychiat.* **44**, 493–555, (Eng. Abstr.) (Ger.)

POMEROY, W. (1975) The diagnosis and treatment of transvestites and transsexuals. *J. Sex Marital Ther.* **1**, 215–24.

POULSEN, H. (1976) [Transsexualism in childhood.] *Ugeskr. Laeger* **138**, 1154–8 (Eng. Abstr.) (Dan.)

PREDESCU, V. *et al.* (1976) Some considerations on transsexualism. *Neurol. Psychiat. (Bucar)* **14**, 111–17 (Eng. Abstr.)

PRICE, V. *et al.* (1972) Survey of 504 cases of transvestism. *Psychol. Rep.* **31**,

903–17.

RANDELL, J. (1975) Transvestism and transsexualism. *Br. J. Psychiat.* Spec. No. **9**, 201–5.

REITER, E. O. *et al.* (1977) The not-so-simple nature of sexuality [editorial]. *J. Pediatr.* **90**, 861–8.

REKERS, G. A. *et al.* (1974) The behavioural treatment of a 'transsexual' preadolescent boy. *J. abnorm. Child. Psychol.* **2**, 99–116.

ROBACK, H. *et al.* (1975) Gender identification and the female impersonator. *South. med. J.* **68**, 459–62.

—— *et al.* (1976) Psychopathology in female sex-change applicants and two help-seeking controls. *J. abnorm. Psychol.* **85**, 430–2.

—— *et al.* (1977) Self-concept and psychological adjustment differences between self-identified male transsexuals and male homosexuals. *J. Homosex.* **3**, 15–20.

ROE, T. F. *et al.* (1977) Ambiguous genitalia in XX male children: report of two infants. *Pediatrics* **60**, 55–9.

ROSENBAUM, J. B. (1977) Gender-specific problems in the treatment of young women. *Am. J. Psychoanal.* **37**, 215–21.

ROTHNIE, N. G. *et al.* (1973) Letter: Pulmonary embolism in a man taking an oral contraceptive. *Lancet* **2**, 799.

SABALIS, R. F. *et al.* (1974) The three sisters: transsexual male siblings. *Am. J. Psychiat.* **131**, 907–9.

—— *et al.* (1977) Transsexualism: alternate diagnostic and etiological considerations. *Am. J. Psychoanal.* **37**, 223–8.

SALDANHA, P. H. *et al.* (1976) [Value of cytogenetic study in transsexualism.] *Arq. Neuropsiquiat.* **34**, 251–7 (Eng. Abstr.) (Por.)

SAMUELS, R. M. *et al.* (1977) A gender dysphoria program in New Jersey. *J. med. Soc. N. J.* **74**, 35–9.

SAUCIER, J. L. (1975) [Note on transsexualism.] *Union Med. Can.* **104**, 1240–2 (Fre.)

SCHACHTER, M. (1972) [Clinico-psychological study of transvestism in male children and adolescents.] *Pediatric.* **27**, 369–79 (Fre.)

SCHERRER, P. *et al.* (1972) [From transsexualism to schizophrenia.] *Ann. Med. Psychol. (Paris)* **2**, 609–35 (Fre.)

SCHROEDER, L. O. (1973) Renaissance for the transsexual: a new birth certificate. *J. forensic Sci.* **18**, 237–45.

SHAVE, D. (1976) Transsexualism as a concretized manifestation of orality. *Am. J. Psychoanal.* **36**, 57–66.

SILINK, M. (1977) Sexual differentiation and genital anomalies. *Med. J. Aust.* **1**, 660–2.

SIMPSON, J. L. *et al.* (1976) The relationship of neoplasia to disorders of abnormal sexual differentiation. *Birth Defects* **12**, 15–50.

SIPOVA, I. (1975) [Intellectual standard of transsexual subjects (author's transl.).] *Cesk. Psychiat.* **71**, 131–6 (Eng. Abstr.) (Cze.)

—— *et al.* (1977) [Androgens and the menstrual cycle in transsexual women (author's transl.).] *Cas. Lek. Cesk.* **116**, 1026–8 (Eng. Abstr.)

SPERBER, M. A. (1973) The 'as if' personality and transvestitism. *Psychoanal. Rev.* **60**, 605–12.

SPIOVA, I. *et al.* (1977) Plasma testosterone values in transsexual women. *Arch. sex. Behav.* **6**, 477–81.

STEINER, B. W. *et al.* (1974) A gender identity project. The organization of a multidisciplinary study. *Can. psychiat. Ass. J.* **19**, 7–12.

STOLLER, R. J. (1968) *Sex and gender: on the development of masculinity and femininity.* Aronson.

—— (1972) Male transsexualism: uneasiness. *Dan. med. Bull.* **19**, 301–6.

—— (1972) Etiological factors in female transsexualism: a first approximation. *Arch. sex. Behav.* **2**, 47–64.

—— *et al.* (1973) Two male transsexuals in one family. *Arch. sex. Behav.* **2**, 323–8.

—— (1973) The male transsexual as 'experiment'. *Int. J. Psychoanal.* **54**, 215–25.

—— (1973) Male transsexualism: uneasiness. *Am. J. Psychiat.* **130**, 536–9.

—— (1976) Two feminized male American Indians. *Arch. sex. Behav.* **5**, 529–38.

—— (1976) *Sex and gender Vol. 2: the transsexual experiment.* Aronson.

STONE, C. B. (1977) Psychiatric screening for transsexual surgery. *Psychosomatics* **18**, 25–7.

STRAIT, J. (1973) The transsexual patient after surgery. *Am. J. Nurs.* **73**, 462–3.

STRAUSS, S. A. (1974) Official re-registration of a female transsexual following medical treatment. *Forensic Sci.* **3**, 19–29.

STÜRUP, G. K. (1976) Male transsexuals: a long-term follow up after sex reassignment operations. *Acta Psychiat. scand.* **53**, 51–63.

TROP, J. L. *et al.* (1975) Rhinoplasty in transsexuals. Psychological considerations. *Plast. reconst. Surg.* **55**, 593–5.

TSOI, W. F. *et al.* (1977) Male transsexualism in Singapore: a description of 56 cases. *Br. J. Psychiat.* **131**, 405–9.

VAN DER SCHOOT, P. *et al.* (1976) Masculinization in male rats is inhibited by neonatal injections of dihydrostestosterone. *J. Reprod. Fertil.* **48**, 385–7.

VAN KAMMEN, D. P. *et al.* (1977) Erotic imagery and self-castration in transvestism/transsexualism: a case report. *J. Homosex.* **2**, 359–6.

VAN PUTTEN, T. *et al.* (1976) Sex conversion sugery in a man with severe gender dysphoria. A tragic outcome. *Arch. gen. Psychiat.* **33**, 751–3.

VESELY, K. (1975) [Risk of gynaecologists participating in operations of transsexualism (author's transl.).] *Cesk. Gynekol.* **40**, 720 (Cze.)

VIDELA, E. *et al.* (1976) Female transsexualist with abnormal karyotype (letter). *Lancet* **2**, 1081.

VIETZE, G. Z. (1975) [Transsexualism.] *Aerztl. Fortbild. (Jena)* **69**, 939–43 (Ger.)

VOLKAN, V. D. *et al.* (1973) Dreams of transsexuals awaiting surgery. *Compr. Psychiat.* **14**, 269–79.

WAGNER, B. (1974) [Transsexualism with XYY-syndrome.] *Nervenarzt* **45**, 548–51 (Ger.)

WÅLINDER, J. *et al.* (1976) A law concerning sex reassignment of transsexuals in Sweden. *Arch. sex. Behav.* **5**, 255–8.

——*et al.* (1977) A study of consanguinity between the parents of transsexuals. *Br. J. Psychiat.* **131**, 73–4.

WELSE, W. (1973) [Diagnostic errors in transvestism and organic inter-sexuality.] *Zentralbl. Gynaekol.* **95**, 1825–30 (Eng. Abstr.) (Ger.)

Western Journal of Medicine (1974) Editorial: Gender dysphoria syndrome—the conceptualization that liberalizes indications for total gender reorientation and implies a broadly based multi-dimensional rehabilitative regimen. Fisk, N. M. *West. J. Med.* **120**, 386–91.

WICKS, L. K. (1977) Transsexualism: a social work approach. *Health soc. Work* **2**, 179–93.

WIEDEKING, C. *et al.* (1977) Plasma noradrenalin and dopamine-beta-hydroxylase during behavioural testing of sexually deviant XYY and XXY males. *Hum. Genet.* **37**, 243–7.

WILLIAMS, G. (1973) An approach to transsexual surgery. *Nurs. Times* **69**, 787.

WOLFORT, F. G. *et al.* (1975) Laryngeal chondroplasty for appearance. *Plast. reconst. Surg.* **56**, 371–4.

YARDLEY, K. M. (1976) Training in feminine skills in a male transsexual: a pre-operative procedure. *Br. J. med. Psychol.* **49**, 329–39.

ZAVITZIANOS, G. (1972) Homeovestism: perverse form of behaviour involving wearing clothes of the same sex. *Int. J. Psychoanal.* **53**, 471–7.

Exhibitionism, scopophilia, and voyeurism

BODENHEIMER, A. R. (1977) [The symbol as eye-catcher. An interpretation of the symbol and a suggestion regarding therapy for exhibitionism (Author's Transl.).] *Psychother. Med. Psychol. (Stuttg.)* **27**, 125–35 (Eng. Abstr.) (Ger.)

CABANIS, D. (1972) [Female exhibitionism.] *Z. Rechtsmed.* **71**, 126–33 (Eng. Abstr.) (Ger.)

EBER, M. (1977) Exhibitionism or narcissism? (letter). *Am. J. Psychiat.* **134**, 1053.

EVANS, W. N. (1974–5) Pseudostupidity: a study in masochistic exhibitionism. *Psychoanal. Rev.* **61**, 619–32.

HACKETT, T. P. (1971) The psychotherapy of exhibitionists in a court clinic setting. *Semin. Psychiat.* **3**, 297–306.

HOLLENDER, M. H. *et al.* (1977) Genital exhibitionism in women. *Am. J. Psychiat.* **134**, 436–8.

JEROTIC, V. (1973) On a case of exhibitionism successfully treated by psycho-therapy. *Psihoterapija* **1**, 73–85.

JONES, I. H. *et al.* (1977) Provoked anxiety as a treatment of exhibitionism. *Br. J. Psychiat.* **131**, 295–300.

KENTSMITH, D. K. *et al.* (1974) Obscene telephoning by an exhibitionist during therapy: a case report. *Int. J. Group Psychother.* **24**, 352–7.

KORDYS, S. *et al.* (1976) [Early stage of exhibitionism.] *Psychiat. Pol.* **10**, 699–701 (Pol.)

KUTCHINSKY, B. (1976) Deviance and criminality: the case of voyeur in a peeper's paradise. *Dis. nerv. Syst.* **37**, 145–51.

MALETZKY, B. M. (1974) 'Assisted' covert sensitization in the treatment of exhibitionism. *J. Consult. clin. Psychol.* **42**, 34–40.

MEYHÖFER, W. (1976) [Exhibitionism.] *Z̧. Hautkr.* **51**, 773–6 (Ger.)

PRAZIC, B. *et al.* (1976) [Exhibitionism.] *Neuropsihijatrija* **24**, 129–35 (Eng. Abstr.) (Scr.)

ROOTH, G. (1973) Exhibitionism, sexual violence and paedophilia. *Br. J. Psychiat.* **122**, 705–10.

—— (1973) Exhibitionism outside Europe and America. *Arch. sex. Behav.* **2**, 351–63.

—— *et al.* (1974) Persistent exhibitionism: short-term response to aversion, self-regulation, and relaxation treatments. *Arch. sex. Behav.* **3**, 227–48.

—— (1975) Indecent exposure and exhibitionism. *Br. J. Psychiat.* Spec. No. **9**, 212–22.

ROTEN, E. (1976) [Contribution to the psychoanalytic theory of exhibitionism.] *Z̧. psychosom. Med. Psychoanal.* **22**, 305–35 (Eng. Abstr.) (Ger.)

SMITH, R. S. (1976) Voyeurism: a review of literature. *Arch. sex. Behav.* **5**, 585–608.

SMUKLER, A. J. *et al.* (1975) Personality characteristics of exhibitionists. *Dis. nerv. Syst.* **36**, 600–3.

STREITBERG, G. (1973) [Adolescent exhibitionism. A case study based on the Rorschach test and the TAT.] *Z̧. klin. Psychol. Psychother.* **21**, 317–28 (Ger.)

WAGNER, E. E. (1974) Projective test data from two contrasted groups of exhibitionists. *Percept. Mot. Skills* **39**, 131–40.

ZAVITZIANOS, G. (1977) More on exhibitionism in women (letter). *Am. J. Psychiat.* **134**, 820.

Homosexuality

ABEL, G. G. *et al.* (1975) Measurement of sexual arousal in male homosexuals: effects of instructions and stimulus modality. *Arch. sex. Behav.* **4**, 623–9.

ABRAMSON, H. A. (1977) Reassociation of dreams. III. LSD analysis of a threatening male–female dog dream and its relation to fear of lesbianism. *J. Asthma Res.* **14**, 131–58.

ACOSTA, F. X. (1975) Etiology and treatment of homosexuality: a review. *Arch. sex. Behav.* **4**, 9–29.

ADAMS, H. E. *et al.* (1977) Status of behavioural reorientation techniques in the modification of homosexuality: a review. *Psychol. Bull.* **84**, 1171–81.

ADELMAN, M. R. (1977) A comparison of professionally employed lesbians and heterosexual women on the MMPI. *Arch. sex. Behav.* **6**, 193–201.

—— (1977) Sexual orientation and violations of civil liberties. *J. Homosex.* **2**, 327–30.

ALEXANDER, G. L. (1975) Homosexuality:— the psychoanalytic point of view. *Psychiat. Commun.* **16**, 19–23.

ALTSHULER, K. Z. (1976) Some notes and an exercise with regard to male homosexuality. *J. Am. Acad. Psychoanal.* **42**, 237–48.

ALVAREZ, W. C. and MARCH, S. (1974) *Homosexuality vs. gay liberation: a confrontation doublebook*. Moonachie, New Jersey.

ANDRESS, V. R. *et al.* (1974) A comparison of homosexual and heterosexual responses to the Menninger Word Association Test. *J. clin. Psychol.* **30**, 205–7.

—— *et al.* (1974) A comparison of homosexual and heterosexual responses to the Menninger Word Association Test. *J. clin. Psychol.* **30**, 205–7.

ATKINS, M. *et al.* (1976) Brief treatment of homosexual patients. *Compr. Psychiat.* **17**, 115–24.

AWAD, G. A. (1976) Father–son incest: a case report. *J. nerv. ment. Dis.* **162**, 135–9.

BAARS, C. (1976) *Homosexual's search for happiness.* Chicago, Illinois.

BADER, M. *et al.* (1977) Venereal transmission of shigellosis in Seattle-King county. *Sex Transm. Dis.* **4**, 89–91.

BAILEY, D. S. (1975) *Homosexuality and the western Christian tradition.* Hamden, Connecticut.

BANCROFT, J. (1975) Homosexuality and the medical profession: a behaviourist's view. *J. med. Ethics* **1**, 176–80.

BANCROFT, J. H. (1975) Homosexuality in the male. *Br. J. Psychiat.* **9**, 173–84.

BARGUES, J. F. (1974) [Sodom: clinic, mythology, metapsychology of homosexuality.] *Ann. Med. Psychol. (Paris)* **2**, 711–31 (Fre.)

BARLOW, D. H. *et al.* (1972) The contribution of therapeutic instruction of covert sensitization. *Behav. Res. Ther.* **10**, 411–15.

—— *et al.* (1974) Plasma testosterone levels and male homosexuality: a failure to replicate. *Arch. sex. Behav.* **3**, 571–5.

—— *et al.* (1975) Case histories and shorter communications. Biofeedback and reinforcement to increase heterosexual arousal in homosexuals. *Behav. Res. Ther.* **13**, 45–50.

BARNETT, L. (1975) *Homosexuality: time to tell the truth to young people, their families and friends.* London.

BARR, R. *et al.* (1976) Autonomic responses of transsexual and homosexual males to erotic film sequences. *Arch. sex. Behav.* **5**, 211–22.

BARR, R. F. (1973) Responses to erotic stimuli of transsexual and homosexual males. *Br. J. Psychiat.* **123**, 579–85.

—— *et al.* (1974) Homosexuality and psychological adjustment. *Med. J. Aust.* **1**, 187–9

BARTHOLOMEW, A. A. *et al.* (1978) Homosexual necrophilia. *Med. Sci. Law.* **18**, 29–35.

BARTOVA, D. *et al.* (1977) [A comment on psychiatric aspects of homosexuality (author's transl.).] *Cas. Lek. Cesk.* **116**, 1029–30 (Eng. Abstr.) (Cze.)

BAVIDGE, K. J. (1976) Changing pattern of male homosexual registrations in a venereal disease clinic, 1964–1974. *Br. J. vener. Dis.* **52**, 165–7.

BEGELMAN, D. A. (1977) Homosexuality and the ethics of behavioural intervention. *J. Homosex.* **2**, 213–19.

BELL, A. P. (1975) Research in homosexuality: back to the drawing board. *Arch. sex. Behav.* **4**, 421–31.

BELOTE, D. *et al.* (1976) Demographic and self-report characteristics of lesbians. *Psychol. Rep.* **39**, 621–2.

BERC, K. M. (1974) Letter: wives of homosexual men. *Am. J. Psychiat.* **131**, 832–3.

BERENT, I. (1973) Original sin: 'I didn't mean to hurt you, mother'—a basic fantasy epitomized by a male homosexual. *J. Am. psychoanal. Ass.* **21**, 262–84.

BERGLER, E. (1962) *Homosexuality—disease or way of life.* Basingstoke.

BIEBER, I. (1976) A discussion of 'homosexuality: the ethical challenge'. *J. Consult. clin. Psychol.* **44**, 163–6.

BIEBER, I. *et al.* (1962) *Homosexuality: a psychoanalytic study.* New York.

BINDER, C. V. (1977) Affection training: an alternative to sexual reorientation. *J. Homosex.* **2**, 251–9.

BIRK, L. (1974) Group psychotherapy for men who are homosexual. *J. Sex. Marital Ther.* **1**, 29–52.

—— *et al.* (1973) Serum testosterone levels in homosexual men. *N. Engl. J. Med.* **289**, 1236–8.

BLOCH, D. (1975–76) The threat of infanticide and homosexuality identity. *Psychoanal. Rev.* **62**, 579–99.

BRAVERMAN, S. J. (1973) Homosexuality. *Am. J. Nurs.* **73**, 652–5.

British Journal of Venereal Diseases (1973) Homosexuality and venereal disease in the United Kingdom. *Br. J. vener. Dis.* **49**, 329–34.

BRODIE, H. K. *et al.* (1974) Plasma testosterone levels in heterosexual and homosexual men. *Am. J. Psychiat.* **131**, 82–3.

BROWN, D. F. (1976) The health service and gay students. *J. Am. Coll. Health Ass.* **24**, 272–3.

BROWN, H. J. (1974) Letter: problems in homosexuality. *J. Am. med. Ass.* **228**, 978.

BROWN, M. *et al.* (1975) Attitudes toward homosexuality among West Indian male and female college students. *J. soc. Psychol.* **97**, 163–8.

BUDA, B. (1973) Homosexuality. *Ther. Hung.* **21**, 11–22.

BURDICK, J. A. *et al.* (1974) Cardiac activity and verbal report of homosexuals and heterosexuals. *J. psychosom. Res.* **18**, 377–85.

—— *et al.* (1974) Differences between 'show' and 'no show' volunteers in a homosexual population. *J. soc. Psychol.* **92**, 159–60.

CANTON-DUTARI, A. (1974) Combined intervention for controlling unwanted homosexual behaviour. *Arch. sex. Behav.* **3**, 367–71.

—— (1976) Combined intervention for controlling unwanted homosexual behaviour: an extended follow-up. *Arch. sex. Behav.* **5**, 269–74.

CARR, G. *et al.* (1977) Anal warts in a population of gay men in New York City. *Sex. Transm. Dis.* **4**, 56–7.

CARRIER, J. M. (1975) Letter to the editor: comments on 'a neuroendocrine predisposition for homosexuality in men'. *Arch. sex. Behav.* **4**, 667

—— (1976) Cultural factors affecting urban Mexican male homosexual behaviour. *Arch. sex. Behav.* **5**, 103–24.

—— (1977) 'Sex-role preference' as an explanatory variable in homosexual behaviour. *Arch. sex. Behav.* **6**, 53–65.

CAUKINS, S. E. *et al.* (1976) The psychodynamics of male prostitution. *Am. J. Psychother.* **30**, 441–51.

CHAPEL, T. A. *et al.* (1977) *Neisseria meningitidis* in the anal canal of homosexual men. *J. infect. Dis.* **136**, 810–12.

CHEVALIER-SKOLNIKOFF, S. (1976) Homosexual behaviour in a laboratory group of stumptail monkeys (*Macaca arctoides*): forms, contexts, and possible social functions. *Arch. sex. Behav.* **5**, 511–27.

CHILES, J. A. (1972) Homosexuality in the United States Air Force. *Compr. Psychiat.* **13**, 529–32.

CHYATTE, C. (1974) Letter: official status of homosexuality. *J. Am. med. Ass.* **227**, 1262.

WAINWRIGHT CHURCHILL (1971) *Homosexual behaviour among males.*

CLARK, T. R. (1975) Homosexuality and psychopathology in nonpatient males. *Am. J. Psychoanal.* **35**, 163–8.

CLIMENT, C. E. *et al.* (1977) Epidemiological studies of female prisoners. IV. Homosexual behaviour. *J. nerv. ment. dis.* **164**, 25–9.

COCHRANE, R. (1974) Values as correlates of deviancy. *Br. J. soc. clin. Psychol.* **13**, 257–67.

COLEMAN, J. C. *et al.* (1977) Hepatitis B antigen and antibody in a male homosexual population. *Br. J. vener. Dis.* **53**, 132–4.

CONDINI, A. *et al.* (1974) [Homosexual delusions in young psychotic patients at the time of their first hospitalization (author's transl.).] *Riv. Patol. Nerv. Ment.* **95**, 35–46 (Eng. Abstr.) (Ita.)

COOMBS, N. R. (1974) Male prostitution: a psychosocial view of behaviour. *Am. J. Orthopsychiat.* **44**, 782–9.

COONS, F. W. (1972) Ambisexuality as an alternative adaptation. *J. Am. Coll. Health Ass.* **21**, 142–4.

CORBETT, S. L. *et al.* (1977) Tolerance as a correlate of experience with stigma: the case of the homosexual. *J. Homosex.* **3**, 3–13.

CORY, D. W. (1975) *Homosexual in America: a subjective approach.* New York.

COV, L. (1972) A group psychotherapy approach to the treatment of neurotic symptoms in male and female patients of homosexual preference. *Psychother. Psychosom.* **20**, 176–80.

CROMPTON, L. (1976) Homosexuals and the death penalty in colonial America. *J. Homosex.* **1**, 277–93.

CUBITT, G. H. *et al.* (1972) Assessing the diagnostic utility of MMPI and 16 PF indexes of homosexuality in a prison sample. *J. Consult. clin. Psychol.* **39**, 342.

DANNELS, J. C. (1972) Homosexual panic. *Perspect. psychiat. Care* **10**, 106–22.

DAVISON, G. C. (1975) Homosexuality: the ethical challenge. *J. Consult. clin. Psychol.* **44**, 157–62.

—— (1977) Homosexuality and the ethics of behavioural intervention: Homosexuality, the ethic challenge. *J. Homosex.* **2**, 195–204.

—— (1978) Not can but ought: the treatment of homosexuality. *J. Consult. clin. Psychol.* **46**, 170.

—— *et al.* (1974) Goals and strategies in behavioural treatment in homosexual pedophilia: comments on a case study. *J. abnorm. Psychol.* **83**, 196–8.

DE CECCO, J. P. (1977) Studying violations of civil liberties of homosexual men and women. *J. Homosex.* **2**, 315–22.

DEFRIES, Z. (1976) Pseudohomosexuality in feminist students. *Am. J. Psychiat.* **133**, 400–4.

—— (1978) Political lesbianism and sexual politics. *J. Am. Acad. Psychoanal.* **6**, 71.

DE LA BALSE, F. A. (1976) [Etiopathogenesis of true male homosexuality (androgenic insufficiency?).] *Rev. Iber. Endocrinol.* **23**, 225–43 (Eng. Abstr.) (Spa.)

DEMARET, G. (1973). [Study of personality change during a therapy centered on the patient.] *Ann. med. Psychol. (Paris)* **2**, 625–36 (Fre.)

DIETZMAN, D. E. *et al.* (1977) Hepatitis B surface antigen (HBsAg) and antibody to HBsAg. Prevalence in homosexual and heterosexual men. *J. Am. med. Ass.* **238**, 2625–6.

DOERR, P. *et al.* (1973) Plasma testosterone, estradiol, and semen analysis in male homosexuals. *Arch. gen. Psychiat.* **29**, 829–33.

—— *et al.* (1976) Further studies on sex hormones in male homosexuals. *Arch. gen. Psychiat.* **33**, 611–14.

DOMINO, G. (1977) Homosexuality and creativity. *J. Homosex.* **2**, 261–7.

DONNELLY, F. C. (1976) The doctor and the homosexual. *N. Z. Med. J.* **83**, 322–4.

DORNER, G. *et al.* (1972) [Release of a positive estrogen feedback effect in homosexual men.] *Endokrinologie* **60**, 297–301 (Eng. Abstr.) (Ger.)

—— *et al.* (1975) A neuroendocrine predisposition for homosexuality in men. *Arch. sex. Behav.* **4**, 1–8.

DRITZ, S. K. *et al.* (1977) Patterns of sexually transmitted enteric diseases in a city. *Lancet* **2**, 3–4.

—— *et al.* (1977) Sexually transmitted typhoid fever [letter]. *N. Engl. J. Med.* **296**, 1359–60.

DUEHN, W. D. *et al.* (1976) The use of stimulus/modeling videotapes in assertive training for homosexuals. *J. Homosex.* **1**, 373–81.

DUNBAR, J. *et al.* (1973) Attitudes toward homosexuality among Brazilian and Canadian college students. *J. soc. Psychol.* **90**, 173–83.

—— *et al.* (1973) Some correlates of attitudes toward homosexuality. *J. soc. Psychol.* **89**, 271–9.

ELLIS, H. and SYMONDS, J. A. (1975) *Sexual inversion.* New York.

ENRIGHT, M. F. *et al.* (1976) Training crisis intervention specialists and peer group counselors as therapeutic agents in the gay community. *Community ment. Health J.* **12**, 383–91.

FARRELL, R. A. *et al.* (1974) Social interaction and stereotypic responses to homosexuals. *Arch. sex. Behav.* **3**, 425–42.

FEINBLOOM, D. H. *et al.* (1976) Lesbian/feminist orientation among male-to-female transsexuals. *J. Homosex.* **2**, 59–71.

FELDMAN, M. P. (1972) Homosexual behaviour: therapy and assessment. *Br. J. Psychiat.* **121**, 456–7.

—— and MACCULLOCH, M. J. (1971) *Homosexual behaviour: therapy and assessment.* Oxford.

FELDMAN, P. (1977) Helping homosexuals with problems: a commentary and a personal view. *J. Homosex.* **2**, 241–9.

FELMAN, Y. M. *et al.* (1977) Examining the homosexual male for sexually transmitted diseases. *J. Am. med. Ass.* **239**, 2046–7.

FINK, P. J. (1975) Homosexuality—illness or life-style? *J. Sex. Marital Ther.* **1**, 225–33.

FITZGERALD, T. K. (1977) A critique of anthropological research on homosexuality. *J. Homosex.* **2**, 385–97.

FLUKER, J. L. (1976) A 10-year study of homosexually transmitted infection. *Br. J. vener. Dis.* **52**, 155–60.

FRANCHER, J. S. *et al.* (1973) The menopausal queen: adjustment to aging and the male homosexual. *Am. J. Orthopsychiat.* **43**, 670–4.

FREEDMAN, M. (1971) *Homosexuality and psychological functioning.* Monterey, California.

FREUND, K. (1977) Should homosexuality arouse therapeutic concern? *J. Homosex.* **2**, 235–40.

—— *et al.* (1973) Heterosexual aversion in homosexual males. *Br. J. Psychiat.* **122**, 163–9.

—— *et al.* (1974) The transsexual syndrome in homosexual males. *J. nerv. ment. Dis.* **158**, 145–54.

—— *et al.* (1974) The phobic theory of male homosexuality. *Arch. gen. Psychiat.* **31**, 495–9.

—— *et al.* (1974) Measuring feminine gender identity in homosexual males. *Arch. sex. Behav.* **3**, 249–60.

—— *et al.* (1974) Femininity and preferred partner age in homosexual and heterosexual males. *Br. J. Psychiat.* **125**, 442–6.

—— *et al.* (1974) Heterosexual aversion in homosexual males. A second experiment. *Br. J. Psychiat.* **125**, 177–80.

—— *et al.* (1974) Parent–child relations in transsexual and non-transsexual homosexual males. *Br. J. Psychiat.* **124**, 22–3.

—— (1975) Heterosexual interest in homosexual males. *Arch. sex. Behav.* **4**, 509–18.

—— *et al.* (1976) Bisexuality in homosexual pedophilia. *Arch. sex. Behav.* **5**, 415–23.

FRIEDBERG, R. L. (1975) Early recollections of homosexuals as indicators of their life styles. *J. individ. Psychol.* **3**, 196–204.

FRIEDMAN, R. C. *et al.* (1976) Psychological development and blood levels of sex steroids in male identical twins of divergent sexual orientation. *J. nerv. ment. Dis.* **163**, 282–8.

—— *et al.* (1976) Reassessment of homosexuality and transsexualism *Ann. Rev. Med.* **27**, 57–62.

—— *et al.* (1977) Plasma prolactin levels in male homosexuals. *Horm. Behav.* **9**, 19–22.

—— *et al.* (1977) Hormones and sexual orientation in men. *Am. J. Psychiat.* **134**, 571–2.

GARFIELD, S. L. (1974) Values: an issue in psychotherapy: comments on a case study. *J. abnorm. Psychol.* **83**, 202–3.

GARTRELL, N. *et al.* (1974) Psychiatrists' attitudes toward female homosexuality. *J. nerv. ment. Dis.* **159**, 141–4.

GARTRELL, N. K. *et al.* (1977) Plasma testosterone in homosexual and heterosexual women. *Am. J. Psychiat.* **134**, 1117–18.

GEIS, G. *et al.* (1976) Reported consequences of decriminalization of consensual adult homosexuality in seven American states. *J. Homosex.* **1**, 419–26.

GERSHAM, H. (1975) The effect of group therapy on compulsive homosexuality in men and women. *Am. J. Psychoanal.* **35**, 303–16.

GIANSANTI, J. S. *et al.* (1975) Palatal erythema: another etiologic factor. *Oral Surg.* **40**, 379–81.

GLASSER, M. (1977) Homosexuality in adolescence. *Br. J. med. Psychol.* **50**, 217–25.

GLUCKMAN, J. B. *et al.* (1974) Primary syphilis of rectum. *N. Y. State J. Med.* **74**, 2210–11.

GLUCKMAN, L. K. (1974) Transcultural consideration of homosexuality with special reference to the New Zealand Maori. *Aust. N.Z. J. Psychiat.* **8**, 121–5.

GOLDBERG, S. (1975) What is 'normal'? Logical aspects of the question of homosexual behaviour. *Psychiatry* **38**, 227–43.

GOLDMEIER, D. *et al.* (1977) Isolation of *Chlamydia trachomatic* from throat and rectum of homosexual men. *Br. J. vener. Dis.* **53**, 184–5.

GOOD, R. S. (1976) The gynecologist and the lesbian. *Clin. Obstet. Gynecol.* **19**, 473–82.

GOODHART, C. B. (1972) Female homosexuality. *Nature (Lond.)* **239**, 174.

GREEN, R. (1972) Homosexuality as a mental illness. Critical evaluation. Author's reply. *Int. J. Psychiat.* **10**, 126–8.

—— (1972) Homosexuality as a mental illness. *Int. J. Psychiat.* **10**, 77–96.

—— (1978) Sexual identity of 37 children raised by homosexual or transsexual parents. *Am. J. Psychiat.* **135**, 692–7.

GREENBERG, J. (1973) A study of male homosexuals (predominantly college students). *J. Am. Coll. Health Ass.* **22**, 56–60.

GREENBERG, J. S. (1973) A study of the self-esteem and alienation of male homosexuals. *J. Psychol.* **83**, 137–43.

—— (1975) A study of personality change associated with the conducting of a high school unit on homosexuality. *J. Sch. Health* **45**, 394–8.

—— (1976) The effects of a homophile organization on the self-esteem and alienation of its members. *J. Homosex.* **1**, 313.

GRIFFITHS, P. D. *et al.* (1974) Homosexual women: an endocrine and psychological study. *J. Endocrinol.* **63**, 549–56.

GUILMOT, P. H. (1972) [New perspectives in medicopsychological aid for homosexuals.] *Acta Psychiat. Belg.* **72**, 265–315 (Eng. Abstr.)

GUNDLACH, R. H. (1977) Birth order among lesbians: a new light on an 'only child'. *Psychol. Rep.* **40**, 250.

GUTSTADT, J. P. (1976) Male psuedoheterosexuality and minimal sexual dysfunction. *J. sex. marital Ther.* **2**, 297–302.

HADDEN, S. B. (1971) Group psychotherapy with homosexual men. *Int. Psychiat. Clin.* **8**, 81–94.

HALLECK, S. L. (1976) Another response to 'homosexuality: the ethical challenge'. *J. Consult. clin. Psychol.* **44**, 167–70.

HALBREICH, U. (1975) [Editorial: Hormonal aspects of homosexuality.] *Harefuah* **89**, 380–1 (Heb.)

HAMMERSMITH, S. K. *et al.* (1973) Homosexual identity: commitment, adjustment, and significant others. *Sociometry* **36**, 56–79.

HARRIS, B. S. (1977) Lesbian mother child custody: legal and psychiatric aspects. *Bull. Am. Acad. Psychiat. Law* **5**, 75–89.

HARRY, J. (1976–77) On the validity of typologies of gay males. *J. Homosex.* **2**, 143–52.

HASSELL, J. *et al.* (1975) Female homosexuals' concepts of self, men, and women. *J. Pers. Assess.* **39**, 154–9.

HATTERER, L. J. (1972) Homosexuality as a mental illness. A critique. *Int. J. Psychiat.* **10**, 103–4.

HATTERER, M. S. (1974) The problems of women married to homosexual men. *Am. J. Psychiat.* **131**, 275–8.

HAYNES, S. N. *et al.* (1976) Homosexuality: behaviours and attitudes. *Arch. sex. Behav.* **5**, 269–74.

HEDBLOM, J. H. (1973) Dimensions of lesbian sexual experience. *Arch. sex. Behav.* **2**, 329–41.

HENDERSON, R. H. (1977) Improving sexually transmitted disease health services for gays: a national prospective. *Sex. Transm. Dis.* **4**, 58–62.

HENDLIN, S. J. (1976) Homosexuality in the Rorschach: a new look at the old signs. *J. Homosex.* **1**, 303–12.

HENLEY, N. M. *et al.* (1978) Interrelationship of sexist, racist, and anti-homosexual attitudes. *Psychol. Rep.* **42**, 83–90.

HERMAN, S. H. *et al.* (1974) An experimental analysis of exposure to 'explicit' heterosexual stimuli as an effective variable in changing arousal patterns of homosexuals. *Behav. Res. Ther.* **12**, 335–45.

HIDALGO, H. A. *et al.* (1976–77) The Puerto Rican lesbian and the Puerto Rican community. *J. Homosex.* **2**, 109–21.

HOENIG, J. *et al.* (1974) Sexual and other abnormalities in the family of a transsexual. *Psychiat. Clin. (Basel)* **7**, 334–46.

HOFFMAN, M. (1972) Homosexuality as a mental illness. Philosophic, empirical, and ecologic remarks. *Int. J. Psychiat.* **10**, 105–7.

HOGAN, R. A. *et al.* (1977) Attitudes, opinions and sexual development of 205 homosexual women. *J. Homosex.* **3**, 123–36.

HOLDER, W. R. *et al.* (1972) Preliminary report on spectinomycin HCl in the treatment of gonorrhoea in homosexual men. *Br. J. vener. Dis.* **48**, 274–5.

HUMPHREYS, L. (1974) [Tearoom trade. Impersonal sex in public places.] *Beitr. Sexualforsch.* **54**, 1–138 (Ger.)

HUNT, S. P. (1978) Homosexuality from a contemporary perspective. *Conn. Med.* **42**, 105–8.

HURWITZ, A. L. *et al.* (1978) Venereal transmission of intestinal parasites. *West. J. Med.* **128**, 89.

IMIELINSKI, K. *et al.* (1976) [Transsexualism and partnership. A clinical case.] *Psychiat. Pol.* **10**, 565–9 (Pol.)

International Journal of Psychiatry (1973) Homosexuality in the male: a report of a psychiatric study group. *Int. J. Psychiat.* **11**, 460–79.

IRWIN, P. *et al.* (1977) Acceptance of the rights of homosexuals: a social profile. *J. Homosex.* **3**, 107–21.

JACOBS, S. (1973) Homosexuality, gonorrhea, jaundice. *J. La. State med. Soc.* **125**, 133–7.

JAMES, S. *et al.* (1977) Significance of androgen levels in the aetiology and treatment of homosexuality. *Psychol. Med.* **7**, 427–9.

JANZEN, W. B. *et al.* (1975) Clinical and sign prediction: the draw-a-person and female homosexuality. *J. clin. Psychol.* **31**, 757–65.

JEFFERISS, F. J. (1976) Venereal disease and the homosexual. *Practitioner* **217**, 741–5.

JONES, C. R. (1974) *Homosexuality and Counseling.* Queen Lane, Philadelphia.

Journal of the Americal Psychoanalytical Association (1977) The psychoanalytic treatment of male homosexuality. Payne, E. C. (Panel Report). *J. Am. psychoanal. Ass.* **25**, 183–99.

JUDSON, F. N. (1977) Sexually transmitted disease in gay men [editorial]. *Sex. Transm. Dis.* **4**, 76–8.

—— *et al.* (1977) Screening for gonorrhea and syphilis in the gay baths— Denver, Colorado. *Am. J. public Health* **67**, 740–2.

KANZER, M. (1972) Freud's views on bisexuality and therapy. Clinical notes (Freud, S.). *Int. J. Psychiat.* **10**, 66–9.

KARLEN, A. (1971) *Sexuality and homosexuality: a new view.* New York.

KARLEN, A. (1972) A discussion of 'Homosexuality as a mental illness'. *Int. J. Psychiat.* **10**, 108–13.

KATZ, J. (Ed.) (1975) *Homosexual emancipation miscellany. 1835–1952: an original anthology.* Arno.

—— (Ed.) (1975) *Homosexuality: lesbians and gay men in society, history and literature.* New York.

KAZAL, H. L. *et al.* (1976) The gay bowel syndrome: clinico-pathologic correlation in 260 cases. *Ann. clin. Lab. Sci.* **6**, 184–92.

KELLY, J. (1977) The aging male homosexual. Myth and reality *Gerontologist* **17**, 328–32.

KENYON, F. E. (1975) Homosexuality in the female. *Br. J. Psychiat.* **9**, 185–200.

KLIMMER, R. (1972) [Report on a masochist with homosexual disposition.] *Z. Aerztl. Fortbild. (Jena)* **66**, 782–5 (Ger.)

KNUTSON, D. C. (1977) The civil liberties of gay persons: present status. *J. Homosex.* **2**, 337–42.

KOHLENBERG, R. J. (1974) Treatment of a homosexual pedophiliac using *in vivo* desensitization: a case study. *J. abnorm. Psychol.* **83**, 192–5.

KOLODNY, R. C. *et al.* (1973) Editorial: Hormones and homosexuality. *Ann. intern. Med.* **79**, 897.

KOPTAGEL, G. (1972) The pictorial expressions as a means of self-satisfaction for a young man with homosexual transvestite tendencies. *Confin. Psychiat.* **15**, 71–6.

KOSLACZ, A. *et al.* (1975) [Follow-up studies of the effectiveness of treatment of homosexuals.] *Psychiat. Pol.* **9**, 241–5 (Eng. Abstr.) (Pol.)

KRELL, L. *et al.* (1975) [Relations between clinically manifested homosexuality and the estrogen-feedback effect.] *Dermatol. Monatsschr.* **161**, 567–72 (Eng. Abstr.) (Ger.)

KRICH, A. M. (1962) *Homosexuals: as seen by themselves and thirty authorities.* Secausus, New Jersey.

KUETHE, J. L. (1975) Children's schemata of man and woman: a comparison with the schemata of heterosexual and homosexual populations. *J. Psychol.* **90**, 249–58.

KUSCHNER, H. *et al.* (1977) The homosexual husband and physician confidentiality. *Hastings Cent. Rep.* **7**, 15–17.

KWAWER, J. S. (1977) Male homosexual psychodynamics and the Rorschach test. *J. Pers. Assess.* **41**, 10–18.

LACHMANN, F. M. (1975) Homosexuality: some diagnostic perspectives and dynamic considerations. *Am. J. Psychother.* **29**, 254–60.

LANAHAN, C. C. (1976) Homosexuality: a different sexual orientation. *Nurs. Forum* **15**, 314–19.

LANER, M. R. (1977) Permanent partner priorities: gay and straight. *J. Homosex.* **3**, 21–39.

LATIMER, P. (1977) A case of homosexuality treated *in vivo* desensitization and assertive training. *Can. psychiat. Ass. J.* **22**, 185–9.

LAWRENCE, J. C. (1975) Homosexuals, hospitalization, and the nurse. *Nurs. Forum* **14**, 305–17.

—— (1977) Gay peer counseling. *J. psychiat. Nurs.* **15**, 33–7.

LEDJRI, *et al.* (1974) [From latent homosexuality to generalized homosexuality.] *Tunis. Med.* **52**, 199–205 (Fre.)

LEE, J. A. (1976) Forbidden colors of love: patterns of gay love and gay liberation. *J. Homosex.* **1**, 401–18.

—— (1977) Going public: a study in the sociology of homosexual liberation. *J. Homosex.* **3**, 49–78.

LESSE, S. (1973) The current confusion over homosexuality. *Am. J. Psychother.* **27**, 151–4.

—— (1974) Editorial: to be or not to be an illness? That is the question— or—the status of homosexuality. *Am. J. Psychother.* **28**, 1–3.

LESTER, D. (1975) The relationship between paranoid delusions and homosexuality. *Arch. sex. Behav.* **4**, 285–94.

—— *et al.* (1977) Sex-deviant hand writing, femininity and homosexuality. *Percept. Mot. Skills* **45**, (3 Pt 2), 1156.

LEVINE, E. M. (1976) Male transsexuals in the homosexual subculture. *Am. J. Psychiat.* **133**, 1318–21.

LEWIS, M. A. *et al.* (1973) Developmental-interest factors associated with homosexuality. *J. Consult. clin. Psychol.* **41**, 291–3.

LEWIS, T. H. (1973) Oglala (Sioux) concepts of homosexuality and the determinants of sexual identification. *J. Am. med. Ass.* **225**, 312–13.

LIMENTANI, A. (1976) Object choice and actual bisexuality. *Int. J. Psychoanal. Psychother.* **5**, 205–17.

—— (1977) The differential diagnosis of homosexuality. *Br. J. med. Psychol.* **50**, 209–16.

LISS, J. L. *et al.* (1973) Change in homosexual orientation. *Am. J. Psychother.* **27**, 102–4.

LONEY, J. (1973) Family dynamics in homosexual women. *Arch. sex. Behav.* **2**, 313–50.

LOPEZ IBOR, J. J. (1974) [Editorial: referendum on homosexuality.] *Actas. Luso. Esp. Nerol. Psiquiat.* **2**, 165–8 (Spa.)

LUMBY, M. E. (1976) Homophobia: the quest for a valid scale. *J. Homosex.* **2**, 39–47.

—— (1976) Code switching and sexual orientation: a test of Bernstein's sociolinguistic theory. *J. Homosex.* **1**, 383–99.

LYNCH, V. P. (1972) Parasite transmission. *J. Am. med. Ass.* **222**, 1309–10.

McCAFFREY, J. A. (1972) *Homosexual dialect*. Englewood Cliffs, New Jersey.

McCAULEY, E. A. (1977) Role expectations and definitions: a comparison of female transsexuals and lesbians. *J. Homosex.* **3**, 137–47.

McCONAGY, N. (1973) The doctor and homosexuality. *Med. J. Aust.* **1**, 68–70.

—— (1975) Aversive and positive conditioning treatments of homosexuality. *Behav. Res. Ther.* **13**, 309–19.

—— (1976) Is a homosexual orientation irreversible? *Br. J. Psychiat.* **129**, 556–63.

—— (1977) Behavioural intervention in homosexuality. *J. Homosex.* **2**, 221–7.

—— *et al.* (1972) Subjective and penile plethysmography response to aversion therapy for homosexuality: a partial replication. *Arch. sex. Behav.* **2**, 65–78.

—— *et al.* (1973) Classical, avoidance and backward conditioning treatments of homosexuality. *Br. J. Psychiat.* **122**, 151–62.

MacDONALD, A. P., Jr. *et al.* (1973) Attitudes toward homosexuality: preservation of sex morality or the double standard? *J. Consult. clin. Psychol.* **40**, 161.

McMILLAN, A. (1978) Threadworms in homosexual males. *Brit. med. J.* **1**, 367.

—— *et al.* (1977) Sexually-transmitted diseases in homosexual males in Edinburgh. *Health Bull. (Edinb.)* **35**, 266–71.

MALETZKY, B. M. *et al.* (1973) The treatment of homosexuality by 'assisted' covert sensitization. *Behav. Res. Ther.* **11**, 655–7.

MARGOLESE, M. S. *et al.* (1973) Androsterone–etiocholanolone ratios in male homosexuals. *Br. med. J.* **3**, 207–10.

MARMOR, J. (Ed.) (1965) *Sexual inversion: the multiple roots of homosexuality*. New York.

—— (1972) Homosexuality—mental illness or moral dilemma? *Int. J. Psychiat.* **10**, 114–17.

MAURER, R. B. (1975) Health care and the gay community. *Post-grad. Med.* **58**, 127–30.

MAVISSAKALIAN, M. *et al.* (1975) Responses to complex erotic stimuli in homosexual and heterosexual males. *Br. J. Psychiat.* **126**, 252–7.

MERINO, H. I. *et al.* (1977) An innovative program of venereal disease case-finding, treatment and education for a population of gay men. *Sex. Transm. Dis.* **4**, 50–2.

MEYER, R. G. (1977) Legal and social ambivalence regarding homosexuality. *J. Homosex.* **2**, 281–7.

—— *et al.* (1976–7) A social episode model of human sexual behaviour. *J. Homosex.* **2**, 123–31.

MEYER-BAHLBURG, H. F. (1977) Sex hormones and male homosexuality in comparative perspective. *Arch. sex. Behav.* **6**, 297–325.

MEYERS, J. D. *et al.* (1977) *Giardia lamblia* infection in homosexual men. *Br. J. vener. Dis.* **53**, 54–5.

MILDVAN, D. *et al.* (1977) Venereal transmission of enteric pathogens in male homosexuals. Two case reports. *J. Am. med. Ass.* **238**, 1387–9.

MILLER, R. D. (1978) Pseudohomosexuality in male patients with hysterical psychosis: a preliminary report. *Am. J. Psychiat.* **135**, 112–13.

MILLHAM, J. *et al.* (1976) A factor-analytic conceptualization of attitudes toward male and female homosexuals. *J. Homosex.* **2**, 3–10.

MINNIGERODE, F. A. (1976) Age-status labelling in homosexual men. *J. Homosex.* **1**, 273–6.

—— (1977) Rights or repentance. *J. Homosex.* **2**, 323–6.

MONEY, J. (1972) Editorial: Strategy, ethics, behaviour modification, and homosexuality. *Arch. sex. Behav.* **2**, 79–81.

—— (1976–77) Statement on antidiscrimination regarding sexual orientation. *J. Homosex.* **2**, 159–61.

—— (1977) Bisexual, homosexual, and heterosexual: society, law, and medicine. *J. Homosex.* **2**, 229–33.

MORAN, P. A. (1972) Familial effects in schizophrenia and homosexuality. *Aust. N. Z. J. Psychiat.* **6**, 116–19.

MORIN, S. F. (1977) Heterosexual bias in psychological research on lesbianism and male homosexuality. *Am. Psychol.* **32**, 629–37.

MORRIS, P. A. (1973) Doctors' attitudes to homosexuality. *Br. J. Psychiat.* **122**, 435–6.

MUNTER, P. A. (1973) Some observations about homosexuality and prejudice. *J. Am. Coll. Health Ass.* **22**, 53–5.

MYRICK, F. (1974) Attitudinal differences between heterosexuality and homosexually oriented males and between covert and overt male homosexuals. *J. abnorm. Psychol.* **83**, 81–6.

NATTERSON, J. M. (1976) The self as a transitional object: its relationship to narcissism and homosexuality. *Int. J. Psychoanal. Psychother.* **5**, 131–43.

NAZEMI, M. M. *et al.* (1975) Syphilitic proctitis in a homosexual. *J. Am. med. Ass.* **231**, 389.

NICOLIS, G. L. *et al.* (1974) Letter: Homosexuals in Boston and St. Louis, *N. Engl. J. Med.* **290**, 411–12.

NORRIS, L. (1974) Comparison of two groups in a Southern state women's prison: homosexual behaviour versus non-homosexual behaviour. *Psychol. Rep.* **34**, 75–8.

NORTON, R. H. (1974) *Homosexual literary tradition*. New York.

NYBERG, K. L. (1976) Sexual aspirations and sexual behaviors among homosexually behaving males and females: the impact of the gay community. *J. Homosex.* **2**, 29–38.

—— *et al.* (1976–7) Analysis of public attitudes toward homosexual behaviour. *J. Homosex.* **2**, 99–107.

—— *et al.* (1977) Homosexual labelling by university youths. *Adolescence* **12**, 541–6.

ORWIN, A. *et al.* (1974) Sex chromosome abnormalities, homosexuality and psychological treatment. *Br. J. Psychiat.* **124**, 293–5.

OSTROW, D. G. *et al.* (1977) The experience of the Howard Brown

Memorial Clinic of Chicago with sexually transmitted diseases. *Sex. Transm. Dis.* **4**, 53–5.

OVESEY, L. (1969) *Homosexuality and pseudohomosexuality.* New York.

PANIKIEWSKA, W. *et al.* (1975) [Homosexuality with transvestism in a mentally retarded person.] *Psychiat. Pol.* **9**, 465–6 (Pol.)

PAPAEVENGELOU, G. (1973) Hepatitis-associated antigen in V.D. clinic patients. *Br. med. J.* **3**, 172.

PAPATHEOPHILOU, R. *et al.* (1975) Electroencephalographic findings in treatment-seeking homosexuals compared with heterosexuals: A controlled study. *Br. J. Psychiat.* **127**, 63–6.

PARKER, W. (1971) *Homosexuality: a selective bibliography of over three thousand items.* Millbrae, California.

PARKS, G. A. *et al.* (1974) Variation in pituitary–gonadal function in adolescent male homosexuals and heterosexuals. *J. clin. endocrinol. Metab.* **39**, 796–801.

PATTISON, E. M. (1974) Confusing concepts about the concept of homosexuality. *Psychiatry* **37**, 340–9.

PERETTI, P. O. *et al.* (1976) Self-image and emotional stability of Oedipal and non-Oedipal male homosexuals. *Acta Psychiat. Belg.* **76**, 46–55.

PERKINS, M. W. (1973) Homosexuality in female monozygotic twins. *Behav. Genet.* **3**, 387–8.

PERSON, E. *et al.* (1974) The transsexual syndrome in males. II. Secondary transsexualism. *Am. J. Psychother.* **28**, 174–93.

PERZYNSKI, J. (1977) [Case of symptomatic sexual inversion at an early stage of schizophrenia.] *Psychiat. Pol.* **11**, 101–3 (Pol.)

PHILLIPS, D. *et al.* (1976) Alternative behavioural approaches to the treatment of homosexuality. *Arch. sex. Behav.* **5**, 223–8.

PILLARD, R. C. *et al.* (1974). Plasma testosterone levels in homosexual men. *Arch. sex. Behav.* **3**, 453–8.

PISCICELLI, U. (1973) [Onto-analysis and therapy of homosexuality in autogenic training.] *Minerva. Med.* **64**, 2221–30.

POLLACK, S. *et al.* (1976) The dimensions of stigma: the social situation of the mentally ill person and the male homosexual. *J. abnorm. Psychol.* **85**, 105–12.

PORTER, J. F. (1976) Homosexuality treated adventitiously in a stuttering therapy program: a case report presenting a heterophobic orientation. *Aust. N. Z. J. Psychiat.* **10**, 185–9.

RAYCHAUDHURI, M. *et al.* (1971) Rorschach differentials of homosexuality in male convicts: an examination of Wheeler and Schafer signs. *J. Pers. Assess.* **35**, 22–6.

RATNATUNGA, C. S. (1972) Gonococcal pharyngitis. *Br. J. vener. Dis.* **48**, 184–6.

REKERS, G. A. *et al.* (1977) Assessment of childhood gender behaviour change. *J. Child Psychol. Psychiat.* **18**, 63–5.

RHODES, R. J. (1973) Homosexual aversion therapy. Electric shock technique. *J. Kans. med. Soc.* **74**, 103–5.

RITCHEY, M. G. (1977) Venereal disease among homosexuals [letter]. *J. Am. med. Ass.* **237**, 767.

——— *et al.* (1975) Venereal disease control among homosexuals; an outreach program. *J. Am. med. Ass.* **232**, 509–10.

ROBACK, H. B. *et al.* (1974) Sex of free choice figure drawings by homosexual and heterosexual subjects. *J. Pers. Assess.* **38**, 154–5.

——— *et al.* (1977) Self-concept and psychological adjustment differences between self-identified male transsexuals and male homosexuals. *J. Homosex.* **3**, 15–20.

ROBERTS, L. A. (1977) Female homosexuality. *Nurs. Times* **74**, 1426–9.

ROBERTSON, G. (1972) Parent–child relationships and homosexuality. *Br. J. Psychiat.* **121**, 525–8.

RODIN, P. *et al.* (1972) Gonococcal pharyngitis. *Br. J. vener. Dis.* **48**, 182–3.

ROEDELL, R. F. Jr (1976) Affirmative gay material in a hospital library collection [letter]. *Bull. Med. Libr. Ass.* **64**, 423.

ROGERS, C. *et al.* (1976) Group psychotherapy with homosexuals: a review. *Int. J. Group Psychother.* **26**, 3–27.

ROSENFELS, P. (1971) *Homosexuality: the psychology of the creative process.* New York.

ROY, D. (1972–3) Lytton Strachey and the masochistic basis of homosexuality. (Strachey, L.) *Psychoanal. Rev.* **59**, 579–84.

RUITENBECK, H. (1965) *Homosexuality and creative genius.* New York.

RUITENBECK, H. M. (Ed.) (1974) *Homosexuality a changing picture: a contemporary study and interpretation.* Atlantic Highlands, New Jersey.

RUPP, J. C. (1973) The love bug. *J. forensic Sci.* **18**, 259–62.

RUSSELL, A. *et al.* (1977) Evaluation of assertive training and homosexual guidance service groups designed to improve homosexual functioning. *J. Consult. clin. Psychol.* **45**, 1–13.

SABA, P. *et al.* (1973) [Hormonal changes in male homosexuality. Preliminary study.] *Folia endocrinol. (Roma)* **26**, 126–33 (Eng. Abstr.)

SAGARIN, E. (1976) Prison homosexuality and its effect on post-prison sexual behaviour. *Psychiatry* **39**, 245–57.

SAN MIGUEL, C. L. *et al.* (1976) The role of cognitive and situational variables in aggression toward homosexuals. *J. Homosex.* **2**, 11–27.

SATORI, O. *et al.* (1974) [Removal of large foreign bodies from the rectum.] *Orv. Hetil.* **115**, 1718–21 (Hun.)

SCHÄFER, S. (1977) Sociosexual behaviour in male and female homosexuals: a study in sex differences. *Arch. sex. Behav.* **6**, 355–64.

SCHATZBERG, A. F. *et al.* (1975) Effeminacy. I. A quantitative rating scale. *Arch. sex. Behav.* **4**, 31–41.

SCHERMANN, J. (1975) [Homosexuality. Evolution of its etiopathogenic concepts. Correlation with endocrinology.] *Rev. Ass. Med. Bras.* **21**, 28–34.

SCHMERIN, M. J. *et al.* (1977) Amebiasis. An increasing problem among homosexuals in New York City. *J. Am. med. Ass.* **238**, 1386–7.

SCHMIDT, G. (1978) Letter: Childhood indications of male homosexuality. *Arch. sex. Behav.* **7**, 73–5.

SCHNELLE, J. F. *et al.* (1974) Pupillary response as indication of sexual preference in a juvenile correctional institution. *J. clin. Psychol.* **30**, 146–50.

SCHROCK, R. A. *et al.* (1976) Homosexuality and the medical profession: a behaviourist's view. A commentary. *J. med. Ethics* **2**, 24–7.

SCOTT, J. M. *et al.* (1977) Male homosexual behaviour and ego function strategies in the group encounter. *J. clin. Psychol.* **33**, 1079–84.

SEGAL, B. *et al.* (1972) Covert sensitization with a homosexual: a controlled replication. *J. Consult. clin. Psychol.* **39**, 259–63.

SEITZ, F. C. *et al.* (1974) A comparative analysis of Rorschach signs of homosexuality. *Psychol. Rep.* **35**, 1163–9.

SHARMA, R. P. (1977) Light-dependent homosexual activity in males of a mutant of *Drosophilia melanogaster. Experientia* **33**, 171–3.

SHOHAM, S. G., WEISSBROD, L., GRUBVER, B., and STEIN, Y. (1978) Personality core dynamics and predisposition towards homosexuality. *Br. J. Med. Psychol.* **51**, 161.

SIEGELMAN, M. (1973) Birth order and family size of homosexual men and women. *J. consult. clin. Psychol.* **41**, 164.

—— (1974) Parental background of male homosexuals and heterosexuals. *Arch. sex. Behav.* **3**, 3–18.

—— (1974) Parental background of homosexual and heterosexual women. *Br. J. Psychiat.* **124**, 14–21.

SILVERMAN, L. H. *et al.* (1973) An experimental study of aspects of the psychoanalytic theory of male homosexuality. *J. abnorm. Psychol.* **82**, 178–88.

SILVERSTEIN, C. (1977) Homosexuality and the ethics of behavioural intervention. *J. Homosex.* **2**, 205–11.

SIMMONS, P. D. *et al.* (1977) Antigen among male homosexual patients. *Br. med. J.* **2**, 1458.

Singapore Medical Journal (1972) De Clerambault's syndrome: a review of 4 cases. *Tech. Jl Singapore med. J.* **13**, 227–34.

SIPOVA, I. (1974) [The therapy with lsd in homosexual males and transsexual females (author's transl.).] *Cas. Lek. Cesk.* **113**, 1491–3 (Eng. Abstr.) (Cze.)

SKENE, R. A. (1973) Construct shift in the treatment of a case of homosexuality. *Br. J. med. Psychol.* **46**, 287–92.

SIEGELMAN, M. (1972) Adjustment of male homosexuals and heterosexuals. *Arch. sex. Behav.* **2**, 9–25.

—— (1978) Psychological adjustment of homosexual and heterosexual men: a cross-national replication. *Arch. sex. Behav.* **7**, 1–11.

SMALL, E. L. Jr *et al.* (1977) Counselling homosexual alcoholics. Ten case histories. *J. Stud. Alcohol.* **38**, 2077–86.

SOBEL, H. J. (1976) Adolescent attitudes toward homosexuality in relation to self concept and body satisfaction. *Adolescence* **11**, 443–53.

SOCARIDES, C. W. (1972) Homosexuality—basic concepts and psychodynamics. *Int. J. Psychiat.* **10**, 118–25.

SOHN, N. *et al.* (1977) The gay bowel syndrome. A review of colonic and rectal conditions in 200 male homosexuals. *Am. J. Gastroenterol.* **67**, 478–84.

SOHN, N. *et al.* (1977) Social injuries of the rectum. *Am. J. Surg.* **134**, 611–12.

STAHL, F. *et al.* (1976) Significantly decreased apparently free testosterone levels in plasma of male homosexuals. *Endokrinologie* **68**, 115–17.

STEAKLEY, J. D. (1975) *Homosexual emancipation movement in Germany*. New York.

STEKEL, W. *Homosexual neurosis*. New York.

STEPHAN, W. G. (1973) Parental relationships and early social experiences of activist male homosexuals and male heterosexuals. *J. abnorm. Psychol.* **82**, 506–13.

STOLLER, R. J. *et al.* (1973) A symposium: Should homosexuality be in the APA nomenclature? *Am. J. Psychiat.* **130**, 1207–16.

STONE, N. M. (1976) On the assessment of sexual orientation: a reply to Anderson. *J. Pers. Assess.* **40**, 54–6.

—— *et al.* (1975) Concurrent validity of the Wheeler signs of homosexuality in the Rorschach: P(Ci/Rj) *J. Pers. Assess.* **39**, 573–9.

STRINGER, P. *et al.* (1976) Male homosexuality, psychiatric patient status, and psychological masculinity and femininity. *Arch. sex. Behav.* **5**, 15–27.

STRUPP, H. H. (1974) Some observations on the fallacy of value-free psycho-therapy and the empty organism: comments on a case study. *J. abnorm. Psychol.* **83**, 199–201.

STURGIS, E. T. *et al.* (1978) The right to treatment: issues in the treatment of homosexuality. *J. Consult. clin. Psychol.* **46**, 165.

SUHONEN, R. *et al.* (1975) [Rate of homosexuals among syphilitic patients in Helsinki.] *Duodecim* **91**, 351–3 (Eng. Abstr.) (Fin.)

—— *et al.* (1976) Syphilis, homosexuality and legislation. *Dermatologica* **152**, 363–6.

TANNER, B. A. (1978) Shock intensity and fear of shock in the modification of homosexual behaviour in males by avoidance learning. *Behav. Res. Ther.* **11**, 213–18.

TAYLOR, C. C. (1972) Identical twins: concordance for homosexuality? *Am. J. Psychiat.* **129**, 486–7.

TEWFIK, G. I. (1974) Letter: Homosexuality. *Aust. N. Z. J. Psychiat.* **8**, 207–8.

THIN, R. N. *et al.* (1976) Some characteristics of homosexual men. *Br. J. vener. Dis.* **52**, 161–4.

THOMPSON, N. L. Jr. *et al.* (1973) Parent–child relationships and sexual identity in male and female homosexuals and heterosexuals. *J. consult. clin. Psychol.* **41**, 7.

TOPIAR, A. *et al.* (1975) [A case of sodomy (author's transl.).] *Cesk. Psychiat.* **71**, 386–8 (Eng. Abstr.) (Cze.)

—— *et al.* (1976) [A disorder of psychosexual identity in epilepsy and endocraniosis.] *Bratisl. Lek. Listy.* **66**, 202–6 (Eng. Abstr.) (Cze.)

TOURNEY, G. *et al.* (1973) Androgen metabolism in schizophrenics, homo-sexuals, and normal controls. *Biol. Psychiat.* **6**, 23–36.

—— *et al.* (1975) Hormonal relationships in homosexual men. *Am. J. Psychiat.* **132**, 288–90.

TOWNES, B. D. *et al.* (1976) Differences in psychological sex, adjustment, and familial influences among homosexual and nonhomosexual populations. *J. Homosex.* **1**, 261–72.

TRIPP, C. A. (1975) *Homosexual matrix*. New York.

TURNER, R. K. *et al.* (1974) Personality characteristics of male homosexuals referred for aversion therapy: a comparative study. *Br. J. Psychiat.* **125**, 447–9.

—— *et al.* (1974) A note on the internal consistency of the sexual orientation method. *Behav. Res. Ther.* **12**, 273–8.

TYLER, P. (1972) *Homosexuality in the movies.*

VAISRUB, S. (1977) Homosexuality—a risk factor in infectious disease [editorial]. *J. Am. med. Ass.* **238**, 1402.

VERSTRAETE, B. C. (1977) Homosexuality in ancient Greek and Roman civilization: a critical bibliography. *J. Homosex.* **3**, 79–89.

WARREN, C. A. (1976) Women among men: females in the male homosexual community. *Arch. sex. Behav.* **5**, 157–69.

WAUGH, M. A. (1972) Threadworm infestation in homosexuals. *Trans. St. John's Hospital dermatol. Soc.* **58**, 224–5.

—— (1974) Letter: Sexual transmission of intestinal parasites. *Br. J. vener. Dis.* **50**, 157–8.

WEEKS, R. B. *et al.* (1975) Two cases of children of homosexuals. *Child Psychiat. hum. Dev.* **6**, 26–32.

WEINBERG, M. and BELL, A. (Ed.) (1972) *Homosexuality: an annotated bibliography.* Philadelphia.

WEISSBACH, T. A. *et al.* (1975) The effect of deviant group membership upon impressions of personality. *J. soc. Psychol.* **95**, 263–6.

WEST, D. J. (1968) *Homosexuality.* Chicago.

WESTFALL, M. P. *et al.* (1975) Effeminacy. II. Variation with social context. *Arch. sex. Behav.* **4**, 43–51.

WHITAM, F. L. (1977) Childhood indicators of male homosexuality. *Arch. sex. Behav.* **6**, 89–96.

WHITE, E. *et al.* (1974) Letter: Hepatitis and a venereal disease in homosexuals. *N. Engl. J. Med.* **290**, 1384.

WILLIAM, D. C. *et al.* (1977) Sexually transmitted enteric pathogens in male homosexual population. *N. Y. State J. Med.* **77**, 2050–2.

WILLIAMS, A. H. (1975) Problems of homosexuality. *Br. med. J.* **3**, 426–8.

WILSON, W. P. *et al.* (1973) Arousal from sleep of male homosexuals. *Biol. Psychiat.* **6**, 81–4.

WOODWARD, R. *et al.* (1973) A comparison of two scoring systems for the Sexual Orientation Method. *Br. J. soc. clin. Psychol.* **12**, 411–14.

ZLOTLOW, M. (1972) Religious rationalization of a homosexual. *N.Y. State J. Med.* **72**, 2775–9.

ZUGER, B. (1974) Effeminate behaviour in boys. Parental age and other factors. *Arch. gen. Psychiat.* **30**, 173–7.

—— (1976) Monozygotic twins discordant for homosexuality report of a pair and significance of the phenomenon. *Compr. Psychiat.* **17**, 661–9.

Aggression in the perversion; sadism and masochism

BARBARA, D. A. (1974) Masochism in love and sex. *Am. J. Psychoanal.* **34**, 73–9.

BARRY, D. J. *et al.* (1975) Use of depo-provera in the treatment of aggressive sexual offenders: preliminary report of three cases. *Bull. Am. Acad. Psychiat. Law* **3**, 179–84.

CAPPON, A. (1977) Masochism: a trait in the Mexican national character. *J. Psychoanal. Rev.* **64**, 163–71.

CHASSEQUET-SMIRGEL, J. (1978) Reflexions on the connexions between perversion and sadism. *Int. J. Psychoanal.* **59**, 27.

DRVOTA, S. *et al.* (1975) [Dangerous sexual aggressors (Author's Transl.).] *Cesk. Psychiat.* **71**, 33–7 (Eng. Abstr.) (Cze.)

EVANS, W. N. (1974–5) Pseudostupidity: a study in masochistic exhibitionism. *Psychoanal. Rev.* **61**, 619–32.

FRIED, C. (1971) Icarianism, masochism, and sex differences in fantasy. *J. Pers. Assess.* **35**, 38–55.

FRIEDMAN, H. J. (1973) The masochistic character in the work of Edith Wharton. (Wharton E.). *Semin. Psychiat.* **5**, 313–29.

GRAND, H. G. (1973) The masochistic defence of the 'double mask': its relationship to imposture. *Int. J. Psychoanal.* **54**, 445–54.

GROTH, A. N. *et al.* (1976) Aggressive sexual offenders: diagnosis and treatment. In *Community mental health: target populations*, Burgess, A. W. and Lazare, A. (Eds).

HERMAN, D. *et al.* (1973) The treatment of psychosocial masochism. *Psychoanal. Rev.* **60**, 333–72.

HERMANN, I. (1976) Clinging-going-in-search. A contrasting pair of instincts and their relation to sadism and masochism. *Psychoanal. Q.* **45**, 5–36.

HUNT, W. (1973) Beating fantasies and daydreams revisited; presentation of a case. *J. Am. Psychoanal. Assoc.* **21**, 817–32.

LAX, R. F. (1977) The role of internalization in the development of certain aspects of female masochism: ego psychological considerations. *Int. J. Psychoanal.* **58**, 289–300.

MONTI, P. M. *et al.* (1977) Testosterone and components of aggressive and sexual behaviour in man. *Am. J. Psychiat.* **134**, 692–4.

M'UZAN, M. DE (1973) A case of masochistic perversion and an outline of a theory. *Int. J. Psychoanal.* **54**, 455–67.

NEDOMA, K. (1972) [Recidivist sex aggressor in psychiatric and sexologic expert opinion.] *Cesk. Psychiat.* **68**, 308–11 (Eng. Abstr.) (Cze.)

O'DONNELL, T. J. (1977) The confessions of T. E. Lawrence: the sado-masochistic hero. *Am. Imago* **34**,(2), 115.

OBER, W. B. (1973) Carlo Gesualdo. Prince of Venosa: murder, madrigals, and masochism. (Gesualdo, C.) *Bull N. Y. Acad. Med.* **49**, 634–45.

—— (1975) Swinburne's masochism: neuropathology and psychopathology. *Bull. Menninger Clin.* **39**, 501–55.

RAZAVI, L. (1975) Cytogenetic and dermatoglyphic studies in sexual offenders, violent criminals, and aggressively-behaved temporal lobe epileptics. *Proc. Am. psychopathol. Ass.* **63**, 75–94.

REEVES, D. L. *et al.* (1977) Influence of amygdaloid on self-punitive behaviour in rats. *Physiol. Behav.* **18**, 1089–93.

RIBON, J. F. (1974) [The marquis de Sade: patient or precursor?] (Sade, D.A.) *Nouv. Presse Med.* **3**, 899–901 (Fre.)

SACK, R. L. *et al.* (1975) Masochism: a clinical and theoretical overview. *Psychiatry* **38**, 244–57.

SCHOTT, G. (1973) [Self castration due to sadistic impulsive perversion, simultaneously a contribution to anti-androgen therapy.] *Psychiat. Neurol. Med. Psychol. (Leipz)* **25**, 435–42 (Eng. Abstr.) (Ger.)

SIOMOPOULOS, V. *et al.* (1976) Sadism revisited. *Am. J. Psychother.* **30**, 631–40.

SPENGLER, A. (1977) Manifest sadomasochism of males: results of an empirical study. *Arch. sex. Behav.* **6**, 441–56.

STAAK, M. (1972) [Situations of homicide in heterosexual and homosexual transient partnerships.] *Z. Rechtsmed.* **71**, 39–46 (Eng. Abstr.) (Ger.)

STEPANSKY, P. S. (1977) On passive seductions and precocious desire: the etiology of obsessional neurosis and Freud's earliest theory of 'aggression'. *Psychol. Issues* **10**, 25–56.

STERNBACH, O. (1975) Aggression, the death drive and the problem of sado-masochism. A reinterpretation of Freud's second drive theory. *Int. J. Psychoana.* **56**, 321–33.

STOLOROW, R. D. (1975) The narcissistic function of masochism (and sadism). *Int. J. Psychoanal.* **56**, 441–8.

USHER, A. (1975) Sexual violence. *Forensic Sci.* **5**, 243–55.

Psychotherapy of sex-offenders

BLUMBERG, M. L. (1978) Child sexual abuse. Ultimate in maltreatment syndrome. *N. Y. state J. Med.* **78**, 612–16.

BRANCALE, R. *et al.* (1971) The New Jersey program for sex-offenders. *Int. Psychiat. Clin.* **8**, 145–64.

CARNEY, F. L. (1977) Outpatient treatment of the aggressive offender. *Am. J. Psychother.* **31**, 265–74.

COSTELL, R. *et al.* (1971) Treatment of the sex-offender: institutional group therapy. *Int. Psychiat. Clin.* **8**, 119–44.

GARFIELD, S. L. (1974) Values: an issue in psychotherapy: comments on a case study. *J. abnorm. Psychol.* **83**, 202–3.

GREENLAND, C. (1977) Psychiatry and the dangerous sexual offender. *Can. psychiat. Ass. J.* **22**, 155–9.

GROMSKA, J. (1973) [Problems of sexual psychophysiology and psychotherapy in children.] *Psychiat. Pol.* **7**, 461–8 (Pol.)

HALLECK, S. (1971) Treatment of the sex-offender: the therapeutic encounter. *Int. Psychiat. Clin.* **8**, 1–20.

HYNIE, J. (1973) [Preventive custodial therapy of sex delinquents serving their sentence.] *Cesk. Psychiat.* **69**, 29–31 (Eng. Abstr.) (Cze.)

KEITER, R. H. (1975) Psychotherapy of moral masochism. *Am. J. Psychother.* **29**, 56–65.

KERR, N. (1972) Special handling for sex-offenders. *Perspect. psychiat. Care* **10**, 160–2.

KIRKPATRICK, M. *et al.* (1976) Treatment of requests for sex-change surgery with psychotherapy. *Am. J. Psychiat.* **133**, 1194–6.

LARGE, R. G. (1976) The use of the role construct repertory grid in studying changes during psychotherapy. *Aust. N. Z. J. Psychiat.* **10**, 315–20.

LARSON, D. *et al.* (1974) A group treatment program for masochistic patients. *Hosp. Community Psychiat.* **25**, 525–8.

MARSHALL, W. L. *et al.* (1975) An integrated treatment program for sexual-offenders. *Can. psychiat. Ass. J.* **20**, 133–8.

—— *et al.* (1977) The clinical value of boredom. A procedure for reducing inappropriate sexual interests. *J. nerv. ment. Dis.* **165**, 283–7.

PARFENT'EVA, O. V. (1978) [Forensic psychiatric expertise of crime victims who suffer from oligophrenia]. *Sud. Med. Ekspert* **21**, 39–43. (Eng. Abstr.) (Rus.)

PETERS, J. J. *et al.* (1971) Group psychotherapy for probationed sex-offenders. *Int. Psychiat. Clin.* **8**, 69–80.

SALZMAN, L. (1971) The psychodynamic approach to sex deviations. *Int. Psychiat. Clin.* **8**, 21–40.

SCHUMANN, H. J. VON. (1972) [Resocialization of sexually abnormal patients by a combination of anti-androgen administration and psychotherapy.] *Psychother. Psychosom.* **20**, 321–32 (Eng. Abstr.) (Ger.)

SINGER, V. *et al.* (1977) [A regimen ward for treatment of sexual delinquents (author's transl.).] *Cesk. Psychiat.* **73**, 39–45 (Eng. Abstr.) (Cze.)

VAN MOFFAERT, M. (1976) Social reintegration of sexual delinquents by a combination of psychotherapy and anti-androgen treatment. *Acta Psychiat. scand.* **53**, 29–34.

Behaviour therapy and drug therapy for sexual deviations

APPELT, M. *et al.* (1974) [The effect on sexuality of cyproterone acetate.] *Int. Pharmacopsychiat.* **9**, 61–76 (Eng. Abstr.) (Ger.)

BANCROFT, J. *et al.* (1974) The control of deviant sexual behaviour by drugs. I. Behavioural changes following oestrogens and anti-androgens. *Br. J. Psychiat.* **125**, 310–15.

BANCROFT, J. H. (1975) The treatment of sexual problems. *Ir. med. J.* **68**, 465–9.

BANCROFT, J. H. J. (1976) Evaluation of the effects of drugs on sexual behaviour. *Br. J. clin. Pharmacol.* **3** (Suppl. 1), 83–90.

BANIEWICZ, K. (1977) [Atropine coma treatment in a case of personality disorder with intrusions and sex deviation.] *Psychiat. Pol.* **11**, 591–4 (Pol.)

BARON, D. P. *et al.* (1977) A clinical trial of cyproterone acetate for sexual deviancy. *N. Z. med. J.* **85**, 366–9.

BARRY, D. J. *et al.* (1975) Use of depo-provera in the treatment of aggressive sexual offenders: preliminary report of three cases. *Bull. Am. Acad. Psychiat. Law* **3**, 179–84.

BASTANI, J. B. (1976) Treatment of male genital exhibitionism. *Compr. Psychiat.* **17**, 769–74.

BEBBINGTON, P. E. (1977) Treatment of male sexual deviation by use of a vibrator: case report. *Arch. Sex. Behav.* **6**, 21–4.

BEMPORAD, J. R. *et al.* (1976) Case reports the treatment of a child foot fetishist. *Am. J. Psychother.* **30**, 303–16.

BOAS, C. VAN E. (1973) Cyproteronacetate in sexualogical outpatient practice. *Psychiat. Neurol. Neurochir.* **76**, 151–4.

BRANCALE, R. *et al.* (1971) The New Jersey program for sex offenders. *Int. Psychiat. Clin.* **8**, 145–64.

BROTHERTON, J. (1974) Effect of oral cyproterone acetate on urinary and serum FSH and LH levels in adult males being treated for hypersexuality. *J. Reprod. Fertil.* **36**, 177–87.

BROWNELL, K. D. *et al.* (1977) Patterns of appropriate and deviant sexual arousal: the behavioural treatment of multiple sexual deviations. *J. Consult. clin. Psychol.* **45**, 1144–55.

CALLAHAN, E. J. *et al.* (1973) Aversion therapy for sexual deviation: contingent shock and covert sensitization. *J. abnorm. Psychol.* **81**, 60–73.

CHAMBERS, W. M. *et al.* (1976) The eclectic and multiple therapy of a shoe fetishist. *Am. J. Psychother.* **30**, 317–26.

CORNU, F. (1972) [Catamneses of castrated sex delinquents from the forensic and psychiatric viewpoint.] *Fortschr. Med.* **90**, 1035–6 (Ger.)

—— (1973) [Case histories of castrated sex offenders from a forensic psychiatric viewpoint.] *Bibl. Psychiat.* **149**, 1–132 (Ger.)

COSTELL, R. *et al.* (1971) Treatment of the sex offender: institutional group therapy. *Int. Psychiat. clin.* **8**, 119–44.

DELALOYE, R. (1974) [Sex deviations and their chemical treatment.] *Rev. Med. Suisse Romande* **94**, 565–73 (Fre.)

DIECKMANN, G. *et al.* (1975) Unilateral hypothalomotomy in sexual delinquents. Report on six cases. *Confin. Neurol.* **37**, 177–86.

Drug Therapy Bulletin (1974) Benperidol—a drug for sexual offenders? *Drug Ther. Bull.* **12**, 12.

Drug Therapy Bulletin (1977) Cyproterone to reduce male sex drive? *Drug. Ther. Bull.* **15**, 55–6.

FÄHNDRICH, E. (1974) [Cyproterone acetate in the treatment of sexual deviation in men (Author's Transl.).] *Dtsch. Med. Wochenschr.* **99**, 234–8 passim (Eng. Abstr.) (Ger.)

FENSTERHEIM, H. (1974) Behaviour therapy of the sexual variations. *J. sex. marital Ther.* **1**, 16–28.

FIELD, L. H. (1973) Benperidol in the treatment of sexual offenders. *Med. Sci. Law* **13**, 195–6.

FREY, H. (1975) [Androcur (cyproterone acetate)—a drug with antiandrogen effect.] *Tidsskr. Nor. Laegeforen.* **95**, 1368–9 (Nor.)

GAENSBAUER, T. J. (1973) Castration in treatment of sex offenders: an appraisal. *Rocky Mt. med. J.* **70**, 23–8.

HALLECK, S. (1971) Treatment of the sex offender: the therapeutic encounter. *Int. psychiat. clin.* **8**, 1–20.

HALVORSEN, K. A. *et al.* (1972) [Antiandrogenic treatment of 2 psychiatric patients.] *Ugeskr. Laeger* **134**, 2206–7 (Dan.)

HARBERT, T. L. *et al.* (1974) Measurement and modification of incestuous behaviour: a case study. *Psychol. Rep.* **34**, 79–86.

HIOB, J. (1977) [Treatment of sex offenders.] *Ther. Ggw.* **116**, 593–626 (Ger.)

HYNIE, J. (1973) [Preventive custodial therapy of sex delinquents serving their sentences.] *Cesk. Psychiat.* **69**, 29–31 (Eng. Abstr.) (Cze.)

INCE, L. P. (1973) Behaviour modification of sexual disorders. *Am. J. Psychother.* **17**, 446–51.

JANCZEWSKI, Z. *et al.* (1977) [Cyproterone acetate in the treatment of hypersexuality in men.] *Endokrynol. Pol.* **28**, 541 (Pol.)

JOB, J. C. *et al.* (1977) The use of luteinizing hormone-releasing hormone in pediatric patients. *Horm. Res.* **8**, 171–87.

JOHNSEN, S. G. *et al.* (1974) Therapeutic effectiveness of oral testosterone. *Lancet* **2**, 1473–5.

JOST, F. (1974) [The treatment of sexual deviants with the antiandrogen cyproteron-acetate (1971–1974) (Author's Transl.).] *Praxis* **63**, 1318–25 (Eng. Abstr.) (Ger.)

KOCKOTT, G. *et al.* (1973) [Behaviour therapy of sexual disorders: diagnosis and methods of treatment.] *Nervenarzt* **44**, 173–83 (Ger.)

LASCHET, U. *et al.* (1975) Antiandrogens in the treatment of sexual deviations of men. *J. Steroid Biochem.* **6**, 821–6.

LEDERER, J. (1974) [Treatment of sex deviations with cyproterone acetate.] *Probl. Actuels. Endocrinol. Nutr. Serie* **18**, 249–60 (Fre.)

LEHRMAN, K. L. (1976) Pulmonary embolism in a transsexual man taking diethylstilbestrol. *J. Am. med. Ass.* **235**, 532–3.

LENTON, E. A. *et al.* (1977) Episodic secretion of growth hormone in a male transsexual during treatment with oestrogen both before and after orchidectomy. *J. Endocrinol.* **74**, 337–8.

LEVIN, S. M. *et al.* (1977) Variations of covert sensitization in the treatment of pedophilic behaviour: a case study. *J. consult. clin. Psychol.* **45**, 896–907.

MACCULLOCH, M. J. *et al.* (1974) Sexual interest latencies in aversion therapy: a preliminary report. *Arch. sex. Behav.* **3**, 289–99.

MARSHALL, W. L. (1973) The modification of sexual fantasies: a combined treatment approach to the reduction of deviant sexual behaviour. *Behav. Res. Ther.* **11**, 557–64.

—— *et al.* (1975) An integrated treatment program for sexual offenders. *Can. psychiat. Ass. J.* **20**, 133–8.

MELCHIODE, G. A. (1974) Trends in sex therapy—the Philadelphia plan. *Pa. Med.* **77**, 43–5.

MIES, R. *et al.* (1974) [Treatment with anti-androgens.] *Dtsch Med. Wochenschr.* **99**, 255–7 (Ger.)

MILLER, H. L. *et al.* (1976) Behaviour and traditional therapy applied to pedophiliac exhibitionism: a case study. *Psychol. Rep.* **39**, 1119–24.

MOHR, J. W. (1971) Treatment of the sex offender: evaluation of treatment. *Int. Psychiat. clin.* **8**, 227–42.

MONEY, J. (1971) The therapeutic use of androgen-depleting hormone. *Int. Psychiat. clin.* **8**, 165–74.

—— *et al.* (1976) Combined antiandrogenic and counseling program for treatment of 46, XY and 47, XYY sex offenders. In Sachar, E. J. (ed.) *Hormones, behaviour, and psychopathology*, pp. 105–20. New York.

MOTHES, C. (1976) Cyproterone acetate (letter). *Lancet* **2**, 1020.

MURRAY, M. A. *et al.* (1975) Endocrine changes in male sexual deviants after treatment with anti-androgens, oestrogens or tranquillizers. *J. Endocrinol.* **67**, 179–88.

NEWMAN, L. E. (1976) Treatment for the parents of feminine boys. *Am. J. Psychiat.* **133**, 683–7.

NADVORNIK, P. *et al.* (1975) [Sterotactic approach to sexual deviation treatment (Author's Transl.).] *Cesk. Psychiat.* **71**, 230–3 (Eng. Abstr.) (Slo.)

OATES, W. E. (1971) Treatment of the sex offender: religious attitudes and pastoral counseling. *Int. Psychiat. clin.* **8**, 41–52.

PIETRANTONIO, C. (1976) [Possibilities of drug treatment in some sex behaviour anomalies.] *Ateneo Parmense [Acta biomed.]* **47**, 613–33 (Eng. Abstr.) (Ita.)

PINARD, G. *et al.* (1976) [Treatment of a case of fetishism with masochism by behaviour therapy.] *Union Med. Can.* **105**, 1863–5 (Eng. Abstr.) (Fre.)

PISCICELLI, U. (1975) [Autogenic training in sexology.] *Minerva Med.* **66**, 252–6 (Eng. Abstr.) (Ita.)

REKERS, G. A. *et al.* (1974) Behavioural treatment of deviant sex-role behaviours in a male child. *J. appl. behav. Anal.* **7**, 173–90.

RHODES, R. J. *et al.* (1977) Sexual deviancy. Treatment: a case study for a child molester. *J. Kans. med. Soc.* **78**, 122–4.

ROGNANT, J. (1973) [Behaviour therapy in neurotic exhibitionism.] *Encephale* **62**, 332–44 (Fre.)

ROSE, R. M. (1976) Antiandrogen therapy of sex offenders. In *Hormones, behaviour, and psychopathology*, (ed. E. J. Sacher) pp. 121–4). New York.

ROSEN, R. C. *et al.* (1977) Penile plethysmography and biofeedback in the treatment of a transvestite-exhibitionist. *J. consult. clin. Psychol.* **45**, 908–16.

ROSENTHAL, T. L. (1973) Response-contingent versus fixed punishment in aversion conditioning of pedophilia: a case study. *J. nerv. ment. Dis.* **156**, 440–3.

SERBER, M. *et al.* (1971) Treatment of the sex offender: behaviour therapy techniques. *Int. Psychiat. clin.* **8**, 53–68.

SINGER, V. *et al.* (1977) [A regimen ward for treatment of sexual delinquents (Author's Transl.).] *Cesk. Psychiat.* **73**, 39–45 (Eng. Abstr.) (Cze.)

SIPOVA, I. (1974) [The therapy with lsd in homosexual males and transsexual females (Author's Transl.).] *Cas. Lek. Cesk.* **113**, 1491–3 (Eng. Abstr.) (Cze.)

STEVENSON, J. *et al.* (1972) Behaviour therapy technique for exhibitionism. A preliminary report. *Arch. gen. Psychiat.* **27**, 839–41.

STÜRUP, G. K. (1971) Treatment of the sex offender. Castration: the total treatment. *Int. Psychiat. clin.* **8**, 175–96.

TAUS, L. *et al.* (1973) [5-year follow-up study of 5 sexual deviants after therapeutic operation.] *Cesk. Psychiat.* **69**, 51–5 (Eng. Abstr.) (Cze.)

TENNENT, G. *et al.* (1974) The control of deviant sexual behaviour by drugs: a double-blind controlled study of benperidol, chlorpromazine, and placebo. *Arch. sex. Behav.* **3**, 261–71.

UNGER, H. R. (1977) Cyproterone and hypersexuality (letter). *N. Z. med. J.* **86**, 39–40.

VIRDIS, R. *et al.* (1978) Endocrine studies in a pubertal male pseudohermaphrodite with 17-ketosteroid reductase deficiency. *Acta Endocrinol. (Kbh.)* **87**, 212–24.

VOGT, H. J. (1973) [Therapy of exhibitionism.] *Med. Klin.* **68**, 129 (Ger.)

WARD, N. G. (1975) Successful lithium treatment of transvestism associated with maniic depression. *J. nerv. ment. Dis.* **16,** 204–6.

WERFF TEN BOSCH, J. J. VAN. (1973) Manipulation of sexual behaviour by anti-androgens. *Psychiatr. Neurol. Neurochir.* **76**, 147–9.

Sexual deviation and the law

Committee on Psychiatry and Law. (1977) Psychiatry and sex psychopath legislation: the 30s to the 80s. *Publ. Group Adv. Psychiat.* **9**, 827–959 (Eng. Abstr.)

CRYER, L. *et al.* (1978) Payment procedures for medical examinations of rape victims in Houston. *Tex. Med.* **74**, 59–62.

DEBARGE, A. *et al.* (1973) [Medicolegal examination of the hymen. Analytical study of 384 medicolegal expertises of sexual assaults.] *Med. Leg. Dommage Corpor.* **6**, 298–300 (Fre.)

EISENMENGER, W. *et al.* (1977) [Medicolegal findings following sex offences.] *Beitr. Gerichtl. Med.* **35**, 13–16 (Eng. Abstr.) (Ger.)

FEHLOW, P. (1973) [Causes and forensic assessment of sexual offences.] *Psychiat. Neurol. med. Psychol. (Leipz.)* **25**, 535–44 (Eng. Abstr.) (Ger.)

FINEMAN, (1977) Fratricide and cuckoldry: Shakespeare's doubles. *J. Psychoanal. Rev.* **64**, 409–53.

FORBES, G. (1972) Sexual offences. *Practitioner* **209**, 287–93.

FORST, M. L. (1977) The psychiatric evaluation of dangerousness in two trial court jurisdictions. *Bull. Am. Acad. Psychiat. Law* **5**, 98–110.

FRÖHLICH, H. H. (1974) [Significance of sexual knowledge, interests, and previous experience for the special credibility of witnesses.] *Psychiat. Neurol. med. Psychol. (Leipz.)* **26**, 25–32 (Eng. Abstr.) (Ger.)

GIGEROFF, A. K. (1968) *Sexual deviations in the criminal law: homosexual, exhibitionist, and pedophilic offences in Canada.* Toronto.

GOODRICH, M. (1976) Sodomy in medieval secular law. *J. Homosex.* **1**, 295–302.

—— (1976) Sodomy in ecclesiastical law and theory. *J. Homosex.* **1**, 427–34.

GRANT, J. H. (1973) Pornography. *Med. Sci. Law.* **13**, 232–8.

GREENAWALT, K. (1976) Restricting the right of privacy. The Burger court and claims of privacy. *Inquiry* **6**, 19–20.

HARTLAND, J. (1974) An alleged case of criminal assault upon a married woman under hypnosis. *Am. J. clin. Hypn.* **16**, 188–98.

HENN, F. A. *et al.* (1976) Forensic psychiatry: profiles of two types of sex offenders. *Am. J. Psychiat.* **133**, 694–6.

HINDERER, H. (1973) [Evaluation and differentiation of the penal responsibility of the sex offender.] *Psychiat. Neurol. med. Psychol. (Leipz.)* **25**, 257–65 (Eng. Abstr.) (Ger.)

HOLZER, F. J. (1971) [Sex murderer Zingerle.] *Arch. Kriminol.* **148**, 14–23 contd. (Ger.)

—— (1971) [Sex murderer Zingerle.] *Arch. Kriminol.* **148**, 94–105 concl. (Ger.)

HUNTINGTON, K. (1976) Forensic gynaecology. *Practitioner* **216**, 519–28.

KERR, N. (1972) Special handling for sex offenders. *Perspect. psychiat. Care* **10**, 160–2.

KNIGHT, B. (1976) Forensic problems in practice VIII—Sexual offences. *Practitioner* **217**, 288–93.

KOSA, F. (1971) [False accusations to camouflage autoerotic acts.] *Arch. Kriminol.* **148**, 106–10 (Ger.)

L'EPEE, P. *et al.* (1973) [Use of expert testimony.] *Med. Leg. Domm. Corpor. (Paris)* **6**, 85–93 (Fre.)

LINDABURY, V. A. (1975) Editorial: The Criminal Code and rape and sex offences. *Can. Nurse* **71**, 3.

MAGYAR, I. *et al.* (1975) [Criminal psychiatry evaluation of sexual aberrations.] *Arch. Kriminol.* **156**, 85–94 (Ger.)

Medical Trials Technical Quarterly (1972) Medical testimony in a case of trauma and nymphomania (AKA, 'San Francisco cable car case'), showing the cross-examination of the defendant's neuropsychiatrist by the plaintiff's lawyer. I. *Med. Trial. Tech. Q.* **19**, 83–120.

—— (1972) Medical testimony in a case of trauma and nymphomania (AKA, 'San Francisco cable car case'), showing the cross-examination of the defendant's neuropsychiatrist by the plaintiff's lawyer. II. *Med. Trial. Tech. Q.* **19**, 205–40.

—— (1973) Medical testimony in a case of trauma and nymphomania (AKA 'San-Francisco cable car cas'), showing the cross-examination of the defendant's neuropsychiatrist by the plaintiff's lawyer. II. *Med. Trial. Tech. Q.* **19**, 317–60.

MELLAN, J. *et al.* (1972) [Forensic evaluation of sex offenders.] *Cesk. Psychiat.* **68**, 218–22 (Eng. Abstr.) (Cze.)

MONEY, J. (1977) Bisexual, homosexual, and heterosexual: society, law, and medicine. *J. Homosex.* **2**, 229–33.

PAUL, D. M. (1975) The medical examination in sexual offences. *Med. Sci. Law* **15**, 154–62.

—— (1977) The medical examination in sexual offences against children. *Med. Sci. Law* **17**, 251–8.

PETIT, G. *et al.* (1973) [Statistical and criminological studies of sexual violence.] *Med. Leg. Dommage Corpor.* **6**, 386–9 (Fre.)

POLE, K. F. (1976) Letter to the editor: The medical examination in sexual offences. *Med. Sci. Law* **16**, 73–4.

POWER, D. J. (1976) Sexual deviation and crime. *Med. Sci. Law* **16**, 111–28.

PRESSER, C. S. (1977) Legal problems attendant to sex reassignment surgery. *J. Leg. Med.* **5**, 17–24.

RADER, C. M. (1977) MMPI profile types of exposers, rapists, and assaulters in a court services population. *J. consult. clin. Psychol.* **45**, 61–9.

RESNIK, H. L. and WOLFGANG, M. E. (Eds) (1972) *Sexual behaviours: social, clinical, and legal aspects.* Boston.

SASS, F. A. (1975) Sexual asphyxia in the female. *J. forensic Sci.* **20**, 181–5.

SAURY, H. (1973) [Medical expert testimony in child abuse, indecent behaviour and drug addiction (excluding psychiatric expert testimony). Viewpoint of the magistrate.] *Med. Leg. Domm. Corpor. (Paris)* **6**, 82–4 (Fre.)

SCHMAIZ, K. (1973) [Medical sex transformation from the legal viewpoint.] *Med. Monatsschr.* **27**, 142–3 (Ger.)

SIDLEY, N. T. *et al.* (1973) A proposed 'dangerous sex offender' law. *Am. J. Psychiat.* **130**, 765–8.

SLOVENKO, R. (1973) Everything you wanted to have in sex laws. *J. forensic Sci.* **18**, 118–24.

STILL, A. (1975) Police enquiries in sexual offences. *J. forensic Sci. Soc.* **15**, 183–8.

SWIGERT, V. L. *et al.* (1976) Sexual homicide: social, psychological, and legal aspects. *Arch. sex. Behav.* **5**, 391–401.

TREMBLAY, R. R. *et al.* (1975) [Endocrine and psychiatric anomalies observed in a man with an XYYY karyotype.] *Union Med. Can.* **104**, 418–22 (Eng. Abstr.) (Fre.)

UHLENBRUCK, W. (1977) [Transsexualism and legal status.] *Ther. Ggw.* **116**, 2357–61 (Ger.)

WAHLSTRÖM, J. *et al.* (1976) A man with presumptive Y/Y translocation, observed in a forensic psychiatric department. *Clin. Genet.* **10**, 82–8.

WALSH, F. M. *et al.* (1977) Autoerotic asphyxial deaths: a medicolegal analysis of forty-three cases. *Leg. med. Ann.* 155–82.

WILLOTT, G. M. (1975) The role of the forensic biologist in cases of sexual assault. *J. forensic Sci. Soc.* **15**, 269–76.

WILSON, P. (1971) *Sexual dilemma: aborton, homosexuality, prostitution and the criminal threshold.* Queensland.

WRIGHT, R. K. *et al.* (1976) Homicidal hanging masquerading as sexual asphyxia. *J. forensic Sci.* **21**, 387–9.

Sexual deviation: general and miscellaneous

ABEL, G. G. *et al.* (1974) The role of fantasy in the treatment of sexual deviation. *Arch. gen. Psychiat.* **30**, 467–75.

—— *et al.* (1975) Identifying specific erotic cues in sexual deviations by audiotaped descriptions. *J. appl. behav. Anal.* **8**, 247–60.

BANCROFT, J. (1977) Hormones and sexual behaviour. *Psychol. Med.* **7**, 553–6.

BARTHOLOMEW, A. A. (1973) Two features occasionally associated with intravenous drug users: a note. *Aust. N. Z. J. Psychiat.* **7**, 206–7.

BEIGEL, H. G. (1976) Changing sexual problems in adults. *Am. J. Psychother.* **30**, 422–32.

BELL, A. P. (1972) Human sexuality—a response. *Int. J. Psychiat.* **10**, 99–102.

BENEZECH, M. M. (1972) [Sexual delinquency.] *Bord. Med.* **5**, 2649–58 (Eng. Abstr.) (Fre.)

BERNSTEIN, I. (1976) Masochistic reactions in a latency-age girl. *J. Am. psychoanal. Ass.* **24**, 589–607.

BEYER, C. (1976) [Neuroendocrinal factors and behaviour.] *Bol. Estud. Med. Biol.* **29**, 181–5 (Spa.)

BLOMQUIST, C. (1973) [The ethics of torture.] *Lakartidningen* **70**, 4148–9 (Swe.)

BORNEMAN, E. (1976) [Language and sex. Empirical studies of a subculture.] *Bibl. Psychiat.* **154**, 80–4 (Ger.)

BOURGUIGNON, A. (1977) [Status of vampirism and autovampirism.] *Ann. Med. Psychol. (Paris)* **1**, 181–96 (Eng. Abstr.) (Fre.)

BOWMAN, E. P. (1977) Sexual and contraceptive attitudes and behaviour of single attenders at a Dublin family planning clinic. *J. biosoc. Sci.* **9**, 429–45.

BRANDON, S. (1975) Management of sexual deviation. *Br. med. J.* **3**, 149–51.

BRANT, R. S. *et al.* (1977) The sexually misused child. *Am. J. Orthopsychiat.* **47**, 80–90.

BROWN, J. J. *et al.* (1977) Correlates of females' sexual fantasies. *Percept. Mot. Skills* **45**, 819–25.

BRZEK, A. (1977) [Male sexuality and alcohol (Author's Transl.).] *Cas. Lek. Cesk.* **116**, 1024–6 (Eng. Abstr.) (Cze.)

BURGESS, A. W. *et al.* (1975) Sexual trauma of children and adolescents. *Nurs. Clin. North Am.* **10**, 551–63.

—— *et al.* (1976) The sexually abused. In Burgess, A. W. and Lazare, A. (eds) *Community mental health: target populations*, pp. 239–63. Englewood Cliffs, New Jersey.

BUSH, M. (1975) Sex offenders are people. *J. psychiat. Nurs.* **13**, 38–40.

CAVENAR, J. O., Jr *et al.* (1977) Autofellatio: a power and dependency conflict. *J. nerv. ment. Dis.* **165**, 356–60.

CHAPMAN, J. D. (1977) New horizons in sex therapy. *J. Am. Obstet. Ass.* **77**, 133–9.

CHASSEGUET-SMIRGEL, J. (1974) Perversion, idealization and sublimation. *Int. J. Psychoanal.* **55**, 349–57.

CHEE, K. T. (1974) A case of bestiality. *Singapore med. J.* **15**, 287–8.

CHROMY, K. (1974) [To relations between delinquent sexual behaviour and the type of sexual deviation (Author's Transl.).] *Cesk. Psychiat.* **70**, 192–4 (Eng. Abstr.) (Cze.)

—— *et al.* (1977) [A case of unusual sexual behaviour in senium (Author's Transl.).] *Cesk. Psychiat.* **73**, 195–8 (Eng. Abstr.)

CORNTHWAITE, S. A. *et al.* (1974) Oral and rectal coitus amongst female gonorrhoea contacts in London. *Br. J. clin. Pract.* **28**, 305–6.

DAVIDSON, J. M. (1977) Neurohormonal bases of male sexual behaviour. *Int. Rev. Physiol.* **13**, 225–54.

DE BACKER, E. *et al.* (1977) [Adenomectomy and virility.] *Acta Urol. Belg.* **45**, 354–64 (Eng. Abstr.) (Fre.)

—— *et al.* (1977) Sexual behaviour after prostatectomy. *Eur. Urol.* **3**, 295–8.

DIECKMANN, G. *et al.* (1975) Unilateral hypothalomotomy in sexual delinquents. Report on six cases. *Confin. Neurol.* **37**, 177–86.

—— Treatment of sexual violence by stereotactic hypothalomotomy. In *Neurosurgical treatment in psychiatry, pain, and epilepsy*, Sweet, W. H. *et al.* (eds) pp. 451–62. Baltimore.

EASSON, G. A. (1977) Adolescent sexuality in the Soviet Union—a personal perspective. *J. Sch. Health* **47**, 610–12.

EDMONDSON, J. S. (1972) A case of sexual asphyxia without fatal termination. *Br. J. Psychiat.* **121**, 437–8.

ERIKSSON, N. E. (1973) [Physicians and torture.] *Nord. Med.* **88**, 217–18 (Swe.)

ETCHEGOYEN, R. H. (1978) Some thoughts on transference perversion. *Int. J. Psychoanal.* **59**, 45.

FEHLOW, P. (1974) [Causes of sex crimes in adolescents.] *Aerztl. Jugendkd.* **65**, 219–24 (Ger.)

—— (1975) [The female sexual delinquent.] *Psychiat. Neurol. Med. Psychol. (Leipz.)* **27**, 612–18 (Eng. Abstr.) (Ger.)

FINANCE, F. *et al.* (1974) [A case of cruelty towards animals.] *Ann. Med. Psychol. (Paris)* **2**, 557–76 (Fre.)

FLAXMAN, N. (1972) Nymphomania—a symptom. I. *Med. Trial Tech. Q.* **19**, 183–95.

—— (1973) Nymphomania—a symptom. II. Psychoses. *Med. Trial. Tech. Q.* **19**, 305–16.

FLYNN, R. J. *et al.* (1977) Normative sex behaviour and the person with a disability: assessing the effectiveness of the rehabilitation agencies. *J. Rehabil.* **43**, 34–6.

FOERSTER, K. *et al.* (1976) [Necrophilia in a 17 year old girl.] *Schweiz. Arch. Neurol. Neurochir. Psychiat.* **119**, 97–107 (Eng. Abstr.) (Ger.)

FONG, R. (1977) Talking to patients in special clinics. *Nurs. Times* **73**, 1648–9.

FORAKER, A. G. (1976) The romantic necrophiliac of Key West. *J. Fla. med. Ass.* **63**, 642–5.

FREUND, K. *et al.* (1972) The female child as a surrogate object. *Arch. sex Behav.* **2**, 119–23.

—— (1977) Psychophysiological assessment of change in erotic preferences. *Behav. Res. Ther.* **15**, 297–301.

FRÖHLICH, H. H. (1973) [Some methodical aspects of psychological opinion on juvenile sexual delinquents.] *Psychiat. Neurol. Med. Psychol. (Leipz.)* **25**, 53–9 (Eng. Abstr.) (Ger.)

GAGNON, J. H. and Simon, W. (1967) *Sexual deviance.* London.

GERSON, A. (1974) The delilah syndrome (or the father's role in female promiscuity). *J. Am. vet. med. Ass.* **165**, 74–9.

GIAMBRA, L. M. *et al.* (1977) Sexual daydreams and quantitative aspects of sexual activity: some relations for males across adulthood. *Arch. sex Behav.* **6**, 497–505.

GIZA, J. S. *et al.* (1974) [Sexual disorders in women former inmates of concentration camps as an element of KZ-syndrome.] *Przegl. Lek.* **31**, 65–75 (Pol.)

GODLEWSKI, J. (1977) [Sex deviation and atypical sexual behaviour.] *Pol. Tyg. Lek.* **32**, 377–8 (Pol.)

—— 1977) [Classification of psychosexual disorders.] *Psychiat. Pol.* **11**, 219–25 (Pol.)

—— (1977) [A contribution to the problem of sex norms.] *Psychiat. Pol.* **11**, 567–71 (Pol.)

GOLDBERG, A. (1975) A fresh look at perverse behaviour. *Int. J. Psychoanal.* **56**, 335–42.

GOLDSTEIN, M. (1975) Antonioni's Blow-up: from crib to camera. *Am. Imago.* **32**, 240–63.

GOODE, E. and TROIDEN, R. (1975) *Sexual deviance and sexual deviants.*

GOODMAN, J. D. (1976) The behaviour of hypersexual delinquent girls. *Am. J. Psychiat.* **133**, 662–8.

HARTLEY, A. I. *et al.* (1975) Reporting child abuse. *Tex. Med.* **71**, 84–6.

HARJANIC, B. *et al.* (1978) Sexual abuse of children. *J. Am. med. Ass.* **239**, 331–3.

HITCHENS, E. W. (1972) Denial: an identified theme in marital relationships of sex offenders. *Perspect. Psychiat. Care* **10**, 152–9.

HOENIG, J. (1976) Sigmund Freud's views on sexual disorders in historical perspective. *Br. J. Psychiat.* **129**, 193–200.

HOFFDING, P. (1973) [Torture—a symptom of sick societies.] *Ugeskr. Laeger.* **135**, 2311–12) (Dan.)

—— (1974) [Letter: Torture.] *Yngre. Laeger.* **4**, 297 (Dan.)

HOLDEN, T. E. *et al.* (1973) Bestiality, with sensitization and anaphylactic reaction. *Obstet. Gynecol.* **42**, 138–40.

HOLROYD, J. C. *et al.* (1977) Psychologists' attitudes and practices regarding erotic and nonerotic physical contact with patients. *Am. Psychol.* **32**, 843–9.

HOLZER, D. (1976) [Sexually pathologic development as a result of early childhood brain damage.] *Prax. Kinderpsychol. Kinderpsychiat.* **25**, 173–5 (Eng. Abstr.) (Ger.)

JACOBS, S. (1972) The diabetic's complicated life. *Med. Times* **100**, 88–90.

JAFFE, A. C. *et al.* (1975) Sexual abuse of children. An epidemiologic study. *Am. J. Dis. Child.* **129**, 689–92.

JAMES, J. *et al.* (1977) Early sexual experience and prostitution. *Am. J. Psychiat.* **134**, 1381–5.

JOHNSON, J. (1973) 'Psychopathia Sexualis.' *Br. J. Psychiat.* **122,** 211–16.

KALES, J. D. *et al.* (1977) Patients may need basic sex education even today. *Pa. Med.* **80**, 48–50.

Kentsmith, D. K. (1975) Sexual deviation-diagnosable disorder or variant of normal behaviour. *Nebr. med. J.* **60**, 225–8.

KING, F. (1972) *Sexuality, magic, and perversion.* New York.

KINSEY, A. C. *et al.* (1953) *Sexual behaviour in the human female.* Philadelphia.

KIRK, J. (1974) Four questions about sex in our society. *Med. Times* **102**, 68–80.

KIRK, S. A. (1975) The sex offences of blacks and whites. *Arch. sex. Behav.* **4**, 295–302.

KOLARSKY, A. *et al.* (1975) [Strange woman as object of deviant male and biology of phases of sexual behaviour (Author's Transl.).]. *Cesk. Psychiat.* **71**, 291–4 (Eng. Abstr.) (Cze.)

KÖRNER, H. (1977) [Sex offenses in old age.] *Beitr. Sexualforsch.* **56**, 81–253 (Ger.)

KOSKA, W. (1973) [Comparative analysis of harlotry acts committed with juveniles and adults.] *Przegl. Lek.* **30**, 401–5 (Pol.)

LANCASTER, N. P. (1978) Necrophilia, murder, and high intelligence: a case report. *Br. J. Psychiat.* **132**, 605.

LANHAM, D. A. (1974) Editorial: The dangerous sex offender. *Med. Ann. D. C.* **43**, 6–7.

LEIBBRAND, A. *et al.* (1974) [Change in medical concepts as illustrated by hysteria and perversion.] *Med. Klin.* **69**, 761–5 (Ger.)

LESNIAK, R. *et al.* (1972) Case report: multidirectional disorders of sexual drive in a case of brain tumour. *Forensic. Sci.* **1**, 333–8.

LESTER, L. F. *et al.* (1977) Dimensions of college student behaviour. *J. Am. Coll. Health Ass.* **26**, 90–3.

DE LOCHT, P. (1976) [Morals and sex deviations.] *Acta Psychiat. Belg.* **76**, 882–92 (Eng. Abstr.) (Fre.)

LONDON, L. S. and CAPRIO, F. S. (1950) *Sexual deviations.* London.

LUSSIER, A. (1974) A discussion of the paper by J. Chasseguet-Smirgel on 'Perversion, idealization and sublimation'. *Int. J. Psychoanal.* **55**, 359–63.

McCARTHY, B. W. (1977) Strategies and techniques for the reduction of sexual anxiety. *J. Sex Marital Ther.* **3**, 243–8.

McCREARY, C. P. (1975) Personality profiles of persons convicted of indecent exposure. *J. clin. Psychol.* **31**, 260–2.

—— (1975) Personality differences among child molesters. *J. Pers. Assess.* **39**, 591–3.

McCUBBIN, J. H. *et al.* (1973) Management of alleged sexual assault. *Tex. Med.* **69**, 59–73.

McCULLY, R. S. (1976) A Jungian commentary on Epstein's case wet-shoe fetish. *Arch. sex. Behav.* **5**, 185–8.

McDOUGALL, J. (1972) [Creativeness and sex deviation.] *Rev. Fr. Psychoanal.* **36**, 535–56 (Fre.)

McEWEN, J. L. (1977) Survey of attitudes toward sexual behaviour of institutionalized mental retardates. *Psychol. Rep.* **41**, 874.

MARCUS, E. H. (1974) Letter: 'Dangerousness' of sex offenders. *Am. J. Psychiat.* **131**, 105–6.

MASSON, J. M. (1976) Perversions: some observations. *Isr. Ann. Psychiat.* **14**, 354–61.

Medical Journal of Australia. Dr. Kinsey and the Institute for Sex Research. (Kinsey, A.). *Med. J. Aust.* **1**, 720.

Medical Letters on Drug Therapy (1977) Clonidine (catapres) and other drugs causing sexual dysfunction. *Med. Lett. Drugs Ther.* **19**, 81–2.

Medical Times (1974) The problem of the manipulating patient. *Med. Times* **102**, 76–91.

MELLAN, J. *et al.* (1977) [Sexual socialization in Klinefelter's syndrome (Author's Transl.).] *Cesk. Psychiat.* **73**, 150–4 (Eng. Abstr.) (Cze.)

MELLAN, J. (1977) [The HTVM (heterosexual male development) and PAM (male sexual activity) questionnaires in sexological practice.] *Cas. Lek. Cesk.* **116**, 1030–3 (Eng. Abstr.) (Cze.)

MELLER, J. (1972) Determinants of sexual behaviour in the assessment of sexual deviations. *S. Afr. med. J.* **46**, 2013–16.

MINTZ, I. L. (1975) Parapraxis and the mother–child relationship. *Psychoanal. Q.* **44**, 460–1.

MOLINA DE HARO, A. M. *et al.* (1974) [Sociologic and cultural facts on the sexuality-pathology (Author's Transl.).] *Foila. Clin. Int. (Barc)* **24**, 238–9 (Spa.)

MOORE, W. T. (1974) Promiscuity in a 13-year-old girl. *Psychoanal. Study Child.* **29**, 301–18.

MORGENTHALER, F. (1974) [The position of perversions in metapsychology and technic.] *Psyche (Stuttg.)* **28**, 1077–98 (Eng. Abstr.) (Ger.)

MOSTHER, D. L. (1977) The Gestalt awareness-expression cycle as a model for sex therapy. *J. Sex marital Ther.* **3**, 229–42.

MÜLLER, D. *et al.* (1973) Further results of stereotaxis in the human hypothalamus in sexual deviations. First use of this operation in addiction to drugs. *Neurochirurgia (Stuttg.)* **16**, 113–26.

MÜLLER-SUUR, H. (1974) [Valuation aspects in the concept 'perversion' (Author's Transl.).] *Fortschr. Neurol. Psychiat.* **42**, 213–23 (Eng. Abstr.) (Ger.)

MURRAY, J. E. (1975) Assuring accountability for the poor: patient advocates. *J. Psychiat. Nurs.* **13**, 33–7.

NAEVE, W. (1974) [Suicides and homocides under the disguise of an autoerotic accident.] *Arch. Kriminol.* **154**, 145–9 (Ger.)

Nursing Times (1973) 'I was nineteen and I wanted to die.' *Nurs. Times* **69**, 178.

OLIVER, B. J., Jr. (1967) *Sexual deviation in American society: a social-psychological study of sexual nonconformity.* Coil and U. Pr.

PACSA, A. S. *et al.* (1977) Presence of herpes simplex virus-specific antigens in exfoliated cervical cells of virgins and sexually active women. *Eur. J. Cancer* **13**, 1197–9.

PAITICH, D. *et al.* (1976) The Clarke Parent–Child Relations Questionnaire: a clinically useful test for adults. *J. Consult. clin. Psychol.* **44**, 428–36.

—— *et al.* (1977) The Clarke SHQ: a clinical sex history questionnaire for males. *Arch. sex Behav.* **6**, 421–36.

PARR, D. (1976) Sexual aspects of drug abuse in narcotic addicts. *Br. J. Addict.* **71**, 261–8.

PARRA, A. *et al.* (1978) Plasma gonadotropins and gonadol steroids in children treated with cyclophosphamide. *J. Pediatr.* **92**, 117–24.

PETERS, J. J. (1976) Children who are victims of sexual assault and the psychology of offenders. *Am. J. Psychother.* **30**, 398–421.

PIERONI, N. A. (1976) Amorous lingual motions (letter). *J. Am. dent. Assoc.* **93**, 517.

PITMAN, R. K. (1975) Letter: More on dominance, Freud, and sex. *Am. J. Psychiat.* **132**, 568–9.

POWER, D. J. (1977) Paedophilia. *Practitioner* **218**, 805–11.

PRANDONI, J. R. *et al.* (1973) Selected Rorschach response characteristics of sex offenders. *J. Pers. Assess.* **37**, 334–6.

PREDESCU, V. *et al.* (1978) [Normal and pathological human psychosexuality and its determining factors.] *Rev. Med. Int.* [*Neurol. Psihiatr.*] **23**, 59–73.

RABOCH, J. *et al.* (1977) Adult cryptorchids: sexual development and activity. *Arch. sex Behav.* **6**, 413–19.

RADA, R. T. (1976) Alcoholism and the child molester. *Ann. N. Y. Acad. Sci.* **273**, 492–6.

RESNIK, H. L. *et al.* (1971) New directions in the treatment of sex deviance. *Int. Psychiat. Clin.* **8**, 211–26.

ROSEN, A. C. (1974) Brief report of MMPI characteristics of sexual deviation. *Psychol Rep.* **35**, 73–4.

Rozovsky, L. E. (1973) Sex and the single hospital. *Can. Hospital* **50**, 29–31.

Russell, J. K. (1974) Sexual activity and its consequences in the teenager. *Clin. Obstet. Gynaecol.* **1**, 683–98.

Sachs, S. B. (1977) Sex and the psychiatrist. *S. Afr. med. J.* **51**, 83–4.

Sauri, J. J. (1974) [On perverse transgression.] *Acta Psiquiat. Psicol. Am. Lat.* **20**, 387–94 (Eng. Abstr.) (Spa.)

Scharfman, M. A. (1976) Perverse development in a young boy. *J. Am. Psychoanal. Ass.* **24**, 499–524.

Schier, E. (1978) [Significance of sex education for the prevention of sex deviation in children and adolescents.] *Z. Gesamte Hyg.* **24**, 207–9.

Schlesinger, B. (1977) From A to Z with adolescent sexuality. *Can. Nurse* **73**, 34–7.

Schlesinger, S. L. *et al.* (1975) Petechial hemorrhages of the soft plate secondary to fellatio. *Oral Surg.* **40**, 376–8.

Schneck, J. M. (1974) Zooerasty and incest fantasy. *Int. J. clin. exp. Hypn.* **22**, 299–302.

Schneider, H. (1977) Psychic changes in sexual delinquency after hypothalomotomy. In *Neurosurgical treatment in psychiatry, pain, and epilepsy*, Sweet, W. H. *et al.* (eds) pp. 463–8. Baltimore.

Schorsch, E. (1970) [Problem of the so-called sex deviation.] *Beitr. Sexualforsch.* **49**, 88–103 (Ger.)

Schultz, L. G. (1973) The child sex victim: social, psychological and legal perspectives. *Child Welfare* **52**, 147–57.

Schürch, J. (1972) [Development of sex deviations in advanced age. Catamnestic study.] *Schweiz Arch. Neurol. Neurochir. Psychiat.* **110**, 331–63 (Fre.)

Schuster, R. (1976) [Statistical study of sexual delinquents under the influence of alcohol in Middle Hesse.] *Beitr. Gerichtl. Med.* **34**, 229–34 (Eng. Abstr.) (Ger.)

Sed'ova, A. *et al.* (1977) [Sexual abuse of under-age girls.] *Cesk. Pediat.* **32**, 181–2 (Eng. Abstr.) (Slo.)

Sgroi, S. M. (1975) Sexual molestation of children. The last frontier in child abuse. *Child. Today* **4**, 18–21, 44.

Shalness, N. (1972) Nymphomania and Don Juanism. *Med. Trial Tech. Q.* **19**, 1–6.

Simpson, M. *et al.* (1977) Patrons of massage parlors: some facts and figures. *Arch. sex. Behav.* **6**, 521–5.

Socarides, C. W. (1976) Beyond sexual freedom: clinical fallout. *Am. J. Psychother.* **30**, 385–97.

Soloff, L. A. (1977) Sexual activity in the heart patient. *Psychosomatics* **18**, 23–8.

Stekel, W. (1971) *Sexual aberrations.* 2 Vols. Liveright.

Stephens, G. J. (1978) Creative contraries: a theory of sexuality. *Am. J. Nurs.* **78**, 70–5.

Stoller, R. J. (1974) The Samuel Novey Lecture. Does sexual perversion exist? *Johns Hopkins med. J.* **134**, 43–57.

—— (1974) Hostility and mystery in perversion. *Int. J. Psychoanal.* **55**, 425–34.

STRUPP, H. H. (1974) Some observations on the fallacy of value-free psychotherapy and the empty organism: comments on a case study. *J. Abnorm. Psychol.* **83**, 199–201.

SYKORA, E. (1977) [Female sexual activity (Author's Transl.).] *Cas. Lek. Cesk.* **116**, 1017–18 (Eng. Abstr.) (Cze.)

SZEWCZYK, H. (1972) [Studies and follow-up studies on aged sex-offenders.] *Z. Alternsforsch.* **26**, 307–15 (Ger.)

—— et al. (1975) [Problem of the damage in children and adolescents due to sexual delinquency.] *Aerztl. Jugendkd.* **66**, 54–63 (Ger.)

TALLENT, N. (1977) Sexual deviation as a diagnostic entity: a confused and sinister concept. *Bull. Menninger Clin.* **41**, 40.

TAYLOR, B. (1976) Motives for guilt-free pederasty: some literary considerations. *Sociol. Rev.* **24**, 97–114.

TENNENT, T. G. (1975) The dangerous offender. *Br. J. Psychiat.* Spec. No. **9**, 308–15.

TERRELL, M. E. (1977) Identifying the sexually abused child in a medical setting. *Health soc. Work* **2**, 112–30.

TINKLENBERG, J. R. et al. (1974) Drug use among youthful assaultive and sexual offenders. *Res. Publ. Assoc. Res. nerv. ment. Dis.* **52**, 209–24.

TROSMAN, H. (1975) Letter: More on dominance, Freud, and sex. *Am. J. Psychiat.* **132**, 568.

TURELL, R. (1974) Sexual problems as seen by proctologist. *N. Y. State J. Med.* **74**, 697–8.

TWARDY, S. (1976) Sexual malpractice. *Med. Trial Tech. Q.* **23**, 173–86.

OCHÔA, D. M. (1974) A discussion of the paper by Robert J. Stoller on 'Hostility and mystery in perversion'. *Int. J. Psychoanal.* **55**, 435–8.

VIRKKUNEN, M. (1976) The paedophilic offender with antisocial character. *Acta Psychiat. scand.* **53**, 401–5.

WATSON, G. T. (1977) Alcohol and human sexual behaviour. *Behav. Res. Ther.* **15**, 239–52.

WATSON, J. P. et al. (1977) Aspects of the psychopathology of sexual behaviour. *Proc. R. Soc. Med.* **70**, 789–92.

WEEKS, R. B. (1976) The sexually exploited child. *South. med. J.* **69**, 848–52.

WHITE, C. M. (1977) Human sexuality: model program, Letterman Army Medical Center. *Milit. Med.* **142**, 939–41.

WILSON, G. T. (1977) Alcohol and human sexual behaviour. *Behav. Res. Ther.* **15**, 239–52.

ZINKIN, L. (1977) 'Death in Venice'—a Jungian view. *J. Anal. Psychol.* **22**, 354–66.

Rape

ABEL, G. G. et al. (1977) The components of rapists' sexual arousal. *Arch. gen. Psychiat.* **34**, 895–903.

BASSUK, E. et al. (1975) Organizing a rape crisis program in a general hospital. *J. Am. med. Wom. Assoc.* **30**, 486–90.

BAUER, G. (1971) [The series rapist Bernhard N. Report on a murderer released from prison.] *Arch. Kriminol.* **147**, 65–73 (Ger.)

BENNETT, J. R. (1977) A model for evaluation design for a rape counseling program. *Child Welfare* **56**, 395–400.

BEST, C. L. *et al.* (1977) Psychological profiles of rape crisis counselors. *Psychol. Rep.* **40**, 1127–34.

BOWDEN, P. (1978) Rape. *Br. J. Hosp. Med.* **20,** 286.

British Medical Journal (1975) Editorial: Victims of rape. *Br. med. J.* 171–2.

—— (1975) Letter: Victims of rape. *Br. med. J.* 453–4.

—— (1978) Rape and the laboratory. *Br. med. J.* **6131**, 154.

BURGESS, A. W. *et al.* (1973) The rape victim in the emergency ward. *Am. J. Nurs.* **73**, 1740–5.

—— (1974) Crisis and counseling requests of rape victims. *Nurs. Res.* **23**, 196–202.

—— (1974) Rape trauma syndrome. *Am. J. Psychiat.* **131**, 981–6.

—— (1975) Accountability: a right of the rape victim. *J. psychiat. Nurs.* **13**, 11–16.

—— (1976) Coping behaviour of the rape victim. *Am. J. Psychiat.* **133**, 413–18.

—— (1977) Courtroom use of hospital records in sexual assault cases. *Am. J. Nurs.* **77**, 64–8.

CALHOUN, L. G. *et al.* (1978) The effects of victim physical attractiveness and sex of respondent on social reactions to victims of rape. *Br. J. soc. clin. Psychol.* **17**, 191.

CLARK, T. P. (1976) Primary health care: counseling victims of rape. *Am. J. Nurs.* **76**, 1964–6.

COHEN, M. L. *et al.* (1971) The psychology of rapists. *Semin. Psychiat.* **3**, 307–27.

COTTRAUX, J. (1977) [Treatment of rape behaviour by internal sensitization. Deconditioning by mental imagery (letter).] *Nouv. Presse Med.* **6**, 1973 (Fre.)

CREMERS, H. T. (1975) [Battery and rape; medico-ethical problems in the examination and reporting to the police (court).] *Ned. Tijdschr. Geneeskd.* **119**, 1259–62 (Dut.)

CRYER, L. *et al.* (1976) Rape evidence kit: simplified procedures for the emergency department. *JACEP* **5**, 890–3.

DAHLKE, M. B. *et al.* (1977) Identification of semen in 500 patients seen because of rape. *Am. J. clin. Pathol.* **68**, 740–6.

DAVIS, J. H. (1974) Editorial: Medical care for the sexually assaulted. *J. Fla. med. Assoc.* **61**, 588.

DE LA VIGNE, A. R. (1972) [Young girl chasers with motor cycles. Medicolegal study.] *Rev. Neuropsychiat. Infant.* **20**, 591–8 (Eng. Abstr.)

DONADIO, B. *et al.* (1974) Seven who were raped. *Nurs. Outlook* **22**, 245–7.

ENOS, W. F. *et al.* (1972) The medical examination of cases of rape. *J. forensic Sci.* **17**, 50–6.

—— *et al.* (1974) Standard rape investigation form. *Va. Med. Mon.* **101**, 43–4.

EVERETT, R. B. *et al.* (1977) The rape victim: a review of 117 consecutive cases. *Obstet. Gynecol.* **50**, 88–90.

FACER, W. A. (1977) Rape (letter). *N. Z. med. J.* **86**, 152.

FEILD, H. S. (1978) Attitudes towards rape: a comparative analysis of police, rapists, crisis counselors, and citizens. *J. Pers. Psychol.* **36**, 156.

FERTEL, J. H. (1977) Health and support services for rape victims on Oahu. *Hawaii med. J.* **36**, 385–91.

GAGER, N. and SCHURR, C. (1976) *Sexual assault, confronting rape in America.*

GIBBENS, T. C. *et al.* (1977) Behavioural types of rape. *Br. J. Psychiatry* **130**, 32–42.

GIVEN, B. W. (1976) Sex-chromatin bodies in penile washings as an indicator of recent coitus. *J. forensic Sci.* **21**, 381–6.

GLOVER, D. *et al.* (1976) Diethylstilbestrol in the treatment of rape victims. *West J. Med.* **125**, 331–4.

GOTTESMAN, S. T. (1977) Police attitudes towards rape before and after a training program. *J. psychiat. Nurs.* **15**, 14–18.

GREENBERG, M. I. (1974) Letter: Serological tests for syphilis in rape cases. *J. Am. med. Ass.* **227**, 1381.

GROTH, A. N. *et al.* (1977) Rape: a sexual deviation. *Am. J. Orthopsychiat.* **47**, 400–6.

—— *et al.* (1977) Rape: power, anger, and sexuality. *Am. J. Psychiat.* **134**, 1239–43.

—— *et al.* (1977) Sexual dysfunction during rape. *N. Engl. J. Med.* **297**, 764–6.

GUNDLACH, R. H. (1977) Sexual molestation and rape reported by homosexual and heterosexual women. *J. Homosex.* **2**, 367–84.

HANSS, J. W. Jr. (1975) Another look at the care of the rape victim. *Ariz. Med.* **32**, 534–5.

HARTMAN, R. (1974) Rape. *Ill. med. J.* **145**, 518–19.

HAYMAN, C. R. *et al.* (1973) What to do for victims of rape. *Med. Times* **101**, 47–51.

Health and Social Work (1976) Rape—a personal account. *Health Soc. Work* **1**, 83–95.

HOLMSTROM, L. L. *et al.* (1975) Assessing trauma in the rape victim. *Am. J. Nurs.* **75**, 1288–91.

Hospitals (1976) City-county hospital contract provides free care for rape victims. *Hospitals* **50**, 44–6.

HUERD, D. (1977) How a rape advocacy service works. *Hosp. Prog.* **58**, 70–7.

HUNT, G. R. (1977) Rape: an organized approach to evaluation and treatment. *Am. Fam. Physician* **15**, 154–8.

JOE, V. C. *et al.* (1977) Religiousness and devaluation of a rape victim. *J. clin. Psychol.* **33**, 64.

JOHNSON, S. C. *et al.* (1976) Examination of the alleged rape victim. *J. Iowa med. Soc.* **66**, 447–50.

JONES, C. *et al.* (1973) Attribution of fault to a rape victim as a function of respectability of the victim. *J. pers. soc. Psychol.* **26**, 415–19.

Journal of Reproductive Medicine (1974) Alleged rape. An invitational symposium. *J. reprod. Med.* **12**, 133–44, passim.

Journal of the American Medical Association (1974) Letter: Serological tests for syphilis in rape cases. *J. Am. med. Ass.* **228**, 1227–8.

KANIN, E. J. *et al.* (1977) Sexual aggression: a second look at the offended female. *Arch. sex. Behav.* **6**, 67–76.

KAUFMAN, A. *et al.* (1975) Total health needs of the rape victim. *J. Fam. Pract.* **2**, 225–9.

—— *et al.* (1976) Follow-up of rape victims in a family practice setting. *South. med. J.* **69**, 1569–71.

—— *et al.* (1977) Impact of a community health approach to rape. *Am. J. Public Health* **67**, 365–7.

KERCHER, G. A. *et al.* (1973) Reactions of convicted rapists to sexually explicit stimuli. *J. Abnorm. Psychol.* **81**, 46–50.

LALONDE, C. (1976) [Physicians and society: confronted by rape.] *Can. med. Assoc. J.* **115**, 278–80 (Fre.)

LeBOURDAIS, E. (1976) Rape victims: the unpopular patients. *Dimens Health Serv.* **53**, 12–14.

LeFORT, S. (1977) Care of the rape victim in emergency. *Can. Nurs.* **73**, 42–5.

LINDABURY, V. A. (1975) Editorial: The Criminal Code and rape and sex offences. *Can. Nurs.* **71**, 3.

McCOMBIE, S. L. *et al.* (1976) Development of a medical center rape crisis intervention program. *Am. J. Psychiat.* **133**, 418–21.

McGUIRE, L. S. *et al.* (1976) Survey of incidence of and physicians' attitudes towards sexual assault. *Public Health Rep.* **91**, 103–9.

MAEHLY, A. C. *et al.* (1977) [Zinc sulfate under the prepuce. Criminal trace in a sexual murder.] *Arch. Kriminol.* **159**, 139–43 (Ger.)

MAREK, Z. *et al.* (1974) [Victimology of rape (Authors' Transl.).] *Przegl. Lek.* **31**, 578–82 (Pol.)

MARSHALL, W. L. *et al.* (1977) The clinical value of boredom. A procedure for reducing inappropriate sexual interests. *J. nerv. ment. Dis.* **165**, 283–7.

Medical and Scientific Law (1976) Submission to Mrs. Justice Heilbron's Advisory Group on the Law of Rape. *Med. Sci. Law.* **16**, 154–8.

Medico-Legal Journal (1976) Editorial: Rape. *Med. Leg. J.* **44**, 1–5.

METZGER, D. (1976) It is always the woman who is raped. *Am. J. Psychiat.* **133**, 405–8.

Modern Health Care (1975) Rape victim guidelines. *Mod. Hth Care* **3**, 74.

NADELSON, C. C. (1977) Rapist and victim [editorial]. *N. Engl. J. Med.* **297**, 784–5.

New England Journal of Medicine (1978) Rape (letter) *N. Engl. J. Med.* **298**, 167–8.

NG, A. Y. (1974) The pattern of rape in Singapore. *Singapore med. J.* **15**, 49–50.

NOTMAN, M. T. *et al.* (1976) The rape victim: psychodynamic considerations. *Am. J. Psychiat.* **133**, 408–13.

PAUL, D. M. (1977) The medical examination of the live rape victim and the accused. *Leg. Med. Ann.* 137–53.

PERDUE, W. C. *et al.* (1972) Personality characteristics of rapists. *Percept. Mot. Skills* **35**, 514.

PETERS, J. J. (1975) Social, legal and psychological effects of rape on the victim. *Pa. Med.* **78**, 34–6.

Philadelphia Medicine (1976) Treatment of suspected victims of sexual assault. *Pa. Med.* **79**, 73–5.

PLANT, J. *et al.* (1977) E. D. involvement grows in audit activities, rape treat-ment. *Hospitals* **51**, 107–8; 110–12.

PRICE, V. (1975) Rape victims—the invisible patients. *Can. Nurse* **71**, 29–34.

RADA, R. T. (1975) Alcoholism and forcible rape. *Am. J. Psychiat.* **132**, 444–6.

—— *et al.* (1976) Plasma testosterone levels in the rapist. *Psychosom. Med.* **38**, 257–68.

—— (ed.) (1978) *Clinical aspects of the rapist.* Grune and Stratton, New York.

RADER, C. M. (1977) MMPI profile types of exposers, rapists, and assaulters in a court services population. *J. Consult. clin. Psychol.* **45**, 61–9.

RINGROSE, C. A. (1977) Pelvic reflexes in rape complaints *Can. J. Public Health* **68**, 31.

ROBINSON, G. E. (1976) Management of the rape victim. *Can. med. Assoc. J.* **115**, 520–2.

ROCK, W. J. (1978) Comments on rape therapy procedure (letter). *Hosp. Prog.* **59**, 7.

ROOT, I. *et al.* (1974) The medical investigation of alleged rape. *West. J. Med.* **120**, 329–33.

RUFF, C. F. *et al.* (1976) The intelligence of rapists. *Arch. sex. Behav.* **5**, 327–9.

RUMSEY, M. G. *et al.* (1977) A case of rape: sentencing judgements of males and females. *Psychol. Rep.* **41**, 459–65.

SCHÄFER, J. *et al.* (1972) [Genital injuries in childhood caused by rape.] *Orv. Hteil.* **113**, 2245–6 (Hun.)

SCHIFF, A. F. (1973) Rape in foreign countries. *Med. Trial. tech. Q.* **20**, 66–74.

—— (1973) A statistical evaluation of rape. *Forensic Sci.* **2**, 339–49.

—— (1974) Rape in foreign countries. *Med. Trial tech. Q. Annual* 66–74.

—— (1975) An unusual case of pseudo-rape *J. forensic Sci.* **20**, 637–42.

—— (1975) Sperm identification—acid phosphate test. *Med. Trial tech. Q.* **21**, 467–74.

—— (1975) The new Florida 'rape' law. *J. Fla. med. Assoc.* **62**, 40–2.

SCHNECK, J. M. (1977) Hypnotic elucidation of isolation and displacement following a sexual assault. *Dis. nerv. Syst.* **38**, 934–5.

SCHUMANN, G. B. *et al.* (1976) Prostatic acid phosphatase. Current assessment in vaginal fluid of alleged rape victims. *Am. J. clin. Pathol.* **66**, 944–52.

SELIGMAN, C. *et al.* (1977) Rape and physical attractiveness: assigning responsibility to victims. *J. Pers.* **45**, 554–63.

SHAINESS, N. (1976) Psychological significance of rape. Some aspects. *N. Y. State J. Med.* **76**, 2044–8.

SILVERMAN, D. (1977) First do no more harm: female rape victims and the male counselor. *Am. J. Orthopsychiat.* **47**, 91–6.

—— (1978) Sharing the crisis of rape: counselling the mates and families of victims. *Am. J. Orthopsychiat.* **48**, 166–73.

SINGH, A. (1977) Note on rape and social structure. *Psychol. Rep.* **41**, 134.

SLOAN, D. (1976) Rape: the gynecologist's role. *J. reprod. Med.* **17**, 324–6.

SOLVSKA, M. *et al.* (1975) [Gynaecological findings in sexual offences (Author's Transl.).] *Cesk. Gynekol.* **40**, 721–3 (Slo.)

SOOTHILL, K. L. *et al.* (1976) Rape: a 22-year cohort study. *Med. Sci. Law* **16**, 52–9.

Soules, M. R. *et al.* (1978) The forensic laboratory evaluation of evidence in alleged rape. *Am. J. Obstet. Gynecol.* **130**, 142–7.

—— *et al.* (1978) The spectrum of alleged rape. *J. reprod. Med.* **20**, 33–9.

Symonds, M. (1976) The rape victim: psychological patterns of response. *Am. J. Psychoanal.* **36**, 27–34.

Van Dyke, C, (1977) Why a catholic hospital provides rape relief. *Hosp. Prog.* **58**, 64–9.

Walker, M. J. and Brodsky, S. L. (1976) *Sexual assault: the victim and the rapist*. Lexington Books.

Weiss, E. H. *et al.* (1972) The mental health committee: report of the Sub-committee on the Problem of Rape in the District of Columbia. *Med. Ann. D. C.* **41**, 703–4.

West, D. J., Roy, C., and Nichols, F. L. (1978) *Understanding sexual attacks*. Heinemann, London.

Western Journal of Medicine (1975) Guidelines for the interview and examinations of alleged rape victims. *West J. Med.* **123**, 420–2.

Williams, C. C. *et al.* (1973) Rape: a plea for help in the hospital emergency room. *Nurs. Forum* **12**, 388–401.

Wolfgang, M. E. *et al.* (1975) Rape, race, and the death penalty in Georgia. *Am. J. Orthopsychiat.* **45**, 658–68.

Woodling, B. A. *et al.* (1977) Sexual assault: rape and molestation. *Clin. Obstet. Gynecol.* **20**, 509–30.

Author Index

Entries in *italic* refer to the reference lists at the end of each chapter where bibliographic details may be found. Note that only page numbers in the text and references at the end of each chapter are given; see also the Bibliography (pp. 481–529).

Reich, W., *63*, 72, *78*
Reifenstein, E. C., 445, *478*
Reiss, A., 383, *437*
Rekers, G. A., 116, 117, *138*
Reynolds, E. J., 118, *137*
Reynolds, J., 397, *437*
Rhue, T., 7, *26*
Richards, P. G., 415, 416, *437*
Richardson, H., *434*
Richart, R. M., *62*
Richter, M., 469, *479*
Rickles, N. K., 140, 141, 142, 146, *193*
Rifkin, A. H., 8, 12, *26*, 50, *62*, 129, *137*, 247, 262, *275*, 363, 369, *373*, 430, *432*
Rioch, D. M., 460, *476*, 477
Riviere, J., 48, *63*, 238, *241*
Robbins, E., 12, *28*
Roberts, J. B., 458, *476*
Roberts, R. W., *437*
Robertson, J., 455, *480*
Robertson, L. L., 458, *476*
Robin, K. D., 383, 414, *434*
Robinson, K., 415, *437*
Robinson, T. J., 458, *479*
Rock, P., 382, *437*
Rogers, A. J., 383, *437*
Rognant, J., 157, *193*
Roiphe, H., 51, *62*, *63*, 85, 86, *107*
Root, W. S., 459, *480*
Rooth, F. G., 140, 143, 156, 157, *193*, 359, *374*
Rose, R. M., 7, *27*, *28*, 471, 477
Rosen, A. C., 116, 117, *138*
Rosen, I., 33, *62*, *63*, *64*, 74, 77, *78*, *137*, *138*, *194*, 211, 236, *241*, 245, 293, *305*, 312, *350*, *375*, 421, 422, *435*, *437*, *438*
Rosenbluth, D., 455, *480*
Rosenfeld, H. A., 262, *276*
Rosenfeld, R., 200, 201, *205*, *241*
Rosenthal, D., 5, *28*
Rothman, G., 424, *437*
Rotman, D. B., 142, *192*
Roy, J. R., 444, *478*
Rubenstein, D., *350*
Rubinstein, L. H., 310, *350*, 421, *437*
Rubinstein, M., *438*
Russell, D., 403, *438*
Rycroft, C., 368, *374*

Saayman, G. S., 467, 468, *479*
Sachs, H., 40, 55, *64*, 247, 249, 250, *276*
Sadger, J., 140, *193*, 243, *276*
Sadock, B. J., 197, *204*
Sagarin, E. C., 383, 413, 414, *438*
Saghit, M., 12, *28*
Sandler, J., 66, *78*, 282, *305*
Sartorius, N. H., 365, *374*
Sawyer, C. H., 453, 477
Sayler, G. O., *434*

Schleidt, M., 469, *478*
Schlien, J. M., 365, *374*
Schmideberg, M., 236, *241*, 385, *438*
Schmidt, E., *375*
Schofield, M., 415, *438*
Schur, E., 378, 382, 383, 396, *438*
Schwendinger, H., 397, 399, *438*
Schwendinger, J., 397, 399, *438*
Scott, J. P., 455, *480*
Scott, P. D., 3, *28*, 346, *350*, 363, *375*, 384, *438*
Scott, P. P., 459, 460, *478*, *480*
Seemanova, E., 392, *438*
Segal, S. J., 453, *480*
Seligman, M. E. P., *375*
Sellar, D., 390, *438*
Selzer, A. L., 365, *374*
Senn, M. J. E., *107*
Serber, M., 157, *194*
Sherwin, R. V., 417, *438*
Sherwood, M., 7, *28*
Shields, J., 5, *26*
Shirley, J., 384, *433*
Short, M., 384, *433*
Sidley, N., *438*
Siegelman, M., 9, *28*
Siirala, M., 334, *350*
Silverman, D., *63*, 162, *194*
Silverstone, T., *62*, *63*, *193*, *375*
Simmons, J., 414, *438*
Simon, W., 409, 413, 414, 418, *433*, *434*
Sion, A., 413, *438*
Skolnick, J., 383, 406, *438*
Slavson, S. R., 179, *194*
Slovenko, R., *63*, *350*, 376, 414, 429, *433*, *436*, *437*, *438*, *439*
Smith, D. K., 427, *438*
Smith, J. C., 397, 398, 400, 410, *438*
Socarides, C. W., 50, 57, *64*, 116, 118, *138*, 202; *205*, 211, 232, 234, *242*, 245, 246, 247, 262, 270, 271, *276*, 277, 280, *305*, 418, *439*
Solat, M., 397, *439*
Solyom, L., 361, *375*
Southill, K., 401, *439*
Sperling, M., 34, *64*, 83, 84, 100, *108*, 140, 150, *194*, 232, 237, *242*
Spiegel, N. T., 84, *108*
Spitz, R. A., 86, 455, *480*
Stabile, G. D., 383, 414, *434*
Stafford-Clark, D., 116, *138*
Stärcke, A., 152, *194*
Stekel, W., *138*, 140, *194*
Stempfel, R. S., 454, *480*
Stephen, J., 387, 390, *439*
Stephens, E., 419, *439*
Stephenson, J., 157, *194*
Sterba, R., *63*

Subject Index